Preface

Over the past few years there has been a fundamental revolution in the field of ophthalmic lasers. New and better types of lasers have been developed; new and better applications of those lasers have emerged for the diagnosis and treatment of many ocular diseases. On a daily basis, our practices have been changed because we now use some of these new techniques or because we refer to specialists who use them. Our ability to diagnose and treat many ocular diseases has improved tremendously during the past ten years, to say nothing of the past 40 years since the laser was invented. In fact, one of the very first uses of lasers in the early 1960s was for the treatment of ocular disorders.

This book responds to the need for a current, comprehensive, practical understanding of clinical ophthalmic lasers and their diagnostic and therapeutic uses. It emphasizes the important new diagnostic uses of lasers for both the anterior segment and posterior segment and the therapeutic uses for the anterior segment. The therapeutic uses of lasers in the posterior segment are not covered.

The basic outline of the book has emerged from lectures I have given for the Ophthalmic Laser Course at the Pennsylvania College of Optometry and for continuing education programs sponsored by the college or by the Light and Laser Institute. In the mid-1980s Dr. Felix Barker and I started putting together educational programs for practitioners in the United States. Since then we have expanded the programs to include the lectures and laboratories for the college's laser course and international lectures.

Chapter 1 covers the basics of lasers: how they work, what components are necessary, how their output is described, and the characteristics of laser radiation. It also covers the way lasers and tissues interact, as well as the damage mechanisms that account for the clinical uses of the ophthalmic lasers. This chapter lays the foundation for understanding the uses of all the available clinical lasers, as well as any future laser systems. Chapter 2 covers the different types of ophthalmic lasers available. For each laser system, there is a description of the active medium, excitation mechanism, laser cavity configuration, output characteristics (e.g., wavelength(s), power range, temporal and spatial modes), operating characteristics, damage mechanism(s), and the various ophthalmic applications.

There is also a summary table of ophthalmic lasers with their primary characteristics and applications.

Chapter 3 provides fairly comprehensive coverage of the new ophthalmic diagnostic uses of lasers. For each use, the laser system and the technique are described, the clinical uses are listed, and the advantages and disadvantages are explained. Some of the diagnostic laser systems are commercially available and some are still in the research-and-development stage. The recent development of laser-based retinal imaging systems has been exciting, and these systems are evolving with better hardware, software, and analysis parameters. These are nascent technologies, much like visual field systems were 10 to 20 years ago.

Chapters 4 through 9 are devoted to therapeutic uses of ophthalmic lasers in the anterior segment. Each chapter includes descriptions of the indications, contraindications, pre-procedure management, clinical technique, post-procedure management, and complications. Those techniques that are most frequently employed are highlighted and explained in more detail than the less frequently employed techniques. Chapter 4, by Dr. David Gubman, briefly covers the use of lasers for vision correction. There are many recently-published, full-length books on laser-based refractive surgery. Chapter 5 covers the most-used ophthalmic laser technique: laser posterior capsulotomy. Chapters 6 to 8 cover uses of the laser in glaucoma treatment. Chapter 6 describes laser iridotomy, Chapter 7 covers laser trabeculoplasty, and Chapter 8 covers other laser techniques for the treatment of the glaucomas. Chapter 9 treats other anterior segment therapeutic uses of lasers, including oculoplastic surgery and photodynamic therapy. The therapeutic use chapters contain helpful tables of indications, contraindications, and complications for the various therapeutic uses of ophthalmic lasers. Many of the chapters also contain unique tables of the occurrence of various complications of therapeutic laser use. Chapter 7 has thorough tables of the short-term and long-term effectiveness of ALT for different types of glaucoma. In the last chapter, Chapter 10, Dr. Felix Barker describes the issues of clinical laser safety.

The intent is that the book will be useful for both the novice and the experienced eyecare practitioner (optometrists and ophthalmologists), as well as for students and residents in training programs. All eyecare practitioners need to be knowledgeable about the advances and uses of ophthalmic laser systems. This book will be especially useful for those practitioners who refer patients for laser treatment. The practitioner should know when to refer, what the specialist will do, and what complications can occur. This will allow for better care and for better patient education. The book will also be useful for practitioners who want to know more about the diagnostic uses of lasers. The book will help practitioners decide which type of system will be useful for their practice, their patients, or referral of their patients.

Acknowledgments

I wish to thank PCO for providing me with two mini-sabbaticals to spend dedicated time for writing portions of this book.

I wish to thank the two contributors to this book, Dr. David Gubman and Dr. Felix Barker, for taking time away from their teaching, research, and clinical activities to share their knowledge and insights.

I wish to thank my family, especially my wife Jan, for their patience and understanding. Writing a book takes an enormous amount of time and effort.

Finally, I thank the editorial and production staff of Butterworth-Heinemann for their encouragement, advice, and assistance.

Contents

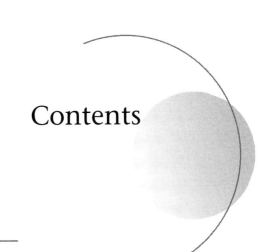

Chapter 4. **Clinical Laser Vision Correction**   *183*
David Gubman

Chapter 5. **Laser Posterior Capsulotomy**   *209*
Charles M. Wormington

Chapter 6. **Laser Iridotomy**   *257*
Charles M. Wormington

Chapter 10. **Laser Eye Safety**   *499*
Felix Barker

Index   *519*

Contributors

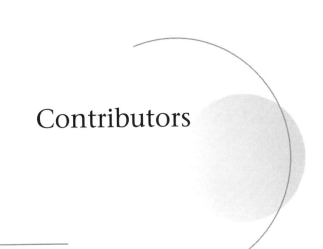

Felix M. Barker, II, OD, MS, FAAO
Director of Research
Director of Affiliated Residency Programs
Clinical Educator at The Eye Institute
Course Director, Anterior Segment Eye Disease
Course Director, Ophthalmic Lasers
Pennsylvania College of Optometry
Elkins Park, Pennsylvania

David Gubman, OD, MS, FAAO
Private Practice
Vorhees, New Jersey

Chapter 1
Ophthalmic Lasers: Basics and Tissue Interactions

Charles M. Wormington

I. Laser Theory

A. Introduction to Laser Theory

Because of the ability of a laser to generate an intense, collimated beam of radiation at a given wavelength, the laser is a unique instrument for ophthalmic use. Using the theories of Planck and Einstein, Townes and Schawlow laid down the basic principles of the laser (Schawlow & Townes, 1958). This was followed by the construction of the first visible laser by Maiman in 1960 (Maiman, 1960). Laser theory involves understanding three basic concepts: energy levels, population inversion, and stimulated emission.

B. *Principles of Laser Theory* (Hecht, 1994; Silfvast, 1996; Sliney & Wolbarsht, 1980).

1. **Energy Levels.** Atoms and molecules have distinct energy levels (Figure 1–1). Electrons can occupy one or more of these energy levels and move from one to another. Most electrons occupy the lowest or ground energy level. Electrons can move from one energy level (e.g., E_0) to a higher one (e.g., E_2) by the absorption of energy from an external source. Photons with an energy equal to the difference in energy between the two levels ($h\nu = E_2 - E_0$, where h is Planck's constant and ν is the frequency of the radiation) can be absorbed by electrons in the E_0 state and thus raise them to the E_2 state. Once raised to this higher energy level, the electrons are said to be in an "excited state." The excited states of interest are metastable where the electrons remain for relatively long periods of time. As shown in the diagram, the metastable state is reached by an intersystem crossing where the electron moves from level E_2 to level E_1.

2. **Population Inversion.** For laser action to occur, it is necessary to excite a majority of the electrons in the ground state to an excited metastable state. This leads to a condition known as "population inversion" in which there are more electrons in the higher energy level than in the ground state, the inverse of the usual condition. Once in this excited condition, the electrons are primed and ready for the next process known as "stimulated emission."

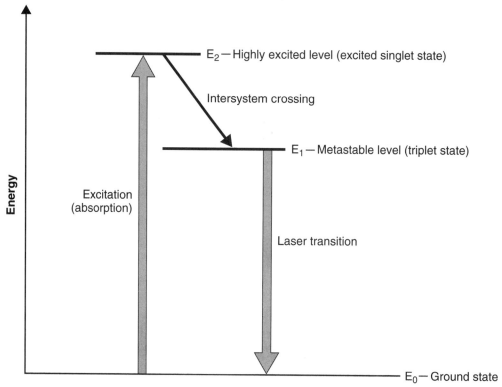

Figure 1–1 Simplified diagram of energy levels in a three-level laser.

3. **Stimulated Emission.** Once an electron has been excited to a higher metastable energy level, it can fall to a lower level in one of two different ways. First, it could spontaneously return to a lower level giving off a photon in a random direction. This is called "**spontaneous emission**." It can be in the form of **fluorescence** in which the electron falls from an excited singlet state or in the form of **phosphorescence** in which an electron falls from an excited triplet state (Figure 1–2). The second way an electron can move to a lower energy level is to have an incident photon stimulate the excited atom to emit a photon (Figure 1–3). The energy of the incident photon must be equal to the energy of the photon released when the excited electron drops to the lower energy level. Since the energy of the photons is equal to $h\nu$ (which is equal to hc/λ where c is the speed of light and λ is the wavelength of the radiation), the wavelength of the two photons is identical. Thus the incident photon stimulates the emission of another photon of the same wavelength and hence the process produces **monochromatic** radiation. The two photons are also in phase with each other, so this process also produces **coherent** radiation.

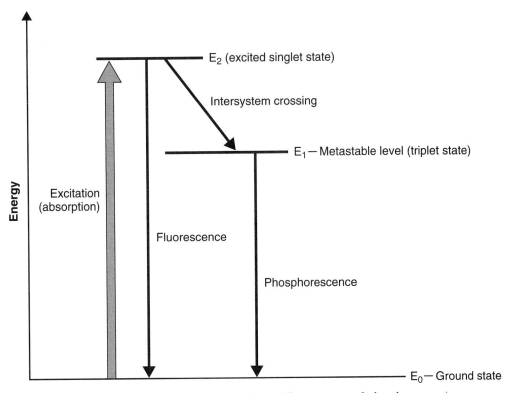

Figure 1–2 Simplified diagram of spontaneous emission (fluorescence and phosphorescence).

II. Laser Components

A. Introduction to Laser Components

In order to apply the principles of laser theory and construct a laser, three components must be present: a laser medium, an excitation mechanism, and a feedback mechanism.

B. Laser Medium

The active medium is the type of atom or molecule whose electrons are involved in producing the laser action. Lasers are named after their active medium. Three types of media can be used:

1. **Gas** (e.g., helium-neon (HeNe), argon (Ar), krypton (Kr), carbon dioxide (CO_2), excimer (ArF)).
2. **Liquid** (e.g., Rhodamine dye used in a tunable dye laser).
3. **Solid** (e.g., neodymium (Nd), GaAlAs diode laser).

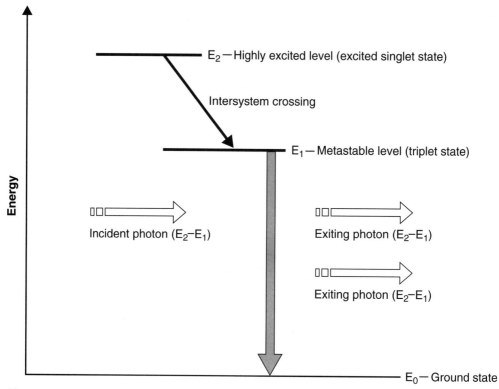

Figure 1–3 Simplified diagram of stimulated emission. An incident photon stimulates the emission of another photon that has the same wavelength and which is in phase with the incident photon.

C. Excitation Mechanism (Pump)

To raise electrons in the active medium to a higher energy level and produce the population inversion, lasers use a pumping system. This system pumps energy into the laser medium to increase the number of electrons in the excited metastable energy level. A number of different pumping systems are available.

1. **Electrical Pumping.** Electrons can be excited by passing an electric current through a gas or a semiconductor. An arc or a glow discharge can be produced and maintained by a cathode and an anode at opposite ends of a tube filled with gas. This can lead to electron collisions that excite the electrons in the lasing medium. In a diode laser, an electric current is induced at a junction of the semiconductor and leads to excitation.

2. **Optical Pumping.** In most dye lasers and solid state lasers, the electrons are excited by the absorption of photons from an intense light source. This source can be a flashlamp wrapped around the laser tube, or it can be another laser.

3. **Chemical Pumping.** The energy released in the breaking or making of chemical bonds during a chemical reaction can also be used to excite lasers. However, this is not a commonly used mechanism.

D. Feedback Mechanism (Resonance Cavity)

1. **Resonance Mirrors.** An optical cavity is produced by placing a mirror at each end of the laser so that the photons may be reflected back and forth from one mirror to the other (Figure 1–4). One mirror is a high reflectance mirror that reflects essentially all the photons that hit it. The other mirror is a partially transmissive mirror that reflects most of the photons but allows some to pass through. The latter mirror is thus the **output coupler** that provides a means to form the external laser beam.

2. **Cascade Process (Amplification).** Some of the excited electrons spontaneously fall to a lower energy level and emit photons in random directions. The lasing process is begun when one of these spontaneous photons emerges along the axis between the mirrors and hits another excited atom, producing stimulated emission. There are now two photons with the same wavelength, in phase with each other, traveling in the same direction toward one of the mirrors. Each of these photons can strike another atom and stimulate the emission of another photon as they bounce back and forth between the two mirrors. In this way a chain reaction begins. A single photon produces two photons, which produce four, which produce eight, and so on. Thus, as

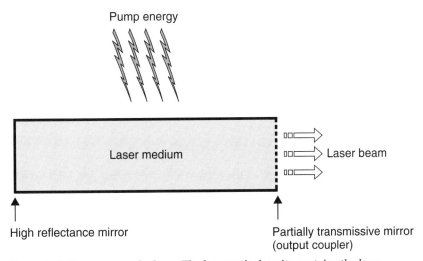

Figure 1–4 Components of a laser. The laser optical cavity contains the laser medium and the two resonance cavity mirrors. The excitation mechanism (pump) pumps energy into the laser cavity to produce a population inversion.

the photons are fed back into the active medium by the mirrors, this photon cascade leads to amplification of the laser energy.

3. **Laser.** The term laser is an acronym for *Light Amplification by Stimulated Emission of Radiation*. This summarizes the principles involved in the production of laser radiation.

III. Excitation Sources

A. Electrical Current in Gas

Many of the ophthalmic lasers are excited by passing an electrical current through a gas leading to a glow discharge or an arc. Table 1–1 lists the major gas lasers and their most significant output wavelengths.

Table 1–1 Some Typical Ophthalmic Lasers

Laser	Active Medium	Wavelength(s)
Lasers pumped by an electrical current in a gas		
Argon (Ar)	Ionized Ar gas	488 nm (blue), 514.5 nm (green)
Carbon dioxide (CO_2)	CO_2 gas	10,600 nm (far infrared)
Excimer		
Argon fluoride (ArF)	ArF	193 nm (UV-C)
Xenon chloride (XeCl)	XeCl	308 nm (UV-B)
Helium-neon (HeNe)	Neon gas	543.5 nm (green), 632.8 nm (red)
Krypton (Kr)	Ionized Kr gas	531 nm (green), 568 nm (yellow), 647 nm (red)
Lasers pumped by an electrical current in a solid		
Gallium Aluminum Arsenide (GaAlAs)	GaAlAs	600–900 nm (red and IR-A)
Optically pumped lasers		
Dye lasers	Various organic dyes	Tunable around the major wavelength for a given dye (dyes are available to span the entire spectrum from UV to IR)
Er:YAG	Er	2940 nm (IR-B)
Holmium (THC:YAG)	ThHoCr	2140 nm (IR-B)
Nd:YAG	Nd	1064 nm (IR-A)
Nd:YAG frequency-doubled	Nd	532 nm (green)
Nd:YLF	Nd	1053 nm (IR-A)

B. Electrical Current in Solid

Laser action takes place when an electrical current is passed through the flat junction in a semiconductor or diode laser (see Table 1–1).

C. Optical Pumps

Flash lamps or lasers can be used to achieve population inversion in a number of ophthalmic solid state and dye lasers (see Table 1–1).

IV. Temporal Modes of Operation

A. Introduction to Temporal Modes

The rate at which the laser energy is delivered is important because it helps determine the type of interaction of the laser radiation with the exposed tissue. The rate of delivery depends on how the excitation energy is applied to the active medium and on how the resonance cavity is configured. The temporal output can be either continuous or pulsed (Sliney and Trokel, 1993) (Figure 1–5).

Figure 1–5 Temporal patterns of laser pulses. Pulses from lasers can vary over a tremendous range of durations from femtoseconds (10^{-15} s) to seconds. Laser outputs can be described by different terms such as mode-locked, Q-switched, free-running, and continuous wave. Typical patterns of laser output are shown here. (Reprinted with permission from Sliney DH, Trokel SL. Medical lasers and their safe use. New York: Springer-Verlag, 1993, p. 16.)

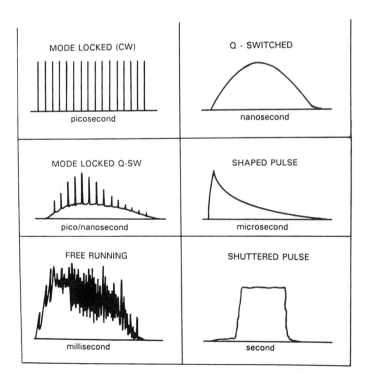

B. Continuous Wave (CW)

Some lasers operate in a continuous mode where the emerging flow of photons is constant. In this CW mode, the power output is constant with time, and therefore the peak power output is equal to the average power output. For safety purposes, a laser is considered CW if the output lasts longer than 250 ms. The typical ophthalmic lasers that operate in the CW mode are the Ar, Kr, HeNe, and diode lasers. The power output of these lasers is typically on the order of milliwatts to watts.

C. Pulsed

Some lasers operate in a pulsed mode where the output lasts from a few milliseconds to a few femtoseconds (10^{-15} s). These pulses can be single or a series of pulses. When there is a series or burst of pulses, the number of pulses emitted per second is called the pulse repetition rate, and this is given in Hertz (i.e., Hertz = pulses/s). In the pulsed mode the power output is not constant with time, and therefore the peak power output is higher than the average power output. As a particular example of a pulsed laser, the Nd:YAG laser can be operated in three different pulsed modes: free-running, Q-switched, or mode-locked.

1. **Free-Running.** In the free-running mode, each pulse lasts from 1 to 100 ms (1 ms = 10^{-3} s).

2. **Q-Switched.** In the Q-switched mode, the pulses last from 3 to 20 ns (1 ns = 10^{-9} s). This pulse duration typically results in power outputs on the order of megawatts. The Q refers to the resonant quality of the laser cavity. A high Q factor indicates that laser emission will occur, whereas a low Q factor indicates that no emission will occur and that the excitation energy will be stored in the laser active medium. That quality or Q factor can be changed by placing a special shutter between one of the mirrors and the laser medium. This shutter prevents laser action until the maximal population inversion has been obtained in the laser medium. Two major types of shutters are used:

   a. **Active Q-Switch.** This switch consists of an electro-optical shutter known as a Kerr cell or a Pockel cell. The laser beam is polarized by a fixed polarizer in the cavity. The polarization of the adjacent Kerr cell can be changed by applying a high-voltage pulse across the cell. When both polarizations are aligned, the beam is transmitted through the transparent Q-switch, and when the polarizations are perpendicular to each other, the beam is stopped by the now opaque Q-switch.

   b. **Passive Q-Switch.** This switch usually consists of a saturable dye cell. When the dye is exposed to a low beam irradiance, the dye is opaque and prevents beam transmission. Once the beam reaches a certain threshold irradiance, the dye bleaches and becomes transparent for a very short period of time.

3. **Mode-Locked.** In the mode-locked mode, the pulses last from 6 femtoseconds (1 fs = 10^{-15} s) to 80 picoseconds (1 ps = 10^{-12} s). This pulse duration results in power outputs

on the order of 100 megawatts (1 MW = 10^6 W) to 1000 GW (1 GW = 10^9 W). A number of closely spaced wavelengths and, hence, temporal frequencies oscillate back and forth in the laser cavity simultaneously. The phases of these oscillations are usually independent and different. By synchronizing these oscillations, the peaks of the waves will occur simultaneously at a given instant and result in a brief series of very short pulses.

V. Spatial Modes of Operation

A. Transverse Electromagnetic Modes (TEM)

1. In the laser's resonance cavity, photons or electromagnetic waves are traveling back and forth between the two mirrors. Constructive interference and, hence, stability of the combination of these electromagnetic fields occurs only for a limited number of conditions or modes, known as TEM modes. In these standing wave patterns or TEM modes, the electric and the magnetic fields are perpendicular or transverse to each other and to the direction of propagation of the beam. The energy distribution perpendicular to the beam axis is described by TEM mode notation.

2. The different modes are designated TEM_{pq}, where p and q are integers denoting the number of nodes in the standing wave pattern along the x and y directions, respectively. In other words, these modes are labeled with the number of minima that occur when the beam is scanned horizontally (p) and then vertically (q). Figure 1–6 shows a number of these modes.

B. Fundamental Mode

1. A single mode or fundamental mode is denoted when p and q are both zero. This TEM_{00} mode therefore has no nodes in the plane perpendicular to the beam axis. This mode is generated when the rays are limited to those around the **central axial path**. The output of a laser operating in this mode is a spherical wave with a **Gaussian intensity distribution** as shown in Figure 1–7. The intensity of this beam is greatest at the beam axis and falls off exponentially with radial distance from the beam axis.

2. This Gaussian beam profile is important for ophthalmic applications because it produces the **smallest possible spot size**.

3. Because the smallest spot size is achieved when focusing this TEM_{00} beam, it also produces the **highest power density** at the focus.

4. The fundamental mode beam is thus **used for delicate work**, such as performing a posterior capsulotomy, because it localizes the damage to the smallest area (Loertscher, 1983).

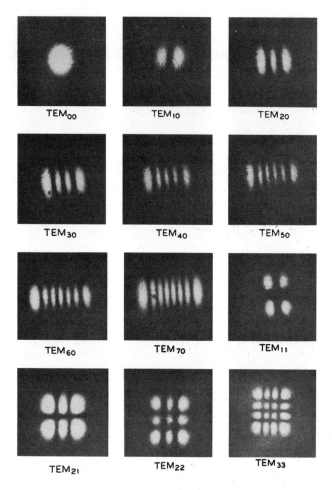

Figure 1–6 Photographs of some of the mode patterns from a gas laser. The modes are designated as TEM_{pq}, where p and q are integers denoting the number of nodes in the standing wave pattern along the x and y directions, respectively. (Reprinted from Kogelnik H, Li T. Laser beams and resonators. Appl Optics 5:1550–1567 (1966), with permission from Optical Society of America.)

C. Multimode

1. Once a laser cavity is made to generate a given higher-order mode, that laser also emits all modes with lower order. Therefore, this type of laser is known as a multimode laser.

2. By using rays in the laser that are at a slight angle to the central axial path, multimode distributions are obtained. These intensity distributions are **non-Gaussian**. This then leads to a **higher total power output** but with a **lower power density** due to a **larger cross-sectional beam area**.

3. Because of the beam characteristics, the multimode laser is **used on thick structures**, such as cutting thick vitreous strands (Loertscher, 1983).

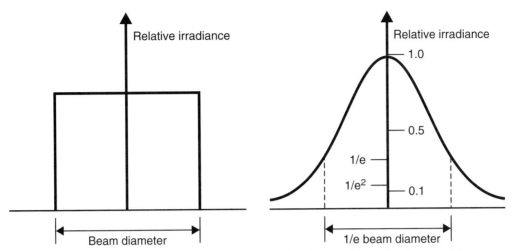

Figure 1–7 Beam profiles. A rectangular beam profile and a theoretical Gaussian beam profile are shown. The diameter of the Gaussian beam can be defined at 1/e (as shown) or at 1/e².

4. The output of a multimode laser may be no more coherent than the output of an appropriately filtered incandescent source (Young, 1992). Highly coherent light is only generated in a single mode laser.

VI. Beam Parameters

When describing laser output, a few terms are important. Although the output of all lasers may be described using any of the parameters, different parameters are characteristically used for pulsed lasers and CW lasers.

A. Radiant Energy

The output of a pulsed laser is normally given in energy terms. The usual unit of energy is a **joule (J)**. For example, the output of an ophthalmic Q-switched Nd:YAG laser is usually given in **millijoules (mJ)**.

B. Radiant Power

The output of a CW laser is normally given in power terms, that is, the rate at which energy is delivered. The unit of power is a **watt (W)**. One watt is equal to one joule emitted per second. For example, the output of an Argon photocoagulation or a HeNe aiming laser is usually given in watts.

C. Radiant Exposure

The ratio of the total emitted energy to the cross-sectional area of the beam is called the radiant exposure or the **fluence**. The usual units are therefore **joules per square centimeter (J/cm²)**.

D. Irradiance

The ratio of the emitted power to the cross-sectional area of the beam is labeled the irradiance. It's also sometimes referred to as the power density. The usual units are **watts per square centimeter (W/cm²)**. For example, an argon laser that emits 2 W in a beam area of 0.5 cm² has an irradiance of 4 W/cm².

VII. Beam Size

A. Introduction

For ophthalmic applications, the beam size is important in defining the exposure parameters and assessing the safety of the beam. Several terms are used to describe and measure the beam size.

B. Beam Waist

The beam waist is the region of the beam that has the smallest diameter. The waist can be located either inside or outside the laser cavity. In an ideal diffraction-free system in which ray tracing analysis applies, the laser focus would be an infinitesimally small spot, a point. In reality, it is a spot with a finite diameter, known as the beam waist.

C. Beam Boundary

The boundary of the beam and, thus, the beam diameter can be denoted in a number of ways:

1. **Solid Angle.** For converging/diverging beams, the solid angle method for determining the beam diameter involves a simple geometrical analysis of the beam and laser parameters: the diameter of the laser aperture and the focal point of the beam. Rays from the edge of the laser aperture to the focal point form a solid angle. The diameter of a cross-section of this solid cone at any given distance from the aperture can be used as a measure of the beam diameter.

2. **1/e Diameter.** For a Gaussian fundamental mode laser beam, the radius, and hence the diameter, can be measured at the 1/e power point (where e = 2.71828). If the intensity of the symmetrical Gaussian beam at the center is normalized to 1, the radius of the beam can be defined as the distance from the center of the beam to the point where the intensity distribution has fallen off to 1/e (see Figure 1–7). When measured in this way, 63% of the total power of the laser beam is contained within

the 1/e beam diameter. This diameter is used for laser safety calculations (Sliney & Wolbarsht, 1980).

3. **1/e² Diameter.** For a Gaussian beam, the diameter can also be measured at the $1/e^2$ power point. In this case, 86.5% of the total power of the beam is contained within the $1/e^2$ diameter. This diameter is often used by laser manufacturers to describe the output of their lasers (Sliney & Wolbarsht, 1980).

D. Beam Divergence

The beam from a collimated laser spreads out as it moves further from the laser. This divergence is measured in radians or milliradians. Figure 1–8 shows a beam emerging from a laser aperture with an initial diameter of d and a beam divergence of ϕ. At a distance L from the aperture, the beam diameter D is made up of the initial beam diameter d plus the vertical legs of an upper and lower right triangle. Each leg is equal to L • sin ($\phi/2$). Thus D is simply:

$$D = d + L \bullet \sin(\phi/2) + L \bullet \sin(\phi/2)$$

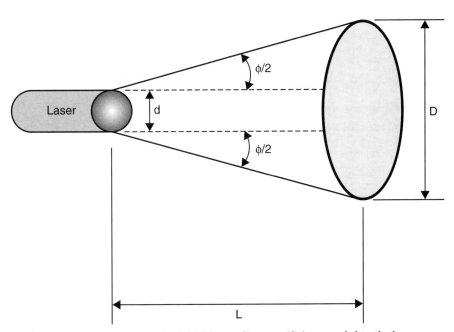

Figure 1–8 Beam divergence. The initial beam diameter (d) is expanded to the beam diameter, D, at a distance L from the laser due to the beam divergence (ϕ).

If the small angle approximation is used (sin α ≈ tan α ≈ α, where α is given in radians), then the diameter can be written as:

$$D = d + L \bullet \phi/2 + L \bullet \phi/2 = d + L\phi$$

For example, a beam having an initial diameter of 1 mm and a divergence of 1 mrad (10^{-3} rad) will have what diameter at 1 meter from the laser?

$$D = 1\,mm + 1000\,mm\,(10^{-3}\,rad)$$
$$D = 2\,mm$$

Thus, the beam divergence is a measure of the rate of increase in beam diameter with distance from the laser. A typical gas laser will have a beam divergence on the order of 1 mrad. Thus, the beam expands about 1 mm for every meter away from the laser. This is orders of magnitude smaller than the divergence of most other sources of radiant energy.

E. Angular Aperture (Cone Angle)

The beam emitted by an ophthalmic Nd:YAG laser converges to a focus (beam waist) and then diverges. The convergence or cone angle is usually 16°. This value is a compromise because of competing criteria.

1. A wider angle will **maximize**
   a. spatial stability of the breakdown region,
   b. decrease in power density at points beyond the focus (e.g., at the retina), and
   c. aiming/focusing accuracy.
2. A smaller angle will **minimize** any beam path obstruction. For example, when aiming at a posterior capsule, a wider beam may intercept and damage the iris unintentionally.

VIII. Laser Light Characteristics

Laser radiation has three unique characteristics that are important in ophthalmic applications.

A. Laser Radiation Is Coherent. This characteristic is a result of the nature of the process of stimulated emission of radiation. As noted previously, the photon that hits the atom and the photon emitted as a result of this stimulation are both in phase with each other and are, hence, coherent.

B. Laser Radiation Is Monochromatic. This characteristic is also a result of the nature of the process of stimulated emission of radiation. As we saw before, each of the photons has the same energy and, hence, the same wavelength. Therefore, the radiation is monochromatic. This feature can be extremely important for ophthalmic applications. This monochromatic output

1. **eliminates chromatic aberration** and

2. **allows selective tissue damage** because of selective tissue absorption (discussion later in this chapter).

C. Laser Radiation Can Be Collimated. The cascade process or amplification only occurs for those photons that move essentially parallel to the long axis of the resonance cavity, bouncing back and forth between the two cavity mirrors. Therefore, the emerging laser beam is collimated (i.e., the emerging rays are nearly parallel to each other). The collimation of most lasers is so good that the divergence of the emitted beam is on the order of 1 mrad.

D. The Monochromatic and Collimated Characteristics Are the Most Important for Ophthalmic Uses. These features together allow the laser output to be focused down to a diffraction-limited spot size, if necessary. This results in a fantastic focusing potential that can be employed to selectively damage tissue. The ability to use monochromatic radiation increases the ability to selectively damage tissue because of the fact that some tissues absorb certain wavelengths better than other wavelengths.

IX. Laser–Tissue Interactions

A. Transmission

Laser radiation may simply pass through and not interact with the tissue at all.

B. Reflection

Laser radiation can be reflected in either a specular or diffuse manner.

C. Scatter

Some radiation is scattered in various directions, including forward scatter (Niemz, 1996).

1. **Elastic Scattering.** In this process, no energy is lost to the tissue and the laser wavelength is unchanged.

2. **Inelastic Scattering.** In this process, a small amount of energy is either lost to the molecules of the tissue or taken up from the molecules. The wavelength of the laser radiation is shifted slightly to the red or the blue, respectively. An example of this is the Doppler effect where the wavelength is shifted by moving particles (e.g., erythrocytes).

D. Absorption

In order for radiation to damage tissue, it must be absorbed by atoms or molecules in the tissue. The energy absorbed per photon is dependent on the wavelength of the photon and is given by:

$$E = h\nu = hc/\lambda$$

where E is the energy of the photon, h is Planck's constant (6.626×10^{-34} J-sec), ν is the frequency of the photon, c is the speed of light, and λ is the wavelength of the photon. For example, a photon from the ArF excimer laser has an energy of:

$$E = (6.626 \times 10^{-34} \text{J-s})(3 \times 10^8 \text{m-s}^{-1})(193 \times 10^{-9} \text{m})$$
$$= 1 \times 10^{-18} \text{J}$$

X. Ocular Absorption

A. Absorbers

There are a number of important chromophores in and around the eye. Laser radiation may be absorbed by one or more of these chromophores. The amount of absorption is a function of the laser wavelength and the tissue properties. Table 1–2 and Figure 1–9 show the customary division of the relevant electromagnetic spectrum. These divisions are based on similar photobiologic responses and tissue absorption properties (CIE: Commission International de l'Eclairage—the International Commission on Illumination, 1970).

1. **UV Region**
   a. **Nucleic acids—deoxyribonucleic acid (DNA) and ribonucleic acid (RNA).** The nucleic acids absorb most in the UV-C region from about 240 to 280 nm. They also absorb in the IR due to their hydrogen bonds (Mellerio, 1991).

Table 1–2 The Photobiologic (CIE) Divisions of the Electromagnetic Spectrum

UV-C (100 to 280 nm)
UV-B (280 to 315 nm)
UV-A (315 to 400 nm)
Light (400 to 760–780 nm)
IR-A (760–780 to 1400 nm)
IR-B (1400 to 3000 nm)
IR-C (3000 to 1,000,000 nm)

These divisions are based on the recommendation of the Committee on Photobiology of the CIE (Commission International de l'Eclairage—the International Commission on Illumination, 1970)

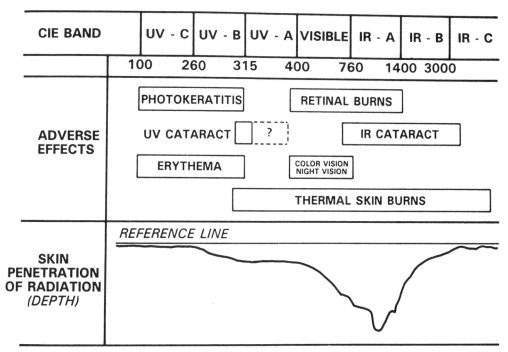

Figure 1–9 The division of the electromagnetic spectrum into photobiological spectral bands. These bands are defined by the International Commission on Illumination. Common adverse effects on skin and ocular tissues are shown. The depth of skin penetration as a function of wavelength is also shown. (Reprinted with permission from Sliney DH, Trokel SL. Medical lasers and their safe use. New York: Springer-Verlag, 1993.)

    b. **Proteins**—most amino acids of the proteins absorb below 200 nm, but the aromatic amino acids can absorb in the upper UV-C region around 270 to 280 nm. Proteins can also absorb in the IR (Mellerio, 1991).

    c. **Melanin** (in the eye and skin).

2. **Visible Region**

    a. **Hemoglobin** (e.g., in the retinal and choroidal blood vessels). Red is absorbed the least (Figure 1–10). Absorption decreases with increasing wavelength except for one peak (555 nm, yellow) in the absorption spectrum of reduced hemoglobin and for two peaks (542 nm, green; 577 nm, yellow) in the spectrum of oxyhemoglobin (Mainster, 1986).

    b. **Xanthophyll** (macular pigment)—blue (400 to 500 nm) is absorbed the most (see Figure 1–10).

    c. **Melanin** (in the eye and skin)—absorption decreases monotonically as wavelength increases (see Figure 1–10).

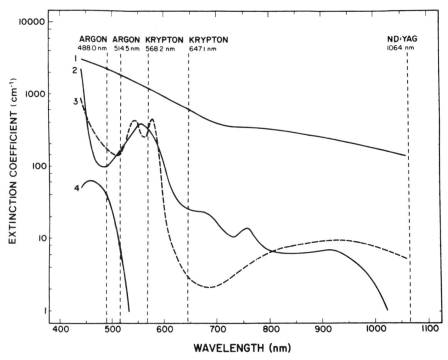

Figure 1–10 Extinction coefficient versus wavelength for melanin (1), oxygenated hemoglobin (2), deoxygenated hemoglobin (3), and xanthophyll (4). The wavelengths for argon, krypton, and Nd:YAG lasers are marked. (Reprinted from Mainster MA. Wavelength selection in macular photocoagulation: tissue optics, thermal effects, and laser systems. Ophthalmology 93:952–958, 1986, with permission from Lippincott Williams & Wilkins.)

    d. **Exogenous chromophores**—there are a number of chromophores that are introduced into the body to increase tissue absorption for certain clinical procedures. For example:

        1) **Psoralens** (used to treat psoriasis)

        2) **Hematoporphyrin derivative** (used to treat tumors)

  3. **Infrared (IR) Region. Water** (all cells and tissues)—there are strong vibrational absorption bands in the IR.

B. Depth of Penetration (Cheong et al., 1990; Jacques, 1992; Mueller et al., 1991; Sliney & Trokel, 1993; Trost, 1991).

  1. The depth of penetration depends on a number of parameters:

    a. **Absorption** by chromophores—this is highly dependent on the laser wavelength. Absorption occurs when a photon collides with an atom and loses its energy to the atom.

    b. **Scattering**—this can also be dependent on the wavelength of the laser and on the size of the scattering centers or particles (Bohren & Huffman, 1983; Van de Hulst, 1981).

1) If the size of the particles is much less than the wavelength of the radiation, then the process is called **Rayleigh scattering**. In this case, the intensity of the scattered radiation depends on $1/\lambda^4$ and thus **scattering increases as the wavelength decreases** (e.g., blue light is scattered more than green or red light). This type of scattering is responsible for the blue sky as well as the red sunset.

2) If the size of the particles is much greater than the wavelength of the radiation, then the process is called **Mie scattering**, and there is **little dependence on the wavelength**. In this kind of scattering, there is a **preferential scattering** of the radiation in the direction of propagation of the radiation (i.e., **in the forward direction**). This type of scattering is responsible for the white light scattered by chalk dust from an eraser.

   c. **Reflection**—the laser beam can be reflected either via specular reflection or by diffuse reflection. In either case, the process of reflection will limit the amount of penetration.

2. In general, the **deepest penetration is in the infrared** (see Figure 1–9). Infrared radiation is scattered less than the visible radiation and so more is transmitted deeper into the tissue.

   a. For laser wavelengths **less than 1400 nm**, the longer the wavelength, the greater the transmission and, hence, the deeper the penetration.

   b. For laser wavelengths **more than 1400 nm**, penetration decreases because of an increase in water absorption.

   c. Table 1–3 shows the approximate tissue penetration depth for a few typical ophthalmic lasers (Cheong et al., 1990; Mueller et al., 1991; Trost, 1991).

3. **Ocular structures** absorb differentially depending on wavelength (Figure 1–11).

   a. **UV**

      1) **Cornea.** In the UV-C (100 to 280 nm) region, the cornea absorbs almost all of the radiation. In the UV-B (280 to 315 nm) and UV-A (315 to 400 nm) regions, the cornea absorbs much of the radiation.

Table 1–3 Typical Tissue Penetration Depths

Laser	Wavelength (nm)	Penetration Depth (mm)
ArF excimer	193	0.002
XeCl excimer	308	0.200
Argon	488	0.300
Nd:YAG/KTP	532	0.800
Dye	630	5.1
Diode	810	2.5
Nd:YAG	1064	10
Ho:YAG	2060	0.29
Er:YAG	2960	0.001
CO_2	10,600	0.019

Data from Cheong et al., 1990; Mueller et al., 1991; Trost, 1991.

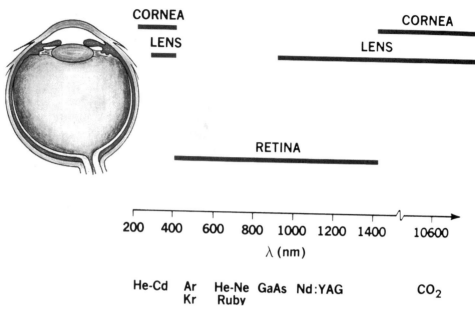

Figure 1–11 Ocular absorbing tissue as a function of laser wavelength. The approximate location of wavelength outputs are shown for a number of ophthalmic lasers.

2) **Lens.** In the UV-B region, the lens absorbs most of the radiation that gets through the cornea. In the UV-A region, the lens absorbs the most.

b. **Visible (400 to 780 nm)**

1) **Cornea and lens.** Most visible radiation is transmitted through the cornea and lens.

2) **Retina.** Most visible radiation is absorbed in the retina by the hemoglobin, xanthophyll, and melanin pigment.

c. **IR**

1) **Retina.** Most of the IR-A (780 to 1400 nm) is absorbed by the retina and choroid, especially by the melanin in the retinal pigmented epithelium (RPE) and the choroidal melanocytes.

2) **Lens and cornea.** Some of the IR-A and a little of the IR-B (1400 to 3000 nm) is absorbed by the lens. Much of the IR-B and most of the IR-C (3000 to 10,000 nm) is absorbed by the cornea.

XI. Damage Mechanisms

A. Photothermal Damage Mechanism

1. **Absorption of Radiation.** Photons from the laser can be absorbed by the molecules of the ocular tissue. An absorbed photon can lead to an electronic excitation or

to a direct increase in the rotational and/or vibrational energy of the molecules. The **wavelength** of the radiation is important in determining the following:

a. **Types of Absorption.** The energy of ultraviolet or visible photons is high enough to cause electronic excitation; whereas, the energy of infrared photons is only high enough to increase the vibrational or rotational energy of molecules.

b. **Selectivity of Absorption.** Selective coagulation can be obtained by matching the laser wavelength to the wavelength of maximum absorption of the tissue chromophore(s). For example, the CO_2 laser wavelength of 10,600 nm in the far-IR (IR-C) is highly absorbed by water, so the first tissue cells hit by the beam will absorb most of the beam.

c. **Penetration Depth.** Penetration depth is highest in the IR-A region of the spectrum and falls off on either side of that region. So an Nd:YAG laser with an output of 1064 nm penetrates much deeper than the CO_2 laser in the IR-C region or than the argon laser at 488 nm (Figure 1–9).

2. **Conversion of Laser Energy into Heat.** If the absorption of a laser photon by a molecule raises an electron to an excited state, energy can be converted from that excited state to the vibrational or rotational states of the molecule (Figure 1–12). This process is called an **internal conversion**. Alternatively, the energy of the absorbed photon can be directly absorbed into the vibrational or rotational states of the molecule. In either case, the average stored kinetic energy of the molecules will be increased. Temperature is a measure of the average kinetic energy of the molecules in the tissue.

3. **Temperature Rise of Tissue.** Therefore, if the absorption of a laser photon increases the average kinetic energy of the molecules, the temperature of the tissue will rise. The threshold for thermal damage depends on the exposure duration. The shorter the exposure duration is, the higher is the irradiance (W/cm^2) necessary to produce thermal damage.

4. **Types of Thermal Damage.** Depending on the rate of energy delivery, at least six types of thermal damage may occur:

a. **Photocoagulation.** The protein molecules of tissues are folded or coiled chains of amino acids. They are held in their native, folded conformation by weak interactions: for example, hydrogen bonds and van der Waals' interactions. Increasing the temperature by as little as 10–20°C can lead to a disruption of these interactions and the consequent unraveling of the protein (Hillenkamp, 1980; Katzir, 1993; Mainster et al., 1970). This process is called **denaturation** and leads to dysfunction. For example, enzymes are inactivated when they become denatured, and cells die when enough of their proteins are denatured. This heating process can also lead to **coagulation** where the fluid tissue is changed to a gel or a solid. This structural change leads to an essentially immediate visible whitening of the irradiated tissue. To obtain photocoagulation then, the laser energy must be delivered at a rate to obtain a tissue temperature in the range of 50–100°C.

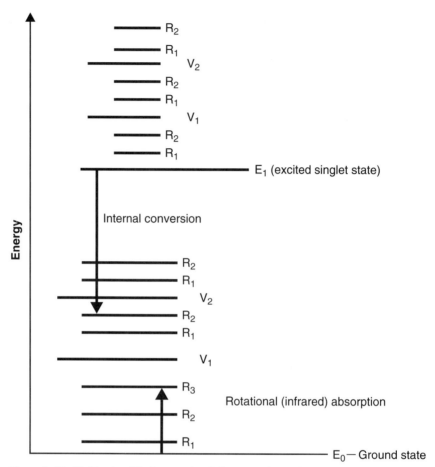

Figure 1–12 *Highly simplified energy level diagram of two electronic states, E_0 and E_1, with vibrational (V) and rotational modes (R). An example of internal conversion is shown where energy is converted from excited state E_1 to a rotational state of the molecule. In addition, an example of rotational absorption is shown where energy from an absorbed photon is directly absorbed into a rotational state. These types of processes can lead to an increase in rotational and vibrational energy and thus to an increase in temperature.*

As an example, this type of damage is used to treat proliferative diabetic retinopathy by performing pan-retinal photocoagulation with an argon or dye laser. Photocoagulation involves a number of histopathologic changes:

1) **Cell Shrinkage.** This shrinkage occurs because of the thermal denaturation as well as the contraction of proteins in the tissue. Most likely, there is also a collapse of the intracellular cytoskeleton (Thomsen, 1991).

2) **Nuclear Pyknosis and Hyperchromatism.** The nuclei and cytoplasm of irradiated cells become more dense due to the condensation of the nuclear chromatin and the cytoplasmic proteins (Thomsen, 1991). At the light microscope level, these processes are reflected in the nuclear pyknosis and the increased uptake of stain (hyperchromatism).

3) **Membrane Rupture.** Membranes of cells and organelles can be ruptured forming membrane fragments (Pearce & Thomsen, 1995).

4) **Birefringence Changes in Collagen and Muscle.** Native birefringence of collagen and muscle can be lost due to the thermal disruption of the regular arrays of collagen molecules and the actin and myosin molecules (Asiyo-Vogel et al., 1997; Thomsen, 1991). This disruption also leads to the appearance of swollen, hyalinized (glassy) collagen fibers.

b. **Photovaporization (Photothermal Ablation).** If the laser energy is delivered at a rate that results in a temperature of 100°C, the water in the tissue will boil and will be vaporized. Just below the surface of the irradiated tissue, hot pockets of superheated steam create vacuoles (bubbles) that rapidly enlarge and then eventually rupture explosively. This series of events is called the **popcorn effect**. The rapid evolution of the steam can result in microscopic particulate removal (Welch et al., 1991). This type of damage is thus used for incision and removal of tissue. For example, a CO_2 laser can be used to remove a basal cell carcinoma on the eyelid.

c. **Photocarbonization.** If the laser energy continues to be delivered after the water boils off, charring or photocarbonization of the tissue occurs. As long as there is water in the tissue, the temperature of the tissue cannot normally climb above 100°C. Once the water has been vaporized, the temperature will rise higher. When the temperature exceeds 150°C, the remaining tissue will begin to vaporize and char (Niemz, 1996).

d. **Melting.** Once the tissue temperature exceeds 300°C, melting can begin (Niemz, 1996). The precise melting temperature depends on the particular type of tissue material.

e. **Photoshortening.** By increasing the temperature of collagen fibrils a small amount, the fibrils will shrink up to one-third of their original length. Heating the collagen to temperatures ranging from 58°C to 76°C will break some of the hydrogen bonds holding the collagen triple helix together and cause a conformational phase transition that shortens the molecule (Koch et al., 1995; Stringer & Parr, 1964). This mechanism is being explored to change the refractive state of the cornea using a holmium laser in a process called laser thermokeratoplasty.

f. **Photowelding.** Soft tissues can be glued together by localized heating (Katzir, 1993). This process has been used to close corneal wounds (Barak et al., 1997;

Burstein et al., 1992). The mechanisms are not fully understood, but they apparently involve the thermal denaturation and adherence of proteins.

g. **Hyperthermia.** By using a relatively long exposure and mildly heating tissue, tumor cells can be stressed and become more susceptible to radiation or other therapeutic modalities (Jacques, 1992).

5. **Thermal Damage Threshold and Heat Conduction**

   a. **Heat Conduction.** The most important way heat is lost from an exposed volume of tissue is by conduction away from that volume into the surrounding tissue.

   b. **Thermal Relaxation Time.** Because heat is conducted away from the exposed tissue, the concept of a thermal relaxation time can be defined as the time, t_r, when the temperature has fallen to 1/e of its initial value (Mellerio, 1991). This is approximated by:

$$t_r \approx C \bullet l^2$$

   where l is the smallest dimension of the exposed tissue volume and C is a constant ($10^6 \, s \, m^{-2}$). As an example, for a typical melanin granule in the RPE with a diameter of $1 \, \mu m$, the t_r is about $1 \, \mu s$; whereas for an arteriole with a diameter of $100 \, \mu m$, the t_r is about $10 \, ms$. Since melanin is the most important chromophore for most retinal photocoagulation exposures, the t_r is essentially determined by the thickness of the melanin layer which is about $5 \, \mu m$. This results in a t_r of about $25 \, \mu s$ even though the laser spot size is larger than $5 \, \mu m$.

   c. **Exposure Duration.** If the exposure time is greater than the thermal relaxation time, then it follows that a significant amount of heat will be conducted from the exposed volume to the surrounding tissue. This means there will be collateral damage, especially if the exposure duration is in the range of about $20 \, \mu s$ to $10 \, s$. So for macular photocoagulation using an argon laser with a duration of $200 \, ms$, the damage will go beyond the laser spot and could involve the fovea if the spot is close to the fovea. For a Q-switched Nd:YAG laser with an exposure time in the nsec region, this means that the exposure is so fast that there is essentially no conduction of heat to the surrounding tissue. However, for this laser, nonthermal effects are more important and will be considered later.

   d. **Spot Size.** Increasing the spot size will result in a greater increase in temperature at the center of the exposed volume because the relative rate of heat loss decreases. This is due to the fact that heat is lost through the surface, and as the laser spot size increases, the volume of the absorbing tissue increases at a faster rate than does the surface area of the absorbing tissue.

   e. **Threshold for Thermal Damage.** The preceding considerations mean that the threshold will decrease as the laser spot size is increased. In the range of 20 μs to $10 \, s$ exposure durations, the threshold will increase as the exposure duration increases. Thus, it is important in laser photocoagulation to adjust the laser beam spot size and duration, as well as the beam irradiance, to produce focal tissue injury and minimize collateral damage.

f. **Selective Photothermolysis.** This is the principle that thermal tissue necrosis (resulting from heat conduction away from the target) is minimized if the laser pulse duration is less than the thermal relaxation time of the target tissue (Anderson & Parrish, 1983). It also involves the concept that a particular target can be selectively destroyed by matching the laser wavelength to the wavelength of maximal absorption by the target.

B. Photochemical Damage

1. **Photochemical Interactions.** Chemical, instead of thermal, changes can also be brought about by the absorption of laser radiation (Mellerio, 1991). Photochemical changes can occur when UV or visible radiation is absorbed by tissue; whereas IR radiation, especially in the IR-B and IR-C range, does not have enough energy to cause a photochemical effect.

   a. **Photosensitizers.** When a sensitizer molecule S is excited, the absorbed photon raises the molecule from its ground state ^0S to an excited singlet state $^1S^*$. In this state the electron spins are paired and the lifetime of the state is very short (10^{-9} to 10^{-6} s). From this state, the molecule may return to the ground state by emitting a long-wavelength photon (about 600–700 nm). The other option is for the electron to change its spin state in a process called **intersystem crossing** and to convert to an excited triplet state $^3S^*$ (see Figure 1–1). In this state the spins are parallel and the lifetime of the state is fairly long (10^{-3} s). In this triplet state the molecule has more time to interact with surrounding molecules and can undergo either of two types of interactions (Foote, 1990).

      1) A **type I** interaction involves a direct interaction of the triplet state (or less commonly, the singlet state) of the photosensitized molecule with a nearby substrate or solvent. This type of reaction results in either electron or hydrogen atom transfer, thus yielding radical ions or radicals.

      2) A **type II** interaction involves the transfer of energy from the triplet (or singlet) state to molecular oxygen ($^3O_2$) to form singlet oxygen ($^1O_2$). Singlet oxygen, in turn, is a reactive molecule that easily interacts with a nearby substrate molecule to form oxidized products. These products are toxic to cells.

   b. **Free Radicals and Toxic Oxygen Species.** These photochemical reactions can create not only singlet oxygen, but also a variety of free radicals (a molecule with one unpaired electron). Free radicals are very reactive and can lead to lipid peroxidation (Halliwell & Gutteridge, 1986). Polyunsaturated fatty acids in membrane lipids are very susceptible to peroxidation and this can lead to the destruction of the membrane and of the cell.

   c. **Photochemical Reactions.** Examples of these reactions include the following:

     1) **Photodissociation.** In this process, the splitting of the molecule can result in free radicals.

     2) **Dimerization.** This involves the linking of two equal monomeric molecules. For example, two adjacent thymine bases on a DNA strand can form a dimer due to absorption of a UV photon (300 to 315 nm). This could then trap the DNA in a nonfunctional conformation.

     3) **Photoinduced Isomerization.** The most obvious example of this type of reaction is the cis-trans isomerization of retinal in photoreceptor transduction.

   d. **Characteristic Features**

     1) **No threshold.** For photons with enough intrinsic energy, that is, those in the UV and blue region, there is no threshold for a photochemical reaction at the molecular level (Mellerio, 1991). For example, with the ArF excimer laser, absorption of even a single photon can lead to the breaking of a molecular bond. Increasing the intensity of the beam merely causes the breaking of more bonds.

     2) **Dose-dependent.** The rate of a photochemical reaction depends on the rate at which photons are incident on the molecule. Each photon has enough energy to excite a molecule or to break a molecular bond, so the more photons there are that are hitting the molecule, the more likely it is that some of these will be absorbed and be effective.

     3) **Reciprocity between threshold irradiance and exposure duration.** The irradiance (W/cm^2) threshold for producing a just ophthalmoscopically visible retinal lesion is reciprocally related to the exposure duration for photochemical damage (Mellerio, 1991). This means the irradiance for a threshold lesion decreases as the exposure duration increases. In other words, if you are using an argon laser and you double the exposure duration (e.g., from 50 ms to 100 ms), the threshold irradiance will decrease by a factor of two.

     4) **Delayed onset.** Another characteristic of photochemical damage is that it often takes time to become manifest. Familiar examples include sunburn and welder's flash or photokeratitis. In both cases, there is usually a delay of hours between the time of the exposure and the time the pain develops.

     5) **Thermal enhancement.** Increasing the temperature of the tissue can increase the rate of destructive processes compared to the rate of repair processes.

  2. **Types of Photochemical Therapies**

   a. **Photoradiation (Photodynamic Therapy, PDT).** In this type of therapy, a photosensitizing drug can be used to treat a tumor (Oleinick & Evans, 1998). The drug is injected into the patient and is selectively taken up by the tumor. Then a laser tuned to the wavelength of maximum absorption of the drug is focused on the tumor. The absorption of the laser radiation by the drug leads to the generation of a toxic species, like singlet oxygen or free radicals. The toxic species then destroys the tumor. Hematoporphyrin derivative and other photosensitizers are being explored using dye lasers to selectively kill ocular tumors, like choroidal melanomas.

b. **Photoablation (Photochemical Ablation, Photoablative Decomposition, Ablative Photodecomposition)**

1) The energy of a single photon (6.4 eV) of an argon fluoride excimer laser is enough to break a carbon-carbon (3.6 eV) or carbon-nitrogen (3.0 eV) bond in a protein. By exposing the cornea to a series of these photons, molecular fragments are created and these fragments leave the surface of the cornea at supersonic velocities, creating a laser plume (Keyes et al., 1985; Krauss et al., 1986; Srinivasan, 1983, 1986). The ejection of the fragments occurs because of the large increase in tissue volume due to the decomposition and to the transfer of the excess photon energy into kinetic energy of the fragments (Garrison & Srinivasan, 1985; Srinivasan & Mayne-Banton, 1982).

2) Controversy has surrounded the issue of whether photoablation with an excimer laser is to be categorized as a photochemical or a photothermal process. A chemical transition (dissociation of molecules) does occur during photoablation, but many distinguish photoablation as a process different from pure photochemical or thermal processes (Niemz, 1996). Others prefer to use terms like photochemical ablation to refer to excimer ablation and photothermal ablation to refer to photovaporization. In reality there is no "pure" photoablation. The ArF excimer laser generates very little thermal energy, whereas the longer-wavelength XeCl excimer laser generates a significant thermal component (Sutcliffe & Srinivasan, 1986).

c. **Photobiostimulation (Biostimulation, Low-Intensity Laser Therapy, Monochromatic Light Therapy).** This process involves the use of a low-level HeNe or diode laser to produce stimulatory or inhibitory effects such as analgesia, reduction of edema, or enhancement of wound healing. In spite of wide clinical usage, especially in Asia and Europe, this process has provoked skepticism (Basford, 1995; Devor, 1990; Lowe et al., 1998). The possible mechanisms are currently being investigated (Belkin & Schwartz, 1994; Belkin et al., 1988; Tuner & Hode, 1998, 1999).

d. **Photodynamic Biologic Tissue Glue.** This process involves crosslinking of a protein solder (fibrinogen) with tissue collagen using a photosensitive singlet oxygen generator (Goins et al., 1997, 1998; Khadem et al., 1994; Oz et al., 1990; Wright et al., 1998). The argon blue-green laser and diode lasers have been used to generate the reactive oxygen species. These oxygen species then produce cross linkages between the ocular tissue and the fibrinogen. Possible uses of the glue include closing bleb leaks after filtration surgery and assisting in wound closure in corneal transplantation.

e. **Photothrombosis.** This process involves the intravenous administration of a photosensitizer dye (e.g., rose bengal or phthalocyanine) with subsequent exposure of blood vessels to laser radiation (Gohto et al., 1998; Joussen et al., 1998; Nanda et al., 1987; Peyman et al., 1997; Primbs et al., 1998; Royster et al., 1988). The photochemical reaction creates reactive singlet oxygen molecules that then cause peroxidation of lipids, proteins, and other macromolecules. This then leads to vessel endothelial damage and platelet aggregation (i.e., thrombus formation). The result is the occlusion of the irradiated blood vessels. Because this is a photochemical process (as opposed to photocoagulation), less laser energy is necessary, and therefore thermal effects are minimized. In addition, recanalization is minimized since the thrombus is formed by platelet aggregation without activation of the extrinsic or intrinsic coagulation system. Possible uses of photothrombosis include treatment of subretinal, iris, and corneal neovascularization as well as lipid keratopathy (Chapter 9).

C. *Photodisruption (Photomechanical; Non-Linear, Ionizing Damage)*

1. **Dielectric Breakdown.** When the output of an Nd:YAG laser is focused to a small spot and the energy is delivered in a very short period of time, dielectric breakdown may occur. In this process, the high irradiance (on the order of 10^{10} to 10^{11} W/cm^2) of the laser beam strips off the electrons of the exposed atoms or molecules, leaving positive ions and free electrons (Mainster et al., 1983). This mixture of ions and electrons is called a **plasma**. It is the fourth state of matter, i.e., there are gas, liquid, solid, and plasma states. It has some characteristics of a gas and some characteristics of a metal; for example, it conducts electrons.

2. **Plasma Formation**
   a. **Initiation.** A plasma can be initiated in two ways:
      1) **Thermionic emission.** This process occurs with high irradiance laser pulses with a duration on the order of a nanosecond (Ready, 1971). The electric field in the pulse can produce focal heating of the exposed tissue and thereby free a bound electron. This process is enhanced by impurities in the tissue because these impurities contain a few free electrons and can act as sites for focal heating (Bass & Barrett, 1972). This is the dominant mechanism in Q-switched lasers.
      2) **Multiphoton absorption.** This mechanism occurs with high irradiance pulses with a duration on the order of a picosecond or shorter (Ready, 1971). A single photon from an Nd:YAG laser at 1064 nm is not energetic enough to ionize an atom. However, if one of the atoms of the tissue absorbs many photons at once, the combined energy can be enough to strip an electron out of orbit. This is the dominant mechanism in mode-locked lasers.

b. **Growth of the Plasma.** A free electron generated by either process is then accelerated by the strong electric field of the laser beam. This fast electron then hits another atom and knocks out one of its outer electrons, thus producing ionization. Then both free electrons are accelerated by the field and hit two other atoms and generate two other free electrons. This process continues and produces a cascade or avalanche of free electrons and, hence, a plasma (Bass & Barrett, 1972).

c. **Plasma High Temperature.** The laser beam greatly increases the average kinetic energy of the tissue atoms and molecules and, therefore, heats the tissue to extremely high temperatures. The temperature of the focal spot where the plasma is created can reach up to **15,000°C**, that is, more than twice the surface temperature of the sun (Barnes & Rieckhoff, 1968)! However, because the energy of the beam only lasts a nanosecond or shorter, the heat does not diffuse into the surrounding tissue. Thus, thermal damage is not clinically significant.

d. **Plasma Shielding**

1) Once the plasma is formed, it absorbs some of the rest of the laser beam (Capon et al., 1988; Nahen et al., 1996; Steinert et al., 1983a,b). This absorption is accomplished by the high density of free electrons in the plasma, which can in turn absorb some of the laser beam photons.

2) This enhanced absorption leads to a shielding effect for structures behind the plasma. For example, when a posterior capsulotomy is performed, the plasma formed just behind the capsule will absorb some of the beam and, thus, decrease the number of photons reaching the retina.

3) This increased absorption by the induced plasma also accounts for the ability of the Nd:YAG laser to be used in nonpigmented tissue. Energy can be deposited in relatively weakly absorbing media (e.g., vitreous or aqueous fluids) creating a plasma and the resultant photodisruption.

e. **Non-Linear Effect.** The formation of a plasma does not occur when the irradiance is low, only when it reaches a certain threshold value. In other words, plasma formation is an all-or-none phenomenon.

f. **Multiple Plasmas.** Due to the statistical nature of plasma formation, there is a finite probability that multiple plasmas may be formed (Capon et al., 1987, 1988). To minimize this probability, the cone angle can be increased by use of a contact lens and the output energy can be minimized.

3. **Plasma-Mediated Ablation (Plasma-Induced Ablation).** Plasma ionization itself results in ablation of tissue, but this damage is confined to the region of dielectric breakdown (Niemz et al., 1991; Stern et al., 1989; Teng et al., 1987). This is to be distinguished from the mechanism of photodisruption which is a result of the secondary effects of the plasma. These secondary effects include the shock waves, cavitation, and jet formation. These latter forces mechanically disrupt the tissue, and at

higher laser pulse energies, this disruption is even more significant than the plasma-mediated ablation damage (Niemz, 1996).

4. **Pressure Waves (Hypersonic and Acoustic Transients).** These waves are produced by:
   a. **Plasma Expansion.** The plasma expands at a supersonic velocity creating a **shock wave** (Barnes & Rieckhoff, 1968; Bell & Landt, 1967; Noack & Vogel, 1995; Vogel et al., 1993). This can then lead to mechanical damage to the tissue and is an important damage mechanism with the Nd:YAG laser. This shock wave results in an audible "snap," a miniature version of the thunder that follows a lightning strike. The shock wave loses energy to the surrounding medium and quickly decelerates to sonic velocities within about $100\,\mu m$ from the center of the plasma (Fujimoto et al., 1985).
   b. **Stimulated Brillouin Scattering.** The high field strength at the focus of the laser beam can also generate a supersonic shock wave and be scattered by that same wave (Brewer & Rieckhoff, 1964; Ready, 1971). In this form of scattering, some of the energy of the laser beam is transferred to the phonons in the acoustic wave, and this then leads to a longer wavelength scattered beam. By increasing the irradiance of the beam, alterations of optical density can be created by the laser radiation itself, and then these alterations can scatter the beam.
   c. **Phase Change.** The high temperature at the laser focus leads to a boiling of the liquid and a vaporization of the tissue. This phase change from solid or liquid to gas can produce acoustic waves and can also lead to the generation of a bubble, that is, to cavitation (Cleary & Hamrick, 1969; Fujimoto et al., 1985; Hu, 1969).
   d. **Thermal Expansion.** The generation of so much heat also leads to the thermal expansion of the tissue which can generate an acoustic wave (Cleary & Hamrick, 1969; Hu, 1969; Venugopalan et al., 1996). This wave or pressure pulse travels at the speed of sound in the tissue and creates a positive pressure region. Once the wave reaches the tissue surface, it is reflected by the air-tissue or water-tissue boundary as a negative pressure region that propagates into the tissue just behind the leading positive pressure region. If the pressure becomes too negative and generates a steep gradient between the two regions, the tissue can break and be ejected as ablated mass. This process is called **spallation** (Dingus & Scammon, 1991).
   e. **Ablation Recoil.** When tissue fragments are rapidly ejected by ablation, the recoil transmits an impulse of momentum back into the tissue (Jacques, 1992). This impulse propagates as a stress wave.

5. **Cavitation.** After the shock wave, an unstable vapor bubble is formed. This formation is called "cavitation."
   a. This bubble oscillates through a series of expansions and contractions (Capon et al., 1986; Mellerio et al., 1987; Vogel et al., 1993). For a 5-mJ Nd:YAG pulse in

saline solution, the maximum diameter of the bubble reaches about 2 mm (Vogel et al., 1986). The diameter of the bubble then decreases with each oscillation due to energy loss to the tissue.

b. Shock waves and high-speed **liquid jets** can also be formed during this action leading to possible tissue damage (Vogel et al., 1986, 1990; Mainster et al., 1983). An example would be corneal endothelial damage during an iridotomy with a Q-switched Nd:YAG laser. Here the damage may be due to jet formation occurring when a gas bubble from an earlier exposure lodges against the cornea and is then hit by acoustic transients from subsequent exposures (Vogel et al., 1990).

c. Liquid jet formation can also occur when a cavitation bubble collapses in the vicinity of a solid boundary, like the posterior surface of an IOL (Tomita & Shima, 1986). This can lead to damage to the IOL due to the high impact pressure of the jet.

d. Since this whole process occurs in about 300 μs, the cavitation bubble is not seen during the laser procedure. What is seen are the debris and microbubbles that are produced by the process (Sherrard & Kerr Muir, 1985; Vogel et al., 1990).

e. Cavitation bubbles generated by femtosecond laser pulses develop more rapidly and have a smaller maximum diameter than the bubbles generated by longer pulses (Juhasz et al., 1996). This results in more localized tissue damage. A similar relationship exists for picosecond pulses versus nanosecond pulses (Vogel et al., 1994).

6. **Spark Emission.** Once the electrons are stripped off the atoms, some of them recombine with the positive ions and emit visible photons, just like the process that occurs to produce a lightning flash. The output is primarily in the ultraviolet and visible wavelengths (Steinert & Puliafito, 1985).

7. **Photospallation**

a. Photospallation is a photomechanical process that differs from photodisruption. After strong absorption of short pulse radiation, thermoelastic stress transients are generated in the tissue and then this leads to tissue cleavage (Hoffman & Telfair, 2000).

b. First, the surface of the target material is heated by the laser beam with a pulse duration much shorter than the thermal relaxation time of the target. This leads to rapid compression followed by dynamic expansion. A positive, compressive stress pulse is created at the site of energy deposition, and this pulse propagates away from the initial site. When the stress wave hits the tissue interface, a negative tensile stress wave is reflected back into the tissue. A bipolar stress pulse is created since the negative pulse trails the positive pulse. If the stress created is greater than the tensile tissue strength, the target tissue will fracture. Fragments or whole layers of tissue may be split off and ejected. Because "spall" means to break up into fragments or chips, this process is called spallation.

c. Precise ablation coupled with submicron, collateral thermal damage results when short pulses (nanosecond), mid-infrared wavelength, and low fluences (less than

$200\,mJ/cm^2$) are used. The shock waves generated by photospallation have peak magnitudes that are about two orders of magnitude less than those created by photodisruption, and thus there is less collateral damage.

d. The photoelastic waves in the photospallation process have potential for use in corneal ablation for refractive surgery (Hoffman & Telfair, 1999, 2000; Telfair et al., 2000a,b). The results appear to be similar to those obtained when using a 193-nm excimer laser, without the high costs of the laser system.

XII. Type and Extent of Damage

The type and extent of damage is a function of a number of parameters:

A. Specific Body Organ or Tissue Exposed

The eye is the most susceptible to damage because of its variety of chromophores and because of the focusing ability of the cornea and lens.

B. Wavelength

As discussed earlier, selective wavelength absorption allows the target tissue to be chosen by the selection of a particular wavelength (see Figure 1–11). The depth of penetration is also selectable.

C. Duration of Exposure

The dominant type of tissue damage can be selected primarily by picking a particular exposure duration (Figure 1–13).

1. For exposures lasting **longer than about 10 s** that have an irradiance near threshold, the predominant damage is **photochemical**. This is especially true for near-UV and blue exposures.

2. For exposures in the region of **microseconds to 10 s**, the predominant damage mechanism is **photothermal**. The ophthalmic argon, krypton, dye, CO_2, CW doubled Nd:YAG, and diode lasers operate in this region.

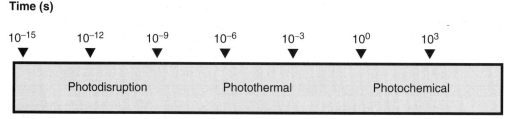

Time (s)

| 10^{-15} | 10^{-12} | 10^{-9} | 10^{-6} | 10^{-3} | 10^{0} | 10^{3} |

| Photodisruption | Photothermal | Photochemical |

Figure 1–13 Laser pulse duration largely determines the laser damage mechanism. This is a continuum with overlap between the mechanisms.

3. For exposures that last for **less than 10µs**, the primary damage mechanism is **photodisruption**. The Nd:YAG and Nd:YLF ophthalmic lasers operate in this region. For lasers that emit in the UV-C region, like the ArF excimer, the damage mechanism can also be photochemical because of the highly energetic photons.

D. Energy Absorbed

The energy absorbed by the tissue is a function of the following parameters:

1. **Energy incident on the cornea**—how much energy actually reaches the eye is obviously important in determining how much energy is finally absorbed.

2. **Beam size**—the larger the beam size is, the more likely it is that the iris or the angle structures may "clip" part of the beam. Also, increasing the beam size, while keeping the energy constant, will decrease the number of photons absorbed per unit area.

3. **Pupil size**—the pupil may be small enough that the iris may stop a portion of the beam.

4. **Spot size**—the smaller the spot size to which the laser beam is focused, the higher is the energy density and, hence, the higher is the number of photons absorbed in a given small area.

References

Anderson RR, Parrish JA. Selective photothermolysis: Precise microsurgery by selective absorption of pulsed radiation. Science 220:524–527 (1983).

Asiyo-Vogel MN et al. Histologic analysis of thermal effects of laser thermokeratoplasty and corneal ablation using Sirius-red polarization microscopy. J Cataract Refract Surg 23:515–526 (1997).

Barak A et al. Temperature-controlled CO_2 laser tissue welding of ocular tissues. Surv Ophthalmol 42 Suppl:S77–S81 (1997).

Barnes PA, Rieckhoff KE. Laser induced underwater sparks. Appl Phys Lett 13:282–284 (1968).

Basford JR. Low intensity laser therapy: still not an established clinical tool. Lasers Surg Med 16:331–342 (1995).

Bass M, Barrett HH. Avalanche breakdown and the probabilistic nature of laser-induced damage. IEEE J Quantum Electron QE-8:338–343 (1972).

Belkin M, Schwartz M. Ophthalmic effects of low-energy laser irradiation. Surv Ophthalmol 39:113–122 (1994).

Belkin M, Zaturunsky B, Schwartz M. A critical review of low energy laser bioeffects. Lasers and Light in Ophthalmol 2:63–71 (1988).

Bell CE, Landt JA. Laser-induced high pressure shock waves in water. Appl Phys Lett 10:46–48 (1967).

Bohren CF, Huffman DR. Absorption and scattering of light by small particles. New York: Wiley, 1983.

Brewer RJ, Rieckhoff KE. Stimulated Brillouin scattering in liquids. Phys Rev Lett 13:334–336 (1964).

Burstein NL et al. Corneal welding using hydrogen fluoride lasers [letter]. Arch Ophthalmol 110:12–13 (1992).

Capon MRC, Docchio F, Mellerio J. Investigations of multiple plasmas from ophthalmic Nd:YAG lasers. Lasers in Ophthalmol 1:147–153 (1987).

Capon MRC, Docchio F, Mellerio J. Nd:YAG laser photodisruption: an experimental investigation on shielding and multiple plasma formation. Graefes Arch Clin Exp Ophthalmol 226:362–366 (1988).

Capon MRC, Mellerio J. Nd:YAG lasers: plasma characteristics and damage mechanisms. Lasers in Ophthalmol 1:95–106 (1986).

Cheong WF, Prahl SA, Welch AJ. A review of the optical properties of biological tissues. IEEE J Quant Electon 26:2166–2185 (1990).

Cleary SF, Hamrick PE. Laser-induced acoustic transients in the mammalian eye. J Acoust Soc Am 46:1037–1044 (1969).

Commission Internationale de l'Eclairage (International Commission on Illumination). International lighting vocabulary. 3rd ed. Publication CIE No. 17 (E-1.1). Paris:CIE, 1970.

Devor M. What's in a laser beam for pain therapy [editorial]? Pain 43:139 (1990).

Dingus RS, Scammon RJ. Grueneisen stress-induced ablation of biological tissue. Proc SPIE 1427:45–54 (1991).

Foote CS. Chemical mechanisms of photodynamic action. In: Gomer CJ, ed. Future directions and applications in photodynamic therapy. Vol. SPIE Institutes for Advance Optical Technologies, Vol. IS6. Bellingham, WA: SPIE Optical Engineering Press, 1990.

Fujimoto JG et al. Time-resolved studies of Nd:YAG laser-induced breakdown. Plasma formation, acoustic wave generation, and cavitation. Invest Ophthalmol Vis Sci 26:1771–1777 (1985).

Garrison BJ, Srinivasan R. Laser ablation of organic polymers: microscopic models for photochemical and thermal processes. J Appl Phys 57:2909–2914 (1985).

Gohto Y et al. Photodynamic effect of a new photosensitizer ATX-S10 on corneal neovascularization. Exp Eye Res 67:313–322 (1998).

Goins KM et al. Photodynamic biologic tissue glue to enhance corneal wound healing after radial keratotomy. J Cataract Refract Surg 23:1331–1338 (1997).

Goins KM, Khadem J, Majmudar PA. Relative strength of photodynamic biologic tissue glue in penetrating keratoplasty in cadaver eyes. J Cataract Refract Surg 24:1566–1570 (1998).

Halliwell B, Gutteridge JM. Free Radicals in Biology and Medicine. Oxford: Oxford University Press, 1986.

Hecht J. Understanding lasers. An entry-level guide. 2nd edition. New York: IEEE Press, 1994.

Hillenkamp F. Interaction between laser radiation and biological systems. In: Hillenkamp F, Pratesi R, Sacchi CA, eds. Lasers in Biology and Medicine. New York: Plenum, 1980; 3:37–68.

Hoffman HJ, Telfair WB. Minimizing thermal damage in corneal ablation with short pulse mid-IR lasers. J Biomed Optics 4:465–473 (1999).

Hoffman HJ, Telfair WB. Photospallation: a new theory and mechanism for mid-infrared corneal ablations. J Refract Surg 16:90–94 (2000).

Hu C-L. Spherical model of an acoustic wave generated by rapid laser heating in a liquid. J Acoust Soc Am 46:728–736 (1969).

Jacques SL. Laser-tissue interactions. Photochemical, photothermal, and photomechanical. Surg Clin North Am 72:531–558 (1992).

Joussen AM et al. Photothrombosis of corneal neovascularization with photosensitizers coupled to macromolecules. Lasers Light Ophthalmol 8:211–219 (1998).

Juhasz T et al. Time-resolved observations of shock waves and cavitation bubbles generated by femtosecond laser pulses in corneal tissue and water. Lasers Surg Med 19:23–31 (1996).

Katzir A. Lasers and Optical Fibers in Medicine. San Diego: Academic Press, Inc, 1993.

Keyes T, Clarke RH, Isner JM. Theory of photoablation and its implications for laser phototherapy. J Phys Chem 89:4194–4196 (1985).

Khadem J, Truong T, Ernest JT. Photodynamic biologic tissue glue. Cornea 13:406–410 (1994).

Koch DD et al. Noncontact holmium:YAG laser thermal keratoplasty. In: Salz JJ, ed. Corneal laser surgery. St. Louis: Mosby-Year Book, 1995; 17:247–254.

Kogelnik H, Li T. Laser beams and resonators. Appl Optics 5:1550–1567 (1966).

Krauss JM, Puliafito CA, Steinert RF. Laser interactions with the cornea. Surv Ophthalmol 31:37–53 (1986).

Loertscher H. Laser-induced breakdown for ophthalmic applications. In: Trokel SL, ed. YAG laser ophthalmic microsurgery. Norwalk: Appleton-Century-Crofts, 1983; 4:39–66.

Lowe AS et al. Effect of low intensity monochromatic light therapy (890 nm) on a radiation-impaired, wound-healing model in murine skin. Lasers Surg Med 23:291–298 (1998).

Maiman TH. Stimulated optical radiation in ruby. Nature 187:493–494 (1960).

Mainster MA. Wavelength selection in macular photocoagulation: tissue optics, thermal effects and laser systems. Ophthalmology 93:952–958 (1986).

Mainster MA et al. Retinal-temperature increases produced by intense light sources. J Opt Soc Am 60:264–270 (1970).

Mainster MA et al. Laser photodisruptors: Damage mechanisms, instrument design and safety. Ophthalmology 90:973–991 (1983).

Mellerio J. The interaction of light with biological tissues and the potential for damage. In: Marshall J, ed. The susceptible visual apparatus. Boca Raton: CRC Press, Inc, 1991; 3:30–53.

Mellerio J, Capon M, Docchio F. Nd:YAG lasers—A potential hazard from cavitation bubble behavior in anterior chamber procedures? Lasers in Ophthalmol 1:185–190 (1987).

Mueller G, Doerschel K, Kar H. Biophysics of the ablation process. Lasers Med Sci 6:241–254 (1991).

Nahen K, Noack J, Vogel A. Plasma formation in water by picosecond and nanosecond Nd:YAG laser pulses: transmission, scattering, and reflection. Proc SPIE Lasers in Ophthalmology IV 2930:38–49 (1996).

Nanda SK et al. A new method for vascular occlusion. Photochemical initiation of thrombosis. Arch Ophthalmol 105:1121–1124 (1987).

Niemz MH. Laser-tissue interactions. Fundamentals and applications. New York: Springer Verlag, 1996.

Niemz MH, Klancnik EG, Bille JF. Plasma-mediated ablation of corneal tissue at 1053 nm using a Nd:YLF oscillator/regenerative amplifier laser. Lasers Surg Med 11:426–431 (1991).

Noack J, Vogel A. Streak-photographic investigation of shock-wave emission after laser-induced plasma formation in water. Proc SPIE Laser-Tissue Interaction VI 2391:284–293 (1995).

Oleinick NL, Evans HH. The photobiology of photodynamic therapy: cellular targets and mechanisms. Radiat Res 150 (Suppl.):S146–S156 (1998).

Oz MC et al. Tissue soldering by use of indocyanine green dye-enhanced fibrinogen with the near infrared diode laser. J Vasc Surg 11:718–725 (1990).

Pearce J, Thomsen S. Rate process analysis of thermal damage. In: Welch AJ, Van Gemert MJC, eds. Optical-thermal response of laser-irradiated tissue. New York: Plenum Press, 1995; 17:561–606.

Peyman GA et al. Photodynamic therapy for choriocapillaris using tin ethyl etiopurpurin (SnET2). Ophthalmic Surg Lasers 28:409–417 (1997).

Primbs GB et al. Photodynamic therapy for corneal neovascularization. Ophthalmic Surg Lasers 29:832–838 (1998).

Ready JF. Effects of high-power laser radiation. New York: Academic Press, 1971.

Royster AJ et al. Photochemical initiation of thrombosis: Fluorescein angiographic, histologic, and ultrastructural alterations in the choroid, retinal pigment epithelium, and retina. Arch Ophthalmol 106:1608–1614 (1988).

Schawlow AL, Townes CH. Infrared and optical lasers. Phys Rev 112:1940–1949 (1958).

Sherrard ES, Kerr Muir MG. Damage to the corneal endothelium by Q-switched Nd:YAG laser posterior capsulotomy. Trans Ophthalmol Soc UK 104:524–528 (1985).

Silfvast WT. Laser fundamentals. New York: Cambridge University Press, 1996.

Sliney DH, Trokel SL. Medical lasers and their safe use. New York: Springer-Verlag, 1993.

Sliney D, Wolbarsht M. Safety with Lasers and Other Optical Sources: A Comprehensive Handbook. New York: Plenum Press, 1980.

Srinivasan R. Kinetics of the ablative photodecomposition of organic polymers in the far ultraviolet (193 nm). J Vac Sci Technol B 1:923–926 (1983).

Srinivasan R. Ablation of polymers and biological tissue by ultraviolet lasers. Science 234:559–565 (1986).

Srinivasan R, Mayne-Banton V. Self-developing photoetching of poly (ethylene terephthalate) films by far-ultraviolet excimer laser radiation. Appl Phys Lett 41:576–578 (1982).

Steinert RF, Puliafito CA. The Nd-YAG laser in ophthalmology. Principles and clinical applications of photodisruption. Philadelphia: WB Saunders Company, 1985.

Steinert RF, Puliafito CA, Kittrell C. Plasma shielding by Q-switched and modelocked Nd-YAG lasers. Ophthalmology 90:1003 (1983a).

Steinert RF, Puliafito CA, Trokel S. Plasma formation and shielding by three ophthalmic Nd:YAG lasers. Am J Ophthalmol 96:427–434 (1983b).

Stern D et al. Corneal ablation by nanosecond, picosecond and femtosecond lasers at 532 nm and 625 nm. Arch Ophthalmol 107:587–592 (1989).

Stringer H, Parr J. Shrinkage temperature of eye collagen [letter]. Nature 204:1307 (1964).

Sutcliffe E, Srinivasan R. Dynamics of UV laser ablation of organic polymer surfaces. J Appl Phys 60:3315–3322 (1986).

Telfair WB et al. Healing after photorefractive keratectomy in cat eyes with a scanning mid-infrared Nd:YAG pumped optical parametric oscillator laser. J Refract Surg 16:32–39 (2000a).

Telfair WB et al. Histological comparison of corneal ablation with Er:YAG laser, Nd:YAG optical parametric oscillator laser, and excimer laser. J Refract Surg 16:40–50 (2000b).

Teng P et al. Acoustic studies of the role of immersion in plasma-mediated laser ablation. IEEE J Qu Electron QE-23:1845–1852 (1987).

Thomsen S. Pathologic analysis of photothermal and photomechanical effects of laser-tissue interactions. Photochemistry and Photobiology 53:825–835 (1991).

Tomita Y, Shima A. Mechanism of impulsive pressure generation and damage pit formation by bubble collapse. J Fluid Mech 169:535–564 (1986).

Trost D. Holmium:YAG lasers improve knee surgery. Photonics Spectra August:111 (1991).

Tuner J, Hode L. It's all in the parameters: a critical analysis of some well-known negative studies on low-level laser therapy. J Clin Laser Med Surg 16:245–248 (1998).

Tuner J, Hode L. Low level laser therapy: clinical practice and scientific background. Sweden: Prima Books, 1999.

Van de Hulst HC. Light scattering by small particles. NewYork: Dover Publications, 1981.

Venugopalan V, Nishioka NS, Mikic BB. Thermodynamic response of soft biological tissues to pulsed infrared-laser irradiation. Biophys J 70:2981–2993 (1996).

Vogel A, Busch S, Asiyo-Vogel M. Time-resolved measurements of shock-wave emission and cavitation-bubble generation in intraocular laser surgery with ps- and ns-pulses and related tissue effects. Proc SPIE Ophthalmic Technologies III 1877:312–322 (1993).

Vogel A et al. Cavitation bubble dynamics and acoustic transient generation in ocular surgery with pulsed neodymium:YAG lasers. Ophthalmology 93:1259–1269 (1986).

Vogel A et al. Intraocular Nd:YAG laser surgery: light-tissue interaction, damage range, and reduction of collateral effects. IEEE J Quantum Electron 26:2240–2260 (1990).

Vogel A et al. Intraocular photodisruption with picosecond and nanosecond laser pulses: tissue effects in cornea, lens, and retina. Invest Ophthalmol Vis Sci 35:3032–3044 (1994).

Welch AJ et al. Laser thermal ablation. Photochem Photobiol 53:815–823 (1991).

Wright MM et al. Laser-cured fibrinogen glue to repair bleb leaks in rabbits. Arch Ophthalmol 116:199–202 (1998).

Young M. Optics and Lasers: Including Fibers and Optical Waveguides. 4th rev ed, New York: Springer-Verlag, 1992.

Chapter 2
Clinical Instrumentation

Charles M. Wormington

I. Introduction

A. General References. A number of books and articles summarize the different types of lasers and accessories used to diagnose and treat ocular diseases (Bloom & Brucker, 1997; Hecht, 1992, 1994; Karlin, 1995; L'Esperance, 1989; Silfvast, 1996; Sliney & Trokel, 1993).

B. The following information is intended to give an outline of the different ophthalmic lasers in terms of their characteristics, operating requirements, damage mechanisms, and ophthalmic applications. Table 2–1 summarizes the primary information.

II. Gas Lasers

A. Helium-Neon (HeNe) Laser

1. **Active Medium.** The active medium in a HeNe laser is a mixture of helium and neon gases. The mixture contains more helium than neon gas (about 5 to 12 times more).

2. **Excitation Mechanism.** The HeNe laser uses an **electric discharge** to excite the electrons.
   a. An ignition voltage of approximately 10 kilovolts (kV) is used to start the lasing, and a maintenance voltage of about 2 kV is used to keep the laser in continuous operation.
   b. The electrons in the discharge pass from the cathode at one end of the laser to the anode at the other end. The electrons collide with both the helium and neon atoms. This process raises both types of gas to higher excited states.
   c. Most of the excited energy in the helium atoms is transferred to the neon atoms. The movements of the excited electrons in the neon gas from higher to lower energy states result in a number of laser emission wavelengths (Figure 2–1).

Table 2–1 Summary of Ophthalmic Lasers: Primary Characteristics and Applications

Laser Type	Wavelength (nm)	Active Medium	Temporal Mode	Primary Damage Mechanism	Possible Applications
HeNe	543.5 (green) 632.8 (red)	Gas: Helium Neon	Continuous (CW)	Low-power	Aiming lasers Laser flare-cell meters Laser pointers
Argon (Ar)	488 (blue) 514.5 (green)	Gas: Argon	CW	Photothermal Photochemical	Laser trabeculoplasty Laser iridotomy Laser iridoplasty Retinal photocoagulation Photodynamic therapy (PDT) Oculoplastic surgery Scanning laser ophthalmoscopy Laser suture lysis Laser sclerostomy
Krypton (Kr)	531 (green) 568 (yellow) 647 (red)	Gas: Krypton	CW	Photothermal	Laser iridotomy Laser trabeculoplasty Oculoplastic surgery Retinal photocoagulation PDT
Carbon dioxide (CO_2)	10600 (far-IR)	Gas: CO_2	CW	Photothermal	Oculoplastic surgery Laser phacolysis Laser sclerostomy
Excimer (ArF)	193 (UV)	Gas: Argon Fluoride	Pulsed	Photochemical	Laser in-situ keratomileusis (LASIK) Photorefractive keratectomy (PRK) Phototherapeutic keratectomy (PTK) Laser epithelial keratomileusis (LASEK) Laser trabecular ablation Laser sclerostomy
Nd:YAG	532 (green) 1064 (near-IR)	Solid state: Neodymium ions in yttrium, aluminum, garnet matrix	CW Pulsed: Q-switched	Photodisruption (pulsed) Photothermal (CW)	Posterior capsulotomy Laser iridotomy Laser trabeculoplasty Laser phacolysis Laser sclerostomy Cyclophotocoagulation Retinal photocoagulation Oculoplastic surgery

Table 2–1 Summary of Ophthalmic Lasers: Primary Characteristics and Applications *Continued*

Laser Type	Wavelength (nm)	Active Medium	Temporal Mode	Primary Damage Mechanism	Possible Applications
Nd:YLF	527 (green) 1053 (near-IR)	Solid state: Neodymium ions in yttrium, lithium, fluoride matrix	CW Pulsed: Q-switched Mode-locked	Photodisruption (pulsed) Photothermal (CW)	Intrastromal PRK Laser iridotomy Laser phacolysis Laser sclerostomy Posterior capsulotomy
Er:YAG	2940 (mid-IR)	Solid state: Erbium ions in yttrium, aluminum, garnet matrix	CW Pulsed	Photothermal	Oculoplastic surgery Laser phacolysis Laser iridotomy Laser sclerostomy Posterior capsulotomy
THC:YAG (holmium)	2127 (mid-IR)	Solid state: Thulium, holmium, chromium ions in yittrium, aluminum, garnet matrix	Pulsed	Photothermal	Laser thermal keratoplasty (LTK) Laser phacolysis Laser sclerostomy Oculoplastic surgery
Diode	620–895 red-IR	Solid state: GaAlAs Gallium Aluminum Arsenide	CW	Photothermal	Retinal photocoagulation Laser iridotomy Laser iridoplasty Laser sclerostomy Laser suture lysis Laser trabeculoplasty Oculoplastic surgery Cyclophotocoagulation Laser pointers Aiming beams Scanning laser ophthalmoscopy Laser Doppler interferometry Optical coherence tomography (OCT) Retinal laser polarimetry
Dye	310–1200 (UV, visible, IR)	Fluorescent dyes	CW Pulsed	Photothermal Photochemical	Retinal photocoagulation Oculoplastic surgery PDT Laser iridotomy Laser sclerostomy Laser suture lysis

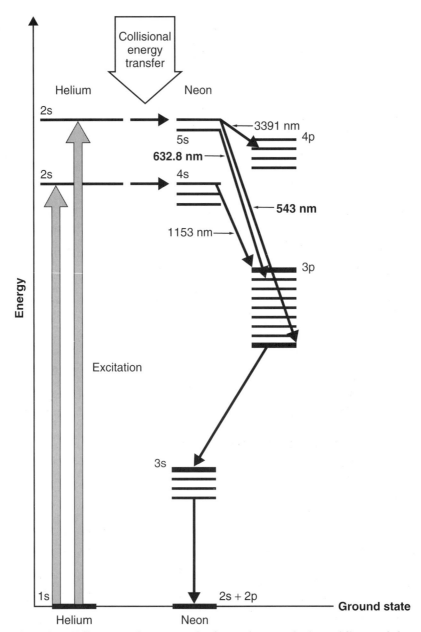

Figure 2–1 Helium–neon laser energy levels are shown as horizontal lines and the laser transitions are indicated by arrows. The energy level heights are only relative and are not shown to scale.

3. **Laser Cavity Configuration.** The laser is typically a gas-filled, linear tube with an internal cathode at one end and an anode at the other end. One of the cavity mirrors is totally reflective, and the other transmits about one percent of the radiation to form the external beam.

4. **Output Characteristics**
   a. **Wavelength.** Table 2–2 shows the wavelengths that can potentially be emitted by a HeNe laser. The standard output is at **632.8 nm** in the red region of the visible spectrum. Most of the HeNe lasers used for ocular applications emit at this wavelength. A HeNe laser configured to emit at **543.5 nm** in the green has been used in a diagnostic ophthalmic laser application.
   b. **Power.** The range of powers typically available from the various HeNe laser lines is from 0.1 to 5 mW. The standard ophthalmic HeNe laser emits on the order of 1 mW of power or less.
   c. **Temporal Modes.** The standard HeNe laser is operated in the **continuous-wave** mode.
   d. **Spatial Modes.** The standard HeNe laser emits a **fundamental mode (TEM_{00})** beam with the typical Gaussian intensity profile. The beam is usually linearly polarized.
   e. **Beam Diameter and Divergence.** The beam diameter of the typical HeNe laser is about 1 mm. The divergence of the typical beam is on the order of 1 milliradian (mrad).

Table 2–2 Major Wavelengths (nm) of Gas Lasers

HeNe	Ar	Kr	CO_2	Excimer
543.5	275.4	219	10,600	193 (ArF)
594.1	300.3	242		222 (KrCl)
604	302.4	266		248 (KrF)
611.9	305.5	337.4		308 (XeCl)
629	334	350.7		350 (XeF)
632.8 (strong)	351.1	356.4		
635	363.8	406.7		
640.1	454.6	413.1		
730.5	457.9	415.4		
1152.6	465.8	468		
1523.5	472.7	476.2		
2396	476.5	482.5		
3392	488 (strong)	520.8		
	496.5	530.9		
	501.7	568.2		
	514.5 (strong)	647.1 (strong)		
	528.7	676.4		
	1090	752.5		
		799.3		

    f. **Lifetime.** HeNe lasers typically have rated lifetimes of 10,000 to 20,000 hours.

    g. **Efficiency.** The overall efficiency of a laser is defined as the ratio of the optical output power divided by the electrical input power. This ratio is usually multiplied by 100 to give a percentage value. A HeNe laser has fairly low efficiency on the order of 0.01% to 0.1%.

5. **Operating Requirements**

    a. **Electrical Input.** The typical ophthalmic HeNe laser requires a normal **115-volt** (V) wall connection. The usual power consumption for a 1-mW HeNe laser is about 20 W.

    b. **Cooling.** Because ophthalmic HeNe lasers are low-power lasers, they employ passive air cooling.

    c. **Maintenance.** The usual laser is essentially maintenance-free and does not normally need to be adjusted.

6. **Damage Mechanism.** Because ophthalmic HeNe lasers are operated at very low powers (1 mW or less), there is no significant risk of damage when they are used as directed by the manufacturers. The maximum permissible retinal exposure time is on the order of an hour, and this involves continuous exposure to the same retinal location for that period of time.

7. **Ophthalmic Applications**

    a. **Aiming.** Many therapeutic lasers use HeNe lasers as aiming devices. The main beam of both ultraviolet and infrared lasers is invisible and so a visible laser beam is necessary to position and focus the main beam. Even some of the visible therapeutic lasers (e.g., some argon lasers) use the safer HeNe laser as an aiming device.

    b. **Illumination.** Many diagnostic lasers and some therapeutic lasers use the HeNe laser to illuminate the object of interest. This includes some scanning laser ophthalmoscopes and laser biomicroscopes, as well as some fiberoptic endoscopes.

    c. **Interferometry and Holography.** Some laser interferometers, laser speckle optometers, blood flow devices, laser Doppler velocimeters/flowmeters, and holographic interferometers use the HeNe also.

    d. **Scattering.** Some forms of laser flare cell meters and photon correlation spectroscopy units have used HeNe lasers.

B. Argon (Ar) Laser

This is the most important ophthalmic ion laser (Hecht, 1992, 1994; L'Esperance, 1989; Mainster, 1986; Pomerantzeff et al., 1976; Sigelman, 1984).

1. **Active Medium.** The Ar laser is an ion laser in which the active medium is a mixture of positive ions of the rare gas, argon. The gas consists of a singly ionized argon ion (Ar^+) species and a doubly ionized argon ion (Ar^{2+}) species.

2. **Excitation Mechanism.** Like the HeNe laser, the argon laser is excited by an **electric discharge.**

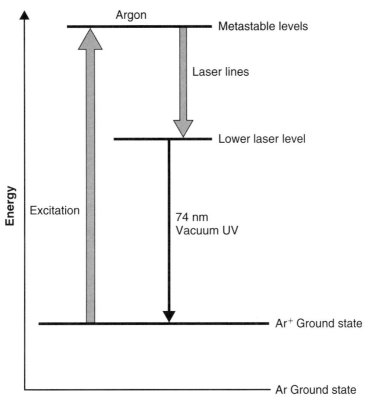

Figure 2–2 Examples of argon energy levels and laser transitions are shown. Visible Ar laser lines are generated by transitions from singly ionized argon atoms (Ar⁺). Lines with wavelengths shorter than 400 nm arise from doubly ionized argon atoms (Ar⁺²). There are a number of metastable upper energy levels and a number of lower laser levels (not shown). Visible laser lines occur by transitions from numerous pairs of upper and lower levels.

a. An ignition voltage of a few kV is used to start the lasing, and then a maintenance voltage of about 90 to 400 V is used for continuous operation.

b. This mechanism involves a high-current (10–70 A) discharge along the length of the laser tube that is concentrated in the center of the tube. This high current results in electron collisions with the argon atoms. This process is used to ionize the gas as well as excite the ions.

c. Spontaneous emission from the higher to the lower energy states produces a number of laser lines (Figure 2–2). When the electrons move from the lower laser energy level to the ground state of the ion, a 74-nm photon is emitted.

3. **Laser Cavity Configuration.** Because of the hot plasma created by the high current densities in the tube, the tube is usually made of high-temperature ceramic

and metal materials. The optics in the laser cavity determine which line or lines are emitted.

4. **Output Characteristics**
   a. **Wavelength.** Table 2–2 shows the wavelengths that can potentially be emitted by an argon laser. Emission from the singly ionized Ar^+ is in the visible and infrared region, and emission from the doubly ionized Ar^{2+} is in the near-ultraviolet region. The standard outputs for ophthalmic uses are the two strongest lines at 488 nm in the blue (70%) and 514.5 nm in the green (30%).
   b. **Power.** Most ophthalmic argon lasers have outputs on the order of a few watts.
   c. **Temporal Modes.** The standard ophthalmic therapeutic argon laser is operated in the continuous-wave mode. Mechanical shutters allow pulse durations from about 0.01 sec up to a few seconds.
   d. **Spatial Modes.** Ophthalmic argon lasers emit a **fundamental mode (TEM$_{00}$)** beam with a Gaussian intensity profile. The beam is usually linearly polarized.
   e. **Beam Diameter and Divergence.** The beam diameter of an argon laser can vary from 0.6 to 2 mm with divergences of 0.4 to 1.2 mrad.
   f. **Spot Size.** The available spot sizes on ophthalmic argon lasers are either continuously variable or selectable in steps from 50 μm to either 1000 or 2000 μm.
   g. **Lifetime.** Argon lasers typically have rated lifetimes of 1000 to 10,000 hours. The lower-power lasers usually have longer lifetimes.
   h. **Efficiency.** The overall efficiency of an ophthalmic argon laser is quite low, on the order of 0.001–0.01%. This results in a large amount of wasted heat.

5. **Operating Requirements**
   a. **Electrical Input.** The ophthalmic argon lasers typically require 220-V, one- or three-phase inputs with up to 60 A per phase. This usually requires rewiring of the laser room. One lower-power ophthalmic laser system only requires 110-V input.
   b. **Cooling.** Argon lasers require either forced-air or water cooling. Water cooling is necessary for the higher-power lasers and can involve continuous tapwater inflow and outflow or an internal circulating water system.
   c. **Maintenance.** The tubes are somewhat sensitive to temperature and mechanical stresses, so realignment of the optics may be necessary at times. The tubes and optics can degrade with time because of contamination and erosion and the argon gas can be depleted and contaminated. The tube can then be replaced or refurbished.

6. **Damage Mechanisms**
   a. Ophthalmic argon lasers generally use a **thermal** damage mechanism. With the 488 nm blue beam there is also a possibility of **photochemical** damage when operating below the thermal damage threshold.
   b. The beam is particularly absorbed by melanin, xanthophyll, and hemoglobin. Using the data compiled by Francois C. Delori, L'Esperance noted the percentage

of various laser lines absorbed by blood in a 140-μm vessel (L'Esperance, 1989). For the 488-nm line, 83% is absorbed by an artery (oxyhemoglobin) and 77% by a vein (deoxyhemoglobin).

c. Employing an in vitro system, Cohen et al. (1995) found that for oxygen-treated blood with a hematocrit of 46%, the transmission of argon green (514 nm) radiation was 15% through a 100-μm-thick sample (i.e., 85% absorption) and 1% through a 200-μm-thick sample (99% absorption). For carbon-dioxide treated blood with a hematocrit of 46%, the transmission was 20% through a 100-μm-thick sample (80% absorption) and 2% for a 200-μm-thick sample (98% absorption).

7. **Ophthalmic Applications** (Figure 2–3 shows a typical ophthalmic argon laser system).

Coagulation around retinal holes and tears
Closure of cyclodialysis clefts
Cyclophotocoagulation
Goniophotocoagulation
Gonioplasty
Holographic interferometry
Laser closure of overfiltering/leaking blebs
Laser iridoplasty
Laser iridotomy
Laser sclerostomy
Laser speckle blood flow measurement
Laser speckle optometer
Laser suture lysis
Laser trabecular ablation
Laser trabeculoplasty
Laser triggered, repetitive angiography
Laser revision of failing filter blebs
Oculoplastic surgery
Panretinal photocoagulation
Photodynamic therapy
Photon correlation spectroscopy
Pupilloplasty and photomydriasis
Scanning laser ophthalmoscopy
Suture lysis
Treatment of angiofibromas
Treatment of central serous chorioretinopathy
Treatment of macular edema
Vascular ablation

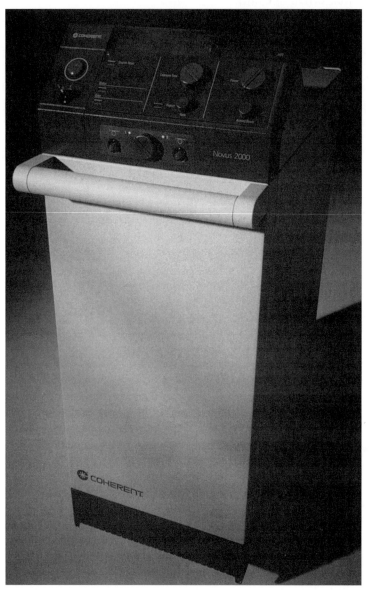

Figure 2–3 Coherent Novus 2000 ophthalmic argon laser. (Courtesy of Lumenis, Santa Clara, CA.)

8. **Advantages**
   a. The 488-nm (blue) and 514.5-nm (green) lines are absorbed well by melanin in the retinal pigment epithelium and choroid, and by hemoglobin in the retinal and choroidal vessels.

9. **Disadvantages**
   a. **Higher Rayleigh Scattering.** The 488-nm (blue) line is scattered more than the 514.5-nm (green) line. In older patients with cataractous changes, more power is needed at the level of the cornea to produce an equivalent retinal burn. In addition there may be more collateral retinal damage due to intraretinal scattering.
   b. **Absorption by the Macular Xanthophyll Pigment.** The 488-nm line is more highly absorbed by the macular xanthophyll pigment than is the 514.5-nm line. This can lead to significant inner retinal damage in the macular area when the blue line is used.

C. Krypton (Kr) Laser (Bird & Grey, 1979; Bloom & Brucker, 1997; L'Esperance, 1989; Marshall & Bird, 1979; Morse, 1985; Peyman et al., 1984; Singerman, 1982; Trempe et al., 1982; Yannuzzi & Shakin, 1982).

1. **Active Medium.** Like the Ar laser, the Kr laser is also an ion laser in which the active medium is a mixture of positive ions of a rare gas, in this case krypton gas. The gas consists of a singly ionized krypton ion (Kr^+) species and a doubly ionized krypton ion (Kr^{2+}) species. A triple ionized (Kr^{3+}) species can also be generated.

2. **Excitation Mechanism.** Like the Ar and HeNe lasers, the krypton laser is excited by an electric discharge in a similar manner.

3. **Laser Cavity Configuration.** The tube in a krypton laser is similar to that in an argon laser.

4. **Output Characteristics**
   a. **Wavelength.** Table 2–2 shows the major wavelengths that can potentially be emitted by a krypton laser. Emission from the singly ionized Kr^+ is in the visible and infrared region, and emission from the doubly ionized Kr^{2+} is in the near-ultraviolet region. The standard output for ophthalmic uses is the 647.1-nm red line. The lines at 530.8 nm (green) and 568.2 nm (yellow) can also be used for ophthalmic application.
   b. **Power.** Most ophthalmic krypton lasers have outputs on the order of a few watts.
   c. **Temporal Modes.** The standard ophthalmic therapeutic krypton laser is operated in the continuous-wave mode. Mechanical shutters allow pulse durations from about 0.01 sec up to a few seconds.

    d. **Spatial Modes.** Ophthalmic krypton lasers emit a **fundamental mode (TEM$_{00}$)** beam with a Gaussian intensity profile. The beam is usually linearly polarized.

    e. **Beam Diameter and Divergence.** Typically, as with the argon lasers, the beam diameter can vary from 0.6 to 2 mm with divergences of 0.4 to 1.2 mrad.

    f. **Spot Size.** The available spot sizes vary from 50 μm to either 1000 or 2000 μm.

    g. **Lifetime.** Krypton lasers typically have rated lifetimes of 1000 to 10,000 hours, like argon lasers. However, krypton lasers usually have shorter lifetimes than argon lasers because of faster gas depletion.

    h. **Efficiency.** Like the argon laser, the krypton laser efficiency is very low (0.0001% to 0.01%).

5. **Operating Characteristics**

    a. **Electrical Input.** The ophthalmic krypton lasers typically require 220-V, one- or three-phase inputs with up to 50 A per phase. Like the situation with argon lasers, this kind of power input usually requires the rewiring of the laser room.

    b. **Cooling.** Also like argon lasers, the ophthalmic krypton lasers require either forced-air or water cooling.

    c. **Maintenance.** As with the argon laser, realignment of optics may be necessary at times. Degradation of the tube and optics, as well as depletion of the gas, occurs with the krypton lasers. Just as with the argon laser, the tube can be either refurbished or replaced.

6. **Damage Mechanism**

    a. Ophthalmic krypton lasers use a **thermal damage** mechanism.

    b. The 530.8-nm (green) line is highly absorbed by both oxyhemoglobin (97%) and deoxyhemoglobin (95%) (L'Esperance, 1989). Similarly, the 568.2-nm (yellow) line is highly absorbed by oxyhemoglobin (96%) and deoxyhemoglobin (96%). The 647.1-nm (red) line is very poorly absorbed by oxyhemoglobin (3%) and poorly by deoxyhemoglobin (12%).

    c. For an in vitro system, Cohen et al. (1995) found that for oxygen-treated blood with a hematocrit of 46%, the transmission of krypton red (647 and 676 nm) radiation was 54% through a 100-μm-thick sample (i.e., 46% absorption) and 27% through a 200-μm-thick sample (73% absorption). For carbon-dioxide-treated blood with a hematocrit of 46%, the transmission was 60% through a 100-μm-thick sample (40% absorption) and 30% for a 200-μm-thick sample (70% absorption).

    d. Because melanin absorption decreases as the wavelength increases, melanin absorbs the green line best, followed by the yellow line, and then the red line.

7. **Ophthalmic Applications**

    Cyclophotocoagulation
    Holographic interferometry

Laser iridotomy
Laser suture lysis
Laser trabeculoplasty
Oculoplastic surgery
Photodynamic therapy
Retinal and macular photocoagulation

8. **Advantages**
   a. The green line is absorbed well by hemoglobin in the blood. This is good for photocoagulation of vessels.
   b. The green line is absorbed well by melanin. This allows excellent chorioretinal photocoagulation.
   c. The yellow line is useful for retinal photocoagulation because of its high absorption by hemoglobin and melanin and because of its low absorption by xanthophyll pigment.
   d. The red line is good for photocoagulation in the avascular zone of the fovea. This results from the absorption by melanin and the low absorption by macular xanthophyll pigment.
   e. The red line can be used for photocoagulation of subretinal neovascularization. It penetrates deeper in the choroid than the argon beam and is adequately absorbed if there is sufficient melanin in the choroid and retinal pigment epithelium.
   f. The red line is scattered less than either the green or the yellow lines. This allows the red line to penetrate mildly cataractous lenses better than the green and yellow lines.
   g. The red line can be used for retinal photocoagulation when there is a vitreal, preretinal, or retinal hemorrhage because of its low absorption by hemoglobin.

9. **Disadvantages**
   a. For a given electrical input power, the output power of krypton lasers is lower than for argon lasers.
   b. The yellow line is not useful for photocoagulation of the inner retinal layer due to its relatively poor absorption.
   c. The yellow line is not ideal for retinal photocoagulation when there is a vitreal, preretinal, or retinal hemorrhage. This is because of the high absorption by hemoglobin.
   d. The red line is not good for inner retinal layer photocoagulation due to its poor absorption.
   e. The red line is not useful for chorioretinal applications when the melanin level is low (i.e., in lightly pigmented fundi).
   f. The red line is less effective than the green or yellow line for treating vascular abnormalities because of its low absorption by hemoglobin.

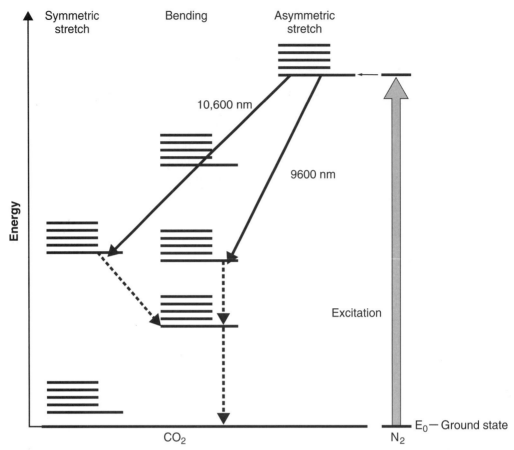

Figure 2–4 The energy level diagram for a carbon dioxide laser. The two noted laser transitions occur between vibrational levels of the molecule.

D. Carbon Dioxide (CO_2) Laser

1. **Active Medium.** The gaseous active medium is a mixture of carbon dioxide (CO_2), nitrogen (N_2), and an inert gas, usually helium (He). Each gas serves a distinct role.

    a. **CO_2 is the radiation emitter**, making this a **molecular gas laser** (Figure 2–4).

    1) Electron collisions excite the molecules to higher vibrational states. They then decay to a metastable vibrational level (an asymmetric stretching mode).

    2) From there it can drop to one of two other **vibrational modes** resulting in the two principal laser transitions:

    a) the main transition is to a symmetric stretching mode yielding a **10.6-μm line**, or

    b) another major transition is to a bending mode yielding a **9.6-μm line**.

3) Superimposed on these two vibrational transitions is a complex set of closely spaced **rotational transitions.** This results in about 100 possible distinct lines.

  b. **N_2 increases efficiency** by capturing energy from the pumping source and transferring it to CO_2. This helps excite the CO_2 to the upper laser level.

  c. **Helium also helps increase the laser efficiency.** It is a buffer gas that aids in heat transfer, and it helps the CO_2 drop from the lower laser vibrational levels to the ground state.

2. **Excitation Mechanism.** Excitation can occur via either of two pumping modes:

  a. a **direct-current electric discharge** between electrodes near each end of the tube (discharge-excited), or

  b. a **radio-frequency discharge** perpendicular to the axis of the tube (RF-excited).

3. **Laser Cavity Configuration**

  a. **Sealed-Tube Lasers.** These have a classic glass tube filled with the gases and with mirrors at both ends of the tube.

  b. **Waveguide Lasers.** These lasers have a small cavity lined with metal and/or dielectric materials and formed into a waveguide.

  c. **Axial (Longitudinal) Slow-Flowing–Gas Lasers.** These lasers are not sealed. They pass the gas slowly in one end of the tube and out the other end.

  d. **Fast Axial-Flow Lasers.** As the name implies, these lasers involve gas pumped rapidly through the length of the laser tube.

  e. Other configurations are used for even higher power CO_2 lasers (e.g., transverse-flow, gas-dynamic, and transversely excited atmospheric (pressure) lasers).

4. **Output Characteristics**

  a. **Wavelength.** The nominal **operating wavelength is 10.6 μm (far-IR)**. The actual output is multiline radiation between 9 and 11 μm that peaks strongly where the gain is highest at 10.6 μm.

  b. **Power.** In ophthalmic laser applications, power ranges up to 50 W.

  c. **Temporal Modes.** The standard ophthalmic therapeutic CO_2 laser is operated in the **continuous-wave (CW)** mode. Exposure times can be changed from 0.1 sec to continuous.

  d. **Spatial Modes.** By changing the design and the optics of the laser cavity, four basic transverse modes can be realized in the CO_2 laser:

    1) **TEM_{00} emission** (i.e., the fundamental mode with a Gaussian profile).

    2) **Multimode emission**, in which there are a number of different oscillation modes that result in the largest output power possible.

    3) **Unstable-resonator emission** where the beam has a doughnut-like profile.

    4) **Waveguide lasers** where the mode is determined by the design of the waveguide rather than by the cavity mirrors.

e. **Beam Diameter and Divergence.** A variety of beam diameters and divergences are possible depending on the design of the laser cavity and the mode structure. The beam diameter can range from 1 mm to 200 mm and the divergence can range from 0.5 mrad to 10 mrad.

f. **Spot Size.** A range of spot sizes is available from 1 to 2 mm.

g. **Lifetime.** The lifetimes of CO_2 lasers depend on the cavity design, but the typical CW laser can operate for one to a few thousand hours on a single gas fill.

h. **Efficiency.** The CO_2 laser has an efficiency of from 5% to 20%, higher than any of the other gas lasers.

5. **Operating Characteristics**

a. **Electrical Input.** Input depends on the type of laser, but the typical laser only requires 110-V with a power consumption of up to 15 A.

b. **Cooling.** Forced-air can be used for small lasers, but water cooling is necessary for higher power lasers.

c. **Maintenance.** Occasional or continuous replenishment of the CO_2 gas is necessary, depending on the type of laser, since the gas is broken down by the discharge. At times, optics must be replaced because of degradation.

6. **Damage Mechanism.** Ophthalmic CO_2 lasers use a **photothermal damage** mechanism.

a. The beam is **highly absorbed by water** and, hence, is absorbed at the surface of ocular and adnexal tissues.

b. The depth of the damage is linearly proportional to the laser power output and the duration of exposure. At the usual power and duration levels, very superficial tissue interaction occurs. **Most of the beam is absorbed in the first 20 μm of tissue** (Sliney & Trokel, 1993).

c. Tissue **absorption is not dependent on tissue color or pigmentation**.

d. **Hemostasis** is aided by the thermal sealing of the cut blood vessels adjacent to the delivery site.

e. The beam is **used to cut via photovaporization when** the spot size is smallest **(focused) and** the **pulse is short**.

1) When the energy density is high, as in a focused beam, the superficial layer of tissue fluid boils, producing an **explosive volume expansion (photovaporization)**.

2) This results in evaporation of the fluid, a **mechanical disintegration** of the tissue cells, and the creation of a **smoke plume**.

3) During this process, the temperature at the edge of the vaporization crater is maintained at about 100°C. Heat conduction (diffusion) results in thermal denaturation and coagulation in adjacent tissue.

f. The beam is **used to coagulate via photocoagulation when** the spot size is larger **(defocused)**. The **longer the duration** of the pulse, **the more photocoagulation** occurs in adjacent tissue by thermal diffusion.

1) When the energy density is low, as in a defocused beam, explosive tissue evaporation will cease, and photocoagulation becomes the dominate damage mechanism.

2) At intermediate energy densities, the tissue fluid may slowly vaporize until the water boils off, and then photocarbonization can occur as the temperature increases to about 300°C (Niemz, 1996).

7. **Ophthalmic Applications** (Figure 2–5 shows a typical ophthalmic carbon dioxide laser system).

Laser phacolysis
Laser sclerostomy
Oculoplastic surgery

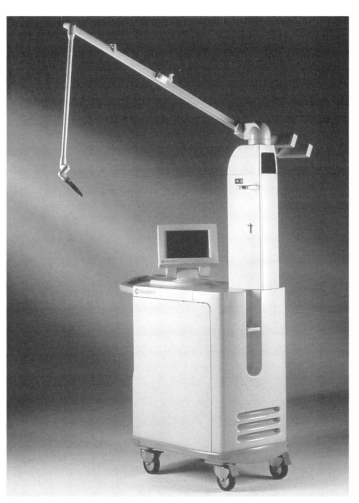

Figure 2–5 Coherent Ultrapulse 5000 L carbon dioxide laser system. (Courtesy of Lumenis, Santa Clara, CA.)

8. **Delivery Systems**
   a. **Aiming** is simplified by a **coaxial**, **visible HeNe** beam.
   b. A hollow, **articulated arm with mirrors** at the joints is used to deliver the beam. Standard optical fibers will not transmit the beam efficiently.
   c. Slit-lamp delivery
   d. Operating microscope delivery
   e. Hand-held probe delivery

E. Excimer Laser Systems (Abad & Krueger, 1997; Seiler & McDonnell, 1995; Stein et al., 1995; Waring, 1989, 1993).

1. **Active Medium.** Excimer lasers form a family of ultraviolet lasers that are made up of a combination of a **rare gas** (e.g., argon, krypton, or xenon) and a **halogen** (e.g., bromine, chlorine, or fluorine). The rare gas makes up 0.5% to 12% of the total gas volume and the halogen makes up about 0.5%.
   a. A buffer rare gas (e.g., helium or neon) makes up the bulk (88% to 99%) of the total gas mixture. This buffer gas does not participate directly in the generation of radiation, but is used to transfer energy.
   b. The term **excimer** comes from the contraction of "**exci**ted di**mer**." This term originally referred to a molecule made up of two identical atoms that came together only in the excited state. The meaning of the term has now been broadened to include any diatomic molecule that is held together only in the excited state.
   c. Table 2–2 lists the most important excimer lasers and their wavelengths. Figure 2–6 shows the energy level diagram for the excimer lasers.
   d. The most important active medium for ophthalmic excimer lasers is **ArF**.

2. **Excitation Mechanism.** Like most of the other gas lasers, the excimer lasers are excited by an **electric discharge**.
   a. The electrons formed by the electric discharge transfer energy to the gases in the mixture. But before the electric discharge occurs, usually the gas mixture is preionized by a pulse of ultraviolet radiation from a row of miniature UV spark discharges. Then the electric discharge excites the rare gas and halogen atoms to form the excimer diatomic molecules.
   b. In the excited state, the two atoms attract each other to form the excimer molecule. When the excimer drops to the ground state, the two constituent atoms repel each other and the excimer molecule falls apart. At the same time, a highly energetic photon is formed.
   c. This is an excellent laser medium with high gain because the population inversion occurs as soon as the excited state (excimer) is formed. There are essentially no molecules in the ground state since a molecular ground state does not exist. The diatomic molecule falls apart as soon as the electrons move to the lower laser level.

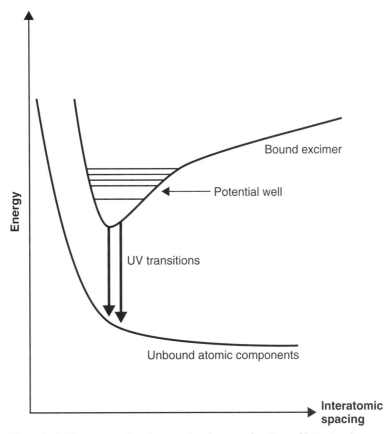

Figure 2–6 The energy of excimer molecules as a function of interatomic spacing is shown for both the excited and the ground states. The excited state has a potential well that helps stabilize it, but the two atoms of the dimer repel each other in the ground state.

    d. The excimer laser pulse duration is determined by the lifetime of the excited molecule. This lifetime and, hence, the pulse are about 10–50 ns long.

3. **Laser Cavity Configuration**
    a. Because of the high gain of the laser, the resonant cavity can consist of a highly reflective mirror on one end and an uncoated optical surface at the other end. In other words, the output coupler is not another mirror; it is an optical window. It transmits 90% to 96% of the radiation and reflects only the normal 4% to 10% of the incident radiation.
    b. In the ArF excimer laser, the optics are usually composed of magnesium fluoride or calcium fluoride because they are more transparent to the 193-nm radiation than quartz or fused-silica. The cavity is a tube that is filled with the gas and

then sealed. Repeated gas fills are necessary because the gas is degraded during use.

c. The electric discharge occurs perpendicular to the long axis of the laser cavity.

4. **Output Characteristics**

a. **Wavelength.** Table 2–2 indicates the major wavelengths of the different types of excimer lasers. The standard excimer laser used for corneal refractive surgery is the **ArF laser** with a line at **193 nm.**

b. **Power.** The average power output is on the order of 2 W. This can be calculated by multiplying the pulse energy in joules by the repetition rate in Hz (i.e., pulses per second). The peak powers are on the order of 10^8 W.

c. **Temporal Modes.** The excimer lasers operate in a pulsed mode. The pulse duration is typically from 10–20 ns, with a repetition rate of 5–15 Hz.

d. **Spatial Modes.** The output of excimer lasers is multimode with fairly poor beam quality. The quality of the beam is improved using a variety of techniques.

e. **Beam Diameter and Divergence.** The typical excimer laser emits a rectangular beam about 10×20 mm across with divergences of 1×3 mrad or 2×3 mrad.

f. **Spot Size.** Once produced in a rectangular form by the laser, the beam is homogenized and shaped by various techniques. Various kinds of apertures can be used to change the size of the beam. For example, an expanding aperture can be used to form a circular beam that expands to 6 or 7 mm in diameter. Alternatively, a scanning laser slit or spot can be used.

g. **Lifetime.** Lifetimes vary and are not usually quoted.

h. **Efficiency.** Excimer lasers have typical wall-plug efficiencies of 1% to 2%.

5. **Operating Characteristics**

a. **Electrical Input.** In general, small excimer lasers require on the order of 110-V, single phase, 10-A input. High-power excimer lasers may require 220-V, three-phase, 20–100-A input.

b. **Cooling.** Ophthalmic ArF lasers are usually air-cooled.

c. **Maintenance.** Early systems required daily gas refills, but the refill period in some of the new systems has been extended up to a year. The optics and some parts of the electrical system must be replaced occasionally. Nitrogen gas is used to purge the system in order to reduce transmission losses, increase the mirror lifetime, precipitate particles in the main gas chamber, and cool the system.

6. **Damage Mechanism.** The mechanism of UV laser ablation has been the subject of some controversy (Cross & Bowker, 1987; Isner & Clarke, 1987; Jacques, 1992; Kitazawa et al., 1997). Some have advocated a **photochemical process** (Hahn et al., 1995; Srinivasan et al., 1987). Others have advocated a combination of **photothermal and photomechanical processes** (Kitai et al., 1991; Lane et al., 1987;

Venugopalan et al., 1995). Some prefer to call the process simply **photoablation** (Niemz, 1996).

a. In the case of the ArF excimer laser used for photorefractive keratoplasty and phototherapeutic keratoplasty, each photon is highly energetic with an energy of 6.4 electron volts (eV).

b. If the corneal tissue absorbs one of these photons, there is enough energy to break a covalent molecular bond. Typical C—C or C—N bonds in proteins, glycosaminoglycans, and nucleic acids have intramolecular bond energies of 3.0 to 3.6 eV. The irradiated molecules then disintegrate into fragments when the bonds are split.

c. Via radiationless relaxation, the majority of the incident energy is subsequently converted into heat. The solid macromolecular corneal tissue is then converted into a gas with a temperature higher than 1000°C (Kermani et al., 1988; Venugopalan et al., 1995). This rapidly expanding hot gas causes the fragments to be ejected from the surface of the tissue at supersonic velocities, forming a **plume** above the cornea (Bor et al., 1993; Puliafito et al., 1987; Srinivasan, 1986). The high temperatures are achieved for only picoseconds as the gas expands and the thermal energy is converted into kinetic energy. The molecular fragments in the plume include breakdown products of collagen and proteoglycans as well as **free radicals** (Ediger et al., 1997; Kahle et al., 1992; Pettit et al., 1996). The free radicals may play a role in the development of the **corneal haze** (Jain et al., 1995). The redeposition of plume particles on the cornea and the partial absorption of subsequent laser pulses by the airborne particles may contribute to the formation of **central islands** (Noack et al., 1997).

d. There is **minimal collateral tissue damage**. Because of the shortness of the pulse duration and the ablative removal of tissue, there is minimal **thermal effect** on the tissue. Using various techniques, the measured increase in corneal temperature during and after excimer ablation varied from 6°–12°C (Bende et al., 1988; Betney et al., 1997; Bilgihan et al., 1996; Kitazawa et al., 1997; Niizuma et al., 1994). In one report, the corneal temperature rose to 53°C (Berns et al., 1988). Because the corneal temperature approaches the denaturation temperature for collagen (40°C and above), the temperature increase may contribute to the formation of corneal subepithelial haze (Kitazawa et al., 1997; Lewis et al., 1967). Adjacent tissue damage is confined to an area of less than 1 μm width (Puliafito et al., 1985; Trokel et al., 1983).

e. A **shock wave** is generated due to the impact of the laser pulse on the cornea (Bor et al., 1993; Srinivasan et al., 1987; Venugopalan et al., 1995). The shock wave produces an audible snap, propagates through the air with a speed of 1.5 to 4 km/s, and creates a pressure transient peak of as high as 90 bar (Bor et al., 1993; Kermani & Lubatschowski, 1991; Siano et al., 1997).

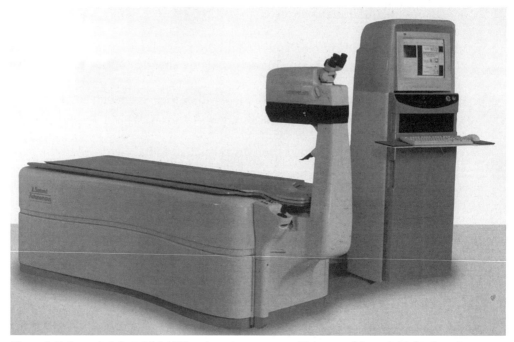

Figure 2–7 Summit InfinityLS LASIK excimer laser system. (Courtesy of Summit Technology, Inc., Waltham, MA.)

    f. A **surface wave** created by the recoil forces of the laser plume spreads out from the laser impact zone (Bor et al., 1993). Initially, the amplitude of the wave is as large as 150 to 200 μm, and it moves along the surface at a rate of several meters per second.

7. **Ophthalmic Applications** (Figure 2–7 shows a typical ophthalmic excimer laser system)

    Laser in situ keratomileusis (LASIK)
    Laser phacolysis
    Laser sclerostomy
    Laser subepithelial keratomileosis or laser-assisted subepithelial keratectomy (LASEK)
    Laser trabecular ablation
    Photorefractive keratoplasty (PRK)
    Phototherapeutic keratoplasty (PTK)

III. Solid-State Lasers

A. Nd:YAG

1. **Active Medium.** The Nd:YAG laser is a solid-state laser in which the active medium is composed of neodymium (Nd^{3+}) ions in a crystal matrix consisting of a mixture of

yttrium, aluminum, and garnet ($Y_3Al_5O_{12}$). The Nd^{3+} ions exist as an impurity (about 1%) or dopant in this hard, garnet-like crystal host. The Nd^{3+} ions take the place of some of the yttrium atoms in the matrix.

2. **Excitation Mechanism.** An external light source is used to pump all Nd:YAG lasers. Ophthalmic Nd:YAG lasers are pumped by pulsed flashlamps, but can also be pumped by diode lasers or even continuous tungsten arc lamps. Figure 2–8 is an energy-level diagram for this laser. Strong absorption occurs at 730 nm and 800 nm, followed by nonradiative decay to a metastable excited state, then decay to a lower laser level along with strong emission at 1064 nm, and finally decay to the ground state.

3. **Laser Cavity Configuration.** The resonator is a rod-shaped cavity with mirrors at both ends. The rod or cylinder is typically a few millimeters in diameter and a few centimeters long. At first a flashlamp was wrapped around the rod in a helical configuration, but now a linear lamp placed parallel to the rod is preferred. The cavity can also contain a pulse switch (e.g., Q-switch or mode-lock switch) and a limiting aperture.

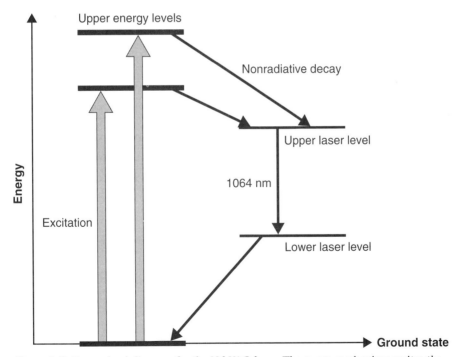

Figure 2–8 Energy level diagram for the Nd:YAG laser. The pump mechanism excites the electrons from the ground state to excited levels. Fast, nonradiative decay occurs to bring the electrons to the metastable upper laser level. The main Nd:YAG laser transition occurs at 1064 nm from the upper to the lower laser level.

Table 2–3 Wavelengths of Major Solid-State Lasers

Material	Wavelengths (nm)
Pulsed quadrupled Nd:YAG	266
Pulsed tripled Nd:YAG	355
Pulsed doubled Nd:YLF	523
CW doubled Nd:YAG	532
Pulsed doubled Nd:YAG	532
Pulsed or CW Nd:YLF	1047; 1053
Pulsed or CW Nd:YAG	1064
CW Nd:YLF	1313
Pulsed or CW Nd:YAG	1319
CW Nd:YLF	1321
CW Nd:YAG	1335
Ho:YAG	2127
Er:YSSG	2796
Er:YLF	2810
Er:YAG	2940

4. **Output Characteristics**
   a. **Wavelength.** The typical ophthalmic Nd:YAG laser emits at **1064 nm** in the near-IR (Table 2–3). The use of a nonlinear crystal (e.g., KTP) can generate harmonics of the fundamental frequency. Thus a frequency-doubled Nd:YAG laser emits at half of the fundamental wavelength, i.e., at **532 nm** in the green. The frequency can also be tripled or quadrupled to generate laser outputs at **355 nm** or **266 nm**.
   b. **Power.** The output power depends on the pumping source, the wavelength, and the resonator configuration. **Q-switched** lasers are capable of outputs on the order of a **million watts** (10^6 W); The energy per pulse is adjustable on the typical ophthalmic laser up to about 10 mJ. **CW** lasers have outputs on the order of **watts**. **Mode-locked** lasers can generate outputs on the order of a **hundred million watts** (10^8 W).
   c. **Temporal Modes.** Most commonly, the temporal mode is **Q-switched pulsed** with durations of 3 to 30 ns. **CW** modes are also available. **Mode-locked** modes have pulse durations of 20 to 200 ps. **Free-running** pulsed modes have durations on the order of milliseconds. The pulsed lasers can also operate in a **burst mode** with from one up to five pulses per burst.
   d. **Spatial Modes.** The typical ophthalmic Nd:YAG laser is operated in the **fundamental mode (TEM$_{00}$)** with a Gaussian profile. Some ophthalmic lasers can be operated in **multiple transverse modes** (multimode).

e. **Beam Diameter and Divergence.** Internally, the beam diameter coming out of the cavity is on the order of a millimeter in diameter with a divergence of about a milliradian. But the beam emerging from a typical ophthalmic laser is a converging beam with a **cone angle of 16°**.

f. **Spot Size.** With a converging beam, the spot size depends on position relative to the focus point. At the focus point, the minimum spot size is about **10 to 15 µm**.

g. **Lifetime.** Being solid-state systems, the Nd:YAG lasers can last for 10 or more years. The limiting component, the one that needs to be replaced occasionally, is the flashlamp. Flashlamps can operate for a few million pulses before they need to be replaced. Diode-pumped lasers can operate for much longer periods (over 20,000 hours).

h. **Efficiency.** The efficiency of flashlamp-pumped lasers is in the region of 0.1% to 1%. For diode-pumped lasers, the efficiency increases to about 10% because more of the output of the diode laser is absorbed.

5. **Operating Characteristics**
   a. **Electrical Input.** Ophthalmic Nd:YAG lasers typically require 115-V inputs and can thus be plugged into an ordinary wall outlet. A maximum of 4 to 8 A is drawn by the laser, so a 15-A outlet with a ground is sufficient.
   b. **Cooling.** Because of its relatively low power output, the typical ophthalmic laser uses **convective air cooling**.
   c. **Maintenance.** Nd:YAG lasers are durable instruments. The most frequent maintenance task is flashlamp replacement after a few million pulses.

6. **Damage Mechanisms.** For Q-switched and mode-locked systems, the damage mechanism is **photodisruption**. For CW systems, the damage mechanism is **photothermal**.

7. **Ophthalmic Applications** (Figure 2–9 shows a typical ophthalmic Nd:YAG laser system).

   Q-switched lasers
   Anterior capsulotomy
   Anterior stromal puncture
   Closure of cyclodialysis clefts
   Cyclophotocoagulation
   Deposit removal
   Intrastromal ablation
   Laser closure of overfiltering/leaking blebs
   Laser goniopuncture
   Laser hyaloidectomy
   Laser peripheral iridotomy
   Laser phacolysis

Laser revision of failing filter blebs
Laser sclerostomy
Laser suture lysis
Laser synechialysis
Laser trabecular ablation
Laser trabeculoplasty
Membranectomy
Oculoplastic surgery
Posterior capsulotomy
Pupilloplasty/sphincterotomy
Selective laser trabeculoplasty
CW lasers
See also the applications of Ar lasers

B. Nd:YLF Laser

1. **Active Medium.** The Nd:YLF is also a solid-state laser where the active medium is composed of neodymium ions, but in this laser the matrix consists of yttrium, lithium, and fluoride ($YLiF_4$; acronym is YLF) instead of YAG.

2. **Excitation Mechanism.** The typical ophthalmic Nd:YLF laser is diode-pumped.

3. **Laser Cavity Configuration.** Same as for Nd:YAG laser.

4. **Output Characteristics**
   a. **Wavelength.** Because the host matrix has a different composition compared to the Nd:YAG laser, the fundamental output wavelength is slightly different, **1053 nm** instead of 1064 nm (see Table 2–3). Harmonics of the fundamental frequency can also be generated with a nonlinear crystal. For example, a frequency-doubled laser emits at **527 nm**.
   b. **Power.** The typical Nd:YLF ophthalmic laser is operated in the mode-locked or Q-switched mode with a peak power output on the order of **10 million watts** (10^7 W). The energy per pulse can range up to about 400 μJ. The laser can also be operated in a CW mode with powers up to about 0.25 W.
   c. **Temporal Modes.** Typically the ophthalmic Nd:YLF laser is operated in the mode-locked or Q-switched mode with a pulse duration of 40 to 60 ps. The maximum repetition rate is typically 1 kHz.
   d. **Spatial Modes.** The typical spatial mode is the fundamental **(TEM_{00})** mode with a Gaussian profile. Because the Nd:YLF crystal is birefringent, the output of the laser is polarized.
   e. **Beam Diameter and Divergence.** Similar to the Nd:YAG laser.
   f. **Spot Size.** The minimum spot size is about 10 to 20 μm.
   g. **Lifetime.** Similar to diode-pumped Nd:YAG laser.
   h. **Efficiency.** Similar to diode-pumped Nd:YAG laser.

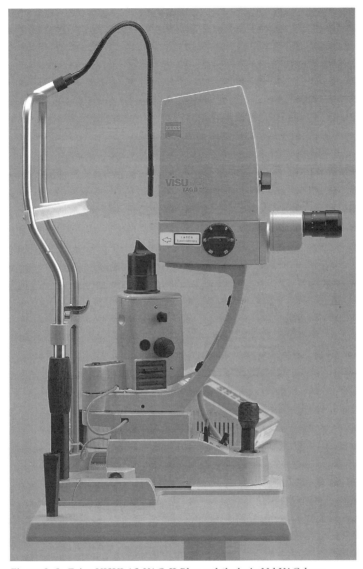

Figure 2–9 Zeiss VISULAS YAG II Plus ophthalmic Nd:YAG laser system. (Courtesy of Zeiss Humphrey Systems, Dublin, CA.)

5. **Operating Characteristics**
   a. **Electrical Input.** Similar to Nd:YAG laser.
   b. **Cooling.** Similar to Nd:YAG laser.
   c. **Maintenance.** Similar to diode-pumped Nd:YAG laser.

6. **Damage Mechanism.** In the picosecond (Q-switched and mode-locked) mode, the damage mechanism is **photodisruptive**. In the CW mode, the damage mechanism is **photothermal**.

7. **Ophthalmic Applications**
   Intrastromal PRK
   Laser iridotomy
   Laser revision of failing filter blebs
   Laser peripheral iridotomy
   Laser phacolysis
   Laser sclerostomy
   Laser vitreolysis (lysis of vitreous membranes and strands)
   Membranectomy
   Posterior capsulotomy
   Pupilloplasty/photomydriasis

C. *Er:YAG Laser* (Bende et al., 1989; Brazitikos et al., 1995; Hecht, 1992).

1. **Active Medium.** The active medium is erbium (Er) ions in a yttrium aluminum garnet (YAG) matrix. Other possible hosts include yttrium scandium gallium garnet (YSGG) and yttrium lithium fluoride (YLF).

2. **Excitation Mechanism.** A flashlamp is typically used to pump an erbium laser. However, like other solid-state lasers, an erbium laser can also be pumped by an external laser.

3. **Laser Cavity Configuration.** The crystal is a cylindrical rod about 80 mm long.

4. **Output Characteristics**
   a. **Wavelength.** The primary output of the Er:YAG laser is at **2.94 μm** in the mid-infrared (see Table 2–3). If the host matrix is changed to YSGG the output is at 2.796 μm, and for YLF it is 2.81 μm.
   b. **Power.** In the pulsed mode, output can be on the order of hundreds of millijoules, and in the CW mode, output can be at the level of watts.
   c. **Temporal Modes.** Depending on the pumping mechanism and the cavity configuration, the Er:YAG can be run in the CW or pulsed mode. Pulse repetition rates of up to 100 Hz have been used. With different pumping systems, the pulse duration can be 0.1 to 200 ms or 75 to 600 μs (free-running mode). Acousto-optic Q switching can be used to generate pulses in the nanosecond region.
   d. **Spatial Modes.** This type of laser can be operated in the fundamental (TEM_{00}) mode and multiple transverse modes (multimode). But it is usually run in a high-order multimode.
   e. **Beam Diameter and Divergence.** Variable with fiber transmission.
   f. **Spot Size.** The spot size is variable.
   g. **Lifetime.** Not available
   h. **Efficiency.** Not available

5. **Operating Characteristics**
    a. **Electrical Input.** The input depends on the particular laser, but it can be 220 V/30 A or 230 V/16 A.
    b. **Cooling.** There is a self-contained water-air heat exchanger cooling system.
    c. **Maintenance.** The flashlamp must be replaced when needed. The filters on the cooling system need to be replaced periodically. The fiberoptic trunk also needs to be replaced after a number of uses.

6. **Damage Mechanism.** Because the primary output is in the mid-infrared region, this laser uses a **photothermal** damage mechanism, especially photovaporization (Berger & D'Amico, 1997). The explosive photovaporization creates a cavitation bubble that can grow to 1 mm diameter within the first 60 μs. Because the laser output is highly absorbed by water, this laser has a very short penetration depth (~1 μm) and thus only acts upon the outer surface of tissue (Lin et al., 1990). This allows it to be used for corneal ablation and sclerostomies. However, there is more collateral tissue damage (up to 3 μm) than there is with the excimer laser (less than 1 μm) (Bende et al., 1989). By increasing the pulse duration from 50 μs to 250 μs, the thermal damage can go from <10 μm to ≤50 μm (Hill et al., 1993). The temperature in the irradiated tissue rises by up to 25°C, which is similar to the rise seen using the ArF excimer laser (Bende et al., 1992).

7. **Ophthalmic Applications** (Figure 2–10 shows a typical ophthalmic Er:YAG laser system).
    Ablation of epiretinal membranes
    Anterior capsulotomy
    Corneal trephination for penetrating keratoplasty
    Laser iridotomy
    Laser phacolysis
    Laser sclerostomy
    Laser trabecular ablation
    Oculoplastic surgery
    Photorefractive keratectomy
    Posterior capsulotomy
    Retinotomy
    Sclerostomy
    Transection of vitreous membranes

D. Holmium:YAG (THC:YAG or CTH:YAG) Laser (Hecht, 1992; Brinkmann et al., 1994; Patel & Wood, 1995).

1. **Active Medium.** The holmium laser is actually a thulium and holmium-doped, chromium-sensitized YAG laser (THC:YAG). The chromium ion (Cr^{3+}) absorbs strongly in the visible wavelength region and can transfer energy to thulium ions (Tm^{3+}), which then transfer the energy to holmium (Ho^{3+}) ions.

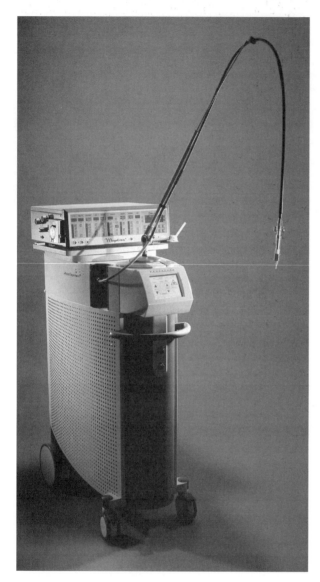

Figure 2–10 Asclepion-Meditec Phacolase ophthalmic Er:YAG laser system. (Courtesy of Asclepion-Meditec AG, Jena, Germany.)

2. **Excitation Mechanism.** The typical holmium laser is flashlamp-pumped. A diode laser can also be used to pump the laser.

3. **Laser Cavity Configuration.** The doped crystal is flanked by two mirrors. The crystal is then excited by the pump source.

4. **Output Characteristics**
   a. **Wavelength.** Holmium in a YAG host emits at a wavelength of 2.127 µm in the mid-infrared (see Table 2–3).
   b. **Power.** The pulsed holmium laser can generate up to 300 mJ per pulse, but is used typically in the region around 20 mJ for ophthalmic purposes.
   c. **Temporal Modes.** Although capable of CW or pulsed modes, the ophthalmic holmium laser typically uses the long-pulsed mode with pulse durations of 250 to 300 µs. Repetition rates are typically 5 to 15 Hz. The laser can also be Q-switched to generate 200 ns pulses. With a diode pump, the laser can also generate CW power on the order of a watt.
   d. **Spatial Modes.** Not available
   e. **Beam Diameter and Divergence.** The beam diameter of one of the lasers is 4 mm.
   f. **Spot Size.** Spot diameters are variable, but have been on the order of 350 to 550 µm. Because this laser's wavelength allows transmission through quartz optical fibers, the diameter of the optical fiber can determine the spot size (often 300 µm).
   g. **Lifetime.** The lifetime of a flashlamp is 500,000 to 1 million pulses.
   h. **Efficiency.** The efficiency is about 0.1% at maximum output.

5. **Operating Characteristics**
   a. **Electrical input.** The input is typically 120/220 V, 10/5 A, single phase.
   b. **Cooling.** Cooling is by water, with a water-to-air heat exchanger.
   c. **Maintenance.** Routine maintenance includes checking the optics and cleaning them if necessary, as well as checking and/or replacing the cooling water.

6. **Damage Mechanism.** The holmium laser uses a **photothermal** damage mechanism. Its output is highly absorbed by water.

7. **Ophthalmic Applications** (Figure 2–11 shows a typical ophthalmic holmium laser system).
   Anterior capsulotomy
   Laser phacolysis
   Laser thermal keratoplasty (LTK)
   Laser sclerostomy
   Laser trabecular ablation
   Oculoplastic surgery

E. Ti:sapphire (Tunable Vibronic Solid-State Laser)

1. **Active Medium.** The active medium is a titanium ion (Ti^{3+}) as an impurity (about 0.1%) in a sapphire (Al_2O_3) crystal matrix. Each titanium atom takes the place of an aluminum atom in the matrix, thus making this a titanium-doped sapphire laser.

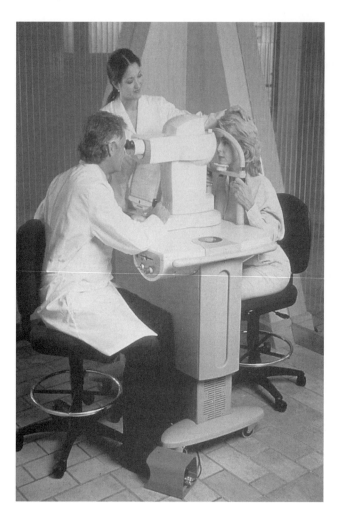

Figure 2–11 Sunrise Hyperion ophthalmic holmium laser system. (Courtesy of Sunrise Technologies, Inc., Fremont, CA.)

2. **Excitation Mechanism**

   a. The electrons are **optically pumped** by another laser or sometimes by a special flashlamp. Because the peak for absorption is around 500 nm, the pumping laser should have an output in that neighborhood. Thus, for example, an argon or frequency-doubled Nd:YAG or Nd:YLF laser could be used to pump the Ti:sapphire laser.

   b. Four levels of transitions are involved. The pumping laser excites the electron to a vibrational sublevel of an excited electronic state. The electron then drops to the bottom of the vibrational band of that electronic state releasing a phonon (a discrete unit of vibrational energy). This state is the upper laser level, and the laser emission occurs when the electron falls from this state to a vibrational sublevel of the ground level electronic state. The electron then relaxes to the bottom of the ground state's vibrational band and consequently releases more vibrational energy.

3. **Laser Cavity Configuration.** The laser crystal is a short (about 1 cm long), red rod arranged between two mirrors.

4. **Output Characteristics**
   a. **Wavelength.** The output of this laser is a tunable wavelength.
      1) Tunability results from the **vibrational sublevels** for different electronic energy levels.
      2) A given electronic energy level is spread out into a "**vibronic band**" of energies due to the superimposed vibrational sublevels.
      3) The laser transitions then occur between a given vibrational sublevel of one electronic state to another vibrational sublevel of another electronic state. Thus a band of laser wavelengths is emitted. The fundamental, tunable wavelength range is from **660 nm to 1180 nm** (Table 2–4). The highest output power occurs between 700 nm to 900 nm.
      4) Even lower wavelengths (e.g., in the near ultraviolet and visible region) can be generated by second, third, or even fourth harmonic production.
   b. **Power.** The output of the laser depends on the wavelength and on the power of the pumping laser. The output is typically on the order of a few watts. Almost 50 W of CW output have been achieved.
   c. **Temporal Modes.** Usually operated in the CW mode, the laser can also be operated in a pulsed mode with a Q-switched pumping laser or even with mode-locking.
   d. **Spatial Modes.** The fundamental **(TEM$_{00}$)** mode is produced. Technically, the laser can be operated in either a single-mode or multi-mode output.
   e. **Beam Diameter and Divergence.** The beam diameter is on the order of 1 mm and the divergence is on the order of 1 mrad.
   f. **Spot Size.** The spot size is variable.

Table 2–4 Wavelengths of Major Vibronic Solid-State Lasers

Material	*Wavelengths (nm)*
Pulsed quadrupled Ti:sapphire	210
Pulsed tripled Ti:sapphire	235–300
Pulsed doubled Ti:sapphire	350–470
Pulsed doubled Alexandrite	360–400
CW Alexandrite	700–830 (strongest room temperature emission)
Pulsed Alexandrite	701–826 (720–800 commercially available)
Pulsed Co:MgF$_2$	1750–2500
Pulsed or CW Ti:sapphire	660–1180 (680–1130 commercially available)

Data from Hecht 1992, 1994.

g. **Lifetime.** The lifetime is limited only by that of the pumping laser.

h. **Efficiency.** Efficiency depends on the power of the pumping laser and the tuned output wavelength. It can be as high as 25% of the power of the pumping laser.

5. **Operating Characteristics**
   a. **Electrical Input.** The input voltage and current depend on the requirements of the pumping laser.
   b. **Cooling.** Forced air, flowing water, or refrigeration can be used to cool the laser.
   c. **Maintenance.** The level and type of maintenance is primarily determined by the type of pumping laser.

6. **Damage Mechanism.** The type of damage mechanism is determined by the output wavelength, duration, and power. Therefore, the mechanism could be photothermal, photodisruptive, or even photochemical.

7. **Ophthalmic Applications.** Theoretically, this type of laser could replace most of the currently available ophthalmic lasers.

IV. Semiconductor (Diode) Lasers (Balles & Puliafito, 1990; Brancato & Pratesi, 1987; Hecht, 1992, 1994; Patel & Wood, 1995; Silfvast, 1996)

A. Introduction. A great variety of semiconductor materials could be employed to create a semiconductor laser (Table 2–5). All of these materials can be characterized as diodes

Table 2–5 Wavelengths of Major Semiconductor (Diode) Lasers

Material	*Wavelengths (nm)*
ZnSSe	447–480
ZnCdSe	490–525
ZnSe	525
AlGaInP	620–680
GaInP	670–680
GaAlAs	620–895
GaAs	904
InGaAs	980–1050
InGaAsP	1100–1650
InGaAsSb	1700–4400
PbCdS	2700–4200
PbEuSeTe	3300–5800
PbSSe	4200–8000
PbSnTe	6300–29,000
PbSnSe	8000–29,000

Data from Hecht 1992, 1994.

(see excitation mechanism section). At the present time, ophthalmic diode lasers are made of **gallium, aluminum, and arsenide (GaAlAs)**.

B. GaAlAs Lasers

1. **Active Medium.** The active medium is gallium, aluminum, and arsenide.

2. **Excitation Mechanism.** Excitation of electrons in a diode laser occurs by the process of **current injection**. This happens when the diode is forward-biased, that is, a negative voltage is applied to the n-type semiconductor layer and a positive voltage is applied to the p-type layer (see the next section).

3. **Laser Cavity Configuration.** In the last few years, there has been an explosive growth in semiconductor laser technology. This has involved an expansion in not only the types of configurations, but also the wavelengths, power levels, and beam quality available.

    a. Two energy bands are created in semiconductor lasers (Figure 2–12). The lower energy band is called the **valence band** and is composed of electrons involved in chemical bonding in the crystal lattice. The higher energy band is called the **conduction band** and is composed of electrons that are freely mobile in the crystal. The energy difference between the two bands is called the **bandgap** and is determined by the composition of the diode.

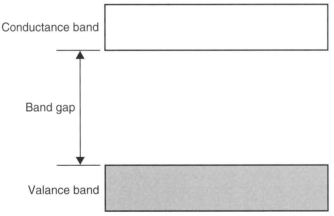

Figure 2–12 The bandgap in a diode laser. The valance band is the energy levels of the bound electrons in a crystal, and the conductance band is the energy levels of the free electrons. The bandgap is the energy difference between the valance and conductance bands. The name is derived from the fact that there are no energy levels between the two bands. The bandgap is determined by the composition of the semiconductor, and its energy is proportional to the wavelength of the laser radiation generated by the diode laser.

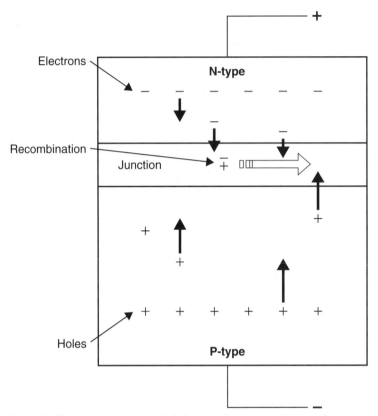

Figure 2–13 A semiconductor diode laser with n-type and p-type layers. Forward-biasing initiates the flow of electrons and holes resulting in the recombination of many of the electrons and holes in the junction. This leads to energy released as photons.

b. The active zone of a diode laser is the junction between two semiconductor layers (Figure 2–13). One layer, the n-type layer, is doped with electron donors like arsenic (As) or phosphorous (P) that have extra electrons. Electrons from this material can be elevated to the conduction band. The other layer, the p-type layer, is doped with electron acceptors like gallium (Ga) or aluminum (Al) that have fewer electrons than the atoms they replace in the crystal lattice. These generate "holes" in the semiconductor crystal, that is, areas where a negatively-charged electron is missing. Thus holes effectively carry a positive charge. There can be apparent motion of the holes when an electron from another atom in the crystal jumps into a hole and thus leaves behind a newly created hole.

c. When the diode is forward-biased, the negative voltage attracts the valance band holes to the junction and the positive voltage attracts the conductance band electrons to the junction. This current injects a high density of holes and electrons into the junction and thereby creates a population inversion.

d. As an excess electron jumps from the conduction band to a hole in the valence band, this electron-hole recombination event generates a photon with an energy equal to the bandgap energy.

e. The resonance cavity is formed by the cleaved, parallel facets or faces of the crystal that act as partially transmissive mirrors. The photons generated by recombination are internally reflected and stimulate emission of other photons in the p-n junction area.

4. **Output Characteristics**

   a. **Wavelength.** The bandgap energy in the diode active layer determines the wavelength of the laser. The bandgap is a function of the composition of the diode laser (see Table 2–5). For example, a GaAs diode laser emits at 904 nm, but by adding various amount of aluminum to the active layer, the bandgap energy is increased and the laser emits at shorter wavelengths, 620 to 895 nm. Most therapeutic ophthalmic diode lasers are composed of **GaAlAs** and operate in the region of **750 to 850 nm**.

   b. **Power.** The typical single-element GaAlAs diode laser generates on the order of 100 mW of power. By using an array of these lasers, powers of up to 25 W have been generated in the CW mode and significantly higher powers in a quasi-CW stacked array.

   c. **Temporal Modes.** Commercially available ophthalmic diode lasers operate in the CW mode currently. Diode lasers are theoretically capable of being mode-locked or Q-switched.

   d. **Spatial Modes.** Most diode lasers emit a single transverse mode and they may generate single or multiple longitudinal modes.

   e. **Beam Diameter and Divergence.** For edge-emitters, the beam is elliptical. It can have dimensions of a few micrometers by a micrometer (for a single-element diode) to a few centimeters (for an array). Beam divergence is on the order of 700 mrad (40°) by 170 mrad (10°) without special collimating optics. Some diode lasers are surface-emitters and have a circular beam.

   f. **Spot Size.** By using special optics, various spot sizes can be selected in ophthalmic diode lasers (e.g., 75 μm to 990 μm).

   g. **Lifetime.** Expected lifetimes for diode lasers are well over 10,000 hours.

   h. **Efficiency.** The overall efficiency of commercially available ophthalmic diode lasers is about 30%. This is much higher than the efficiency (0.001% to 0.01%) of the typical argon ophthalmic laser.

5. **Operating Characteristics**

   a. **Electrical Input.** Low operating voltages and currents are necessary for diode lasers. The typical ophthalmic diode laser uses wall plug inputs of 120 V and 2 A or less. If necessary, the laser can be run on batteries.

   b. **Cooling.** Passive air cooling is used on the commercially available ophthalmic units.

    c. **Maintenance.** Very little maintenance is necessary with diode lasers because they are solid-state devices. The output window may need to be cleaned occasionally.

6. **Damage Mechanism**

    a. The typical ophthalmic diode laser uses a **photothermal** damage mechanism. As wavelength ranges expand, **photochemical** mechanisms may be used. And as output powers increase, thus allowing mode-locking and Q-switching, then **photodisruptive** mechanisms may also be used.

    b. Using an in vitro system, Cohen et al. (1995) found that for oxygen-treated blood with a hematocrit of 46%, the transmission of diode infrared (810 nm) radiation was 62% through a 100-μm-thick sample (i.e., 38% absorption) and 32% through a 200-μm-thick sample (68% absorption). For carbon-dioxide-treated blood with a hematocrit of 46%, the transmission was 62% through a 100-μm-thick sample (38% absorption) and 40% for a 200-μm-thick sample (60% absorption).

7. **Ophthalmic Applications** (Figure 2–14 shows a typical ophthalmic diode laser system).

    Closure of cyclodialysis clefts

    Cyclophotocoagulation

    Laser closure of overfiltering/leaking blebs

    Laser Doppler interferometry

    Laser Doppler velocimetry/flowmetry

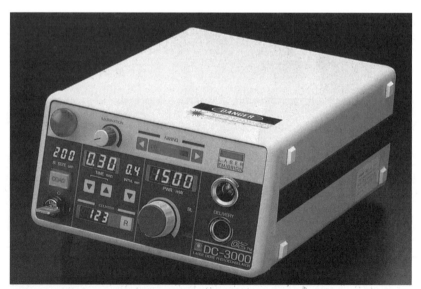

Figure 2–14 Nidek DC-3000 ophthalmic diode laser system. (Courtesy of Nidek Incorporated, Fremont, CA.)

Laser interferometry fundus pulsation measurement
Laser iridoplasty
Laser peripheral iridotomy
Laser revision of failing filter blebs
Laser sclerostomy
Laser speckle blood flow measurement
Laser suture lysis
Laser trabeculoplasty
Oculoplastic surgery
Optical coherence tomography
Photon correlation spectroscopy
Retinal laser polarimetry
Retinal photocoagulation
Scanning laser ophthalmoscopy

V. Dye Lasers (Brancato et al., 1986; Cunha-Vaz & de Abrieu, 1988; Duker et al., 1989; L'Esperance, 1985)

A. Active Medium. The active medium is a **fluorescent organic molecule** (dye). Ophthalmic dye lasers use dyes that are dissolved in liquid solvents. These organic solvents include molecules like dimethyl sulfoxide (DMSO), methanol, and ethylene glycol.

B. Excitation Mechanism. Dye lasers are optically pumped with a flashlamp or another laser. The typical ophthalmic dye laser is pumped with an argon laser. The external light source raises the dye molecule to an excited state (Figure 2–15). Via radiationless decay, the molecule drops to the metastable upper laser level. When the molecule moves to the lower laser level, laser emission occurs and the molecule drops to the ground state via another radiationless decay process. Because dye molecules are large with multiple ring structures, their absorption and emission spectra are complex. This is a result of the fact that each electronic energy level is subdivided into smaller vibrational and rotational energy levels. Therefore laser emission occurs over a broad spectrum of wavelengths that almost form a continuum.

C. Laser Cavity Configuration. Cavity optics and structure can vary depending on the pump source, method of wavelength selection, type of dye, and mode of operation.

D. Output Characteristics

1. **Wavelength.** The output wavelength depends on the type of dye and solvent, the pump, and the configuration of the laser. For a given dye and pump source, the range of output is on the order of 50 nm. To move to another region of the spectrum, another dye is selected. So by changing dyes, the wavelength can be changed from

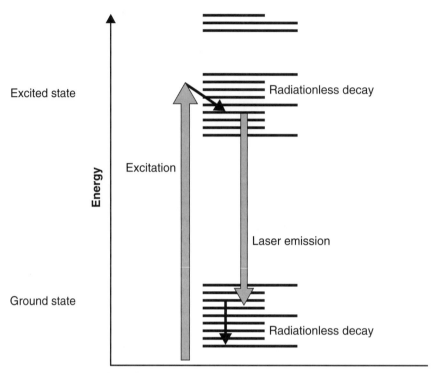

Figure 2–15 Energy level diagram for a dye laser. The electronic energy levels are shown with vibrational (long lines) and rotational (short lines) substates.

about **310 nm to** about **1200 nm**, that is, from the near-ultraviolet to the near-infrared. The lower end of this spectrum can be stretched down to about 200 nm with the use of nonlinear crystals for sum-frequency generation or harmonic generation. In the case of sum-frequency generation, the frequency of the pump source is added to the frequency of the dye laser to generate a lower wavelength. In harmonic generation, the frequency of the dye laser can be added to itself to generate the second harmonic wavelength.

2. **Power.** The output power also depends on the type of dye, the pump source, and the laser configuration. Because a large variety of dyes is available, manufacturers typically quote the maximum output of the laser using Rhodamine 6G, a very efficient dye. Using an argon pumping laser, the typical ophthalmic dye laser can generate outputs on the order of watts.

3. **Temporal Modes.** Depending on the pump source, the output can be CW or pulsed.

4. **Spatial Modes.** Depending on the pump source, the output can be fundamental mode or multimode. The output is typically linearly polarized.

5. **Beam Diameter and Divergence.** Because the typical ophthalmic dye laser is pumped by a CW argon laser, the beam diameter is about 0.5 to 1 mm and the beam divergence is about 0.5 to 2 mrad. If a pulsed laser or a flashlamp is used as a pump, the beam diameters and divergences can be even higher.

6. **Spot Size.** The spot size is variable.

7. **Lifetime.** Because thermal and/or photochemical degradation of the dyes can occur, the dyes themselves have limited lifetimes. This means that the lifetimes depend on the power, wavelength, and temporal output of the pump source. Dyes can last from an hour to over 1000 hours.

8. **Efficiency.** The most often quoted efficiency for dye lasers is the **conversion efficiency**. In other words, the percent of the energy from the pump source that is converted into the dye laser output energy is noted. This value is typically on the order of a **few percent**. This means that the wall plug efficiency is even smaller since it is the percent of electrical input to the pump laser converted into the dye laser output. Thus, in dye lasers the output of the wall plug is degraded twice, by the pump source and by the dye laser itself.

E. Operating Characteristics

1. **Electrical Input.** The electrical input required depends primarily on the pump source. Thus, the input can vary from 110 V and 10 A to 220 V and 100 A.

2. **Cooling.** Cooling requirements also depend on the pump source. The typical ophthalmic dye laser head is cooled by the dye-flow system itself.

3. **Maintenance.** Typical maintenance includes replacement of the dye solution and optical realignment in addition to the maintenance of the pump source.

F. Damage Mechanism. Because of the broad range of output wavelengths, powers, and temporal modes, the damage mechanism can vary. The typical ophthalmic dye laser is used for **photothermal** or, at times, **photochemical** procedures.

G. Ophthalmic Applications (Figure 2–16 shows a typical ophthalmic dye laser system.)

Corneal stromal vascularization treatment

Laser iridotomy

Laser sclerostomy

Laser suture lysis

Oculoplastic surgery

Photodynamic therapy

Retinal photocoagulation

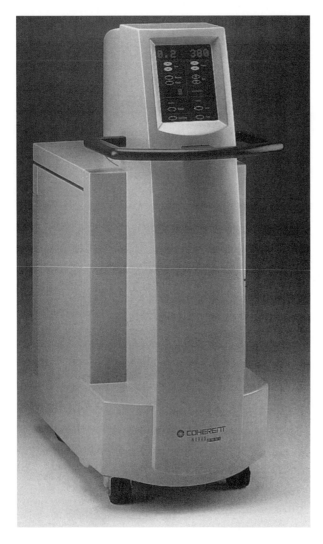

Figure 2–16 Coherent Novus Omni ophthalmic dye laser system. (Courtesy of Lumenis, Santa Clara, CA.)

VI. Free Electron Lasers (Brau, 1988; Bende et al., 1995; Ellis et al., 1999; Hecht, 1992, 1994; Jean & Bende, 1994, 1998; Shen et al., 1999; Silfvast, 1996; Toth et al., 1999; Walker et al., 1995, 1997)

A. Active Medium. The active medium is a beam of free electrons that passes through an alternating magnetic field.

B. Operating Principles

1. A beam of free electrons is generated by an accelerator.

2. The beam is then passed through an alternating magnetic field. This field is typically generated by a wiggler magnetic array consisting of a series of magnets arranged with

their magnetic poles alternating so that the magnetic field reverses every few centimeters. As the electrons travel down the array of alternating magnets, they are bent alternately left and right by interaction with the magnetic field. This leads to a "wiggly" path of oscillatory motion and the radiation of energy, that is, an optical beam.

3. Reflecting this beam back down the wiggler or injecting an external laser beam into the wiggler can lead to amplification of radiation. This situation occurs when the electrons interact with the laser beam and satisfy a resonance condition described by the following equation:

$$\lambda = 0.131p\big/(0.3H + E)^2$$
where
p = the period of the wiggler magnet array
E = the energy of the electrons.

This simplified formula indicates that the laser wavelength can be lengthened by decreasing the electron energy or by increasing the magnet period.

4. The electrons emit their radiation in phase with the laser beam and therefore add coherently to the beam, amplifying it.

C. Components

1. **Magnetic-Field Sources.** The magnetic field can be generated by two major sources:
   a. an array of permanent magnets or electromagnets with alternating polarity or
   b. a powerful electromagnetic wave.

2. **Electron Accelerators.** A number of types of accelerators can be used:
   a. radio-frequency linear accelerators
   b. induction linear accelerators
   c. microtrons
   d. storage rings
   e. electrostatic accelerators (e.g., a van de Graff generator)
   f. pulse line accelerator and modulator

3. **Optical Cavity.** Similar to conventional lasers, free electron lasers use mirrors at both ends of the resonance cavity.

D. Output Characteristics

1. **Wavelength**
   a. A significant advantage of free electron lasers is their tunability. This results from the fact that free electrons are not confined to discrete energy levels.
   b. Theoretically, they can be tuned from the microwave to the soft x-ray region. In practice, they have been operated from the UV (248 nm) to the far infrared region (up to about 8000 μm).

    c. For ophthalmic purposes, the infrared range of wavelengths from 2700 to 6700 nm (2.7 to 6.7 μm) has been explored.

2. **Power.** Small free electron lasers generate on the order of 100 W. Large lasers have the potential for generating tremendous power levels (on the order of 1 GW pulsed).

3. **Temporal Modes.** Ophthalmic experiments carried out with the Vanderbilt University laser used 4 μs macropulses that consisted of 2 ps micropulses with a 2.9 GHz repetition rate.

4. **Spatial Mode.** The laser is operated in the TEM_{00} mode.

E. Damage Mechanism. The damage mechanism in the middle infrared region (2.7 to 6.7 μm) is **photothermal**. The wavelength output is tunable to the vibrational modes of proteins, lipids, and/or water (Edwards et al., 1994).

F. Ophthalmic Applications

    Acute optic nerve sheath fenestration

    Potential for oculoplastic laser resurfacing

    Study of collateral thermal damage from corneal photoablation

    Study of infrared photoablation

VII. Laser Delivery Systems (Bloom & Brucker, 1997; Coscas & Singerman, 1998; Katzir, 1993; Verdaasdonk & van Swol, 1997)

A. Introduction

1. A **laser delivery system** is a system used for controlled transport of laser radiation between a laser and a target.

2. **Aiming systems** are also used for target acquisition and focusing. These are coaxial, visible beams that include the following:
    a. Attenuated treatment beams (e.g., argon green or blue/green)
    b. HeNe lasers (red—632.8 nm)
    c. Diode lasers (visible red)

B. Delivery System (Entrance Optics, Beam Guide, and Target Optics) (Figure 2–17).

1. The **entrance optics** condition the laser beam for transport through the beam guide. This may involve a mirror or it may be a focusing lens to couple the laser beam with a fiberoptic or another kind of waveguide.

2. The **beam guide** can be a waveguide (e.g., a fiberoptic made of silica) or a series of mirrors or prisms (e.g., an articulated arm). For example, silica fibers are often used for lasers that operate in the range from 300 to 2500 nm. Fiberoptic delivery systems

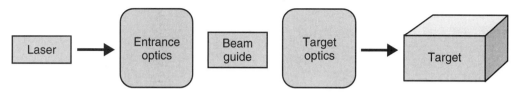

Figure 2–17 Components of a laser delivery system.

can be either contact or noncontact systems (i.e., where the end of the fiberoptic either touches or does not touch the tissue).

3. The **target optics** are used to focus and/or deliver the beam to the target. They can include the following:

   a. **Focusing and collimated handpieces** (e.g., for manual targeting of periocular skin lesions or for laser thermokeratoplasty)

   b. **Slit lamp biomicroscopes** (e.g., for argon laser iridotomy)

   c. **Binocular indirect ophthalmoscopes** (e.g., for argon laser panretinal photocoagulation)

   d. **Scanning systems** (e.g., for CO_2 laser skin resurfacing or for scanning beam excimer laser photorefractive keratectomy)

   e. **Modified fiber tips** (e.g., a sapphire tip used as a contact probe for laser sclerostomy)

   f. **Laser contact lenses** (e.g., a central Abraham lens for Nd:YAG laser posterior capsulotomy)

   g. **Laser noncontact lenses** (e.g., a +78-D lens for laser photocoagulation of the retina)

   h. **Endoscopes or endoprobes** (e.g., for ab interno laser sclerostomy)

   i. **Operating microscopes**

References

Abad JC, Krueger RR. Basic science and principles. In: Talamo JH, Krueger RR, eds. The excimer manual. A clinician's guide to excimer laser surgery. Boston: Little, Brown and Company, 1:3–34 (1997).

Balles MW, Puliafito CA. Semiconductor diode lasers: a new laser light source in ophthalmology. International Ophthalmol Clin 30:77–83 (1990).

Bende T et al. Thermal gradients in the cornea during photoablation with the Er:YAG laser. Lasers Light Ophthalmol 5:79–82 (1992).

Bende T, Kriegerowski M, Seiler T. Photoablation in different ocular tissues performed with an erbium:YAG laser. Lasers Light Ophthalmol 2:263–269 (1989).

Bende T, Seiler T, Wollensak J. Side effects in excimer corneal surgery. Corneal thermal gradients. Graefes Arch Clin Exp Ophthalmol 226:277–280 (1988).

Bende T, Walker R, Jean B. Thermal collateral damage in porcine corneas after photoablation with free electron laser. J Refract Surg 11:129–136 (1995).

Berger JW, D'Amico DJ. Modeling of erbium:YAG laser-mediated explosive photovaporization: implications for vitreoretinal surgery. Ophthalmic Surg Lasers 28:133–139 (1997).

Berns MW et al. An acute light and electron microscopic study of ultraviolet 193-nm excimer laser corneal incisions. Ophthalmology 95:1422–1433 (1988).

Betney S et al. Corneal temperature changes during photorefractive keratectomy. Cornea 16:158–161 (1997).

Bilgihan K et al. Excimer laser corneal surgery and free oxygen radicals. Jpn J Ophthalmol 40:154–157 (1996).

Bird AC, Grey RH. Photocoagulation of disciform macular lesions with the krypton laser. Br J Ophthalmol 63:669–673 (1979).

Bloom SM, Brucker AJ. Laser surgery of the posterior segment. 2nd ed. Philadelphia: Lippincott-Raven Publishers, 1997.

Bor Z et al. Plume emission, shock wave and surface wave formation during excimer laser ablation of the cornea. Refract Corneal Surg 9(2 Suppl):S111–S115 (1993).

Brancato R et al. Clinical applications of the tunable dye laser. Lasers Ophthalmol 1:115–118 (1986).

Brancato R, Pratesi R. Applications of diode lasers in ophthalmology. Lasers Ophthalmol 1:119–129 (1987).

Brau CA. Free-electron lasers. Science 239:1115–1121 (1988).

Brazitikos PD et al. Erbium:YAG laser surgery of the vitreous and retina. Ophthalmology 102:278–290 (1995).

Brinkmann R et al. Investigations on laser thermokeratoplasty. Lasers and Light in Ophthalmology 6:259–270 (1994).

Cohen SM, Shen JH, Smiddy WE. Laser energy and dye fluorescence transmission through blood in vitro. Am J Ophthalmol 119:452–457 (1995).

Coscas G, Singerman L. Current techniques in ophthalmic laser surgery. 3rd ed. Boston: Butterworth-Heinemann, 1998.

Cross FW, Bowker TJ. The physical properties of tissue ablation with excimer lasers. Med Instrum 21:226–230 (1987).

Cunha-Vaz JG, Faria de Abreu JR. The tunable dye laser in the management of retinal vascular disease. Int Ophthalmol 12:193–196 (1988).

Duker JS et al. Semiconductor diode laser endophotocoagulation. Ophthalmic Surg 20:717–719 (1989).

Ediger MN, Pettit GH, Matchette LS. In vitro measurements of cytotoxic effects of 193 nm and 213 nm laser pulses at subablative fluences. Lasers Surg Med 21:88–93 (1997).

Edwards G et al. Tissue ablation by a free-electron laser tuned to the amide II band. Nature 371:416–419 (1994).

Ellis DL et al. Free electron laser infrared wavelength specificity for cutaneous contraction. Lasers Surg Med 25:1–7 (1999).

Hahn DW, Ediger MN, Pettit GH. Dynamics of ablation plume particles generated during excimer laser corneal ablation. Lasers Surg Med 16:384–389 (1995).

Hecht J. The laser guidebook. Blue Ridge Summit, PA: Tab Books, 1992.

Hecht J. Understanding lasers. An entry-level guide. 2nd ed. New York: IEEE Press, 1994.

Hill RA et al. Effects of pulse width on erbium:YAG laser photothermal trabecular ablation (LTA). Lasers Surg Med 13:440–446 (1993).

Isner JM, Clarke RH. The paradox of thermal ablation without thermal injury. Lasers Med Sci 2:165–173 (1987).

Jacques SL. Laser-tissue interactions. Photochemical, photothermal, and photomechanical. Surg Clin North Am 72:531–558 (1992).

Jain S et al. Antioxidants reduce corneal light scattering after excimer keratectomy in rabbits. Lasers Surg Med 17:160–165 (1995).

Jean B, Bende T. Photoablation of gelatin with the free-electron laser between 2.7 and 6.7 microns. J Refract Corneal Surg 10:433–438 (1994).

Jean B, Bende T. Infrared lasers. Therapeutic applications. Ophthalmol Clin North Am 11:243–255 (1998).

Kahle G et al. Gas chromatographic and mass spectroscopic analysis of excimer and erbium: yttrium aluminum garnet laser-ablated human cornea. Invest Ophthalmol Vis Sci 33:2180–2184 (1992).

Karlin DB. Lasers in ophthalmic surgery. Cambridge, MA: Blackwell Science, 1995.

Katzir A. Lasers and optical fibers in medicine. San Diego: Academic Press, Inc., 1993.

Kermani O, Koort HJ, Roth E, Dardenne MU. Mass spectroscopic analysis of excimer laser ablated material from human corneal tissue. J Cataract Refract Surg 14:638–641 (1988).

Kermani O, Lubatschowski H. [Structure and dynamics of photo-acoustic shock-waves in 193 nm excimer laser photo-ablation of the cornea]. Fortschr Ophthalmol 88:748–753 (1991).

Kitai MS et al. The physics of UV laser cornea ablation. IEEE J Quantum Electron 27:302–307 (1991).

Kitazawa Y et al. The efficacy of cooling on excimer laser photorefractive keratectomy in the rabbit eye. Surv Ophthalmol 42 Suppl 1:S82–S88 (1997).

Lane RJ, Wynne JJ, Geronemus RG. Ultraviolet laser ablation of skin: healing studies and a thermal model. Lasers Surg Med 6:504–513 (1987).

L'Esperance FA Jr. Clinical applications of the organic dye laser. Ophthalmology 92:1592–1600 (1985)

L'Esperance FA Jr. Ophthalmic lasers. 3rd ed. St. Louis: C. V. Mosby Company, 1989.

Lewis M, Dubin M, Andahl V. The physical properties of bovine corneal collagen. Exp Eye Res 6:57–69 (1967).

Lin CP, Stern D, Puliafito CA. High-speed photography of Er:YAG laser ablation in fluid. Implication for laser vitreous surgery. Invest Ophthalmol Vis Sci 32:2546–2550 (1990).

Mainster MA. Wavelength selection in macular photocoagulation: tissue optics, thermal effects, and laser systems. Ophthalmology 93:952–958 (1986).

Marshall J, Bird AC. A comparative histopathological study of argon and krypton laser irradiations of the human retina. Br J Ophthalmol 63:657–668 (1979).

McHugh JDA et al. Initial clinical experience using a diode laser in the treatment of retinal vascular disease. Eye 3:516–527 (1989).

Morse PH. Argon vs. krypton laser lesions: is the wavelength more important than the power? Ann Ophthalmol 17:86–91 (1985).

Niemz MH. Laser–tissue interactions. Fundamentals and applications. New York: Springer Verlag, 1996

Niizuma T, Ito S, Hayashi M, Futemma M, Utsumi T, Ohashi K. Cooling the cornea to prevent side effects of photorefractive keratectomy. J Refract Corneal Surg 10:S262–S266 (1994).

Noack J, Toennies R, Hohla K, Birngruber R, Vogel A. Influence of ablation plume dynamics on the formation of central islands in excimer laser photorefractive keratectomy. Ophthalmology 104:823–830 (1997).

Patel CKN, Wood OR II. Fundamentals of lasers. In: Karlin DB, ed. Lasers in ophthalmic surgery. Cambridge, MA: Blackwell Science, 1995; 1:1–29.

Pettit GH et al. Electron paramagnetic resonance spectroscopy of free radicals in corneal tissue following excimer laser irradiation. Lasers Surg Med 18:367–372 (1996).

Peyman GA, Raichand M, Zeimer RC. Ocular effects of various laser wavelengths. Surv Ophthalmol 28:391–404 (1984).

Pomerantzeff O et al. Effect of the ocular media on the main wavelengths of argon laser emission. Invest Ophthalmol Vis Sci 15:70–77 (1976).

Puliafito CA et al. Excimer laser ablation of the cornea and lens. Experimental studies. Ophthalmology 92:741–748 (1985).

Puliafito CA et al. High-speed photography of excimer laser ablation of the cornea. Arch Ophthalmol 105:1255–1259 (1987).

Seiler T, McDonnell PJ. Excimer laser photorefractive keratectomy. Surv Ophthalmol 40:89–118 (1995).

Shen J-H et al. Acute optic nerve sheath fenestration with the free-electron laser. Proc SPIE Ophthalmic Technologies IX 3591:235–240 (1999).

Siano S et al. Intraocular measurements of pressure transients induced by excimer laser ablation of the cornea. Lasers Surg Med 20:416–425 (1997).

Sigelman J. Retinal diseases: pathogenesis, laser therapy, and surgery. Boston: Little Brown, 1984.

Silfvast WT. Laser fundamentals. New York: Cambridge University Press, 1996.

Singerman LJ. Red krypton laser therapy of macular and retinal vascular disease. Retina 2:15–28 (1982).

Sliney DH, Trokel SL. Medical lasers and their safe use. New York: Springer-Verlag, 1993.

Srinivasan R. Ablation of polymers and biological tissue by ultraviolet lasers. Science 234:559–565 (1986).

Srinivasan R, Dyer PE, Braren B. Far-ultraviolet laser ablation of the cornea: photoacoustic studies. Lasers Surg Med 6:514–519 (1987).

Stein HA, Cheskes AC, Stein RM. The excimer. Fundamentals and clinical use. Thorofare, NJ: SLACK Inc, 1995.

Toth CA et al. In-vivo tissue response to the free-electron laser. Proc SPIE Ophthalmic Technologies IX 3591:160–170 (1999).

Trempe CL et al. Macular photocoagulation: optimal wavelength selection. Ophthalmology 89:721–728 (1982).

Trokel SL, Srinivasan R, Braren B. Excimer laser surgery of the cornea. Am J Ophthalmol 96:710–715 (1983).

Venugopalan V, Nishioka NS, Mikic BB. The thermodynamic response of soft biological tissues to pulsed ultraviolet laser radiation. Biophys J 69:1259–1271 (1995).

Verdaasdonk RM, van Swol CFP. Laser light delivery systems for medical applications. Phys Med Biol 42:869–894 (1997).

Walker R et al. Photoablation with the free-electron laser in the far IR in biological soft tissue (cornea). Proc SPIE Laser-Tissue Interaction VI 2391:126–137 (1995).

Walker R et al. Photoablation with the free-electron laser between 10 and 15 μm in biological soft tissue (cornea). J Biomed Opt 2:204–210 (1997).

Waring GO III. Development of a system for excimer laser corneal surgery. Trans Am Ophthalmol Soc 87:854–983 (1989).

Waring GO III. Laser corneal surgery: fundamentals and background. In: Brightbill FS, ed. Corneal surgery. 2nd ed. St. Louis: CV Mosby, 1993; 40:480–511.

Yannuzzi LA, Shakin JL. Krypton red laser photocoagulation of the ocular fundus. Retina 2:1–14 (1982).

Chapter 3
Ophthalmic Diagnostic Uses of Lasers

Charles M. Wormington

I. Introduction to Diagnostic Uses of Lasers

There is a tremendous growth in the application of laser technology to assist in the diagnosis of ophthalmic disorders. Over the past 10 years there has been an explosive, exponential expansion of the numbers of research and development projects designed to explore new diagnostic uses of lasers. There has also been a large increase in the number of commercially available laser diagnostic systems. These innovations range from imaging to detection to measurement systems. The following applications are a sample of the most important new diagnostic systems.

II. Scanning Laser Ophthalmoscopy

A. Introduction

Scanning laser ophthalmoscopy has been around since the early 1980s. In that time, the technique and the applications have been improved and expanded (Mainster et al., 1982; Webb et al., 1980, 1990). Commercially available systems have also been marketed recently.

B. Technique

1. Many **laser sources** have been used in these instruments. **Argon** (blue, 488 nm; green, 514 nm), **helium-neon** (633 nm), **and diode** (780 nm) lasers have been focused to a 10- to 20-μm spot on the retina and are used in one of the commercially available instruments (Webb et al., 1980). Another instrument uses a **frequency-doubled Nd:YAG** laser and a He-Ne laser.

2. A **scanning unit** moves the laser spot on the retina in a raster pattern by pivoting the incident beam about the entrance pupil.

3. A **light detector** measures the radiation scattered by the illuminated point on the retina.
   a. The intensity of the scattered radiation determines the brightness of a corresponding point (pixel) on a video monitor.
   b. As the laser sweeps across the retina, a video image is built up, typically with a 30-Hz frame rate and a 60-Hz field rate.

4. The result is a dynamic, real-time video imaging of the fundus. Each image has a resolution of 256 × 256 pixels resulting in 65,536 individual measurements. Different sizes of grids can be used to record the images: 10° × 10°, 15° × 15°, or 20° × 20° grids.

5. **Infrared illumination** has a number of advantages:
   a. Lower illumination power levels are possible compared to visible illumination since the fundus has a higher reflectivity for IR (Delori & Pflibsen, 1989).
   b. IR penetrates deeper into the fundus and thus allows imaging of the choroid in addition to the retina (Manivannan et al., 1994).
   c. Clearer fundus images are formed compared to IR illumination in conventional fundus cameras (Manivannan et al., 1994). In the conventional system, illumination is not monochromatic, and the film is somewhat sensitive to visible radiation also.

C. Clinical Uses

1. **Ophthalmoscopy**
   a. An undilated pupil can be employed. However, it may be of benefit to dilate the pupils of patients with small pupils and/or cataracts (Zangwill et al., 1997c).
   b. Low light levels can be used. This is more comfortable for the patient.
   c. An increased, high-contrast image is obtained.

2. **Fundus Camera**
   a. Dynamic recording is possible.
   b. Better resolution than video recording through conventional fundus cameras is obtainable.
   c. The SLO is superior to conventional fundus cameras at visualizing the retina in eyes with cataract (Beckman et al., 1995; Kirkpatrick et al., 1995).
   d. Images can be
      1) stored on videotape,
      2) digitized and stored on a computer,
      3) stored on an optical disk, or
      4) computer-enhanced to improve contrast.
   e. The SLO can be used to detect defects in the retinal nerve fiber layer. This can be useful in glaucoma, Leber's hereditary optic neuropathy, and other optic neuropathies (Lindblom & Bond-Taylor, 1998).

    f. Infrared imaging provides better visualization of subretinal structures such as choroidal new vessels, hyperpigmentation, and drusen (Elsner et al., 1996; Hartnett & Elsner, 1996). Shallow detachments of the neuroretina can also easily be detected (Remky et al., 1998).

    g. Using the argon blue laser, a new clinical entity, white dot fovea, has been identified (Yokotsuka et al., 1997). Although the white dots do not produce symptoms, they may play a role in the differential diagnosis of macular holes.

3. **Angiography**

    a. **Fluorescein Angiography** (Duijm et al., 1996; Gabel et al., 1988; Kuck et al., 1993; Mainster et al., 1982; Scheider et al., 1993).

        1) There is better detection of fluorescence which allows a 1/10 smaller bolus of fluorescein.

        2) Low light levels are used.

        3) The generation of 50 images/sec allows rapid changes in fluorescence to be followed (Woon et al., 1990).

        4) Stereoscopic photography using a modified Allen separator can be accomplished which allows better stereo and the ability to display the images on a video monitor, a digital printer, or 35-mm film (Frambach et al., 1993).

        5) Fluorescein angiography of the anterior segment can be performed (Kuckelkorn et al., 1997; Lindblom, 1998).

        6) A new technique has been developed to create functional, parametric images of the retinal circulation that may be useful for early detection and monitoring of retinopathy (Hipwell et al., 1998).

        7) Macular choriocapillary filling time can be determined to assess circulation. This has been performed in eyes with age-related macular degeneration and may help delineate eyes that are at risk for progressive disease (Zhao et al., 1995).

        8) Oral fluorescein angiography can also be accomplished (Garcia et al., 1999).

        9) Retinal montages covering fields of 100° to 140° can be created automatically (Rivero et al., 1999).

    b. **Indocyanine Green (ICG) Angiography** (Kuck et al., 1993; Scheider & Schroedel 1989; Scheider et al., 1992, 1993).

        1) ICG's excitation peak is at 805 nm, and its fluorescence peak is at 835 nm, both in the near-IR region.

        2) Because the excitation and fluorescence of ICG are at longer wavelengths than fluorescein dye, chorioretinal pathology may be seen through overlying RPE detachments, lipid deposits, macular xanthophyll pigment, and hemorrhage (Guyer et al., 1992).

        3) ICG offers enhanced image resolution, hard copy generation, and image archiving (Guyer et al., 1992).

4) Since almost all of the ICG is protein-bound, it leaks more slowly from choroidal vessels and choroidal neovascular membranes than fluorescein does. This allows more distinct visualization of newly formed vessels, as they aren't masked by the dye (Kuck et al., 1993; Scheider et al., 1992).

5) These characteristics allow

   a) choroidal angiograms with high temporal and spatial resolution (Schneider et al., 1995; Scheider & Schroedel, 1989),

   b) enhanced detection of choroidal abnormalities and subretinal neovascular membranes that appear as occult or ill-defined in fluorescein angiography (Gelisken et al., 1998b; Kuck et al., 1993),

   c) quantitative measurements of choroidal circulation,

   d) earlier detection of tumors,

   e) planning and monitoring of laser treatment strategies (e.g., ICG allows earlier detection of persistent or recurring subretinal neovascular membranes),

   f) exploration of the etiology of central serous chorioretinopathy (e.g., abnormal choroidal vascular hyperpermeability is indicated by choroidal hyperfluorescence of ICG) (Scheider et al., 1993),

   g) detection of the feeding vessels of classic choroidal neovascularization (Gelisken et al., 1998a),

   h) detection of aneurysms of the choroidal vasculature (Schneider et al., 1998),

   i) imaging of the microvasculature of choroidal melanomas (Mueller et al., 1998),

   j) investigation of the peripapillary region in glaucoma patients (O'Brart et al., 1997), and

   k) distinguishing of different types of drusen (Arnold et al., 1997).

6) In retinal pigment epithelium detachments, the ICG angiogram of the serous fluid appears dark while it appears bright with a conventional fundus camera (Flower et al., 1998; Wolf et al., 1994). The bright appearance is apparently due to scatter by the fluid of fluorescent light from adjacent fluorescent structures (Flower et al., 1998).

7) ICG angiography using the SLO has been used to guide feeder vessel photocoagulation in a new treatment for subfoveal choroidal neovascularization in age-related macular degeneration (Shiraga et al., 1998). This technique may be an option to treating the whole retinal area.

c. **Simultaneous ICG and Fluorescein Angiography** (Axer-Siegel et al., 1999; Bischoff et al., 1995b; Freeman et al., 1998; Holz et al., 1998). Compared to consecutive administration of the two dyes, simultaneous use involves much less time, only one injection, and enhanced interpretation since the two angiograms have identical magnifications.

d. **Fluorescent (or Fluorescein) and ICG Leukocyte Angiography**

   1) Leukocytes can be stained using ICG, fluorescein, acridine orange, or other dyes (Arend et al., 1995; Hossain, 1999; Kimura et al., 1995; Matsuda et al., 1996; Miyamoto et al., 1996; Nishiwaki et al., 1995, 1996; Yang et al., 1997a). In addition to leukocytes, fluorescent platelets can be detected in the retinal vessels.

   2) Alternatively, a sample of blood can be withdrawn, stained with fluorescein or other dyes, and then only the stained leukocytes reintroduced (Fillacier et al., 1995; Hossain et al., 1998; Khoobehi & Peyman, 1999; Kim et al., 1997; Le Gargasson et al., 1997; Yang et al., 1997b). This technique eliminates the problem of highly fluorescent plasma.

   3) The movement of fluorescently labeled leukocytes can be quantitated in arteries, veins, retinal capillaries, and choroidal vessels.

   4) This method may be useful in studying the inflammatory process (Miyamoto et al., 1996; Parnaby-Price et al., 1998), diabetic retinopathy and retinal ischemia (Hiroshiba et al., 1998; Tsujikawa et al., 1998), or the effects of therapeutic agents (Hiroshiba et al., 1998; Nishiwaki et al., 1997).

   5) Acridine orange leukocyte angiography has been used to evaluate leukocyte dynamics during ischemia reperfusion injury, autoimmune uveitis, and after scatter photocoagulation in rats (Hiroshiba et al., 1998; Kimura et al., 1995; Nishiwaki et al., 1995; Parnaby-Price et al., 1998; Tsujikawa et al., 1998). Because the dye is phototoxic to cellular lysosomes and carcinogenic, its use has been limited to rodents.

e. **Fluorescent Vesicle Angiography** (Khoobehi & Peyman, 1994; Peyman et al., 1996a,b).

   1) Fluorescent dyes can be encapsulated in lipid vesicles and then injected into a vein.

   2) The movement of the vesicles can be quantified using the SLO (Khoobehi & Peyman, 1994).

   3) This method has been used to study photothrombosis using photodynamic therapy in experimental animals (Moshfeghi et al., 1998).

   4) Blood flow in the retinal arteries, veins, and capillaries of the optic nerve and macula can be measured simultaneously (Khoobehi & Peyman, 1994).

   5) The blood velocity in individual choroidal vessels has been measured with this technique in primate eyes (Peyman et al., 1996a). Overall, this technique has not been highly successful.

f. **Fluorescent Microsphere Angiography (FMA)**

   1) Small latex microspheres (1–2 μm diameter) are used to carry a single dye that fluoresces at a single wavelength or several different dyes that fluoresce at different wavelengths. By choosing different excitation wavelengths, differ-

ent layers of the fundus can be assessed, from the anterior retina to the posterior choroid.
2) The SLO can act both as a dye activator and as a fluorescence detector.
3) Blood velocity can be obtained from particle tracking and analysis of results.
4) Unlike with liposome-based systems, this technique allows assessment of blood flow in the choriocapillaris (Khoobehi et al., 1997).
5) So far, this technique has been used in monkeys and rabbits; biodegradable-polymer microspheres may potentially be usable in humans.
6) FMA has been used to study blood velocity in experimental iris tumors (Peyman et al., 1998). It has also been used to study vascular occlusion using photodynamic therapy in rabbits (Moshfeghi et al., 1998).

4. **Psychophysical Testing** (Mainster et al., 1982).
   a. **Retinal Perimetry (Microperimetry) and Retinal Function Mapping** (e.g., Varano & Scassa, 1998).
      1) The SLO can project varied stimuli onto given locations in the retina.
      2) Both static threshold and kinetic perimetry can be performed.
      3) The SLO can define the physical and functional borders of lesions with increased accuracy and reliability compared to standard clinical perimetry.
      4) The SLO can continuously record the location of the fixation target.
      5) The SLO can be used to map macular scotomata before and then after photocoagulation. For example, the SLO has been used to evaluate retinal function around laser scar lesions following laser treatment for juxtafoveal choroidal neovascularization (Oshima et al., 1998). This may help in understanding the visual outcome and rehabilitation potential of such patients. It has also been used before and after laser photocoagulation for clinically significant diabetic macular edema (Rohrschneider et al., 2000).
      6) Microperimetry has been used to assess functional recovery after foveal translocation surgery for age-related macular degeneration (Fujikado et al., 1998).
      7) The SLO has been used to show that macular sparing actually does occur in patients with occipital lesions (Trauzettel-Klosinski & Reinhard, 1998). However, an earlier SLO report suggested that macular sparing may be a perimetric artifact (Bischoff et al., 1995a).
      8) Normal thresholds for fundus perimetry have been evaluated (Rohrschneider et al., 1998). A significant correlation has been shown between increase in age and increase in threshold.
      9) Using the SLO, it has been shown that focal retinal nerve fiber layer defects in glaucoma patients correspond to localized areas of depressed retinal sensitivity (Orzalesi et al., 1998; Uchida et al., 1996b).
      10) Using the SLO, it has been found that large drusen may influence retinal sensitivity (Takamine et al., 1998).

11) Functional assessment before and after surgery for macular holes can be performed (e.g., Amari et al., 2001; Byhr & Lindblom, 1998; Guez et al., 1998). Full-thickness holes can be distinguished from pseudoholes or impending macular holes (Tsujikawa et al., 1997). In addition, full-thickness macular breaks can be differentiated from pseudobreaks via microperimetry (Kakehashi et al., 1996).

12) Functional impairment due to retinal photocoagulation can be assessed quantitatively with the SLO (e.g., Ishiko et al., 1998; Timberlake et al., 1989). In addition, the patient's fixation point and its stability can be determined.

13) The relationship between the sensitivity of the blind spot periphery and the optic disc surface topography has been investigated (Meyer et al., 1997).

14) The pattern of visual loss in age-related geographic atrophy has been explored with microperimetry (Sunness et al., 1995).

15) Angioscotomas (i.e., scotomas due to blood vessel shadows) have been investigated with the SLO using blue-on-yellow and red-on-red microperimetry (Remky et al., 1996).

16) Microperimetry has been used to show that the area of the retina over a choroidal neovascularization can still be functional after submacular surgery (Loewenstein et al., 1998). And it can be used to help plan the site of surgical intervention for submacular surgery (Hudson et al., 1995; Sabates et al., 1996). When combined with ICG angiography, it may also be useful in choosing the appropriate treatment (Schneider et al., 1996).

17) The anatomic and functional abnormalities as well as the location and stability of fixation have been evaluated in cases of subfoveal neovascularization due to various diseases (Tezel et al., 1996).

18) Microperimetry can provide information that may be helpful in the management of central serous chorioretinopathy (Toonen et al., 1995).

19) Combined choroidal and retinal ischemia during interferon therapy was found to be associated with central and paracentral scotomas via microperimetry (Hoerauf et al., 2000a).

b. **Localized Retinal Acuity Testing** (Mainster et al., 1982; Timberlake et al., 1989).

   1) The SLO can place an acuity target on the retinal position to be tested.

   2) Hence, the visual acuity at individual retinal positions can be measured.

   3) For example, visual acuity measurement using the SLO has been performed to help assess function in macular holes before and after surgery (e.g., Guez et al., 1998).

c. **Preferred Retinal Locus Determination** (e.g., Mainster et al., 1982).

   1) The retinal locus of best visual acuity can be determined since the SLO can project any text onto given retinal locations (Fletcher & Schuchard, 1997).

   2) Patients with low vision may then be trained to use their best retinal areas for reading (Fletcher et al., 1994).

3) The preferred retinal locus has been used in functional assessment of macular holes before and after surgery (e.g., Guez et al., 1998).

4) Fixation patterns, reading rates, and prognosis have been investigated in eyes with central and parafoveal scotomas due to age-related macular degeneration and Stargardt disease (Sunness et al., 1996).

d. **Retinal Amsler Grid Testing**

1) For example, with the HeNe laser a red grid on a black background can be projected onto a given retinal area (Mainster et al., 1982).

2) The patient's subjective response can be compared to the locations of visible retinal lesions. This has been used to show that Amsler grid reports have poor validity (Schuchard, 1993).

e. **Contrast Sensitivity Testing**

1) A sine wave grating can be projected onto the retina in a known location.

2) Contrast sensitivity can then be measured at various spatial frequencies (Frambach et al., 1994).

3) This kind of testing has been accomplished with normal, ocular hypertensive, and glaucomatous patients (Horn et al., 1996a).

f. **Photostress Recovery Testing**

1) The SLO can be used to perform photostress recovery testing not only at the fovea but also at extrafoveal locations (Ito et al., 1997).

2) The argon laser green light can be used to bleach selected areas of the retina. Microperimetry threshold testing can then be accomplished with the HeNe laser red light.

3) The recovery time is measured from the end of the bleach to the recognition of the red test spot.

4) This has been used to test inside and outside the areas of idiopathic central serous chorioretinopathy and also inside and outside the scotomatous areas of glaucoma patients (Horiguchi et al., 1998).

g. **Modified Watzke-Allen Test** (Guez et al., 1998).

1) The SLO has been used to project horizontal or vertical lines 2 minutes of arc thick onto the retina. The patient's task is to indicate whether the line is continuous or broken.

2) This test has been applied in the case of macular holes before and after surgery.

3) This method improves on the Watzke-Allen test because the line is sharper with less scattered light and the precise location of the line with respect to the hole can be monitored.

h. **Predictive Visual Acuity Testing** (Cuzzani et al., 1998).

1) By projecting targets of different shapes and sizes as well as allowing visualization of the macula, the SLO can be used to predict the visual outcome of cataract surgery.

2) One of the advantages of the SLO is that its infrared and red laser beams are scattered less than white light by the cataract. This can allow better visualization of the fundus than can be obtained by indirect ophthalmoscopy. It also allows the SLO to penetrate cataracts better than the Potential Acuity Meter.

3) Another advantage is its large depth of focus allowing simultaneous visualization of the lens opacities and the retinal vessels. Thus, the clearest area through a cataract can be determined.

4) The SLO has been used to predict potential visual acuity in cataract patients. It predicted the best corrected visual acuity (BCVA) within two lines of the final BCVA in 97% of 31 eyes compared to 61% of the same eyes for the Potential Acuity Meter.

5. **ERG/VER Stimuli** (e.g., Horn et al., 1996b).
   a. The SLO can project various stimuli onto the retina, including pattern reversal stimuli (Katsumi et al., 1989).
   b. Not only can the precise location of the stimulus on the retina be observed, but the focus of the stimulus can be ensured.

6. **Quantitative Fundus Reflectometry (Imaging Retinal Densitometry; Fundus Reflection Densitometry; Retinal Densitometry)** (e.g., Liem et al., 1996).
   a. The SLO can be used to measure photopigment density, macular pigment density, contrast of retinal vessels, and fundus reflectance (Elsner et al., 1990).
   b. By measuring density differences between dark-adapted and bleached retina, visual pigment levels can be assessed noninvasively. Density maps (e.g., maps of photopigment distribution) can be produced.
   c. Rod and cone visual pigment kinetics have been assessed during the clinical course of multiple evanescent white-dot syndrome (van Meel et al., 1993).
   d. The retinal nerve fiber layer can be objectively assessed in a manner similar to red-free retinal photography (Cooper et al., 1992).
   e. Differences in foveal cone photopigment and macular pigment distribution with age have been assessed (Elsner et al., 1998a).
   f. It has been found with the SLO that foveal visual pigment density is the same in amblyopic and normal eyes (Delint et al., 1998b).
   g. In patients with unexplained visual loss, scanning laser densitometry has been used to assess foveal cone photoreceptor function (DeLint et al., 1996).
   h. Central rod distribution and sensitivity can also be assessed using this technique (Tornow & Stilling, 1998).

7. **Measurement of Eye Movements**
   a. The SLO can be used to specify the rotational state of the eye in three dimensions (e.g., Ott et al., 1990).

    b. Fundus tracking can be performed (Bantel et al., 1991).

    c. Ocular torsion movements can be studied (Schworm et al., 1997).

    d. Vestibulo-ocular and visuo-motor testing can also be accomplished.

    e. Saccade profiles can be assessed (Stetter et al., 1996). Knowledge of saccade pattern while reading can be useful in rehabilitation of visually impaired individuals (Rohrschneider et al., 1996).

    f. Fixational eye movements can be quantified (e.g., Moller et al., 1996).

8. **Retinal Vascular Assessment** (e.g., Harris et al., 1994).

    a. The arterio-venous passage time can be measured (i.e., the time it takes for a dye bolus to go from a specific artery to the corresponding vein).

    b. Retinal capillary blood flow can be measured (e.g., in diabetics versus normal patients of cystoid macular edema) (Ohnishi et al., 1994; Wolf et al., 1991). Quantitative assessment of retinal circulation can be accomplished using digital image analysis (Arend et al., 1999).

    c. Optic nerve head capillary blood flow can be measured (Cantor et al., 1994). In addition, epipapillary blood velocities can be calculated (Arend et al., 1999).

    d. The SLO can be used to determine the foveal avascular zone and perifoveal intercapillary areas (i.e., the density of the capillary beds).

    e. Thus, eyes at risk of developing diabetic retinopathy may be identified.

    f. Prognosis and effect of laser panretinal photocoagulation can be assessed.

    g. Blood flow through iris vessels can also be measured.

    h. Measuring retinal capillary flow and perifoveal intercapillary areas may be useful in assessing the efficiency of hypertensive treatment and may help identify patients at risk for cerebrovascular events (Kutschbach et al., 1998).

    i. Retinal macrocirculation can be measured (Wolf et al., 1994).

9. **Epiretinal Membrane Evaluation** (Ogura & Honda, 1993).

10. **Color Imaging** (Manivannan et al., 2001). By using blue (argon, 488 nm), green (coumarin dye, 547 nm), and red (diode, 670 nm) lasers and combining images, a true color representation of the fundus can be achieved.

11. **Measurement of Stiles–Crawford Effect of the First Kind**

    a. The SLO has been used to measure an optical Stiles-Crawford effect (DeLint et al., 1997). Thus, a rapid and objective method for determining local photoreceptor alignment in the central retina is available.

    b. When compared to retinal densitometric data, this method is a rapid and sensitive way to detect cone photoreceptor disturbances (DeLint et al., 1998a).

   c. When applied to amblyopic and normal eyes, this technique has shown that there is no difference in the effect (DeLint et al., 1998b). This suggests that photoreceptor orientation is normal in amblyopia.

D. *Commercially Available Instruments*

  1. Rodenstock SLO (Rodenstock Instrumente GmbH, Ottobrunn, Germany)—this instrument can be used for fundus photography, angiography, perimetry, and visual acuity testing.

  2. Panoramic200 Non Mydriatic Ophthalmoscope (Optos, Marlborough, MA)—this uses two lasers to obtain a wide-field (200°) fundus photograph (Figure 3–1).

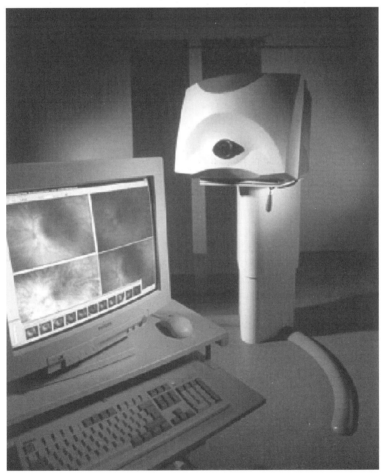

Figure 3–1 Panoramic200 Non Mydriatic Ophthalmoscope. (Courtesy Optos, Marlborough, MA.)

III. Scanning Laser Tomography [Confocal Scanning Laser Ophthalmoscopy (cSLO)]

A. Technique (e.g., Bille et al., 1990).

1. A **laser** is focused on a particular focal plane illuminating a single spot on the retina. Various lasers have been used, including a HeNe laser (632.8 nm) and various diode lasers (670 nm, 780 nm, 830 nm).

2. A **scanning unit** produces a raster-like scan of the beam.

3. **Confocal Detection Unit**
   a. The reflected radiation is focused in a plane optically conjugate to the illuminated plane.
   b. Scattered (stray) radiation and reflections from planes that are not in focus are blocked by a diaphragm at the conjugate plane. This ensures that only radiation originating from the illuminated focal plane is detected.
   c. The reflected radiation at each point in the scan that is detected confocally is displayed as a single pixel on the monitor.
   d. Using this technique, 16 to 24 consecutive image planes are created at 30- to 60-μm intervals.
   e. Data can be acquired in about one second and can be processed and analyzed in about one minute.

4. **Resolution** (e.g., Chauhan et al., 1994; Weinberger et al., 1997).
   a. Horizontal (X–Y axis) = 7–10 μm (vs 400 μm for B-scan ultrasound)
   b. Z-direction (thickness) = 25–50 μm (vs 200 μm for A- and B-scan)

B. SLO Imaging Versatility

The technique of imaging can be varied to filter selectively the clinically pertinent information from unwanted background information (e.g., Elsner et al., 1996; Yoshida et al., 1998b). Three modes are available:

1. **Confocal Imaging Mode**
   a. This mode allows three-dimensional imaging of the fundus via image planes at different depths (e.g., Beausencourt et al., 1997; Hartnett & Elsner, 1996). A **small aperture stop** in the plane of the image blocks light scattered from out-of-focus areas.
   b. Infrared SLO imaging **highlights surface information** and thus improves the visualization of
      1) pores in the lamina cribrosa of the optic nerve head,
      2) RPE abnormalities,
      3) laser photocoagulation scars, and
      4) choroidal vasculature.

2. **Direct Imaging Mode (Nonconfocal Mode)**
   a. In this mode, a **moderate-size aperture stop** is used. Thus, the detected radiation has come from the illuminated object via multiple scattering within the fundus.
   b. Infrared SLO sources allow fundus visualization through nuclear lens opacities.

3. **Indirect Imaging Mode (Dark-Field Mode, Scatter Mode, Tyndall Mode)**
   a. By putting a **central stop** or an occluder in the place of the confocal aperture, most of the reflected light is blocked and a dark background is obtained (Webb and Delori, 1988).
   b. Structures in the fundus will be seen only if they scatter incident radiation sideways (e.g., Elsner et al., 1996). If surrounding structures rescatter this light, it can be detected by the **annular aperture** system. Light from out-of-focus planes can also be detected.
   c. Thus, this mode **highlights tissues that cause significant light scattering** such as the optic nerve head, the choroid, and drusen. For example, the indirect mode enhances significantly the appearance of macular drusen. They appear as discrete raised structures with a higher frequency than in conventional fundus photography. Neurosensory detachments, cystoid macular edema, and subretinal edema in choroidal new vessels can also be detected (Elsner et al., 1996; Remky et al., 1999).

C. *Multiple Scattered Light Tomography (MSLT)*

1. A vertical cavity surface emitting laser (VCSEL) array has been used to develop a prototype instrument for MSLT (Elsner et al., 1998b). The array, with one central and eight peripheral lasers, was used as the light source (850 nm). The instrument was a modification of a TopSS cSLO.

2. With the MSLT, deeper structures are emphasized (e.g., the major choroidal vessels and the choroidal rim of the nerve head). This feature may allow the determination of an objective reference plane for cSLO.

D. *Clinical Uses*

1. **Retinal Topography** (e.g., Bartsch et al., 1990).
   a. The cSLO can be used to quantify the elevation of the retina and changes in the elevation, as well as map irregularities in the retinal surface and the vitreoretinal interface (Varano et al., 1997; Weinberger et al., 1997).
   b. Macular holes can be quantified and evaluated over time with the cSLO (Weinberger et al., 1997). Patients at risk for retinal holes may be detected.
   c. Macular edema can be detected, quantified, and monitored (Hudson et al., 1998; Zambarakji et al., 1999). By using the indirect imaging mode, cystoid macular

edema is highlighted, and this technique may be useful in patients who are sensitive to fluorescein (Ikeda et al., 1998).

d. Three-dimensional, quantitative analysis of macular cysts can be accomplished with the cSLO, providing details of subretinal and intraretinal features not achievable with conventional clinical methods (Beausencourt et al., 2000).

e. Therapeutic trials can be evaluated (e.g., in the treatment of macular edema).

f. The **retinal nerve fiber layer** may be evaluated (Burk et al., 1998). The mean peripapillary slope of the nerve fiber layer may be clinically useful in discriminating between normal subjects and glaucoma patients (Caprioli et al., 1998). The RNFL thickness has been defined as the mean height between the reference plane and the contour line along the same contour line (Gugleta et al., 1999). Even though the RNFL thickness obtained by the cSLO is an indirect measurement, it seems to correlate with the RNFL thickness obtained with optical coherence tomography (Mistlberger et al., 1999). Other methods to estimate RNFL thickness include measuring the full width half height of the axial profile or fitting the axial profile with two Gaussian shapes and calculating the distance between them (Hudson et al., 1998; Sharp et al., 1999; Vieira et al., 1999).

g. The reproducibility of volumetric measurements at the macula is good (Zambarakji et al., 1998).

h. Fine retinal wrinkling around macular holes has been observed with the indirect imaging mode and may be a good marker for repair of the macula after vitreous surgery (Yoshida et al., 1998b).

i. The cSLO may be useful in the differential diagnosis of acute zonal occult outer retinopathy (Nishio et al., 1998).

j. With respect to age-related macular degeneration, the amount of neurosensory detachment can be monitored (Jakkola et al., 1999). It may be useful in assessing change after therapeutic treatment. The spatial extent of pigment epithelial detachments can also be assessed (Kunze et al., 1999).

2. **Optic Nerve Head Topography** (e.g., Anton et al., 1998; Broadway et al., 1998; Burk et al., 1993; Mikelberg, 1998; Zangwill et al., 1997b).

a. The cSLO can be used to measure various parameters (e.g., Saruhan et al., 1998; Mardin & Horn, 1998), including

1) optic disk area (Mardin & Horn, 1998),
2) cup area,
3) neuroretinal rim area,
4) maximum cup depth,
5) mean cup depth,
6) cup volume,
7) cup steepness, and
8) cup-to-disk ratio.

b. **Potential for Earlier Diagnosis of Glaucoma**

    1) Discrimination between normal and glaucomatous eyes has been attempted using various parameters and discriminant functions. In the various studies cited in Table 3–1, the sensitivity varied from 42% to 94%, and the specificity varied from 46% to 100%.

Table 3–1 Discrimination Between Normal and Glaucomatous Eyes for the Heidelberg Retina Tomograph

Sensitivity (%)	Specificity (%)	Parameter	Reference
87	84	Discriminant function analysis	Mikelberg et al., 1995
83	86	Cup shape measure	Uchida et al., 1996a
91	92	Neural network	
77	93	Cup-to-disc area ratio	
87	56	Neural network	Brigatti et al., 1996
74	88	Discriminant function analysis	Iester et al., 1997
62	94	Discriminant function analysis	Bathija et al., 1998
78	88	"Best discriminant function"	
85	80	Mean slope	Caprioli et al., 1998
69	83	Mean height	
84	96	Linear regression	Wollstein et al., 1998
84	95	Multivariate approach	Mardin et al., 1999
83	95	Nonmyopic eyes	Yamazaki et al., 1999
71	96	Myopic eyes	
80	100	Analytic geometric analysis	Iester et al., 1999
75	90	Discriminant function analysis	
70	92	Optic disc sector based discriminant formula	Iester et al., 2000
81	50	Cup shape measure	
84.5	65	Mikelberg formula	
85	75	Bathija formula	
94	46	Mardin formula	
88	89	Mathematical modeling of ONH shape	Swindale et al., 2000
49	98	Discriminant function analysis	
84	96	"HRT analysis"	Wollstein et al., 2000
70	95	Ranked segment analysis	Gundersen & Asman, 2000
85	95	Vertical cup-to-disc ratio	
80	65	Discriminant function analysis	Miglior et al., 2001
52	87	Discriminant function analysis	Sanchez-Galeana et al., 2001
64–75	68–80	Qualitative assessment by 3 graders	
59	90	Linear discriminant function	Zangwill et al., 2001
42	90	Discriminant function analysis	

2) For example, in two studies by the same group, Mikelberg's multivariate discriminant analysis was found to have a fairly high sensitivity (84.5%, 80%) but a fairly low specificity (65%, 65%) for discriminating glaucomatous from normal eyes (Iester et al., 2000; Miglior et al., 2001). This is in contrast to the higher sensitivity (87%) and specificity (84%) found by Mikelberg et al. (1995) in their original study.

3) Ranked segment analysis using the Heidelberg Retina Tomograph software was found to have poor sensitivity (31% to 70%) but high specificity (90% to 95%) for discriminating glaucomatous from normal eyes (Gunderson & Asman, 2000; Miglior et al., 2001).

4) With a new technique that allows analysis without operator input, the sensitivity and specificity of detecting patients with or without glaucoma was 80% and 100%, respectively (Iester et al., 1999). However, one study indicated that ocular hypertensive discs may not be distinguishable from normal discs (Iester et al., 1997).

5) Using a parameter called the normalized rim/disk area ratio, **apparently about 40% of the neuroretinal rim area is lost before the mean defect of the visual field becomes significant** (Bartz-Schmidt et al., 1999). The correlation of the visual field with other cSLO measurements has also been evaluated (Tole et al., 1998).

c. **Potential for Earlier Detection of Progression of Glaucoma**

1) Using an empiric probabilistic approach, a new method for serial analysis of nerve head topographic changes has been suggested (Chauhan et al., 2000). Apparently, this new method has a high level of sensitivity and specificity for the detection of nerve head changes. When this new method was used to follow patients with early glaucomatous visual field defects, it was found that glaucomatous disc changes occurred more frequently than field changes (Chauhan et al., 2001).

2) Two other studies followed early glaucoma patients and their results also suggest that the cSLO is able to measure optic disc changes before visual field changes occur in eyes with progression of glaucoma (Kamal et al., 2000; Mardin et al., 2000a).

d. The cSLO may be capable of detecting different patterns of focal or diffuse optic disc damage (Emdadi et al., 1998).

e. The cSLO can be used to monitor papilledema in cases of idiopathic intracranial hypertension (Mulholland et al., 1998).

f. Imaging of the optic disc at the level of the lamina cribrosa is possible and highly reproducible (Bhandari et al., 1997; Miglior et al., 1998). Changes in lamina cribrosa pore morphometry have been noted with increasing severity of glaucoma (Fontana et al., 1998). The pores become less circular and more elongated with increasing visual field loss.

   g. Regional deformation of the optic nerve head can be detected with the cSLO in response to changes in intraocular pressure (e.g., Kulshrestha et al., 1999; Yan et al., 1998).

   h. The cSLO can be used to quantify the magnitude as well as monitor the resolution of nerve head edema in pseudotumor cerebri (Trick et al., 1998).

   i. Apparently in normal subjects optic nerve head topography does not change significantly with age (Gundersen et al., 1998; Kee et al., 1997). However, one study indicated that significant age related changes occur (Garway-Heath et al., 1997).

   j. Focal optic disc damage and focal defects in short-wavelength automated perimetry are topographically related (Yamagishi et al., 1997).

   k. Diagnosis of optic nerve head drusen can be aided by the cSLO especially in cases of lens opacity (Haynes et al., 1997).

   l. *To increase the accuracy of fundus measurements, the keratometry data from each eye need to be added to the instrument's database (Hosking & Flanagan, 1998). These data are used to correct for magnification errors.*

3. **Corneal Topography** (e.g., Bille et al., 1990).
   a. Corneal curvature may be measured with an accuracy of 0.1 mm (i.e., 0.5 D).
   b. Corneal thickness may be measured with an accuracy of 5 μm.
   c. Incision or ablation depth may be measured in laser refractive surgery.
   d. Anterior chamber angle depth can be measured with a standard deviation of 1.5°.

4. **Vitreous Assessment**
   a. Because of the confocal imaging and monochromatic illumination system, the cSLO is superior to conventional biomicroscopy at visualizing the vitreous (Kakehashi et al., 1995).
   b. The posterior vitreous cortex as well as vitreous opacities can be seen easily (Kakehashi et al., 1995).
   c. Measurements of fluorescein leakage into the vitreous with a cSLO can be used to map retinal leakage and calculate permeability values for the blood-retinal barrier to fluorescein (Lobo et al., 1999).

5. **Scanning Laser Retinoscopy** (Van de Velde et al., 1997).
   a. By using different levels of prefocussing, the SLO can be configured to scan simultaneously the anterior and posterior segments of the eye.
   b. Via patterns of shadows, a portion of the retina is seen superimposed in the pupillary area.
   c. The shadow patterns are due to local variations in refractive error or to wavefront aberrations associated with the cornea and lens.
   d. This can be used to evaluate the optical properties of the cornea after refractive surgery.

6. **Optical Imaging of Nerve Activity** (Stetter & Obermayer, 1999).
   a. Activation of neurons in the brain cortex can be detected by optical imaging.
   b. By illuminating the cortex with visible or infrared radiation, variations in the radiation reflected from the tissue can be used to detect neuronal activation.
   c. Changes in the reflected radiation are due to changes in the oxygenation state of hemoglobin. When a neuron is activated, there is a period of increased oxygen uptake.
   d. For experimental study of the superficial layers of the visual cortex, the cSLO may be useful in detecting neuronal activity with increased resolution, contrast, and depth.

7. **Autofluorescence Imaging**
   a. The cSLO can be used to image the distribution of fundus autofluorescence (e.g., von Rueckmann et al., 1997a). This autofluorescence is most likely due to lipofuscin in the retinal pigment epithelium (Delori et al., 1995).
   b. This technique can also be used to assess macular holes and may become an alternative to fluorescein angiography for differential diagnosis and staging of full thickness macular holes (von Rueckmann et al., 1998).
   c. Autofluorescence imaging may be useful in detection of abnormal phenotypes in early macular dystrophies (von Rueckmann et al., 1997b).
   d. Using the SLO to measure autofluorescence may be useful in identifying eyes at risk for developing exudative age-related macular degeneration (Solbach et al., 1997).

8. **Confocal Tomographic Angiography.** By combining confocal tomography with ICG angiography, it is possible to optically dissect the retinal and optic nerve head vasculature (Bartsch et al., 1995; Melamed et al., 1998). This has been useful, for example, in detecting abnormalities in the retina and choroid in Vogt-Koyanagi-Harada syndrome (Okada et al., 1998).

9. *All of the previously mentioned functions of the SLO are also included.*

E. *Advantages*

1. **Images can be obtained with miotic pupils** (<2 mm). This may allow analysis of glaucoma patients who are on pilocarpine.
2. **Clarity of the ocular media is not that important** (Weinreb et al., 1989). Patients with mild cataractous changes can be analyzed (Zangwill et al., 1997c).
3. **Low light intensity can be used** (Weinreb et al., 1989). For visible light, this means that the patient is more comfortable.
4. A **real-time image** is obtained (Weinreb et al., 1989).
5. This is a **reproducible and reliable** technique (e.g., Chauhan et al., 1994).
   a. Images can be obtained with a reproducibility of about 26–30 μm for depth when averaging three measurements per visit (Lusky et al., 1993; Weinreb et al., 1993).

    b. In one study, only three variables had acceptable reproducibility: average cup depth, half depth area, and volume below (Geyer et al., 1998).

    c. In another study, the parameters that were the most reproducible were volume below, mean depth in contour, and effective area (Azuara-Blanco et al., 1998).

    d. Interobserver and intraobserver agreement can be very good (Garway-Heath et al., 1999; Hatch et al., 1999).

6. Monochromatic illumination makes possible

    a. the **elimination of chromatic aberration**, and

    b. the use of **different wavelengths to highlight different elements of the fundus**.

7. The output of the photodiode is **directly digitized** by a computer. This allows **frame-grabbing** and sophisticated **image processing**.

8. **Three-dimensional information** may be obtained.

9. **Increased image contrast** is obtained due to the reduction of stray and scattered radiation from outside the focal plane or off the optical axis of the system.

F. Disadvantages (Fitzke & Masters, 1993; Rohrschneider et al., 1990).

1. **Ocular optical aberrations** of the cornea and lens, including diffraction effects, limit the resolution of the cSLO.

2. **Lateral and axial measurements are dependent on magnification error correction**.

    a. Lateral magnification error can be corrected by knowing the corneal curvature, refractive error, and axial length (Littmann, 1982).

    b. Axial measurements can be corrected by knowing the axial length of the eye.

3. The cSLO systems are **expensive**.

4. **Eye movement** during measurement can produce an inadequate image.

5. Many of the results are **dependent on** the operator-selected **reference plane**. However, new techniques may allow assessment of the optic nerve head without subjective operator input (Iester et al., 1999; Swindale et al., 2000).

6. A large **normative database** that is age- and race-specific **needs to be established**.

7. **Short- and long-term fluctuation of optic disc topography** exists. Part of this variation depends on intraocular pressure and cardiac pulsation (Chauhan & Mac-Donald, 1995; Lusky et al., 1993). Part is due to misalignment between the patient and the instrument (Orgul et al., 1996).

8. There is **significant variability in size and shape of the optic nerve head among normal subjects** and significant overlap in optic disc parameters between normal and glaucomatous eyes.

9. There is a **need for more longitudinal measurements** of optic disc parameters and a better understanding of the sources of variability in these measurements.

G. *Commercially Available Instruments*

1. Heidelberg Retina Tomograph I and II (Heidelberg Engineering GmbH, Heidelberg, Germany) (Figure 3–2).

2. Heidelberg Retinal Angiograph (Heidelberg Engineering GmbH, Heidelberg, Germany).

3. TopSS CL 2010 (Laser Diagnostic Technologies, San Diego, CA)—no longer available.

4. TopSS XL 2020 (Laser Diagnostic Technologies, San Diego, CA) (Figure 3–3)—no longer available.

5. TopSS with ICG Angiography (Laser Diagnostic Technologies, San Diego, CA)—no longer available.

6. TopSS AngioScan (Laser Diagnostic Technologies, San Diego, CA).

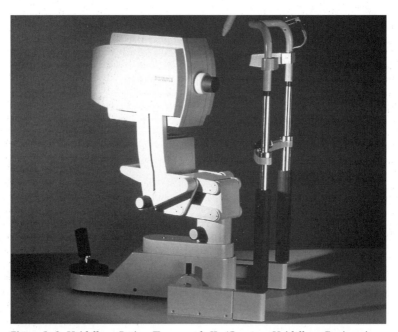

Figure 3–2 Heidelberg Retina Tomograph II. (Courtesy Heidelberg Engineering, Lincoln, RI.)

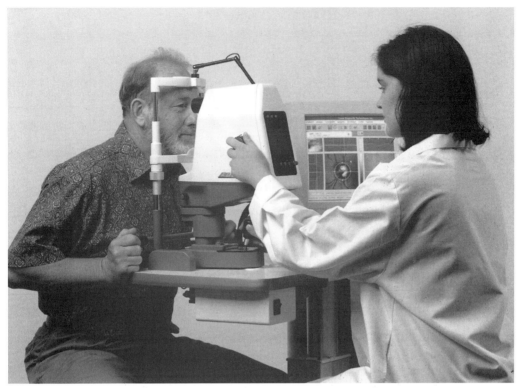

Figure 3–3 TopSS XL 2020. (Courtesy Laser Diagnostic Technologies Inc., San Diego, CA.)

IV. Laser-Triggered, Repetitive Angiography (Targeted Dye Delivery)

A. *Technique* (e.g., Khoobehi et al., 1989, 1992).

  1. The **excitation source** is the blue light (**488 nm**) from an **argon laser**.
  2. Different dyes have been explored.
       a. **Carboxyfluorescein** has an excitation maximum at 490 nm and a fluorescent maximum at 520 nm.
       b. **Calcein** has an excitation maximum at 495 nm and a fluorescent maximum at 515 nm.
  3. Large, **temperature-sensitive liposomes** (spherical lipid shells) encapsulate the dye at high concentrations. This high dye concentration quenches its fluorescence.
  4. The dye-containing liposomes are injected intravenously into the subject.
  5. Exposure to the laser is synchronized to a given point in the cardiac cycle via a heart rate monitor.

6. **Selective Angiography** (Khoobehi et al., 1989).
    a. A specific blood vessel is exposed to the laser radiation.
    b. **Liposomes** in the vessel are **lysed** when the laser beam absorption increases their temperature to 41°C (VanderMeulen et al., 1992).
    c. The dye is released locally and fluoresces intensely as it is diluted in the blood.
    d. Hence, local circulation is visualized in individual vessels.
    e. Laser-targeted delivery choroidal angiography can be performed (Kiryu et al., 1994). This is apparently a safe procedure (Asrani et al., 1995).

7. **Nonselective Angiography**
    a. The optic disk is exposed to the laser beam.
    b. Dye is released into vessels in all four quadrants.
    c. This allows excellent visualization of retinal microcirculation.

8. Although human clinical trials are being pursued, this technique has not yet been approved for human use. Animal studies suggest that the dyes and the laser levels may be safe.

B. *Clinical Uses*

1. Diabetic capillary circulation changes may be evaluated.

2. Tumor blood flow may be monitored during and after laser therapy.

3. Blood velocity and volumetric flow rates may be measured in individual vessels (Khoobehi et al., 1989).

4. Retinal circulation times and mean circulation times may be measured (Khoobehi et al., 1990c).

5. Laser-induced chorioretinal damage can be assessed (Desmettre et al., 1999).

6. **Site-Specific Drug Delivery.** This is a potential method for local drug and dye delivery in the ocular vascular system (Khoobehi et al., 1990a). Selective delivery in either arteries or veins can be accomplished (Ogura et al., 1991). Laser-targeted delivery of a platelet aggregating agent may be useful in occluding retinal and choroidal vessels (Ogura et al., 1993).

7. **Choroidal Angiography.** The response of the choriocapillaris to pathologic and physiologic changes (e.g., flicker stimulation) can be studied (Kiryu et al., 1994, 1995). This technique is better than conventional fluorescein angiography at delineating choroidal neovascularization (Asrani et al., 1996). Selective photocoagulation of feeder vessels in the choroid may be possible.

C. *Advantages*

1. There is **no or minimal background fluorescence** since choroidal fluorescence is quenched by intact liposomes.

2. **Repetitive angiograms can be obtained with one injection** since the dye does not accumulate. Up to 100 angiograms can be performed in 45 min (Zeimer et al., 1990).

3. **Circulation in the arteries and veins is clearly separated.**

4. **Recirculation is not a problem.**

5. **A more distinct dye front is seen.**

D. *Disadvantages*

1. **Some** of the **dyes and** some of the **delivery vehicles can be toxic to humans**.

2. The amount of **laser energy** used in some of the experiments **caused damage** to the retina. Improvements will need to be made in the technique.

V. Retinal Laser Polarimetry (Fourier Ellipsometry; Ellipsometry)

A. *Technique* (Lemij & Tjon-Fo-Sang, 1998; Van Blokland, 1985).

1. A **GaAlAs diode laser** (near-IR–780 nm) is used as the radiation source. HeNe (632.8 nm) and argon (514 nm) lasers have also been used.

2. A **polarization modulator** continuously changes the polarization states of the laser output. The linearly polarized beam from the laser is passed through a rotating quarter-wave retarder.

3. A **scanning unit** moves the beam horizontally and vertically on the retina. This part of the system is the same as in the standard cSLO. The focused beam has a diameter of about 35 μm.

4. The laser beam **double-passes** the retinal nerve fiber layer (RNFL) as the incident beam passes through the RNFL and is then reflected back through it. Because the RNFL is **form-birefringent**, the incident beam undergoes a **phase shift** between the extraordinary beam and the ordinary beam (i.e., the beam is split into two rays with different velocities). This shift is labeled the **retardation**.

5. A **polarization detector** is used to analyze any change in the polarization of the reflected radiation. This element consists of a second synchronously rotating quarter-wave retarder and a linear polarizer in front of a photodetector. The output is then sampled, digitized, and stored by a computer.

6. **Fourier analysis** of the data allows the retardation to be calculated.

7. The **retardation** (i.e., the change in polarization) **is proportional to the RNFL thickness**. A mathematical model was used originally to try to filter out the polarization effects of the cornea (Dreher & Reiter, 1992; Dreher et al., 1992).
   a. There is apparently an **insignificant contribution to the ocular birefringence by the aqueous, crystalline lens, vitreous, and photoreceptor**

outer segments (Bettelheim, 1975; Boehm, 1940; Bour & Lopes Cardozo, 1981; Collur et al., 2000; Brink, 1991; Kremmer et al., 1999; van Blokland & Verhelst, 1987; Weale, 1979).

  1) By comparing a group of phakic eyes to a matched group of pseudophakic and aphakic eyes, there appears to be no significant influence of the lens on the nerve fiber layer thickness using the GDx Nerve Fiber Analyzer (Collur et al., 2000).
  2) RNFL measurements taken after cataract extraction were from 5.35% to 13.4% higher than before the operation depending on the type of intraocular lens implanted (Kremmer et al., 1999).
  3) In another study, the changes in RNFL measurements after cataract extraction were statistically significant when using an Acrysof acrylic intraocular lens, but not significant when using silicon or polymethylmethacrylate lenses (Park et al., 2001). Changes of 15% or greater occurred in about a quarter of the patients.

b. However, the **corneal birefringence is significant**. Form birefringence and, apparently, intrinsic birefringence are both present. One group claimed that the intrinsic birefringence was cancelled out whereas more recent work has shown that it is not cancelled out (Donohue et al., 1995, 1996; McCally & Farrell, 1982; van Blokland & Verhelst, 1987).

c. Under special circumstances, the corneal birefringence can be separated from the retinal birefringence (Brink & van Blokland, 1988).

d. The manufacturer uses an **anterior segment compensating device to compensate for the birefringence** of the anterior ocular structures. The manufacturer has also stated that measurements with the instrument should be taken through an undilated pupil in order to be within the range of the device. One study showed no statistically significant difference between RNFL measurements taken before and after dilation (Hoh et al., 1999a). However, the same study indicated that 22% of the patients had a difference of more than 10% in the measurements before and after dilation. This may be due to misalignments of the beam through the cornea.

e. Although the range of polarization shifts due to the cornea is fairly uniform, some eyes exceed the range of usual compensation by the instrument (Greenfield et al., 1999, 2000). The GDx is designed to compensate for a corneal polarization axis of 15° downward nasally. When the patient's axis falls outside the normal range, the RNFL measurements will be larger than normal (Greenfield et al., 1999, 2000; Kogure et al., 1999a). This variability may account for some of the spread in normative RNFL thickness.

f. The variability in the RNFL data due to corneal polarization axis differences may be corrected by either a revision of the manufacturer's anterior segment compensator or by using the macular GDx data to estimate the corneal axis (Greenfield et al., 2000; Greenfield & Knighton, 2001).

g. Because of stability of the corneal polarization axis, longitudinal comparisons of the RNFL thickness for the same patient should not be affected (Greenfield & Knighton, 2001).

8. Each complete scan yields a retardation map that consists of 256 × 256 pixels (individual retinal positions) or 65,536 total pixels. The value assigned to each pixel is the retardation for that particular position on the retina.

9. The instrument allows for the measurement and graphical depiction of the RNFL thickness in an ellipse/circle around the optic nerve head. This ring has a width of 10 pixels, a diameter of 1.75 disc diameters, and is located concentric to the optic nerve head.

10. In practice, usually three separate scans are obtained and then these are used to create a baseline scan. The baseline scan is then used for subsequent analysis.

11. The computer program also quantitates changes between the current and previous measurements. There is a "Serial Analysis" plot that displays multiple test results on the same page.

12. **Reproducibility** of lateral measurements is 20 μm and of thickness measurements is better than 15 μm.

13. The total **measurement time** is less than 1 sec. This reduces the effects of eye movements on the measurements.

14. Pupil dilation is not necessary. In fact, it is not desirable because of the limitations imposed by the internal birefringence compensation device.

15. A low radiation intensity is used.

16. The commercial instrument has gone through a number of versions and improvements (e.g., NFA, NFA II, and now the GDx). Initially there was fairly large interoperator variability of the data with fair intraoperator variability (Junghardt et al., 1996; Swanson et al., 1995). The variability improved with refinements in analysis and in the second generation instrument (NFA II) (Hoh et al., 1998b; Tjon-Fo-Sang et al., 1997; Zangwill et al., 1997a). To minimize interoperator error when taking measurements on the same patient at different times, a single ellipse should be used for the baseline on all subsequent scans (Hoh et al., 1998b).

17. The coefficients of variation for repeated measurements varied from 3.0% to 9.4% for the NFA II (Hoh et al., 1998b; Hollo et al., 1997b,c; Xu et al., 1998; Zangwill et al., 1997a). For the GDx the mean coefficients of variation for repeated measurements varied from 3.7% to 4.16% for three technicians (Kook et al., 2001b). In normals, 10 of the 14 parameters available on the GDx had an intraclass correlation coefficient

that was greater than 90%; whereas, with glaucoma patients, 13 of the 14 parameters had a coefficient greater than 90% (Colen et al., 2000). To be statistically significant, any change in the retinal nerve fiber layer thickness measured with the GDx would have to be greater than about 7 or 8 μm, at least in the superior or inferior maximum parameters.

18. The first generation instrument's measurements did not correlate very well with photography scores in the same patients (Niessen et al., 1996). This indicates that the information obtained with each may not be equivalent. Using the third generation instrument (the GDx), there was overlap in values although the RNFL thickness values on the whole were significantly higher in relatively healthy eyes compared to eyes with moderate to severe RNFL damage determined photographically (Zangwill et al., 1999).

19. **One of the main problems with the technique is the large range of RNFL thicknesses in normal subjects.** There is a significant overlap between the RNFL thicknesses of normal subjects and patients with glaucoma (Chi et al., 1995; Hoh et al., 2000; Lee & Mok, 1999; Niessen et al., 1996; Tjon-Fo-Sang & Lemij, 1997; Tjon-Fo-Sang et al., 1996; Weinreb et al., 1995b, 1998; Wormington & Alaniz, 1998; Xu et al., 1998).

20. One of the sources of variability has been the presence of blood vessels in the measurement area. Retardation values are lower over the vessels resulting in troughs in the RNFL profile. An algorithm has been developed to remove the vessels from the profiles without oversmoothing the remainder of the profile (Waldock et al., 1998a,b). This algorithm has now been incorporated into the commercial scanning laser polarimeter.

21. Polarimetry measurements taken with and without contact lenses show no statistically significant difference (Bhandari et al., 1999).

22. The GDx version of the instrument has a large normative database. This permits the comparison of the patient's measurements to an age- and race-matched normal group. In the GDx as well as the NFA II, reflectance images are used to adjust the intensity setting of the retardation data. This decreases some of the variability between operators.

23. The GDx uses a neural network to assign a number between 0 and 100 to every patient. The scale is supposed to represent a range from completely normal (0) to very advanced glaucoma (100). For a specificity of 80% and using an unspecified cutoff value, the "Number" parameter had a sensitivity of 82% for detecting perimetric glaucoma patients and a sensitivity of 58% for detecting preperimetric glaucoma patients (Horn et al., 1999). In other studies, the sensitivity and specificity were reported as 82% and 62% (Weinreb et al., 1998), 69% and 77% (Vitale et al., 2000), 92% and 96% (Poinoosawmy et al., 2001), 64% and 82% (Sanchez-Galeana et al., 2001), 54% and

86% (Zangwill et al., 2001), 62% and 96% (Paczka et al., 2001), 43% and 97% (Lauande-Pimental et al., 2001), respectively. Trible et al. (1999) found at a "number" cutoff of 35 and a set specificity of 89%, the sensitivities for early, moderate, and advanced glaucoma were 57%, 71%, and 81%, respectively. Sinai et al. (2000) calculated the sensitivity and specificity using cutoff values from 20 to 40. At a cutoff of 35, they found a sensitivity of 94.1% and a specificity of 76.5%.

B. Clinical Uses—RNFL Analysis

1. **Assessment of Glaucoma Suspects and Patients with Glaucoma** (Chen et al., 1998b; Choplin et al., 1998; de Souza Lima et al., 1997; Hollo et al., 1997c; Marraffa et al., 1997; Reyes et al., 1998; Shirakashi et al., 1997; Weinreb et al., 1995a,b, 1998; Xu et al., 1998).

   a. Discrimination between normal and glaucomatous eyes has been attempted using various parameters and discriminant functions. In the various studies cited in Table 3–2, the sensitivity varied from 54% to 94%, and the specificity varied from 62% to 96%.

      1) A high sensitivity (96%) and specificity (93%) for detecting glaucoma were noted by Tjon-Fo-Sang & Lemij (1997). However, their data were obtained with a group of glaucoma patients whose average mean defect for threshold visual fields was quite high (–10.33 dB with a range of 0.76 to –31.5).

      2) In a later study with the GDx and NFA II, Weinreb et al. (1998) included only early and moderate glaucoma patients (mean deviation of –15 or better only).

Table 3–2 Discrimination Between Normal and Glaucomatous Eyes Using "Number"

Sensitivity (%)	Specificity (%)	"Number" Cutoff	Reference
82	62	17	Weinreb et al., 1998
69	77	20	Vitale et al., 2000
62	96	27	Paczka et al., 2001
84	79	32	Lauande-Pimentel et al., 2001
68	90	32	Yamada et al., 2000
64	82	35	Sanchez-Galeana et al., 2001
94	76	35	Sinai et al., 2000
57	89	35 for early glaucoma	Trible et al., 1999
71		for moderate glaucoma	
81		for severe glaucoma	
92	96	39	Poinoosawmy et al., 2001
54	86	?	Zangwill et al., 2001
82	80	? for perimetric glaucoma	Horn et al., 1999
58	80	? for preperimetric glaucoma	

They tried various parameters and found that with their best discriminant function using three variables they achieved a sensitivity of 74% and a specificity of 92%.

3) Using the GDx, their best algorithm, and a specificity of 89%, Trible et al. (1999) found sensitivities of 57%, 71%, and 81% for early, moderate, and severe glaucoma, respectively.

4) Using their optimal criterion values, Sinai et al. (2000) found that the sensitivity and specificity of the GDx for differentiating glaucoma patients from normals were 94% and 91%, respectively. However, they had a small number of patients and normals, and the average mean defect for the threshold fields of their glaucoma patients was −8.67 dB with a range from −0.36 to −27.5. There was also significant overlap between the GDx parameters for the normals and the glaucoma patients.

b. Neural capacity, as determined by high-pass resolution perimetry, significantly correlates with the NFA-determined RNFL thickness in primary open-angle glaucoma patients, but not in patients with normal-tension glaucoma (Shirakashi et al., 1997, 1999). There was no correlation of total RNFL thickness with the total neural capacity in low tension glaucoma (Shirakashi et al., 1999). However, in low tension glaucoma patients with intraocular pressures between 16 and 21 mm Hg, there appeared to be a significant correlation between the RNFL thickness in each of the inferior and superior quadrants with the corresponding regional neural capacity. No such correlation occurred in low tension glaucoma patients with pressures of 15 and below.

c. In one study the results suggested that the RNFL thickness was reduced more symmetrically in high-tension glaucoma and in a more localized manner in low-tension glaucoma (Kubota et al., 1999).

d. The relationship between RNFL thickness measured with the NFA and visual field data has been investigated (De Natale et al., 2000; Hollo et al., 2001; Kogure et al., 1999b; Kwon et al., 2000; Marraffa et al., 1997; Niessen et al., 1996; Reyes et al., 1998; Serguhn & Gramer, 1996; Shirakashi et al., 1997; Sinai et al., 2000; Tannenbaum et al., 2001; Tjon-Fo-Sang & Lemij, 1997; Weinreb et al., 1995a). There is a weak correlation at best between the visual field indices and the NFA data. Some studies found a significant correlation for certain parameters and other studies found poor correlations.

e. The weak correlation between visual field indices and NFA data may be due to substantial generalized loss of RNFL that does not result in a measurable loss of retinal sensitivity (Kook et al., 2001a; Kwon et al., 2000). This would be consistent with the experimental model of chronic high pressure glaucoma in rhesus monkeys where there is a mixture of localized and diffuse optic neuropathy (Jonas & Hayreh, 1999). Visual field defects may become manifest only after the RNFL thickness has fallen below a certain level. Thus when there is diffuse structural (RNFL) loss that does not result in a decrease in visual field threshold values, a small amount of additional localized structural loss in the superior or inferior quadrants may result in a decrease in the visual field thresholds without being detected by the GDx RNFL parameters.

f. The NFA may be useful in the diagnosis of glaucoma in individuals who have had occipital cortical infarcts (Ong et al., 2000). Possibilities for visual field analysis are limited in these individuals.

g. The GDx may be useful for detecting progression of glaucoma, but more work needs to be done in this area (Hollo et al., 2001; Poinoosawmy et al., 2000).

h. The software and statistical parameters used for data analysis are continuing to evolve and may eventually result in a greater ability to detect glaucoma.

2. **Normals** (Chi et al., 1995; Funaki et al., 1998; Morgan & Waldock, 2000; Tjon-Fo-Sang et al., 1996; Watts et al., 1996; Weinreb et al., 1995b).

a. Discrepancies have been noted in the modulation of retardation values around the optic disk as well as in the change of retardation values with eccentricity from the center of the optic disk when these are compared to anatomic data (Morgan & Waldock, 2000).

b. The correlation between the retardation measurements and the histological measurements of RNFL thickness in two monkey eyecup preparations was good (R = 0.83) (Weinreb et al., 1990). However, these measurements were taken with a prototype instrument using an argon laser (514 nm) instead of the current diode laser (780 nm). In addition, the cornea and lens were removed in order to eliminate polarization artifacts from these birefringent structures. The data taken in this study were then used to convert retardation measurements into units of micrometers with 1° of retardation equal to a RNFL thickness of 7.4 μm.

c. In another study, the overall correlation for histological RNFL thickness and retardation values was R = 0.70 for an adult monkey with the NFA II (Morgan et al., 1998). Regional correlations varied from R = 0.76 to R = 0.06. This study involved an in vivo intact eye for the NFA measurements. The relation between retardation and RNFL thickness was 1° of retardation was equivalent to 16.2 μm instead of the 7.4 μm determined previously. This study along with the study by Weinreb et al. (1990) suggest that **it is better to take the RNFL thickness values of the instrument as relative values of thickness**. Not only is the conversion factor to micrometers approximate, but there may be a scaling difference from the monkey eye to the human eye.

d. The histological study of normal human eyes by Varma et al. (1996) suggests that the difference in RNFL thickness between the temporal quadrant and the superior or inferior quadrants may be exaggerated by the NFA.

    e. Comparing right and left eyes in normal subjects, there is a significant correlation between the total RNFL thickness values in the two eyes of each individual subject (R = 0.90, $P < 0.001$) (Essock et al., 1999). The intraindividual variation was lower than the interindividual variation (7% vs. 21%, respectively). In regions other than the inferior hemiretina, there were significant interocular asymmetries.

    f. A **split nerve fiber layer bundle** is thought to be a clinically normal structural finding with the GDx that can lead to abnormal parameters on the GDx (Colen & Lemij, 2001). In about 12% of normal subjects there is a split bundle in either or both of the eyes. This can lead to an abnormal "superior maximum" or "inferior maximum" parameter as well as to an abnormal "symmetry" parameter.

3. **Aging Effects** (Chi et al., 1995; Choplin et al., 1998; Horn et al., 1999; Lee & Mok, 2000; Poinoosawmy et al., 1997; Tjon-Fo-Sang et al., 1996; Tjon-Fo-Sang & Lemij, 1998; Toprak & Yilmaz, 2000; Weinreb et al., 1995a). The RNFL thickness apparently decreases with age (0.2 to 0.76 μm/year), although this trend was not always statistically significant.

4. **Ethnic Differences** (Funaki et al., 1998; Poinoosawmy et al., 1997; Tjon-Fo-Sang & Lemij, 1998). On the average, the RNFL thickness in whites appears to be thicker than in people of African descent.

5. **Ocular Hypertension.** On the average, RNFL measurements in patients with ocular hypertension are significantly lower than in normals in some studies (Anton et al., 1997; Tjon-Fo-Sang et al., 1996). Another study was unable to identify differences between the two populations (Hoh et al., 2000).

6. **Effect of Corneal Haze After Excimer Refractive Surgery** (Hollo et al., 1997b).

7. **Effect of Refractive Surgery**
    a. In two studies, the difference between RNFL measurements before and after excimer laser photorefractive keratectomy was not statistically significant (Choplin & Schallhorn, 1999; Ozdek et al., 1999).
    b. However, in four other studies there were a statistically significant difference between the measured RNFL thickness before and after laser-assisted in situ keratomileusis (LASIK) (Gurses-Ozden et al., 2000, 2001; Tsai & Lin, 2000; Vetrugno et al., 2000). This discrepancy is probably due to a change in the corneal birefringence or its compensation by the GDx device. This is supported by the fact that RNFL thickness differences were not found by optical coherence tomography or scanning laser tomography and by the unlikelihood that the short increase in intraocular pressure during the procedure could damage the RNFL (Gurses-Ozden et al., 2001).

8. Potentially other **optic neuropathies** may also be detected and monitored (Steel & Waldock, 1998). In patients with previous demyelinating optic neuritis, 94% showed a loss of RNFL with the NFA.

C. Advantages of the Instrument

1. **Noncontact** assessment can be accomplished.
2. **No pupil dilation** is necessary.
3. **Data** are **not dependent on** the choice of a **plane of reference** (Weinreb et al., 1995b)
4. **Data** are **not dependent on a magnification correction** (Weinreb et al., 1995b).
5. **Rapid measurement** occurs in about 0.7 sec.
6. **Low light levels** are used.
7. **Objective and quantitative data** are obtained.
8. A **normative database** exists in the third generation GDx instrument.
9. The NFA II and GDx measurements have **good reproducibility** (Colen et al., 2000; Hoh et al., 1998; Kook et al., 2001b; Zangwill et al., 1997a).

D. Disadvantages of the Instrument

1. **Spuriously high RNFL measurements occur in some eyes**, especially in areas of peripapillary atrophy or chorioretinal scars where the sclera is visible (Zangwill et al., 1998).
2. **For patients with difficulty maintaining fixation, it may be difficult to acquire a well-centered image**. This would include patients that have nystagmus, strabismus, decreased visual acuity, and decreased visual field. Changes of accommodation and, hence, phoria during testing can also disturb fixation.
3. **Anterior and posterior segment pathology may create spurious polarimetry results** (Hoh et al., 1998a, 1999b; Hollo, 1999; Pons et al., 2001; Weinreb et al., 1995b). Pathologies that can generate spurious results include: corneal edema, corneal grafts, keratic precipitates, posterior subcapsular cataracts, anterior uveitis, vitreous opacities, and posterior staphyloma. In addition, dense cataracts may degrade image quality (Hollo, 1999). However, if the visual acuity is 20/200 or better, useful images may be obtained (Kremmer et al., 1999; Lemij, 2001).
4. **Other polarizing structures (e.g., the cornea) may affect the polarization due to the retinal nerve fiber layer** (American Academy of Ophthalmology, 1999). There is a need for better compensation for the polarization of the cornea. Alternatives to address the problem are currently being explored.
5. There is **significant variability in RNFL thickness among normal subjects and significant overlap between normal and glaucomatous eyes** (see preceding discussion).
6. The instrument is **expensive**.
7. There is a **need for more longitudinal measurements** of the nerve fiber layer and a **better understanding of the sources of variability** in the measurements.

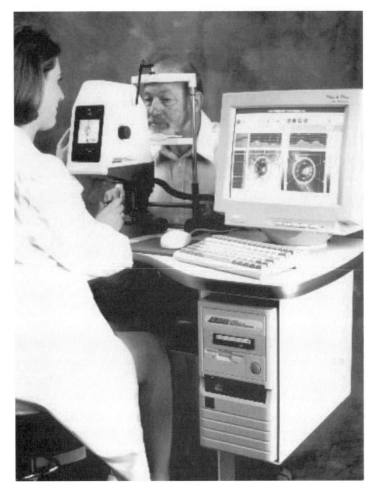

Figure 3–4 GDx Nerve Fiber Analyzer. (Courtesy Laser Diagnostic Technologies Inc., San Diego, CA.)

E. *Commercially Available Instruments*

1. GDx Nerve Fiber Analyzer (Laser Diagnostic Technologies, Inc., San Diego, CA) (Figure 3–4).

2. GDx Access (Laser Diagnostic Technologies, San Diego).

VI. Optical Coherence Tomography (OCT)

A. *Technique* (e.g., Puliafito et al., 1996).

1. OCT is an optical imaging technique based on the principle of low-coherence interferometry (see Laser Doppler Interferometry section). It is analogous to ultrasound B mode imaging except that light is used instead of sound (Huang et al., 1991).

2. A **superluminescent diode laser (843 nm)** is used as a radiation source.

3. A **high-speed, fiber-optic Michelson interferometer** is mounted in a modified slit-lamp biomicroscope.
   a. The radiation from the diode is transmitted along an optical fiber and is split into a **reference arm** and a **sample arm**.
   b. The ocular tissue is illuminated by the beam in the sample arm.
   c. Reflections from the sample travel backwards through the sample arm and are combined with the radiation reflected back from the reference arm mirror.
   d. The two reflections are combined and are detected by a **photodetector**.
   e. The reference arm mirror is longitudinally scanned back and forth with a stepper motor at 160 mm/s, thus generating a **Doppler shift**.
   f. The photodetector measures the intensity of the two interfering beams. The high frequency modulation of the signal due to the Doppler modulation is then demodulated by frequency filtering to extract the signal from the noise.
   g. The signal is most intense when the group delay (time-of-flight) of the two reflections is nearly matched (i.e., when the reference and sample path lengths are essentially equal).
   h. The low coherence ensures that the signal amplitude falls off rapidly as the delay becomes mismatched.
   i. The interferometer signal is then digitized and stored on a computer.

4. The beam is moved laterally after each longitudinal (thickness) scan so that a two dimensional image is formed. A single longitudinal scan is called **optical coherence domain reflectometry** and is analogous to an ultrasound A-scan (Swanson et al., 1992). By laterally moving the beam, the technique becomes **optical coherence tomography** which is analogous to ultrasound B-mode imaging, except with better resolution (Swanson et al., 1993).

5. The precision (standard deviation) of retinal thickness measurements has been determined to be from 5 to 9 μm in one study (Schuman et al., 1996) and from 9 to 16 μm in another study (Baumann et al., 1998). In an earlier study the precision of RNFL thickness measurements was about 10 to 20 μm (Schuman et al., 1996).

6. Thus, optical coherence tomography uses light reflected back from tissue to form images that have a resolution close to that of microscopy. It uses the coherent properties of radiation to generate these images and is therefore an example of a coherence domain technique of time-resolved imaging. Slit-lamp biomicroscopic viewing allows the scan to be placed in the area of interest.

7. Measurements of retinal thickness can be made by measuring the tomograms manually or with computer image processing techniques.

8. The lateral resolution is limited by the separation between adjacent scans on the retina. This means in practice that the **lateral resolution** is **about 70 μm** (Hee

et al., 1998). A new technique called **dynamic coherent focus** can apparently improve the **lateral resolution** to **less than 5 μm** (Lexer et al., 1998).

9. The **axial resolution** of conventional OCT has been claimed to be **about 10 μm** (Hee et al., 1995; Huang et al., 1991). Ultrahigh-resolution OCT has been achieved using a solid-state Ti:sapphire laser (Drexler et al., 2001). The axial resolution obtained was about 3 μm for the retina and about 2 μm for the cornea. The images appeared to detect the RNFL more clearly than conventional OCT.

10. **Image acquisition** takes about **1 sec**.

11. One study that attempted to correlate the OCT images with histology concluded that the layers of high reflectivity were associated with the nerve fiber layer, plexiform layers, retinal pigment epithelium, and the choroid (Toth et al., 1997b). The layers of relative low reflectivity were thought to be associated with the nuclear layers and the photoreceptor inner and outer segments. Another study contradicted the idea of tissue-specific signals (Chauhan & Marshall, 1999). It was concluded that the inner band seen in OCT images is not RNFL specific and that it is not possible to measure precisely specific retinal layers using the OCT. Other limitations to the OCT resolution include noise, image processing, light source bandwidth and wavelength, and the effect of overlying tissues. A recent study suggested that the OCT underestimates the histological RNFL thickness by an average of 37% (Jones et al., 2001).

12. RNFL thickness measured with the OCT is correlated with the visual field mean defect and the corrected pattern standard deviation in glaucoma patients (Mistlberger et al., 1999).

13. Recently, a technique for measuring flow velocity distribution was proposed using the temporal fluctuations of the interference signal of the backscattered light (Imai & Tanaka, 1999).

B. Potential Clinical Applications

1. **Retinal assessment of** (Huang et al., 1991; Swanson et al., 1993)
   a. aging changes (Schuman et al., 1995);
   b. central serous chorioretinopathy (e.g., Iida et al., 2000). OCT is apparently better than biomicroscopy at detecting shallow foveal detachments in cases of central serous chorioretinopathy (Wang et al., 1999b);
   c. chorioretinal inflammatory diseases (Puliafito et al., 1996);
   d. choroidal tumors (Schaudig et al., 1998);
   e. detachment of the neurosensory retina (Hagimura et al., 2000; Ip et al., 1999; Puliafito et al., 1995; Schaudig et al., 1998);
   f. detachment of the pigment epithelium (Puliafito et al., 1995);
   g. diabetic retinopathy (Imai et al., 2001; Puliafito et al., 1996) (see also *Macular Edema*);

h. epiretinal membranes (Puliafito et al., 1995, 1996). This technique may be useful in preoperative and postoperative evaluation of epiretinal membrane surgery (Massin et al., 2000);

i. focal defects in the RNFL (Pieroth et al., 1999; Puliafito et al., 1996; Schuman, 1997);

j. glaucoma (e.g., Hoh et al., 2000; Mistlberger et al., 1999; Puliafito et al., 1996; Schuman, 1997; Schuman et al., 1995)—OCT may be useful for RNFL assessment for early diagnosis and monitoring of glaucoma (Zangwill et al., 2001);

k. Goldmann-Favre syndrome (Theodossiadis et al., 2000);

l. idiopathic polypoidal choroidal vasculopathy (Iijima et al., 2000);

m. intraretinal exudate (Puliafito et al., 1995);

n. laser retinal lesions (e.g., Puliafito et al., 1996; Toth et al., 1997a);

o. macular degeneration (e.g., Puliafito et al., 1996)—e.g., post-excision of a neovascular membrane and foveal translocation surgery (Fujikado et al., 1998);

p. macular edema (e.g., Imasawa et al., 2001; Puliafito et al., 1995, 1996). OCT may become a test for early macular thickening in patients with diabetic retinopathy. It may also be used to monitor resolution or progression of edema (Antcliff et al., 2001);

q. macular holes (e.g., Chauhan et al., 2000; Puliafito et al., 1995, 1996). OCT may be of use in classification and subsequent management of macular holes (Haouchine et al., 2001);

r. ocular hypertension (Parisi et al., 1999);

s. optic disk pitting (e.g., Lincoff & Kreissig, 1998; Puliafito et al., 1996)—e.g., optic disk pit maculopathy before and after pneumatic displacement;

t. optic nerve head drusen (Roh et al., 1998);

u. papilledema (Puliafito et al., 1996);

v. pseudodefects of the RNFL (Tuulonen & Yalvac, 2000);

w. retinal dystrophies (Jacobson et al., 1998; Puliafito et al., 1996);

x. retinal pigment epithelial tears (Giovannini et al., 2000);

y. retinal thickness (Konno et al., 2001a). An increase in macular thickness was noted in about 25% of eyes days to months after cataract surgery (Sourdille & Santiago, 1999). No change in retinal thickness was noted immediately after (0.5 hr) surgery (Grewing & Becker, 2000);

z. retinal trauma (Puliafito et al., 1996);

aa. retinal vascular occlusion (Christoffersen et al., 1998; Puliafito et al., 1996)—e.g., resolution of intraretinal edema after laser treatment for retinal branch vein occlusion;

bb. retinitis pigmentosa (Jacobson et al., 1997);

cc. retinoschisis (e.g., Ip et al., 1999; Puliafito et al., 1996); and

dd. vitreoretinal adhesions, vitreoretinal interface syndrome, and vitreomacular traction syndrome (e.g., Gallemore et al., 2000; Puliafito et al., 1995, 1996; Uchino et al., 2001).

2. **Anterior segment imaging and measurements** (Hoerauf et al., 2000b; Huang et al., 1991).
   a. Corneal thickness (e.g., Hoerauf et al., 2000b)
      1) Corneal edema (e.g., in contact lens evaluation) (Bechmann et al., 2001)
      2) Corneal incision or ablation depth and corneal profile changes in keratorefractive surgery (e.g., Kamensky et al., 1998)
      3) Evaluation of the corneal cap and stromal bed after laser in situ keratomileusis (Maldonado et al., 2000)
      4) Evaluation of cornea with lesions (Hirano et al., 2001)
   b. Anterior chamber depth (e.g., Hoerauf et al., 2000b)
      1) Diagnosis of angle closure glaucoma
      2) Intraocular lens power calculations
   c. Iris thickness and surface profile (Hoerauf et al., 2000b)
   d. Cataract evaluation (DiCarlo et al., 1995; Hoerauf et al., 2000b)
   e. Lens ablation (e.g., Kamensky et al., 1998)
3. **Tissue spectral property assessment** (Huang et al., 1991). With sources of different wavelength, a number of spectral properties may be measured, including:
   a. size of light scattering structures
   b. hydration
   c. hemoglobin oxygenation
   d. chromophore content

C. *Advantages of OCT*

1. **Noninvasive** evaluation is obtained.
2. **Noncontact** assessment is achieved.
3. **High resolution** is accomplished (<20 μm).
4. **High sensitivity** (<100 dB dynamic range) is necessary due to the low signal from backscattered light.
5. **Topographical imaging** is achieved.
6. **No reference plane is required** (Huang et al., 1991).
7. **Results are not affected by the axial length of eye or by the refractive state** (American Academy of Ophthalmology, 1999).
8. **Reproducibility is good** (Baumann et al., 1998; Schuman et al., 1996). Increasing the sampling density improves the reproducibility of the peripapillary circular scan (Gurses-Ozden et al., 1999).

D. *Disadvantages of OCT*

1. Measurement **requires pupillary dilation** (5 mm or more).
2. **Performance is impaired by cortical and posterior subcapsular cataracts** (Swanson et al., 1993).

3. The instrument is **expensive**.

4. There is **no normative database**.

5. The **software and analysis parameters are still evolving**.

6. **For patients with difficulty maintaining fixation, it can be difficult obtaining good images.**

7. There is **considerable overlap of nerve fiber layer thickness values in normal, ocular hypertensive, and glaucomatous eyes** (Hoh et al., 2000).

8. **Specific retinal layers cannot be precisely delineated.**

E. Commercially Available Instrument. Optical Coherence Tomography Scanner (Humphrey Instruments, Dublin, CA) (Figure 3–5)

VII. Clinical Laser Interferometry (Potential Acuity)

A. Technique (e.g., Campbell & Green, 1965; Cavallerano, 1991; Green & Cohen, 1971; Lotmar, 1980; Thibos & Bradley, 1992).

1. A **coherent light source** is necessary. A **HeNe laser (632.8 nm)** has been used. Some of the clinical interferometers use an incandescent or halogen source configured to produce essentially coherent light (Lotmar, 1980). In any case, **two coherent beams** are generated and made to converge and focus at the pupil plane. Beyond the pupil plane the two beams diverge. In other words, these are Maxwellian-view systems.

2. An **interference pattern on the retina** is generated everywhere the two diverging beams overlap. This is a **sinusoidal** interference pattern characterized by
   a. **fringe spacing**, which is determined by the wavelength of the source and by the distance between the two sources at the pupil plane, and
   b. **fringe contrast**, which is determined by the stray or scattered light and by the relative beam intensities.

3. Usually, **four possible orientations** of the fringes are shown to the patient: 0° (horizontal), 45°, 90° (vertical), and 135°.
   a. The size of the interference pattern on the retina varies from 1.5° to 8°, depending on the instrument used.
   b. The vertical and horizontal orientations have a lower threshold than the oblique orientations (Campbell et al., 1966).

4. **Patient setup** is important.
   a. **Dilate** the pupils, especially if there is a cataract or media opacity.
   b. **Correct or at least partially correct a high ametropia.** In cases of high ametropia, an ellipsoidal pattern will be seen by the patient instead of a circular pattern (Goldmann et al., 1980). Unfortunately, the fringes are parallel to the long

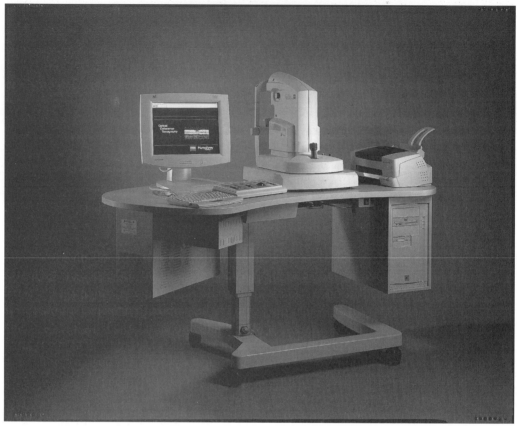

Figure 3–5 Humphrey Optical Coherence Tomography Scanner. (Courtesy Zeiss Humphrey Systems, Dublin, CA.)

    axis of the ellipse, and the patient may cue on the direction of the ellipse axis even if the fringe pattern can't be distinguished.

  c. The **room light should be off or very dim**. Additional light sources can cause light scattering and reduction of fringe contrast on the retina.

  d. **Focus the two beams on the iris and then move them into the pupil and find the clearest path through the opacity.** One technique to enhance your ability to see the clearer paths is to retroilluminate the lens or cornea with a slit lamp biomicroscope.

5. Starting with a low spatial frequency (i.e., a coarse striped pattern), the patient is asked to indicate the orientation of the interference fringes.

  a. If the patient is correct, the spatial frequency is increased, the orientation of the pattern is rotated, and the patient is questioned again.

   b. If the patient is incorrect, the beams may be repositioned and the patient questioned again.
   c. The **endpoint is the highest spatial frequency at which the patient gets more than 50% of the orientations correct (i.e., threshold).**
6. **This threshold spatial frequency in cycles/degree determines the patient's visual acuity.** For example, if the threshold fringe spacing is 30 cycles/degree, the patient can detect fringes that are 2 min apart. This means the patient's minimum angle of resolution is 2 min, and, hence, the visual acuity is equivalent to 20/40.
7. **By varying the target size, additional diagnostic information can be obtained.**
   a. Cystoid macular edema may result in a reduced interference acuity for larger targets.
   b. Macular disease may result in reduced interference acuity for smaller targets.
   c. Amblyopia may result in reduced interference acuity for larger targets (Gstalder & Green, 1971).
8. In some experimental systems, the contrast of the sinusoidal fringes can be varied, and, hence, the patient's **contrast sensitivity function** can be measured (e.g., Campbell & Green, 1965; He & MacLeod, 1996).
9. Other experimental systems have been used as a stimulus for **pattern-reversal visual evoked potentials** (e.g., Simon & Rassow, 1986). Using Fourier analysis and linear regression, an objective visual acuity can be measured.
10. Interferometers have also been used to measure the **modulation transfer function of the eye** (Williams et al., 1994), as well as the **change in vision due to the neurosensory elements associated with age** (Jay et al., 1987).
11. Bypassing the effects of the eye's optics, it has been found that the spacing of the ganglion cells limits peripheral resolution acuity (Anderson et al., 1992).
12. Part of the Stiles-Crawford effects is due to light that passes through some cones before it is absorbed by other cones (Chen & Makous, 1989).
13. The interferometer has been employed to measure the spatial filtering in the visual system after the formation of the retinal image but before a visual nonlinearity fed by single cones (MacLeod et al., 1992). In addition, an interferometer was used to study the nonlinear distortion of interference fringe gratings at the foveal resolution limit (Sekiguchi et al., 1991).

B. *Clinical Uses*
   1. **Amblyopia**
      a. For many patients with amblyopia, the interference acuity is better than the single-letter Snellen acuity (Gstalder & Green, 1971).

b. Interference acuity can be used to predict the outcome of amblyopia therapy. The pretreatment interference acuity is within two lines of the post-treatment Snellen visual acuity in 90% of patients (Selenow et al., 1986).

c. Interference acuity may also play a role in assessing meridional amblyopia (Vernon et al., 1990).

d. Interference fringe patterns appear to be an optimal target for amblyopes.

   1) Since the pattern bypasses the optics of the eye, the amblyope's error or fluctuation of accommodation is obviated.

   2) The very high contrast of the fringes on the retina minimizes the effect of threshold and low suprathreshold contrast abnormalities.

   3) The spatially redundant target minimizes the effects of localization problems and monocular spatial distortion.

e. Laser interferometry suggests that the spatial distortions perceived by strabismic amblyopes may be due to undersampling by cortical neurons (Sharma et al., 1999).

2. **Cataracts** (Angra & Pal, 1990; Bernth-Petersen & Naeser, 1982; Bryant, 1985; Cohen, 1976; Datiles et al., 1987; Enoch et al., 1979; Faulkner, 1983a; Goldmann et al., 1980; Goldstein et al., 1988; Graney et al., 1988; Green, 1970, 1978; Grignolo et al., 1988b; Halliday & Ross, 1983; Kogure & Iijima, 1993; Lasa et al., 1995; Miller et al., 1988; Odom et al., 1988; Sherman et al., 1988; Spurny et al., 1986; Tabbut & Lindstrom, 1986; Thurschwell, 1991).

   a. A positive acuity prediction is usually significant, whereas a negative prediction may be inaccurate (Cohen, 1976; Datiles et al., 1987; Enoch et al., 1979; Graney et al., 1988; Green, 1978; Grignolo et al., 1988b; Lasa et al., 1995; Tabbut & Lindstrom, 1986). The poorer correlation tends to be associated with dense cataracts (Datiles et al., 1987; Goldmann et al., 1980; Grignolo et al., 1988; Lasa et al., 1995; Tabbut & Lindstrom, 1986).

   b. In cataract patients who also have age-related macular degeneration, interferometer acuities are relatively inconsistent in predicting postsurgical Snellen acuities (Bloom et al., 1983; Faulkner, 1983a). In patients with clear media and maculopathy, the interferometer tends to yield more false positive readings than the Potential Acuity Meter (Fish et al., 1986). In cataract patients, the Potential Acuity Meter tends to have better predictive ability than the laser interferometer (Barrett et al., 1995). Although in cataract patients with acuity worse than 20/200 or with glaucoma, the interferometer may be better than the Potential Acuity Meter (Datiles et al., 1987; Lasa et al., 1995; Spurny et al., 1986).

   c. In high myopes with moderate cataracts and poor Snellen acuities, both the laser interferometer and the Potential Acuity Meter appear to be useful in assessing to what extent the vision loss is due to the cataracts (Datiles et al., 1987).

  d. In eyes with posterior subcapsular cataracts, the laser interferometer and the Potential Acuity Meter tend to overestimate the predicted postsurgical acuities (Lasa et al., 1995).

  e. There is apparently no significant difference between interferometer acuities taken before or after pupil dilation (Bosse, 1989).

3. **Posterior Capsule Opacification (Pre-Capsulotomy)**

  a. In one study the white light interferometer was able to predict postsurgical Snellen acuities within two lines in 76% of eyes (Hanna et al., 1989). In another study white light interferometers were able to predict postsurgical acuities to within two lines in 81% (Lotmar interferometer) and 92% (Site interferometer) of eyes (Strong, 1992). In two other studies, the Lotmar interferometer was able to predict postsurgical acuities to within one line in 96.6% of eyes (Faulkner, 1983b) and to within two lines in 80% of eyes (Spurny et al., 1986).

  b. In various studies laser interferometers were able to predict postsurgical Snellen acuities to within two lines in 98% (Strong, 1992) and 63.5% (Lang & Lindstrom, 1985) of eyes.

  c. In the same group of patients, the laser interferometer appears to be better at predicting postsurgical Snellen acuity than the white light interferometers (Strong, 1992).

4. **Corneal Opacification (Pre-Keratoplasty)** (Gstalder & Green, 1972; Steinert et al., 1984). In cases of mild to moderate levels of corneal edema, the Randwal laser interferometer and the Mentor Potential Acuity Meter are useful predictors of retinal function. In cases of severe corneal edema, the interferometer is slightly more accurate.

5. **Cystoid Macular Edema (Clear Media)** (Colvard et al., 1980).

  a. False positive results can occur in cases of macular edema.

  b. These false positives could be due to the ability of the photoreceptors to detect the interference fringes even though the receptors are tilted (Faulkner, 1983a) or to the decreased intraretinal light scattering of the interferometer beam compared to light from a Snellen chart (Guyton, 1987).

6. **Reattached Retinal Detachment.** Early postsurgical interferometer acuities correspond fairly well with the Snellen acuities 6 to 12 months after surgery (Faulkner, 1982).

7. **Uveitis** (Nussenblatt, 1986).

8. **Children** (Richman et al., 1989).

9. **Illiterates**

10. **Malingerers** (Grignolo et al., 1988a).

11. **Genetic Ectopia Lentis** (Guo et al., 1998).

12. **Macular Hole.** The laser interferometer was able to correctly predict postsurgical Snellen acuities within two lines in 70% versus the Potential Acuity Meter in 64% of 17 cases (Barrett & McGraw, 1995; Smiddy et al., 1994).

13. **Intravitreal Hemorrhage (Pre-Vitrectomy)** (Schoenfeld et al., 1994).
    a. In cases of proliferative diabetic retinopathy where there was intravitreal hemorrhage, the laser interferometer was not very useful at predicting visual acuity 6 months after vitrectomy.
    b. Apparently in most cases the lowest spatial frequency could not be projected through the dense intravitreal hemorrhage.

14. **Optic Neuritis.** After staring into an interferometric potential acuity device, many patients with optic neuritis experience a fading of vision with loss of visual acuity after a few minutes (Enoch et al., 1979; Rutgard et al., 1980).

C. Advantages

1. There is **increased light on the retina** as a result of the brightness of the laser and because of the Maxwellian presentation (e.g., Green, 1970).

2. There is **decreased light scatter** with a laser interferometer since the HeNe laser output is in the red end of the spectrum. Rayleigh scattering is proportional to $1/\lambda^4$, so red is scattered less than the white light of conventional acuity charts, which includes light from the more scattered blue end of the spectrum.

3. This technique essentially **bypasses the optics of the eye**.
    a. The interference fringe pattern is not dependent on the patient's ametropia, accommodation, corneal surface irregularities, media opacities, or photoreceptor spatial orientation—at least to a first approximation (Campbell & Green, 1965).
    b. Since the laser is monochromatic, laser interferometer acuity is not affected by pupil entry position. The polychromatic "white-light" interferometers experience decreases in fringe contrast and, hence, acuity due to off-axis chromatic aberration (e.g., Thibos & Bradley, 1992).
    c. This feature makes the interferometer a useful tool for dividing the optical from the neural factors in a patient's vision loss.

4. This technique is a **quantitative measure of macular function**.

5. The technique is also **relatively rapid**.

6. Because **Maxwellian view** is used, **cataracts or other media abnormalities may be avoided** by moving the two beams around in the pupil area.

D. Disadvantages

1. In general, there is **decreased accuracy with increased media density** (Datiles et al., 1987; Goldmann et al., 1980; Grignolo et al., 1988b; Lasa et al., 1995; Tabbut & Lindstrom, 1986). Interferometers tend to work fairly well with mild to moderate

cataracts and when there is no comorbidity. They do not work well with dense cataracts.

2. This technique **requires patient cooperation and understanding**.
3. **False negative predictions can occur.**
   a. A false negative is when the interferometer predicts an improved visual acuity, but the post-treatment visual acuity does not improve.
   b. In general, the accuracy of the interferometers is low when they predict a poor outcome (Cohen, 1976; Datiles et al., 1987; Enoch et al., 1979; Graney et al., 1988; Green, 1978; Grignolo et al., 1988b; Lasa et al., 1995; Tabbut & Lindstrom, 1986). On the other hand, a positive result has good predictive value.
   c. False negatives usually result from
      1) blocked light beam(s) (Faulkner, 1983a),
      2) poor patient responses or understanding, or
      3) failure to dilate the pupil (Faulkner, 1983a).
4. **False positive predictions can occur** (Barrett et al., 1994; Bloom et al., 1983; Faulkner, 1983a,b; Fish et al., 1986; Guyton, 1987; Halliday & Ross, 1983).
   a. A false positive occurs when the interferometer predicts a poor visual acuity, but the post-treatment visual acuity is good.
   b. False positives can occur in cases of
      1) pre-existing amblyopia,
      2) irregular refraction (e.g., irregular corneal astigmatism or scarring and posterior capsule opacification),
      3) macular edema,
      4) macular scotoma (e.g., from age-related macular degeneration or a macular hole),
      5) recent reattached retinal detachment, or
      6) serous detachment of the sensory epithelium of the macula.

E. *Commercially Available Instruments*

   1. Haag-Streit Lotmar Visometer (white light)
   2. Rodenstock Retinometer (laser)

VIII. Laser Biomicroscopy (Retinal Thickness Analyzer)

A. *Technique* (e.g., Zeimer et al., 1996).

   1. This instrument works on the principle of slit-lamp biomicroscopy with a laser source forming a very thin optic section beam (Zeimer et al., 1996). This beam intersects the retina and forms an optic section of the retinal thickness.
   2. A **laser** is used as a slit lamp biomicroscope light source.

a. A **green HeNe laser (543 nm)** is employed to minimize backscatter from the choroid and to enhance the brightness of the beam.

b. A very **narrow beam** is used to optimize depth resolution. The height of the beam is 2 mm and the width is diffraction-limited (approximately 10 to 20 μm). In other words, an extremely thin "optic section" is created.

3. The **biomicroscope** allows a view at an angle of the intersections of the narrow laser beam with the ocular structures. This is similar to a corneal optic section with a conventional slit lamp source. A fluid-filled contact lens is used to improve magnification and resolution by eliminating the refractive power of the cornea.

4. A **microdensitometer** can be used to analyze the image on film or via a computer. However, live visual observation by the clinician results in more information.

5. The **retinal thickness analyzer** is a scanning system (Asrani et al., 1999; Zeimer et al., 1996, 1998).

a. The laser is projected onto the retina at an angle of 15° and scanned across a 2 mm × 2 mm area of the retina. The scan takes either 200 or 400 msec. The retinal thickness is proportional to the observed separation between the intersections of the laser beam with the vitreoretinal interface and the sensory retina–RPE interface.

b. This scan yields 10 optical cross-sections from the light scattered back from the retina at an angle opposite to the incident beam. The scattered light is detected by a CCD camera and then digitally recorded. Another CCD camera is used to provide a fundus image for slit orientation. A third camera is used to image the iris and thus permit easy alignment.

c. Nine different positions of a fixation target are used to produce nine scans. The nine scans thus form a 6 mm × 6 mm map of the central 20° × 20° of the retina made up of 1710 thickness values (Zeimer et al., 1998). The total time for image acquisition is 8 minutes per eye.

d. The software then analyzes the data and produces a topographic map of thickness values (Asrani et al., 1999). The data can be displayed as either a two-dimensional or a three-dimensional color-coded map or as a numeric report. A quality control feature involves the detection of data points that deviate grossly from adjacent points, deletion of those points, and marking the deleted points in black on the final map.

e. The results can be corrected for refractive error and axial length of the eye.

f. Reproducibility was ±11–12 μm for local measurements performed on the same visit and ±13 μm on three different visits (Zeimer et al., 1996, 1998).

g. The **optimal depth resolution is about 50 μm**. This is degraded somewhat by scatter.

h. Limiting factors include the need to dilate the pupil to at least 5 mm and the difficulty in obtaining images in eyes with media opacities and numerous vitreous floaters (Zeimer et al., 1998).

    i. As with all systems that measure retinal thickness, the ability to detect glaucomatous or other losses in nerve fiber layer thickness is limited by the large variation in the number of fibers in the normal population (Curcio & Allen, 1990; Quigley et al., 1990; Repka & Quigley, 1989).

6. **Chorioretinal optical sectioning** is a variant of this technique (Shahidi et al., 1998).
    a. Two lasers are used that have wavelengths near the maximum absorption peaks for fluorescein and indocyanine green (ICG) dyes: **argon green** (488 nm) and a **diode** laser (790 nm). The scanning is performed after injection of a fluorescent dye.
    b. The images have **better contrast** than fluorescein or ICG angiograms because the fluorescence from the underlying or overlapping vasculature is eliminated. As with scanning laser ophthalmoscope angiography, the imaging is hampered by the attenuation of the infrared radiation due to absorption by the retina, pigment epithelium, and the choroid.
    c. The data from a scan are acquired in 660 ms. This minimizes the effect of eye motion.

B. *Clinical Uses*
  1. **Visualization of fine retinal structures** (Ogura et al., 1991).
  2. **Enhanced visualization of vitreal structures and subtle changes in the vitreoretinal interface** (Kiryu et al., 1993).
  3. **Measurement of retinal thickness** (e.g., Asrani et al., 1999; Konno et al., 2001a). The Retinal Thickness Analyzer may be more sensitive than slit-lamp biomicroscopy at detecting changes in retinal thickness. The precise correlation between the different reflective layers in the RTA images and the histological retinal layers has not been established.
  4. **Early diagnosis and/or evaluation of**
      a. **aging changes** (Asrani et al., 1999);
      b. **central serous chorioretinopathy** (Gieser et al., 1997);
      c. **cystoid macular edema** (Asrani et al., 1997; Shahidi et al., 1994a);
      d. **diabetic macular edema** (e.g., Asrani et al., 1997; Gieser et al., 1997; Konno et al., 2001b). This technique may be useful for diagnosis and follow-up of the edema. It may also be useful for evaluation of the efficacy of laser treatment and of postoperative subclinical foveal thickening (e.g., Tsujikawa et al., 1999);
      e. **epiretinal membrane** (Asrani et al., 1997; Kiryu et al., 1993);
      f. **foveal schisis** in X-linked retinoschisis (Tanna et al., 1998);
      g. **glaucoma** (by detecting changes in the RNFL thickness) (e.g., Asrani et al., 1997; Brusini et al., 2000);
      h. **macular cysts** (Folk et al., 1998; Kiryu et al., 1993);

     i. **macular holes, pseudoholes,** and **suspected holes** (e.g., Asrani et al., 1997, 1998; Gieser et al., 1997; Kiryu et al., 1993; Konno et al., 2001b);

     j. **optic disk pit maculopathy** (Oshima & Emi, 1999);

     k. **refractive conditions** (Kremser et al., 1999);

     l. **retinal pigment epithelial detachment** (Asrani et al., 1997; Gieser et al., 1997);

     m. **retinal vein occlusion** (De Geronimo et al., 2001). The RTA can be used for diagnosis of subclinical macular edema and monitoring of treatment; and

     n. **retinitis pigmentosa** (Shahidi et al., 1994).

  5. **Monitoring of therapy**

C. *Commercially Available Instruments*

  1. Retinal Thickness Analyzer (Talia Technology Ltd., Mevaseret Zion, Israel) (Figure 3–6)

  2. Laser Slit (Talia Technology Ltd., Mevaseret Zion, Israel)

IX. Laser Flare Cell Meter (Laser Flare Meter, Laser Cell Meter, Laser Flare Photometry)

A. *Technique* (e.g., Holmer et al., 1994; Sawa et al., 1988).

  1. A **HeNe laser (632.8 nm)** is used for illumination during the measurements. The beam is focused by a condensing lens to a diameter of 20 μm.

  2. A **slit lamp biomicroscope** with a coaxial halogen source is used for observation between measurements.

  3. An **optical scanner** is used to scan the laser beam in the center of the anterior chamber.

  4. A **photomultiplier** measures the intensity of the scattered laser beam in the aqueous. An imaging lens focuses the sampling window (0.3 × 0.5 mm) onto the photomultiplier.

  5. A **computer** accepts patient data, controls the equipment after the initial alignment, calculates the average and standard deviation of the measurements, and displays and prints the data graphically as well as numerically.

  6. **Anterior chamber measurement modes**
    a. **Flare (protein concentration) measurement mode** (Shah et al., 1992).
      1) In this mode, the laser beam is scanned vertically for a distance of 0.6 mm, centered on the sampling window. So the beam scans the area below, in, and finally above the sampling window.
      2) The background scattering intensity is calculated from the mean of the intensity levels below and above the scattering window. This background intensity

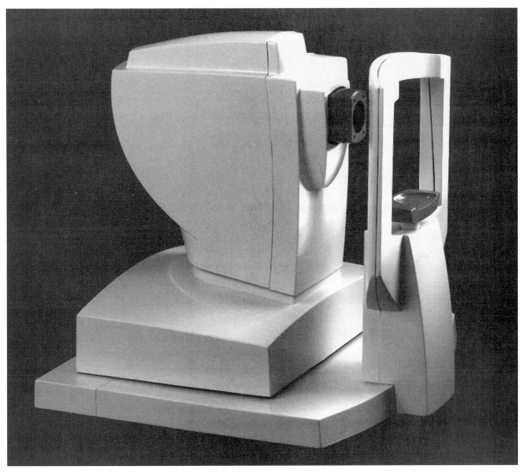

Figure 3–6 Retinal Thickness Analyzer. (Courtesy Talia Technology, Inc., Mevaseret Zion, Israel.)

is subtracted from the scattering intensity in the sampling window, resulting in a flare measurement in photon counts/ms. The photon count/ms is linearly related to the aqueous protein concentration.

   3) A single sampling measurement takes 1 ms. Ten consecutive samplings are averaged together resulting in a total measurement time of 0.5 s in this mode.

b. **Cell count mode** (Sawa et al., 1988).

   1) In this mode, the laser beam is scanned in two dimensions, 0.6 × 0.25 mm, centered on the sampling window. This leads to a sampling volume in the aqueous of 0.075 mm^3 (0.5 × 0.6 × 0.25 mm). This small sampling volume may lead to an underestimation of cells when there are few cells.

2) When the beam strikes a cell in the aqueous, a peak of scattered light is detected, and the computer counts the number of peaks. The cell count is expressed as the number/$0.075\,mm^3$.

3) A single sampling time takes $100\,\mu s$. Ten consecutive samples are taken leading to a total measurement time of $0.5\,s$ in this mode.

7. **Pupil dilation is helpful**, especially in miotic patients. Poor reproducibility results from the constricted iris due to reflections of the laser beam off of the iris (e.g., Oshika, 1991).

B. *Clinical Uses*

The flare value reflects aqueous protein concentration and is thus an index of the extent of blood-aqueous barrier disruption and of the severity of inflammation. This has lead to a number of clinical uses.

1. **Evaluation of blood-aqueous barrier disruption and impairment.** More than 50 articles have been published involving the use of the laser flare-cell meter in more than 16 diseases. Those diseases, with representative articles, include the following:
   a. Diabetic retinopathy (e.g., Zaczek et al., 1999).
   b. Exfoliation (pseudoexfoliation) syndrome (e.g., Wang et al., 1999a).
   c. Uveitis (e.g., Chiou et al., 1998; Oshika, 1991). In addition to objective and quantitative measurement of inflammation, the flare-cell meter may be used to monitor the response, adjust the therapy, detect recurrence, and perform routine follow-up of patients with uveitis (Herbort et al., 1997).
   d. Cytomegalovirus retinitis. Uveitis after the use of HIV protease inhibitors may indicate a good ocular prognosis (Herbort & Chave, 1998).
   e. Pigment dispersion syndrome. Quantification of aqueous melanin granules may be useful for evaluation of eyes with pigment dispersion syndrome and for assessing the effect of various treatments (Mardin et al., 2000b).

2. **Monitoring of post-op inflammation** (including subclinical anterior chamber inflammation). Over 50 articles have appeared describing the use of the laser flare-cell meter in over 15 different procedures. These procedures, with representative articles, include the following:
   a. Argon laser trabeculoplasty (e.g., Moriarty et al., 1993).
   b. Cataract surgery. The flare meter can be useful for objective assessment of surgical technique (e.g., Chee et al., 1999).
   c. Nd:YAG posterior capsulotomy (Altamirano et al., 1992).
   d. Corneal refractive surgery (e.g., El-Harazi et al., 2001).
   e. Panretinal photocoagulation (Larsson & Nuija, 2001).

3. **Assessment of the effects of anti-inflammatory drugs** (e.g., ketorolac, predmisolone) (Flach et al., 1998; Roberts & Brennan, 1995).

4. **Assessment of the effects of drugs on aqueous flow rate** (Mori & Araie, 1991; Oshika & Araie, 1990).

5. **Assessment of the effects of drugs on blood-aqueous barrier permeability** (e.g., latanoprost, timolol) (Diestelhorst et al., 1997).

C. *Advantages*

1. **Rapidity**—The total scan time for both modes together is one sec. Five scans are usually performed, and the results are averaged.

2. **Objectivity**

3. **Noninvasiveness**

4. **Quantifiability**

5. **Simplicity**—Minimal patient cooperation is required.

6. **Accuracy with high reproducibility (8% to 12%) when measuring flare** (e.g., Guillen-Monterrubio et al., 1997).
   a. There is good correlation with clinical grading of flare (e.g., El-Maghraby et al., 1993).
   b. There is good correlation with measured levels of anterior chamber protein (Saari et al., 1997; Shah et al., 1992b).

7. **Higher sensitivity and accuracy than fluorophotometry in assessing blood-aqueous barrier function** (Shah et al., 1993), although an earlier study suggested that fluorophotometry is more sensitive at detecting early changes (Schalnus & Ohrloff, 1992).

D. *Disadvantages*

1. The instrument is **nonlinear** when comparing instrument **cell count** to standard clinical slit-lamp biomicroscope grading of cells (e.g., Ni et al., 1992).
   a. The instrument cell count can **underestimate** when there are few cells, due to the small sampling volume ($0.075 \, mm^3$) and brief sampling time (e.g., Ni et al., 1992).
   b. The instrument can **overestimate** the actual cell count when the protein concentration (flare level) is high (Sawa et al., 1988; Ni et al., 1992).

2. The instrument cell count **cannot discriminate between erythrocytes, leukocytes, or pigment particles** (Sawa, 1990).

3. The instrument is less accurate and repeatable than fluorophotometry in assessing aqueous flow (Maus et al., 1993).

E. *Commercially Available System.* Kowa FC-1000 Laser Flare Cell Meter (Kowa Instrument Corp., Japan)

X. Laser Doppler Velocimetry (LDV)/Flowmetry (LDF)

A. Technique (e.g., Michelson et al., 1996).

1. Various **laser sources** have been used to illuminate blood vessels. They include the red **HeNe** (632.8 nm) and a number of **diode lasers** (670, 750, 757, 780, 783, 785, 810, and 812 nm).

2. A **photomultiplier detector** measures the radiation scattered back from the vessel walls and the moving blood elements.

3. Radiation scattered from the moving particles is shifted in frequency—the classic **Doppler shift**. The frequency shift is proportional to the speed of the red blood cells flowing through the vessels or capillaries.

4. A **spectrum analyzer** is used to obtain the frequency spectrum. A **Fourier transform** identifies the frequencies that constitute the spectrum. The maximum frequency shift corresponds to the maximum speed (V_{max}) of the red blood cells in the center of the blood vessel illuminated by the laser spot.

5. **Volumetric blood flow** can be calculated for a given blood vessel from its cross-sectional area and the mean blood speed. A circular vessel cross section is assumed.

$$\text{retinal blood flow (μl/min)} = V_{mean} \cdot \pi d^2/4$$

where

$$d = \text{vessel diameter}$$
$$V_{mean} = \text{the mean retinal blood speed} = V_{max}/2$$

6. The estimation of total retinal volumetric blood flow has been compared to that derived from radioactively labeled microspheres in animals (Davies et al., 1992). The two methods are in fairly good agreement.

7. **Laser Doppler velocimetry** can be used to measure blood velocity in large retinal blood vessels (e.g., Feke et al., 1989). To do this, the velocimetry data are combined with the vessel size data from fundus photography.

8. **Bidirectional LDV** uses two detectors to obtain the frequency shifts in two directions. This allows an absolute measurement of the blood flow in the larger retinal vessels (e.g., Davies et al., 1992; Riva et al., 1985).

9. Eye-movement artifacts can be minimized by stabilizing the laser illumination spot on the retina and the detected image on the photodetector (Mendel et al., 1993). A **dual-Purkinje-image eye tracker** can be used to stabilize the images in two dimensions.

10. **Laser Doppler flowmetry** involves the use of a spectrum analyzer to calculate blood flow (e.g., Bonner & Nossal, 1981; Chauhan & Smith, 1997).

a. The speed of the red blood cells flowing through the capillaries/vessels is proportional to the broadening of the frequency spectrum.

b. The average blood volume for the illuminated region is proportional to the power spectrum.

c. Flow is derived from the product of the speed and the volume.

d. An improved analysis system can yield results in a few minutes after data acquisition (Yoshida et al., 1998a).

e. Hayreh (1997) believes that the technique essentially measures the retinal circulation in the superficial nerve fiber layer. He thinks that no significant information is obtained about the contribution of the posterior ciliary artery to the optic nerve head. Others have suggested evidence that the technique can measure circulation at the lamina cribrosa, which is mainly supplied by the posterior ciliary arteries (Koelle et al., 1993). The actual depth of measurement is still controversial (e.g., Harris et al., 1997; Hayreh, 1997; Koelle et al., 1993; Michelson et al., 1996).

f. A new device, the compact choroidal laser Doppler flowmeter, is now available (Straubhaar et al., 2000). It allows measurement of choroidal blood flow under the foveal area.

11. **Scanning laser Doppler flowmetry** is a system that combines a scanning laser ophthalmoscope and a laser Doppler flowmeter (e.g., Michelson et al., 1996; 1998b; Piltz-Seymour, 1999).

a. A diode laser (780 nm) is used to scan the retina over an area of 2.7 mm × 0.7 mm, 10° field, with 256 points × 64 lines.

b. The spatial resolution is 10 μm, and the sampling time is 2 s. Satisfactory images are difficult to obtain. A number of factors influence the measurements (Bohdanecka et al., 1998; Kagemann et al., 1998).

c. The Doppler shift for each point is calculated and two-dimensional maps of the retinal perfusion are generated. A topographical image and three corresponding, brightness-coded images are displayed ("volume," "flow," and "velocity" maps).

d. This technique measures only **relative blood flow in capillaries** and not in larger blood vessels. There must be adequate reflectivity of the area and no saccades.

e. The optimal size of the region of interest is 10 pixels × 10 pixels (100 μm × 100 μm).

f. Interobserver evaluation has been improved by a new automatic full field perfusion image analyzer (Michelson et al., 1998b).

g. One of the limitations is the artifacts from eye movements during the data acquisition time (e.g., Hayreh, 1997). Media opacities can also degrade the image making it difficult to obtain adequate images. In addition, errors are introduced by fluctuations in retinal capillary flow due to the cardiac pulse and by differing measurement distances from the eye (Kagemann et al., 1998; Sullivan et al., 1999).

B. Clinical Uses

1. **Measurement of retinal** (e.g., Kagemann et al., 1998), **iris** (e.g., Chamot et al., 2000), and **ciliary body** (e.g., Michelson et al., 1994) **blood flow**.

2. **Detection of blood flow changes in various diseases**. Examples include the following:
   a. **diabetes** (e.g., Grunwald et al., 1996a; Konno et al., 1996; Schocket et al., 1999)
   b. **hypertension** (Grunwald et al., 1999)
   c. **retinal vein occlusion** (e.g., Chen et al., 1998a)

3. **Detection of blood flow changes in response to various drugs and other parameters.** More than 80 journal articles have been published evaluating the blood flow changes due to various parameters. Examples include blood flow changes in response to the following:
   a. **brinzolamide** (Barnes et al., 2000)
   b. **dark adaptation** (e.g., Riva et al., 1983)
   c. **intraocular pressure changes** (e.g., Straubhaar et al., 2000)
   d. **latanoprost** (Seong et al., 1999)
   e. **photocoagulation in diabetic retinopathy** (e.g., Fujio et al., 1994; Grunwald et al., 1989)
   f. **pregnancy** (Schocket et al., 1999)

4. **Evaluation of optic nerve head blood circulation**
   a. **age-related changes** (e.g., Groh et al., 1996). Microcirculation decreases significantly with age.
   b. **glaucoma and ocular hypertension** (e.g., Bohdanecka et al., 1999; Grunwald et al., 1999; Michelson et al., 1998a). Optic nerve head and juxtapapillary blood flow may be significantly reduced. Some controversy exists.
   c. **ischemic optic neuropathy** (e.g., Sebag et al., 1986).
   d. **normal subjects** (e.g., Griesser et al., 1999).
   e. **smokers vs. nonsmokers** (Erb et al., 1999).
   f. **systemic hypertension** (Grunwald et al., 1999).

5. **Evaluation of peripapillary blood flow**
   a. glaucoma (e.g., Hollo et al., 1997a,d)
   b. myopia (Hollo et al., 1997a)

6. **Investigation of choroidal blood flow in animals** (e.g., Kiel & Patel, 1998; Riva et al., 1994b).

7. **Evaluation of choroidal blood flow in humans** (Riva & Petrig, 1995; Riva et al., 1994a, 1995).
   a. age-related macular degeneration (e.g., Spraul et al., 1998)

  b. aging changes (Grunwald et al., 1998a)
  c. glaucoma (Grunwald et al., 1998b)

8. **Investigation of long posterior ciliary arterial blood flow** (Okubo et al., 1990).

C. *Commercially Available Instruments*

1. Bidirectional Laser Doppler Velocimeter (Oculix, Scion, Switzerland)
2. Heidelberg Retina Flowmeter (Heidelberg Engineering GmbH, Heidelberg, Germany) (Figure 3–7)

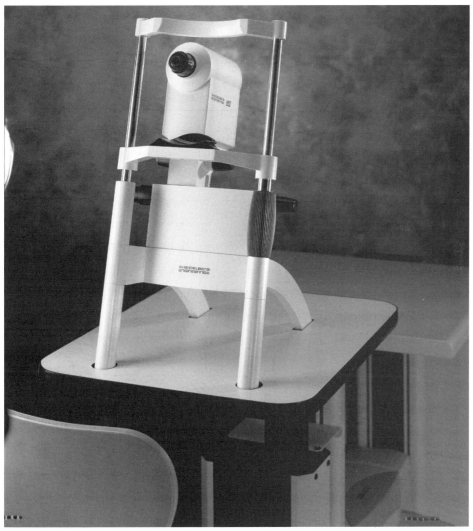

Figure 3–7 Heidelberg Retina Tomograph and Flowmeter. (Courtesy Heidelberg Engineering, Lincoln, RI.)

XI. Laser Doppler Interferometry (LDI; Partial Coherence Interferometry; Optical Coherence Domain Reflectometry; Optical Low-Coherence Reflectometry)

A. *Technique* (e.g., Fercher et al., 1993, 1994; Swanson et al., 1992).

1. A **multimode diode laser (780 nm)** has been used as a radiation source for measurements. More recently, **superluminescent diodes (818 or 830 nm)** have been used to improve precision (e.g., Hitzenberger, 1992).

2. A **Michelson dual-beam interferometer** is used to split the beam into two parallel, coaxial beams that enter the eye. The measuring beam is retarded with respect to the reference beam by twice the difference of the interferometer arm lengths. The mirror associated with the measuring beam is moved back and forth with a constant speed producing a **Doppler shift** of the measuring beam.

3. The two beams are reflected at reflecting structures in the eye. If the path difference of any two reflecting structures is equal to the path difference of the interferometer beams, the **two beams** will **interfere** with each other.

4. A **photodetector** is used to measure the intensity of the two superimposed reflected beams. When the beams interfere with each other, the Doppler frequency will appear in the photodetector signal and the corresponding path length difference will be recorded.

5. The path length difference is the **optical distance between the two reflecting structures** in the eye. The accuracy depends on the coherence length of the laser.

6. The measurement time is about 3 s, following about 20 s for alignment.

7. Improvements in the technique have resulted in a **fully computer-controlled scanning instrument**. This new dual beam version is called a **scanning partial coherence interferometer (SPCI)**. It can perform cross-sectional imaging of the retina as well as function as a biometer (e.g., Drexler et al., 1995a,b, 1998a,b). The longitudinal resolution of this version is about 15 μm. The lateral resolution is limited by microsaccades of the eye and is about 150 μm.

8. Further improvements have included a special diffractive optical element and the use of two spectrally displaced superluminescent diodes (Baumgartner et al., 1998). With these improvements, an **axial resolution of 6–7 μm** has been achieved.

9. Another version of this technique has also been used. The classic **Michelson interferometer** has been used instead of the dual beam interferometer (e.g., Puliafito et al., 1995; Schuman et al., 1995). This version is more sensitive to motion of the eye longitudinally.

B. *Clinical Applications*

1. **Corneal Thickness**
   a. LDI can be used to measure corneal thickness **in refractive surgery** and in cases of **corneal edema**.
   b. For the first attempt at measuring the corneal thickness, the standard deviation (precision) was about 7 µm (Hitzenberger et al., 1992). With a superluminescent diode, the standard deviation was reduced to 1.5 µm and then most recently to 0.3–0.8 µm (Drexler et al., 1997b, 1998b; Findl et al., 1998b; Hitzenberger, 1992).
   c. The accuracy with the multimode diode laser is comparable to that of ultrasound pachometers (about 5 µm) and about half that of optical pachometers (13 µm). The accuracy with the superluminescent diode is much better than either instrument.
   d. Not only the central corneal thickness but the peripheral corneal thickness can also be measured (Hitzenberger et al., 1994). The standard deviation of the geometric thickness increases from about 1.6 µm centrally to about 3.0 µm at 3.3 mm off the corneal apex. This increase is due to the parabolic shape of the corneal profile. More recently, the precision of the central corneal thickness was found to be 0.3 µm, which increased to 0.43 µm at a distance of 2 mm from the apex (Drexler et al., 1997b).
   e. One group has developed a device to measure the corneal thickness continuously for up to one hour with a precision of about 1 µm (Boehnke et al., 1998). This device may be useful in monitoring ablation depths during corneal refractive surgery and possibly for feedback control of the ablation.
   f. Another group has developed what they call an optical low-coherence reflectometer (Waelti et al., 1998). Applying it to the cornea, they achieved thickness measurements with a precision of 3.4 µm.
   g. Still another group calls their technique optical coherence domain reflectometry (e.g., Swanson et al., 1992). In addition to measuring corneal thickness, they have measured the corneal excision depth after using an excimer laser.

2. **Axial Eye Length Measurements** (e.g., Fercher et al., 1994; Hitzenberger et al., 1991a,b).
   a. The axial length of the eye can be accurately measured using this noncontact technique. This length is important in intraocular lens power calculations.
   b. Because of the dual beam technique, motions of the eye parallel to the optic axis do not affect the results.
   c. The standard deviation of the geometric eye length is about 5–9 µm (Drexler et al., 1998b; Findl et al., 1998b). This is more than 10 times better than the conventional ultrasound technique (standard deviation ≈100 to 120 µm). In fact, this technique has been shown to improve the refractive outcome after cataract surgery (Findl et al., 2001).

    d. Eye length can be measured through most cataracts, except for the densest cataracts (Hitzenberger et al., 1993).

    e. Eye length changes during accommodation have been measured (Drexler et al., 1997a, 1998c).

3. **Anterior Chamber Depth** (e.g., Baumgartner et al., 1995; Drexler et al., 1997b, 1998b).

    a. The precision of the measurement in eyes without cycloplegia is about 4.5 μm (Drexler et al., 1998b).

    b. Cycloplegia increases the precision of the measurement to 1.9 μm (Drexler et al., 1997a,b).

4. **Lens Thickness** (e.g., Baumgartner et al., 1995).

    a. The precision of the measurement is about 5 μm (Drexler et al., 1998b).

    b. Cycloplegia increases the precision of the measurement to 1.4 μm (Drexler et al., 1997a,b).

5. **Lens-Capsule Distance** (Findl et al., 1998a,b).

    a. PCI was used to measure the distance between intraocular lenses and the posterior capsule with a precision of 2–4 μm.

    b. This distance is a possible risk factor for posterior capsule opacification.

6. **Retinal Thickness** (e.g., Drexler et al., 1994).

    a. Retinal thickness profiles can be measured by taking measurements at different angles between the visual axis and the measurement direction (Hitzenberger et al., 1991a,b).

    b. The precision of the measurement is about 5 μm (Drexler et al., 1995b; Hitzenberger et al., 1995).

7. **Nerve Fiber Layer Thickness** (Drexler et al., 1995b).

8. **Choroidal Thickness** (e.g., Papastergiou et al., 1998). In chicks and chickens, the choroidal thickness exhibits a diurnal fluctuation and is influenced by visual experience.

9. **Fundus Profile** (Drexler et al., 1994; Fercher et al., 1993). A scanning laser interferometer has been developed to obtain tomographic images of the fundus.

10. **Optic Nerve Head Excavation**

11. **Group Refractive Index Measurement.** The corneal group refractive index can be determined using partial coherence interferometry (Uhlhorn et al., 1998). This measurement can then be used to improve the accuracy of corneal thickness determinations since the index is used to calculate the geometrical thickness from the measured optical thickness. Using two sources with different wavelengths, the group refractive indices and group dispersion of the cornea, aqueous humor, lens, artificial intraocular lenses, and the media along the axial eye length can be determined (Drexler et al., 1998d).

12. **Measurement of Intraocular Lens Movements after Nd:YAG Capsulotomy.** Posterior capsulotomy causes a small backward movement of the IOL (Findl et al., 1999). The hyperopic shift is small and not clinically relevant.

C. Advantages. The advantages of the SPCI include the following:

1. **high precision**
2. **high accuracy**
3. **noncontact**
4. **no pupil dilation**

D. Commercially Available Instrument. Zeiss IOLMaster (Zeiss Humphrey Systems, Dublin, CA) (Figure 3–8)

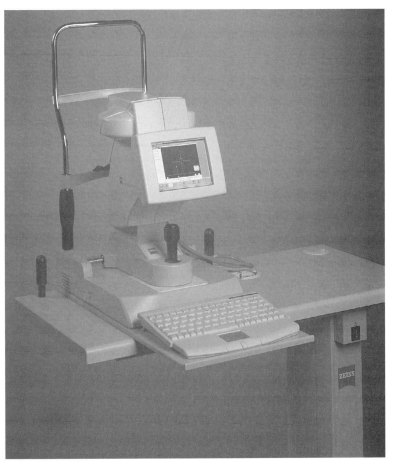

Figure 3–8 Zeiss IOLMaster. (Courtesy Zeiss Humphrey Systems, Dublin, CA.)

XII. Photon Correlation Spectroscopy (PCS)

A. Technique (e.g., Brown, 1993; Bursell et al., 1990; Van Laethem et al., 1991).

1. This technique is also known as **quasi-elastic light scattering** or **dynamic light scattering** or **intensity correlation spectroscopy** or **light-scattering spectroscopy**.

2. The **light source** is a **laser** (e.g., red HeNe (632.8 nm), argon (488 or 514.5 nm), or a doubled diode laser). This is needed because of the coherence and monochromatic properties of lasers.

3. The **spectrometer** includes the optics necessary to deliver the light to the eye and to collect the scattered light from the eye.

4. The **detector** of the scattered light is a **photon-counting photomultiplier**. Both the spectrometer and the detector can be incorporated into a modified slit-lamp biomicroscope (Bursell et al., 1986a; Libondi et al., 1986).

5. Finally, the **signal analyzer** processes the output of the detector. Usually a digital autocorrelator is used to measure the intensity autocorrelation function. Alternatively, the power spectrum of the intensity fluctuations of the scattered light can be measured. This is actually the Fourier transform of the autocorrelation function.

6. Information about the size, shape, and interactions of the scattering molecules can be obtained by measuring the light scattering characteristics of the material. The scattering light produces a pattern of "twinkling" spots that undergo random variations of intensity with time. These fluctuations, the correlation time, are due to the **random thermal (Brownian) motion** of the scattering molecules.

7. The **autocorrelation function** describes the time dependence of these fluctuations and can be used to obtain information about the size and diffusion properties of the scattering molecules. The decay time of the autocorrelation function reflects the particle mobility/diffusivity.

8. A **PCS fiber optic probe** has been developed to study the onset of cataracts (e.g., Ansari et al., 1997; Ansari & Suh, 1996, 1998). The probe uses a laser diode and can be incorporated into a slit-lamp biomicroscope. Topographical contour maps of the lens can be obtained in three dimensions.

9. Another group has developed a **single-mode optical fiber probe** for PCS measurements from the cornea to the retina (e.g., Rovati et al., 1996, 1998).

B. Clinical Applications

1. **Lens**
   a. **Age-related changes and cataractogenesis**
      1) In vivo PCS measurements have identified two molecular classes in the lens. The smaller, faster moving proteins in the nucleus undergo a decrease in

diffusion coefficient with age. The average molecular size of these proteins is comparable to that of α-crystallins. The larger, slower moving particles also undergo a decrease in diffusion coefficient with age. The mean sizes of these particles correspond to protein aggregates (e.g., Ansari & Suh, 1996; Benedek et al., 1987; Bursell et al., 1989b; Dierks et al., 1998; Van Laethem et al., 1991).

2) The technique provides a quantitative assessment of the **pre-cataractous molecular changes** in the in vivo human lens (e.g., Benedek et al., 1987; Dierks et al., 1998; Thurston et al., 1997). The concentration of aggregates increases with age.

3) Studies in vitro have shown the aggregation of lens proteins during the aging process and cataract formation (e.g., Ansari et al., 1998; Ansari & Suh, 1996). PCS can apparently detect the onset of cataractogenesis much earlier than the Scheimpflug system.

4) Studies in aqueous solutions have also been useful in investigating the changes that occur in cataractogenesis (e.g., Andreasi Bassi et al., 1995; Andries & Clauwaert, 1985; Liu et al., 1998).

5) **Galactose cataract development** and **reversal** in rats have been studied (Kaneda et al., 1990). The aggregation of α-crystallin can be detected before the lens opacity develops.

6) A cataract index has been developed to measure quantitatively the intensity autocorrelation of the back scattered light from the lens (Dhadwal & Wittpenn, 2000). This index can help characterize the lens at any age.

b. **Diabetic cataractogenic changes** (e.g., Bursell et al., 1984, 1989a).

1) Diabetics have significantly lower protein diffusion coefficients than age-matched non-diabetics. PCS may be a **useful measure of the risk for cataract development**.

2) **A quantitative measure of early, subclinical cataract development** is possible with PCS. Aggregation of lens proteins leading to opacification can be assessed by measuring the increase in the larger, slower moving aggregates and the decrease in the smaller and faster α-crystallins.

3) In young diabetics (<50), decreased protein diffusion coefficients were found to be significantly associated with increasing duration of the diabetes, use of oral hypoglycemic drugs, and poor control of the diabetes (i.e., increased glycosylated hemoglobin levels).

4) In a 2-year study of diabetics, it was found that for patients with diffusion coefficients greater than the group mean, only 3% showed progression in lens changes, whereas 48% of those with diffusion coefficients below the group mean progressed.

     5) PCS can thus **be used to evaluate preclinical cataractogenic lens changes at the molecular level**. Protein aggregation can be detected and characterized.

     6) PCS may **be useful in assessing the efficacy of therapies to prevent or treat cataracts**.

     7) PCS can also be used **to assess the cataractogenic potential of drugs or radiation used to treat systemic diseases**.

  c. **Effect of acute blood glucose changes on lenses in diabetics** (Bursell et al., 1989c).

2. **Cornea** (e.g., Rovati et al., 1998).

  a. PCS corneal measurements yield a significant change in the scattering from corneas of patients with advanced diabetes.

  b. PCS changes have also been noted in corneal edema (Clayton et al., 1985).

  c. Thus, PCS **may be useful for early detection of corneal pathology**. For example, PCS may be useful in assessing corneal hydration or endothelial pump changes.

  d. The technique may also be useful in early detection of diabetic retinopathy via corneal changes (Rovati et al., 1998).

3. **Aqueous** (Bursell et al., 1986b).

  a. Increased serum cholesterol levels lead to increased light scattering in the aqueous.

  b. Two aqueous protein components have been measured by PCS. The smallest proteins ($\approx$190 A) correspond to low density lipoproteins (LDLs). The larger proteins ($\approx$330 A) correspond to intermediate density lipoproteins (IDLs).

  c. Hence, PCS can be **used to measure cholesterol levels rapidly and non-invasively**.

  d. PCS may thus be useful in **assessing the effectiveness of diet and various cholesterol-lowering drugs**.

4. **Vitreous** (e.g., Rovati et al., 1996, 1998). The use of PCS in the vitreous may be useful in identifying diseases of the posterior chamber, including the detection of early diabetic retinopathy.

C. *Advantages*

1. **Noninvasive/nondestructive**

2. **Objective**

3. **Quantitative**

4. **Rapid**

5. **Sensitive**—preclinical changes in protein diffusivity can be measured (e.g., lens changes can be detected before opacification can be noted).

6. **Molecular probe**

D. Commercially Available Instrument. No instrument is available at this time. SpectRx was developing a new PCS clinical instrument for cholesterol screening but put the project on hold. The instrument was to measure cholesterol levels in the aqueous.

XIII. Fluorescence Spectroscopy

A. Technique (Eppstein & Bursell, 1992; Yu et al., 1996).

1. The **illumination source** can be a **laser** (406.7, 441.6, 488, or 514.5 nm) focused on a small volume in the crystalline lens. Other essentially monochromatic sources can also be used (e.g., a xenon source with appropriate filters).

2. A **confocal optical system** collects the light from the small illuminated volume in the lens. This system can be mounted on a modified slit-lamp biomicroscope, or it can be mounted in a compact handheld device.

3. An **enhanced diode detector array** measures both the excited fluorescent and the backscattered Rayleigh radiation from the small volume.

4. The attenuation of the incident laser beam by lens scattering or lens absorption can vary from individual to individual. For normals, there is essentially a linear relationship between age and fluorescence. For diabetic patients, the lens undergoes an accelerated aging process due to buildup of brown and fluorescence protein adducts and crosslinks.

5. These absorption effects can be taken into account by normalizing the excited fluorescence with respect to the amplitude of the unshifted Rayleigh backscattered excitation light (the **fluorescence/Rayleigh ratio**).

6. Each excitation wavelength results in a fluorescence spectra with an intensity maxima at a given wavelength. The fluorescence/Rayleigh ratio in a 10-nm spectral window centered on the intensity maximum is recorded and analyzed.

7. After correcting for the age-related changes in the fluorescence/Rayleigh ratio, shifts in **hemoglobin A_{1C} (HbA1C) levels** are proportional to shifts in the ratio using the 406.7-nm excitation wavelength (Eppstein & Bursell, 1992). HbA1C is glycosylated hemoglobin, and its levels reflect the mean blood glucose levels over the preceding 6 to 12 weeks. HbA1C levels are taken 2 to 4 times per **year to monitor diabetic control and compliance**.

8. By using the measured Rayleigh profiles to normalize the measured fluorescence, there is a good separation between diabetics and normals (Yu et al., 1996).

B. Clinical Uses

1. Fluorescence spectroscopy can be used **to screen populations for possible undiagnosed diabetes** (Yu et al., 1996).

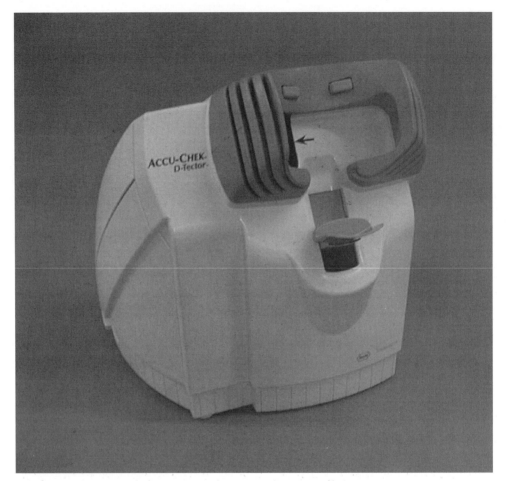

Figure 3–9 Roche Diagnostics Accu-Chek D-Tector. (Courtesy Roche Diagnostics Corporation, Indianapolis, IN.)

2. This technique can also be used **to monitor diabetics** for control and compliance (Eppstein & Bursell, 1992).

C. *Commercially Available Instrument.* Accu-Chek D-Tector (Roche Diagnostics Corporation, IN) (Figure 3–9)

XIV. Holographic Interferometry

A. *Technique* (Baker, 1990; Calkins et al., 1981; Foerster et al., 1994; Friedlander et al., 1991; Kasprzak et al., 1993b, 1995; Matsumoto et al., 1978; Smolek 1988, 1994).

1. A **laser** is employed as the radiation source. Argon, HeNe, and krypton lasers have been used.

2. The laser beam is split into a **reference beam** and an **object beam**. The object beam illuminates the cornea or surface of interest, is reflected off the object, and directed to the film. The reference beam goes directly to the film. These two beams interfere at the film plane.

3. High resolution **holographic interferograms** are formed via electrostatic recording on **thermoplastic film**.

4. A **high-resolution CCD video array** together with image processing produces a **topographical map** of the distortions of the corneal surface. These optical path length deviations can be expressed in microns or in diopters.

5. **Three methods** have been used:
   a. **Double-exposure holographic interferometry** involves recording two holograms of the object in two different positions on the same film. After reconstruction of the image, the object can be seen with an overlay of interference fringes due to the interference of the wavefronts of both positions.
   b. **Real-time holographic interferometry** involves recording a hologram of an object and then, using the object in the same position, reconstructing the image and at the same time have the wavefronts from the image interfere with the wavefronts from the object itself.
   c. **Two wavelength holographic interferometry** involves the use of two laser wavelengths to form an interferogram that is equivalent to one generated by the beat pattern of the combined wavelengths. The product of the two wavelengths divided by the magnitude of their difference yields the equivalent "beat pattern" wavelength.

6. The **accuracy** of the technique is on the **submicron** level, a fraction of a wavelength used to create the hologram.

7. Interferograms of the front and back of the **cornea** and **lens** can be generated. In excised eyes, deformations of the posterior **sclera** due to stresses like intraocular pressure changes can be assessed.

8. This technique can produce a **high-resolution topographic map of the entire surface of the cornea**. The **elastic properties** of the cornea can also be measured. By introducing a stress on the cornea (e.g., a change in the intraocular pressure), the strain or deformation can be evaluated.

B. *Clinical Applications*

1. **Keratorefractive surgery outcomes** may be assessed with this technique.
   a. Corneal wound strength can be evaluated as the wounds are made or postoperatively (Calkins et al., 1981).

b. The effects of different techniques or postoperative treatments can be assessed. For example, radial keratotomy or photorefractive keratectomy effects can be analyzed (Foerster et al., 1993; Smolek, 1994). The corneal asphericity of eyes implanted with the intrastromal corneal ring has been measured (Burris et al., 1993, 1997).

c. Changes of the corneal curvature have been made in response to changes in intraocular pressure (e.g., Kasprzak et al., 1993a, 1994a,b).

2. Knowledge may be gained concerning **numerous ocular degenerative conditions** such as high axial myopia.

C. Previously Commercially Available Instrument. Kerametrics CLAS-1000 laser holographic interferometer (Kera-Metrics Inc., San Diego, CA). This instrument is no longer available.

XV. Laser Speckle Blood Flow Measurement

A. Technique (e.g., Suzuki et al., 1991; Tamaki et al., 1993, 1994, 1995, 1997a; Tomidokoro et al., 1998).

1. Laser speckle is an interference phenomenon. It can be seen when coherent light is scattered from a diffusing surface.

2. A **blue argon** (488 nm), **red HeNe** (632.8 nm) or a **diode** (808 nm) laser have been used as the coherent illumination source. The blue argon source was used to measure blood flow in the retinal circulation, and the diode source was used to measure blood flow in the choroid and the optic nerve head.

3. A **modified fundus camera** can be used to illuminate the retina or optic nerve head with a focused laser beam and to collect and focus the reflected laser radiation.

4. The scattered laser light can be detected and measured with an **area sensor** (100 × 100 pixels, 540 frames/sec) and microcomputer or **a photon-counting photomultiplier and digital correlator**.

5. Using the **area sensor technique**, the difference between data from successive scannings of the speckle pattern is calculated and integrated over the entire pixel area of the sensor. This is called the average difference (AD) value and is an index of the blood flow velocity (Tamaki et al., 1993). More recently another term has been used. The average speckle intensity is measured. The difference between this average intensity and the intensity for successive scans of the speckles in the sensor plane is then calculated. The ratio of the average speckle intensity to this difference is defined as **normalized blur** (NB) (Tamaki et al., 1994, 1995). This NB value is a quantitative index of the tissue blood velocity. These values are color-coded and used to generate a two-dimensional map of tissue blood flow.

6. Using the **photomultiplier technique**, the digital correlator and microcomputer calculate the autocorrelation function. The correlation time is obtained from the autocorrelation function plot as the lag time corresponding to half the correlation function height. The blood flow velocity is calculated using the measured blood vessel diameter and the reciprocal of the correlation time (Suzuki et al., 1991). The measurement time is about 1.05 s and has a coefficient of variation of 12.4%.

7. The coefficients of reproducibility are about 7% in the choroid and 7.5% in the optic nerve head for measurements taken 5 min apart. For measurements taken a day apart, reproducibility was about 11% in the choroid and 12% in the optic nerve head (Tamaki et al., 1995).

8. A new analysis method has been used to compensate for eye movements (Aizu et al., 1998).

9. **Laser speckle photography** has been another technique that was investigated (e.g., Briers & Fercher, 1982). The reciprocal of speckle contrast in the photographic technique is fairly equivalent to NB (Tamaki et al., 1998). However, this technique provided only a semiquantitative estimation of blood flow.

B. Clinical Applications

1. **Retinal Blood Flow.** Blood flow in the retina has been measured in response to intraocular pressure changes (Tamaki et al., 1994) and a number of drugs, including pranidipine (Tamaki et al., 1999c).

2. **Choroidal Blood Flow.** Blood flow in the choroid has been measured in response to intraocular pressure changes (Tamaki et al., 1995) and a number of drugs including carteolol and timolol (Tomidokoro et al., 1999).

3. **Optic Nerve Head Microcirculation Measurement.** Optic nerve head blood flow has been measured in response to intraocular pressure changes (Tamaki et al., 1995), cigarette smoking (Tamaki et al., 1999a) and at least 11 drugs, including betaxolol (Tamaki et al., 1999b), carteolol (Tamaki et al., 1998), and timolol (Tamaki et al., 1997b).

4. **Iris Blood Flow Measurement.** Iris blood flow has been measured in response to changing intraocular pressure (Tomidokoro et al., 1998), betaxolol (Tomidokoro et al., 1998, 1999), carteolol (Tomidokoro et al., 1999), and timolol (Tomidokoro et al., 1998, 1999).

C. No Commercial Instrument Is Available

XVI. Laser Speckle Optometer

A. Technique (Charman, 1979; Charman & Chapman, 1980; Knoll, 1966).

1. The laser speckle generator is a low-power red **HeNe** (632.8 nm) laser. This is used to generate a parallel coherent beam of light.

2. The laser beam is reflected off a **rotating drum** with a granular surface.

3. The reflected wavefronts interfere with each other producing constructive (red spots) and destructive (black spots) interference patterns in space that look like "**speckles**."

4. The patient perceives the speckle phenomenon because of the interference of the wavefronts at the retinal plane. Thus, the speckles are always in focus.

5. The patient perceives **motion** in the speckle pattern that is **dependent on the patient's refractive error and state of accommodation** (e.g., Knoll, 1966; Charman, 1979). The direction of the apparent motion determines the type of refractive error. Motion in the same direction as the rotation of the drum indicates myopia, and the opposite motion indicates hyperopia. The apparent motion can be stopped by appropriately correcting the patient. The small amount of axial chromatic aberration induced by the red laser beam can be accounted for in a number of ways.

6. The speed of laser speckles induced by various levels of refractive defocus and voluntary changes of accommodation has been measured (Richter et al., 1994).

B. Clinical Applications

1. **Refraction**
   a. Measuring the power in multiple meridians can yield the spherical and cylindrical correction with accuracy similar to that of conventional refraction (e.g., Dwyer et al., 1973; Phillips & Sterling, 1975; Whitefoot & Charman, 1980).
   b. Even in cases of finger counting or hand motion acuity due to high ametropia, the laser optometer can be used to refract a patient.
   c. The technique can also be used under low illumination conditions.
   d. Refractive changes during body inversion have been assessed (Lovasik & Kothe, 1989).
   e. Using both red (633 nm) and green (514 nm) speckle patterns simultaneously to refract is feasible but difficult (Morrell & Charman, 1987).
   f. The refractive status of a given meridian of the eye can be determined with a laser optometer (e.g., Phillips et al., 1976).

2. **Night myopia testing and correction** (Fejer & Girgis, 1992). The level of night myopia (e.g., in young drivers) can be measured and an appropriate correction can be given.

3. **Measurement of ocular chromatic aberration** (Morrell et al., 1991).

4. **Measurement of accommodation and the accommodative response** to various stimuli. There have been more than 22 reports using this technique (see e.g., Lovasik et al., 1987; Whitefoot & Charman, 1992).

5. **Measurement of dark focus.** There have been more than 18 studies using this method (see e.g., Jaschinski-Kruza, 1988; Post et al., 1984; Rosenfield, 1989).

C. No Commercial Instrument Is Available. This is presumably due to the fact that laser refraction does not save time over conventional refractive techniques and does not simplify the procedure.

XVII. Laser Interferometry Fundus Pulsation Measurement

A. Technique (Fercher, 1984; Schmetterer et al., 1995, 1998a; Schmetterer & Wolzt, 1998).

1. A single-mode **laser diode (780 nm)** is used as a radiation source to illuminate the eye. The laser power is about 80 μW with a beam diameter of 1 mm at the cornea. The beam is focused to a spot size of 20 to 50 μm on the retina.

2. The laser beam is partially reflected at the anterior surface of the cornea and at the retina.

3. The two reflections produce an **interference pattern** that is imaged on a linear CCD array.

4. The **fundus pulsation amplitude (FPA)** is the maximum distance change between the cornea and retina during the cardiac cycle. This relative distance change is on the order of several micrometers and is due to the rhythmic filling of the ocular blood vessels during systole and diastole.

5. The FPA is a **measure of local pulsatile blood flow** (e.g., Schmetterer et al., 1995). And FPA in the fovea allows assessment of the pulsatile blood flow component in the choroidal vasculature, while FPA in the optic disk is a result of both retinal and choroidal vasculature. Since most of the pulsatile ocular blood flow is due to choroidal blood flow, Hayreh (1997) believes that it does not give information about optic nerve head blood flow.

6. This is a noninvasive, noncontact technique with a total set-up and measurement time of less than 5 min.

7. Reproducibility of the FPA measurements is excellent with an intraclass correlation coefficient between 0.95 and 0.98 (Schmetterer et al., 1998a). This is better than the reproducibility of pneumatonometric and ultrasonographic measurements.

8. There is a strong correlation between FPA and pulse amplitude and pulsatile ocular blood flow measured by pneumotonometry (Schmetterer et al., 2000).

B. Clinical Applications

1. **Blood flow changes in the choroid or optic disk** have been measured in response to more than 33 different drugs and conditions. These include blood flow changes in response to changes in intraocular pressure (Findl et al., 1997), betaxolol, levobunolol, and timolol (Schmetterer et al., 1997b). Significant reductions in FPA have also been measured in the optic nerve head cup and the macula in patients with open-angle glaucoma (Findl et al., 2000a).

2. **Choroidal blood flow in diabetes**
   a. The FPA is significantly smaller in eyes with proliferative retinopathy than in eyes without retinopathy (Schmetterer et al., 1997a). This is consistent with reduced choroidal blood flow in the advanced stage of the disease.
   b. In one study there was no significant difference in FPA in eyes with no retinopathy, background retinopathy, or preproliferative retinopathy (Schmetterer et al., 1997a). However, a later study indicated that choroidal blood flow increases with the progression of diabetic retinopathy (Findl et al., 2000b).

C. No Commercial Instrument Is Available

References

Aizu Y, Asakura T, Kojima A. Compensation of eye movements in retinal speckle flowmetry using flexible correlation analysis based on the specific variance. J Biomed Opt 3:227–236 (1998).

Altamirano D et al. Aqueous humor analysis after Nd:YAG laser capsulotomy with the laser flare-cell meter. J Cataract Refract Surg 18:554–558 (1992).

Amari F et al. Predicting visual outcome after macular hole surgery using scanning laser ophthalmoscope microperimetry. Br J Ophthalmol 85:96–98 (2001).

American Academy of Ophthalmology. Optic nerve head and retinal nerve fiber layer analysis. Ophthalmology 106:1414–1424 (1999).

Anderson RS, Wilkinson MO, Thibos LN. Psychophysical localization of the human visual streak. Optom Vis Sci 69:171–174 (1992).

Andreasi Bassi F et al. Self-similarity properties of alpha-crystallin supramolecular aggregates. Biophys J 69:2720–2727 (1995).

Andries C, Clauwaert J. Photon correlation spectroscopy and light scattering of eye lens proteins at high concentrations. Biophys J 47:591–605 (1985).

Angra SK, Pal BK. Visual acuity testing in cataract—an insight (cataract classification density based). Indian J Ophthalmol 38:153–155 (1990).

Ansari RR et al. In-vivo cataractograms using a compact backscatter dynamic light scattering (DLS) probe. Proc SPIE Medical Applications of Lasers in Dermatology, Ophthalmology, Dentistry, and Endoscopy 3192:202–210 (1997).

Ansari RR et al. Measuring lens opacity: combining quasi-elastic light scattering with Scheimpflug imaging system. Proc SPIE Ophthalmic Technologies VIII 3246:35–42 (1998).

Ansari RR, Suh KI. Three-dimensional scanning of eye (lens and vitreous) using a newly developed dynamic light scattering probe. Proc SPIE Ophthalmic Technologies VI 2673:12–20 (1996).

Ansari RR, Suh KI. Dynamic light scattering particle-size measurements in turbid media. Proc SPIE Coherence Domain Optical Methods in Biomedical Science and Clinical Applications II 3251:146–156 (1998).

Antcliff RJ et al. Intravitreal triamcinolone for uveitic cystoid macular edema: an optical coherence tomography study. Ophthalmology 108:765–772 (2001).

Anton A et al. Mapping structural to functional damage in glaucoma with standard automated perimetry and confocal scanning laser ophthalmoscopy. Am J Ophthalmol 125:436–446 (1998).

Anton A, Zangwill L, Emadadi A, Weinreb RN. Nerve fiber layer measurements with scanning laser polarimetry in ocular hypertension. Arch Ophthalmol 115:331–334 (1997).

Arend O et al. Macular capillary particle velocities: a blue field and scanning laser comparison. Graefes Arch Clin Exp Ophthalmol 233:244–249 (1995).

Arend O et al. Scanning laser ophthalmoscopy-based evaluation of epipapillary velocities: method and physiologic variability. Surv Ophthalmol 44 (Suppl 1):S3–S9 (1999).

Arnold JJ et al. Indocyanine green angiography of drusen. Am J Ophthalmol 124:344–356 (1997).

Asrani S et al. Systemic toxicology and laser safety of laser targeted angiography with heat sensitive liposomes. J Ocul Pharmacol Ther 11:575–584 (1995).

Asrani S et al. Selective visualization of choroidal neovascular membranes. Invest Ophthalmol Vis Sci 37:1642–1650 (1996).

Asrani S et al. Application of rapid scanning retinal thickness analysis in retinal diseases. Ophthalmology 104: 1145–1151 (1997).

Asrani S et al. Serial optical sectioning of macular holes at different stages of development. Ophthalmology 105: 66–77 (1998).

Asrani S et al. Noninvasive mapping of the normal retinal thickness at the posterior pole. Ophthalmology 106:269–273 (1999).

Axer-Siegel R et al. Simultaneous indocyanine green and fluorescein angiography in retinal pigment epithelium tear using the confocal scanning laser ophthalmoscope. Am J Ophthalmol 128:331–339 (1999).

Azuara-Blanco A, Harris A, Cantor LB. Reproducibility of optic disk topographic measurements with the Topcon ImageNet and the Heidelberg Retina. Tomograph. Ophthalmologica 212:95–98 (1998).

Baker PC. Holographic contour analysis of the cornea. In: Masters BR, ed. Noninvasive diagnostic techniques in ophthalmology. New York: Springer-Verlag, 1990; 6:82–98.

Bantel T, Ott D, Rueff M. Global tracking of the ocular fundus pattern imaged by scanning laser ophthalmoscopy. Int J Biomed Comput. 27:59–69 (1991).

Barnes GE et al. Increased optic nerve head blood flow after 1 week of twice daily topical brinzolamide treatment in Dutch-belted rabbits. Surv Ophthalmol 44 (Suppl 2):S131–S140 (2000).

Barrett BT, Davison PA, Eustace PE. Effects of posterior segment disorders on oscillatory displacement thresholds, and on acuities as measured using the Potential Acuity Meter and laser interferometer. Ophthal Physiol Opt 14:132–138 (1994).

Barrett BT, Davison PA, Eustace PE. Clinical comparison of three techniques for evaluating visual function behind cataract. Eye 9:722–727 (1995).

Barrett BT, McGraw PV. Use of the potential acuity meter and laser interferometer to predict visual acuity after macular hole surgery [letter]. Retina 15:528–530 (1995).

Bartsch D-U et al. Analysis of the human macula by confocal laser tomography. In: Nasemann JE, Burk ROW, eds. Scanning laser ophthalmoscopy and tomography. Muenchen: Quintessenz 21:215–223 (1990).

Bartsch D-U et al. Confocal scanning infrared laser ophthalmoscopy for indocyanine green angiography. Am J Ophthalmol 120:642–651 (1995).

Bartz-Schmidt KU et al. Quantitative morphologic and functional evaluation of the optic nerve head in chronic open-angle glaucoma. Surv Ophthalmol 44 (Suppl 1):S41–S53 (1999).

Bathija R et al. Detection of early glaucomatous structural damage with confocal scanning laser tomography. J Glaucoma 7:121–127 (1998).

Baumann M et al. Reproducibility of retinal thickness measurements in normal eyes using optical coherence tomography. Ophthalmic Surg Lasers 29:280–285 (1998).

Baumgartner A et al. Measurement of the anterior structures of the human eye by partial coherence interferometry. Proc SPIE Lasers in Ophthalmology II 2330:146–151 (1995).

Baumgartner A et al. Signal and resolution enhancements in dual beam optical coherence tomography of the human eye. J Biomed Opt 3:45–54 (1998).

Beausencourt E et al. Quantitative analysis of macular holes with scanning laser tomography. Ophthalmology 104:2018–2029 (1997).

Beausencourt E et al. Infrared scanning laser tomography of macular cysts. Ophthalmology 107:375–385 (2000).

Bechmann M et al. Central corneal thickness measurement with a retinal optical coherence tomography device versus standard ultrasonic pachymetry. Cornea 20:50–54 (2001).

Beckman C et al. Confocal fundus imaging with a scanning laser ophthalmoscope in eyes with cataract. Br J Ophthalmol 79:900–904 (1995).

Benedek GB et al. Quantitative detection of the molecular changes associated with early cataractogenesis in the living human lens using quasielastic light scattering. Curr Eye Res 6:1421–1432 (1987).

Bernth-Petersen P, Naeser K. Clinical evaluation of the Lotmar Visometer for macula testing in cataract patients. Acta Ophthalmol 60:525–532 (1982).

Bettelheim FA. On the optical anisotropy of lens fiber cells. Exp Eye Res 21:231–234 (1975).

Bhandari A et al. Quantitative analysis of the lamina cribrosa in vivo using a scanning laser ophthalmoscope. Curr Eye Res 16:1–8 (1997).

Bhandari A, Chen PP, Mills RP. Effects of contact lenses on scanning laser polarimetry of the peripapillary retinal nerve fiber layer. Am J Ophthalmol 127:722–724 (1999).

Bille JF, Dreher AW, Zinser G. Scanning laser tomography of the living human eye. In: Masters BR, ed. Noninvasive diagnostic techniques in ophthalmology. New York: Springer-Verlag, 1990; 28:528–547.

Bischoff P, Lang J, Huber A. Macular sparing as a perimetric artifact. Am J Ophthalmol 119:72–80 (1995a).

Bischoff PM et al. Simultaneous indocyanine green and fluorescein angiography. Retina 15:91–99 (1995b).

Bloom TD, Fishman GA, Traubert BS. Laser interferometric visual acuity in senile macular degeneration. Arch Ophthalmol 101:925–926 (1983).

Boehm G. Ueber maculare (Haidingersche) Polarisation buschel und ueber einen polarizationsoptischen Fehler des Auges. Acta Ophthalmol 18:109–169 (1940).

Boehnke M et al. Continuous non-contact corneal pachymetry with a high speed reflectometer. J Refract Surg 14:140–146 (1998).

Bohdanecka Z et al. Influence of acquisition parameters on hemodynamic measurements with the Heidelberg Retina Flowmeter at the optic disc. J Glaucoma 7:151–157 (1998).

Bohdanecka Z et al. Relationship between blood flow velocities in retrobulbar vessels and laser Doppler flowmetry at the optic disk in glaucoma patients. Ophthalmologica 213:145–149 (1999).

Bonner R, Nossal R. Model for laser Doppler measurements of blood flow in tissue. Appl Opt 20:2097–2107 (1981).

Bosse JC. Potential visual acuity measured with and without pupil dilation. Optom Vis Sci 66:537–539 (1989).

Bour LJ, Lopes Cardozo NJ. On the birefringence of the living human eye. Vision Res 21:1413–1421 (1981).

Briers JD, Fercher AF. Retinal blood-flow visualization by means of laser speckle photography. Invest Ophthalmol Vis Sci 22:255–259 (1982).

Brigatti L, Hoffman D, Caprioli J. Neural networks to identify glaucoma with structural and functional measurements. Am J Ophthalmol 121:511–521 (1996).

Brink HB. Birefringence of the human crystalline lens in vivo. J Opt Soc Am A 8:1788–1793 (1991).

Brink HB, van Blokland GJ. Birefringence of the human foveal area assessed in vivo with Mueller-matrix ellipsometry. J Opt Soc Am A 5:49–57 (1988).

Broadway DC et al. The ability of scanning laser ophthalmoscopy to identify various glaucomatous optic disk appearances. Am J Ophthalmol 125:593–604 (1998).

Brown W, ed. Dynamic light scattering: the method and some applications. Oxford: Clarendon Press, 1993.

Brusini P, Tosoni C, Miani F. Quantitative mapping of the retinal thickness at the posterior pole in chronic open angle glaucoma. Acta Ophthalmol Scand Suppl 78:42–44 (2000).

Bryant WR. The Haag-Streit Lotmar Visometer for determining macular potential prior to cataract surgery. J Am Intraocul Implant Soc 11:581–583 (1985).

Burk ROW et al. Laser scanning tomography and stereogrammetry in three-dimensional optic disc analysis. Graefe's Arch Clin Exp Ophthalmol 231:193–198 (1993).

Burk ROW, Tuulonen A, Airaksinen PJ. Laser scanning tomography of localised nerve fibre layer defects. Br J Ophthalmol 82:1112–1117 (1998).

Burris TE et al. Flattening of central corneal curvature with intrastromal corneal rings of increasing thickness: an eye-bank study. J Cataract Refract Surg 19 Suppl:182–187 (1993).

Burris TE et al. Corneal asphericity in eye bank eyes implanted with the intrastromal corneal ring. J Refract Surg 13:556–567 (1997).

Bursell S-E et al. Clinical photon correlation spectroscopy evaluation of human diabetic lenses. Exp Eye Res 49:241–258 (1989a).

Bursell S-E, Carlyle LR, Rand LI. Progression of cataractogenesis evaluated by quasielastic light scattering. Invest Ophthalmol Vis Sci 30 (Suppl.):328 (1989b).

Bursell S-E, Craig MS, Karalekas DP. Diagnostic evaluation of human lenses. Proc SPIE 605:87–93 (1986a).

Bursell S-E et al. Cholesterol levels assessed with photon correlation spectroscopy. Proc SPIE 712:175–181 (1986b).

Bursell S-E, Karalekas DP, Craig MS. The effect of acute changes in blood glucose on lenses in diabetic and non-diabetic subjects using quasi-elastic light scattering spectroscopy. Curr Eye Res 8:821–834 (1989c).

Bursell S-E, Magnante PC, Chylack LT. In vivo uses of quasi-elastic light scattering spectroscopy as a molecular probe in the anterior segment of the eye. In: Masters BR, ed. Noninvasive diagnostic techniques in ophthalmology. New York: Springer-Verlag, 1990; 18:342–365.

Bursell S-E, Weiss JN, Eichold B. Diagnostic laser light scattering spectroscopy for human eyes. In: Proceedings, 8th international conference on applications of lasers and electrooptics 43:61–67 (1984).

Byhr E, Lindblom B. Preoperative measurements of macular hole with scanning laser ophthalmoscopy. Correlation with functional outcome. Acta Ophthalmol Scan 76:579–583 (1998).

Calkins JL, Hochheimer BF, Stark WJ. Corneal wound healing: holographic stress-test analysis. Invest Ophthalmol Vis Sci 21:322–334 (1981).

Campbell FW, Green DG. Optical and retinal factors affecting visual resolution. J Physiol 181:551–566 (1965).

Campbell FW, Kulikowski JJ, Levinson J. The effect of orientation on the visual resolution of gratings. J Physiol 187:427–436 (1966).

Cantor LB et al. Measurement of superficial optic nerve head capillary blood velocities by scanning laser fluorescein angiography. J Glaucoma 3 (Suppl);S61–S64 (1994).

Caprioli J et al. Slope of the peripapillary nerve fiber layer surface in glaucoma. Invest Ophthalmol Vis Sci 39:2321–2328 (1998).

Cavallerano AA. Potential acuity assessment. In: Eskridge JB, Amos JF, Bartlett JD, eds. Clinical procedures in optometry. Philadelphia: JB Lippincott Co, 1991; 51:470–481.

Chamot SR et al. Iris blood flow response to acute decreases in ocular perfusion pressure: a laser Doppler flowmetry study in humans. Exp Eye Res 70:107–112 (2000).

Charman WN. Speckle movement in laser refraction. I. Theory. Am J Optom Physiol Opt 56:219–227 (1979).

Charman WN, Chapman D. Laser refraction and speckle movement. Ophthalmic Opt 20:41–51 (1980).

Chauhan BC et al. Test-retest variability of topographic measurements with confocal scanning laser tomography in patients with glaucoma and control subjects. Am J Ophthalmol 118:9–15 (1994).

Chauhan BC et al. Technique for detecting serial topographic changes in the optic disc and peripapillary retina using scanning laser tomography. Invest Ophthalmol Vis Sci 41:775–782 (2000).

Chauhan BC et al. Optic disc and visual field changes in prospective longitudinal study of patients with glaucoma: comparison of scanning laser tomography with conventional perimetry and optic disc photography. Arch Ophthalmol 119:1492–1499 (2001).

Chauhan BC, MacDonald CA. Influence of time separation on variability estimates of topographic measurements with confocal scanning laser tomography. J Glaucoma 4:189–193 (1995).

Chauhan BC, Marshall J. The interpretation of optical coherence tomography images of the retina. Invest Ophthalmol Vis Sci 40:2332–2342 (1999).

Chauhan BC, Smith FM. Confocal scanning laser Doppler flowmetry: experiments in a model flow system. J Glaucoma 6:237–245 (1997).

Chauhan DS et al. Papillofoveal traction in macular hole formation. The role of optical coherence tomography. Arch Ophthalmol 118:32–38 (2000).

Chee SP et al. Postoperative inflammation: extracapsular cataract extraction versus phacoemulsification. J Cataract Refract Surg 25:12805 (1999).

Chen B, Makous W. Light capture by human cones. J Physiol 414:89–109 (1989).

Chen E, Gedda U, Landau I. Thinning of the papillomacular bundle in the glaucomatous eye and its influence on the reference plane of the Heidelberg retinal tomography. J Glaucoma 10:386–389 (2001).

Chen H-C et al. Retinal blood flow in nonishchemic central retinal vein occlusion. Ophthalmology 105:772–775 (1998a).

Chen Y-Y et al. Correlation of peripapillary nerve fiber layer thickness by scanning laser polarimetry with visual field defects in patients with glaucoma. J Glaucoma 7:312–316 (1998b).

Chi Q-M et al. Evaluation of the effect of aging on the retinal nerve fiber layer thickness using scanning laser polarimetry. J Glaucoma 4:406–413 (1995).

Chiou AG, Florakis GJ, Herbort CP. Correlation between anterior chamber IgG/albumin concentrations and laser flare photometry in eyes with endogenous uveitis. Ophthalmologica 212:275–277 (1998).

Chiou AG, Mermoud A, Jewelewicz DA. Post-operative inflammation following deep sclerectomy with collagen implant versus standard trabeculectomy. Graefes Arch Clin Exp Ophthalmol 236:593–596 (1998).

Choplin NT, Lundy DC. The sensitivity and specificity of scanning laser polarimetry in the detection of glaucoma in a clinical setting. Ophthalmology 108:899–904 (2001).

Choplin NT, Lundy DC, Dreher AW. Differentiating patients with glaucoma from glaucoma suspects and normal subjects by nerve fiber layer assessment with scanning laser polarimetry. Ophthalmology 105:2068–2076 (1998).

Choplin NT, Schallhorn SC. The effect of excimer laser photorefractive keratectomy for myopia on nerve fiber layer thickness measurements as determined by scanning laser polarimetry. Ophthalmology 106:1019–1023 (1999).

Christoffersen N, Sander B, Larsen M. Precipitation of hard exudate after resorption of intraretinal edema after treatment of retinal branch vein occlusion. Am J Ophthalmol 126:454–456 (1998).

Clayton TL et al. A study of corneal edema using quasielastic light scattering. Invest Ophthalmol Vis Sci 26 (Suppl.):181 (1985).

Cohen MM. Laser interferometry: evaluation of potential visual acuity in the presence of cataracts. Ann Ophthalmol 8:845–849 (1976).

Colen et al. Preproduciblity of measurements with the nerve fiber layer analyzer (NFA/GDx). J Glaucoma 9:363–370 (2000).

Colen TP, Lemij HG. Prevalence of split nerve fiber layer bundles in healthy eyes imaged with scanning laser polarimetry. Ophthalmology 108:151–156 (2001).

Collur S, Carroll AM, Cameron BD. Human lens effect on in vivo scanning laser polarimetric measurements of retinal nerve fiber layer thickness. Ophthalmic Surg Lasers 31:126–130 (2000).

Colvard DM, Kratz RP, Mazzocco TR, Davidson B. Retinal visual acuity and CME [letter]. J Am Intraocul Implant Soc 6:372 (1980).

Cooper RL, Eikelboom RH, Barry CJ. Correlations between densitometry of red-free photographs and reflectometry with the scanning laser ophthalmoscope in normal subjects and glaucoma patients. Intl Ophthalmol 16:243–246 (1992).

Curcio CA, Allen KA. Topography of ganglion cells in human retina. J Comp Neurol 300:5–25 (1990).

Cuzzani et al. Potential acuity meter versus scanning laser ophthalmoscope to predict visual acuity in cataract patients. J Cataract Refract Surg 24:263–269 (1998).

Datiles MB et al. A comparative study between the PAM and the laser interferometer in cataracts. Graefes Arch Clin Exp Ophthalmol 225:457–460 (1987).

Davies EG et al. Validation and reproducibility of bidirectional laser Doppler velocimetry for the measurement of retinal blood flow. Curr Eye Res 11:633–640 (1992).

De Geronimo F et al. A quantitative in vivo study of retinal thickness before and after laser treatment for macular edema due to retinal vein occlusion. Eur J Ophthalmol 11:145–149 (2001).

DeLint PJ, Berendschot TT, van Norren D. Local photoreceptor alignment measured with a scanning laser ophthalmoscope. Vision Res 37:243–248 (1997).

DeLint PJ, Berendschot TT, van Norren D. A comparison of the optical Stiles-Crawford effect and retinal densitometry in a clinical setting. Invest Ophthalmol Vis Sci 39:1519–1523 (1998a).

DeLint PJ et al. Scanning laser densitometry in visual acuity loss of unknown origin. Br J Ophthalmol 80:1051–1054 (1996).

Delint PJ et al. Photoreceptor function in unilateral amblyopia. Vision Res 38:613–617 (1998b).

Delori FC et al. In vivo fluorescence of the ocular fundus exhibits retinal pigment epithelial lipofuscin characteristics. Invest Ophthalmol Vis Sci 36:718–729 (1995).

Delori FC, Pflibsen KP. Spectral reflectence of the human ocular fundus. Applied Optics 28:1061–1077 (1989).

De Natale R et al. Visual field defects and normal nerve fiber layer: may they coexist in primary open-angle glaucoma? Ophthalmologica 214:119–121 (2000).

Desmettre TJ et al. Diode laser-induced thermal damage evaluation on the retina with a liposome dye system. Lasers Surg Med 24:61–68 (1999).

De Souza Lima M, Zangwill L, Weinreb RN. Scanning laser polarimetry to assess the nerve fiber layer. In: Schuman JS, ed. Imaging in glaucoma. Thorofare, NJ: Slack Inc., 1997; 6:83–92.

Dhadwal HS, Wittpenn J. In vivo dynamic light scattering characterization of a human lens: cataract index. Curr Eye Res 20:502–510 (2000).

DiCarlo CD et al. New noninvasive technique for cataract evaluation in the rhesus monkey. Proc SPIE Lasers in Surgery: Advanced Characterization, Therapeutics, and Systems V 2395:636–643 (1995).

Dierks K et al. Protein size resolution in human eye lenses by dynamic light scattering after in vivo measurements. Graefes Arch Clin Exp Ophthalmol 236:18–23 (1998).

Diestelhorst M, Roters S, Krieglstein GK. The effect of latanoprost 0.005% once daily versus 0.0015% twice daily on intraocular pressure and aqueous humour protein concentration in glaucoma patients. A randomized, double-masked comparison with timolol 0.5%. Graefes Arch Clin Exp Ophthalmol 235:20–26 (1997).

Donohue DJ et al. Numerical modeling of the cornea's lamellar structure and birefringence properties. J Opt Soc Am A 12:1425–1438 (1995).

Donohue DJ et al. A numerical test of the normal incidence uniaxial model of corneal birefringence. Cornea 15:278–285 (1996).

Dreher AW, Reiter K. Retinal laser ellipsometry: a new method for measuring the retinal nerve fiber layer thickness distribution? Clin Vision Sci 7:481–488 (1992).

Dreher AW, Reiter K, Weinreb RN. Spatially resolved birefringence of the retinal nerve fiber layer assessed with a retinal laser ellipsometer. Appl Opt 31:3730–3735 (1992).

Drexler W et al. Scanning laser interferometer for fundus profile measurement of the human eye. Proc SPIE Microscopy, Holography, and Interferometry in Biomedicine 2083:363–371 (1994).

Drexler W et al. In vivo optical coherence tomography and topography of the fundus of the human eye. Proc SPIE Lasers in Ophthalmology II 2330:134–145 (1995a).

Drexler W et al. Measurement of the thickness of fundus layers by partial coherence tomography. Opt Eng 34:701–710 (1995b).

Drexler W et al. Biometric investigation of changes in the anterior eye segment during accommodation. Vision Res 37:2789–2800 (1997a).

Drexler W et al. Submicrometer precision biometry of the anterior segment of the human eye. Invest Ophthalmol Vis Sci 38:1304–1313 (1997b).

Drexler W et al. Dual-beam optical coherence tomography: signal identification for ophthalmologic diagnosis. J Biomed Opt 3:55–65 (1998a).

Drexler W et al. Partial coherence interferometry: a novel approach to biometry in cataract surgery. Am J Ophthalmol 126:524–534 (1998b).

Drexler W et al. Eye elongation during accommodation in humans: differences between emmetropes and myopes. Invest Ophthalmol Vis Sci 39:2140–2147 (1998c).

Drexler W et al. Investigation of dispersion effects in ocular media by multiple wavelength partial coherence interferometry. Exp Eye Res 66:25–33 (1998d).

Drexler W et al. Ultrahigh-resolution ophthalmic optical coherence tomography. Nat Med 7:502–507 (2001).

Duijm HF et al. Study of choroidal blood flow by comparison of SLO fluorescein angiography and microspheres. Exp Eye Res 63:693–704 (1996).

Dwyer WO et al. Validity of the laser refraction technique for determining spherical error in different refractive groups. Am J Optom Arch Am Acad Optom 50:222–225 (1973).

El-Harazi SM, Chuang AZ, Yee RW. Assessment of anterior chamber flare and cells after laser insitu keratomileusis. J Cataract Refract Surg 27:693–696 (2001).

El-Maghraby A et al. Reproducibility and validity of laser flare/cell meter measurements of intraocular inflammation. J Cataract Refract Surg 19:52–55 (1993).

Elsner AE et al. Quantitative reflectometry with the SLO. In: Nasemann JE, Burk ROW, eds. Scanning laser ophthalmoscopy and tomography. Muenchen: Quintessenz, 1990; 10:109–121.

Elsner AE et al. Infrared imaging of subretinal structures in the human ocular fundus. Vision Res 36:191–205 (1996).

Elsner AE et al. Foveal cone photopigment distribution: small alterations associated with macular pigment distribution. Invest Ophthalmol Vis Sci 39:2394–2404 (1998a).

Elsner AE et al. Multiply scattered light tomography. Vertical cavity surface emitting laser array used for imaging subretinal structures. Lasers and Light 8:193–202 (1998b).

Emdadi A et al. Patterns of optic disk damage in patients with early focal visual field loss. Am J Ophthalmol 126:763–771 (1998).

Enoch JM, Bedell HE, Kaufman HE. Interferometric visual acuity testing in anterior segment disease. Arch Ophthalmol 97:1916–1919 (1979).

Eppstein JA, Bursell S-E. Non-invasive detection of diabetes mellitus. Proc SPIE Physiological Monitoring and Early Detection Diagnostic Methods 1641:217–226 (1992).

Erb C et al. Confocal scanning laser Doppler flowmetry of the optic nerve in smokers. Neuro-ophthalmology 21:33–37 (1999).

Essock EA, Sinai MJ, Fechtner RD. Interocular symmetry in nerve fiber layer thickness of normal eyes as determined by polarimetry. J Glaucoma 8:90–98 (1999).

Faulkner W. Laser interferometry as a prognostic tool in pseudophakic rhegmatogenous retinal detachment. J Am Intraocul Implant Soc 8:24–26 (1982).

Faulkner W. Laser interferometric prediction of postoperative visual acuity in patients with cataracts. Am J Ophthalmol 95:626–636 (1983a).

Faulkner W. Predicting acuities in capsulotomy patients: interferometers and potential acuity meter. J Am Intraocul Implant Soc 9:434–437 (1983b).

Fejer TP, Girgis R. Night myopia: implications for the young driver. Can J Ophthalmol 27:172–176 (1992).

Feke GT et al. Blood flow in the normal human retina. Invest Ophthalmol Vis Sci 30:58–65 (1989).

Fercher AF. In vivo measurements of fundus pulsations by laser interferometry. IEEE J Quantum Electronics 20:1469–1471 (1984).

Fercher AF, Li HC, Hitzenberger CK. Slit lamp laser Doppler interferometer. Lasers Surg Med 13:447–452 (1993).

Fercher AF, Li HC, Hitzenberger CK. Slit-lamp dual-beam interferometer. Proc SPIE Microscopy, Holography, and Interferometry in Biomedicine 2083:372–377 (1994).

Fillacier K et al. Study of lymphocyte dynamics in the ocular circulation: technique of labeling cells. Curr Eye Res 14:579–584 (1995).

Findl O et al. Effects of changes in intraocular pressure on human ocular haemodynamics. Curr Eye Res 16:1024–1029 (1997).

Findl O et al. Accurate determination of effective lens position and lens-capsule distance with 4 intraocular lenses. J Cataract Refract Surg 24:1094–1098 (1998a).

Findl O et al. High precision biometry of pseudophakic eyes using partial coherence interferometry. J Cataract Refract Surg 24:1087–1093 (1998b).

Findl O et al. Changes in intraocular lens position after neodymium:YAG capsulotomy. J Cataract Refract Surg 25:659–662 (1999).

Findl O et al. Assessment of optic disk blood flow in patients with open-angle glaucoma. Am J Ophthalmol 130:589–596 (2000a).

Findl O et al. Ocular haemodynamics and colour contrast sensitivity in patients with type 1 diabetes. Br J Ophthalmol 84:493–498 (2000b).

Findl O et al. Improved prediction of intraocular lens power using partial coherence interferometry. J Cataract Refract Surg 27:861–867 (2001).

Fish GE et al. A comparison of visual function tests in eyes with maculopathy. Ophthalmology 93:1177–1182 (1986).

Fitzke FW, Masters BR. Three-dimensional vizualisation of confocal sections of in vivo human fundus and optic nerve. Curr Eye Res 12:1015–1018 (1993).

Flach AJ et al. Comparative effects of ketorolac 0.5% or diclofenac 0.1% ophthalmic solutions on inflammation after cataract surgery. Ophthalmology 105:1775–1779 (1998).

Fletcher DC et al. Scanning laser ophthalmoscope macular perimetry and applications for low vision rehabilitation clinicians. Ophthalmol Clinics 7:257–265 (1994).

Fletcher DC, Schuchard RA. Preferred retinal loci relationship to macular scotomas in a low-vision population. Ophthalmology 104:632–638 (1997).

Flower RW, Csaky KG, Murphy RP. Disparity between fundus camera and scanning laser ophthalmoscope indocyanine green imaging of retinal pigment epithelium detachments. Retina 18:260–268 (1998).

Foerster W et al. Qualitative holographic-interferometric analysis of T-incisions of different length in vitro—A preliminary report. Proc SPIE Ophthalmic Technologies III 1877:122–126 (1993).

Foerster W, Kasprzak H, Von Bally G. Measurement of elastic modulus of the central bovine cornea by means of holographic interferometry. Part II. Results. Optom Vis Sci 71:27–32 (1994).

Folk JC, Boldt HC, Keenum DG. Foveal cysts. A premacular hole condition associated with vitreous traction. Arch Ophthalmol 116:1177–1183 (1998).

Fontana L et al. In vivo morphometry of the lamina cribrosa and its relation to visual field loss in glaucoma. Curr Eye Res 17:363–369 (1998).

Frambach DA et al. System to measure contrast-sensitivity function with a scanning laser ophthalmoscope. Proc SPIE Ophthalmic Technologies IV 2126:154–160 (1994).

Frambach DA, Dacey MP, Sadun A. Stereoscopic photography with a scanning laser ophthalmoscope. Am J Ophthalmol 116:484–488 (1993).

Freeman WR et al. Simultaneous indocyanine green and fluorescein angiography using a confocal scanning laser ophthalmoscope. Arch Ophthalmol 116:455–463 (1998).

Friedlander MH et al. Holographic interferometry of the corneal surface. Proc SPIE Ophthalmic Tecnologies 1423:62–69 (1991).

Fujikado T et al. Anatomic and functional recovery of the fovea after foveal translocation surgery without large retinotomy and simultaneous excision of a neovascular membrane. Am J Ophthalmol 126:839–842 (1998).

Fujio N et al. Regional retinal blood flow reduction following half fundus photocoagulation treatment. Br J Ophthalmol 78:335–338 (1994).

Funaki S, Shirakashi M, Abe H. Relation between size of optic disc and thickness of retinal nerve fibre layer in normal subjects. Br J Ophthalmol 82:1242–1245 (1998).

Gabel VP, Birngruber R, Nasemann J. Fluorescein angiography with the scanning laser ophthalmoscope. Lasers Light Ophthalmol 2:35–40 (1988).

Gallemore RP et al. Diagnosis of vitreoretinal adhesions in macular disease with optical coherence tomography. Retina 20:115–120 (2000).

Garcia CR et al. Oral fluorescein angiography with the confocal scanning laser ophthalmoscope. Ophthalmology 106:1114–1118 (1999).

Garway-Heath DF et al., Inter- and intraobserver variation in the analysis of optic disc images: comparison of the Heidelberg Retinal Tomograph and computer-assisted planimetry. Br J Ophthalmol 83:664–669 (1999).

Garway-Heath DF, Wollstein G, Hitchings RA. Aging changes of the optic nerve head in relation to open angle glaucoma. Br J Ophthalmol 81:840–845 (1997).

Gelisken F et al. Indocyanine green angiography in classic choroidal neovascularization. Jpn J Ophthalmol 42:300–303 (1998a).

Gelisken F et al. Indocyanine green videoangiography of occult choroidal neovascularization. A comparison of scanning laser ophthalmoscope with high-resolution digital fundus camera. Retina 18:37–43 (1998b).

Geyer O et al. Reproducibility of topographic measures of the glaucomatous optic nerve head. Br J Ophthalmol 82:14–17 (1998).

Gieser JP et al. Clinical assessment of the macula by retinal topography and thickness mapping. Am J Ophthalmol 124:648–660 (1997).

Giovannini A et al. Optical coherence tomography in the assessment of retinal pigment epithelial tear. Retina 20:37–40 (2000).

Goldmann H, Chrenkova A, Cornaro S. Retinal visual acuity in cataractous eyes. Determination with interference fringes. Arch Ophthalmol 98:1778–1781 (1980).

Goldstein J et al. Clinical comparison of the SITE IRAS hand-held interferometer and Haag-Streit Lotmar visometer. J Cataract Refract Surg 14:208–211 (1988).

Graney MJ et al. A clinical index for predicting visual acuity after cataract surgery. Am J Ophthalmol 105:460–465 (1988).

Green DG. Testing the vision of cataract patients by means of laser-generated interference fringes. Science 168:1240–1242 (1970).

Green DG. Visual acuity: the influence of refraction and diffraction and the use of interference fringes. Int Ophthalmol Clin 18:21–40 (1978).

Green DG, Cohen MM. Laser interferometry in the evaluation of potential macular function in the presence of opacities in the ocular media. Trans Am Acad Ophthalmol Otolayngol 75:629–637 (1971).

Greenfield DS, Knighton RW. Stability of corneal polarization axis measurements for scanning laser polarimetry. Ophthalmology 108:1065–1069 (2001).

Greenfield DS, Knighton RW, Huang X-R. Distribution of corneal polarization axes among normal eyes: implication for scanning laser polarimetry. Invest Ophthalmol Vis Sci 40 (Suppl):2092 (1999).

Greenfield DS, Knighton RW, Huang X-R. Effect of corneal polarization axis on assessment of retinal nerve fiber layer thickness by scanning laser polarimetry. Am J Ophthalmol 129:715–722 (2000).

Grewing R, Becker H. Retinal thickness immediately after cataract surgery measured by optical coherence topography. Ophthalmic Surg Lasers 31:215–217 (2000).

Griesser SM et al. Heidelberg retina flowmeter parameters at the papilla in healthy subjects. Eur J Ophthalmol 9:32–36 (1999).

Grignolo FM et al. Evaluation of macular function by Lotmar's visometer test and blue-field entoptic test in patients with cataract. Ann Ophthalmol 20:247–50, 255 (1988b).

Grignolo FM, Moscone F, Boles-Carenini A. Assessment of malingerers' visual acuity by Lotmar's visometer test. Ann Ophthalmol 20:335–339 (1988a).

Groh MJ et al. Influence of age on retinal and optic nerve head blood circulation. Ophthalmology 103:529–534 (1996).

Grunwald JE, DuPont J, Riva CE. Retinal hemodynamics in patients with early diabetes mellitus. Br J Ophthalmol 80:327–331 (1996).

Grunwald JE, Hariprasad SM, DuPont J. Effect of aging on foveolar choroidal circulation. Arch Ophthalmol 116:150–154 (1998a).

Grunwald JE et al. Optic nerve and choroidal circulation in glaucoma. Invest Ophthalmol Vis Sci 39:2329–2336 (1998b).

Grunwald JE et al. Optic nerve blood flow in glaucoma: effect of systemic hypertension. Am J Ophthalmol 127:516–522 (1999).

Gstalder RJ, Green DG. Laser interferometry in corneal opacification. Preoperative visual potential estimation. Arch Ophthalmol 87:269–274 (1972).

Gstalder RJ, Green DG. Laser interferometric acuity in amblyopia. J Ped Ophthalmol 8:251–256 (1971).

Guez J-E et al. Functional assessment of macular hole surgery by scanning laser ophthalmoscopy. Ophthalmology 105:694–699 (1998).

Gugleta K, Orgul S, Flammer J. Asymmetry in intraocular pressure and retinal nerve fiber layer thickness in normal-tension glaucoma. Ophthalmologica 213:219–223 (1999).

Guillen-Monterrubio OM et al. Quantitative determination of aqueous flare and cells in healthy eyes. Acta Ophthalmol Scand 75:58–62 (1997).

Gundersen KG, Asman P. Comparison of ranked segment analysis (RSA) and cup to disc ratio in computer-assisted optic disc evaluation. Acta Ophthalmol Scand 78:137–141 (2000).

Gundersen KG, Heijl A, Bengtsson B. Age, gender, IOP, refraction and optic disc topography in normal eyes. A cross-sectional study using raster and scanning laser tomography. Acta Ophthalmol Scand 76:170–175 (1998).

Guo X et al. Laser interferometric prediction of postoperative visual acuity in patients with genetic ectopia lentis. J Pediatr Ophthalmol Strabismus 35:225–228 (1998).

Gurses-Ozden R et al. Increasing sampling density improves reproducibility of optical coherence tomography measurements. J Glaucoma 8:238–241 (1999).

Gurses-Ozden R et al. Scanning laser polarimetry measurements after laser-assisted in situ keratomileusis. Am J Ophthalmol 129:461–464 (2000).

Gurses-Ozden R et al. Retinal nerve fiber layer thickness remains unchanged following laser-assisted in situ keratomileusis. Am J Ophthalmol 132:512–516 (2001).

Guyer DR et al. Digital indocyanine-green angiography in chorioretinal disorders. Ophthalmology 99:287–291 (1992).

Guyton DL. Preoperative visual acuity evaluation. Int Ophthalmol Clin 27:140–148 (1987).

Hagimura N et al. Optical coherence tomography of the neurosensory retina in rhegmatogenous retinal detachment. Am J Ophthalmol 129:186–190 (2000).

Halliday BL, Ross JE. Comparison of 2 interferometers for predicting visual acuity in patients with cataract. Br J Ophthalmol 67:273–277 (1983).

Hanna IT et al. The role of white light interferometry in predicting visual acuity following posterior capsulotomy. Eye 3:468–471 (1989).

Haouchine B, Massin P, Gaudric A. Foveal pseudocyst as the first step in macular hole formation: a prospective study by optical coherence tomography. Ophthalmology 108:15–22 (2001).

Harris A, Cantor L, Kagemann L. Imaging of blood flow in glaucoma. In: Schuman JS, ed. Imaging in glaucoma. Thorofare, NJ: Slack, 1997; pp 135–154.

Harris A et al. Physiological perturbation of ocular and cerebral blood flow as measured by scanning laser ophthalmoscopy and color Doppler imaging. Surv Ophthalmol 38 (Suppl):S81–S86 (1994).

Hartnett ME, Elsner AE. Characteristics of exudative age-related macular degeneration determined in vivo with confocal and indirect infrared imaging. Ophthalmology 103:58–71 (1996).

Hatch WV et al. Interobserver agreement of Heidelberg Retina Tomograph parameters. J Glaucoma 8:232–237 (1999).

Haynes RJ et al. Imaging of optic nerve head drusen with the scanning laser ophthalmoscope. Br J Ophthalmol 81:654–657 (1997).

Hayreh SS. Evaluation of optic nerve head circulation: review of the methods used. J Glaucoma 6:319–330 (1997).

He S, MacLeod DI. Local luminance nonlinearity and receptor aliasing in the detection of high-frequency gratings. J Opt Soc Am A 13:1139–1151 (1996).

Hee MR et al. Optical coherence tomography of the human retina. Arch Ophthamol 113:325–332 (1995).

Herbort CP, Chave JP. Cicatrization of cytomegalovirus retinitis following introduction of highly active anti-retroviral therapy: uveitis as a possible indicator of good ocular prognosis. Graefes Arch Clin Exp Ophthalmol 236:795–797 (1998).

Herbort CP et al. Use of laser flare photometry to assess and monitor inflammation in uveitis. Ophthalmology 104:64–71 (1997).

Hipwell JH et al. Quantifying changes in retinal circulation: the generation of parametric images from fluorescein angiograms. Physiol Meas 19:165–180 (1998).

Hirano K et al. Optical coherence tomography for the noninvasive evaluation of the cornea. Cornea 20:281–289 (2001).

Hiroshiba N et al. Alterations of retinal microcirculation in response to scatter photocoagulation. Invest Ophthalmol Vis Sci 39:769–776 (1998).

Hitzenberger CK. Measurement of corneal thickness by low-coherence interferometry. Appl Opt 31:6637–6642 (1992).

Hitzenberger CK, Drexler W, Fercher AF. Measurement of corneal thickness by laser Doppler interferometry. Invest Ophthalmol Vis Sci 33:98–103 (1992).

Hitzenberger CK et al. Measurement of the axial length of cataract eyes by laser Doppler interferometry. Invest Ophthalmol Vis Sci 34:1886–1893 (1993).

Hitzenberger CK et al. Interferometric measurement of corneal thickness with micrometer precision. Am J Ophthalmol 118:468–476 (1994).

Hitzenberger CK et al. Retinal layers located with a precision of 5 μm by partial coherence interferometry. Proc SPIE Ophthalmic Technologies V 2393:176–181 (1995).

Hitzenberger CK, Fercher AF, Juchem M. Measurement of the axial eye length and retinal thickness by laser Doppler interferometry. Proc SPIE Holography, Interferometry, and Optical Pattern Recognition in Biomedicine 1429:21–25 (1991a).

Hitzenberger CK, Fercher AF, Juchem M. Measurement of the axial eye length and retinal thickness by laser Doppler interferometry. Proc SPIE Ophthalmic Technologies 1423:46–50 (1991b).

Hoerauf H et al. Combined choroidal and retinal ischemia during interferon therapy: indocyanine green angiographic and microperimetric findings. Arch Ophthalmol 118:580–582 (2000a).

Hoerauf H et al. Slit-lamp-adapted optical coherence tomography of the anterior segment. Graefes Arch Clin Exp Ophthalmol 238:8–18 (2000b).

Hoh ST et al. Factors affecting image acquisition during scanning laser polarimetry. Ophthalmic Surg Lasers 29:545–551 (1998a).

Hoh ST et al. Peripapillary nerve fiber layer thickness measurement reproducibility using scanning laser polarimetry. J Glaucoma 7:12–15 (1998b).

Hoh ST et al. Effect of pupillary dilation on retinal nerve fiber layer thickness as measured by scanning laser polarimetry in eyes with and without cataract. J Glaucoma 8:159–163 (1999a).

Hoh ST et al. Factors affecting image acquisition during scanning laser polarimetry: author's response [letter]. Ophthalmic Surg Lasers 30:411–412 (1999b).

Hoh ST et al. Optical coherence tomography and scanning laser polarimetry in normal, ocular hypertensive, and glaucomatous eyes. Am J Ophthalmol 129:129–135 (2000).

Hollo G. Factors affecting image acquisition during scanning laser polarimetry [letter]. Ophthalmic Surg Lasers 30:74 (1999).

Hollo G et al. Evaluation of the peripapillary circulation in healthy and glaucoma eyes with scanning laser Doppler flowmetry. Int Ophthamol 20:71–77 (1997a).

Hollo G, Nagymihaly A, Vargha P. Scanning laser polarimetry in corneal haze after excimer laser refractive surgery. J Glaucoma 6:359–362 (1997b).

Hollo G et al. Scanning laser polarimetry of the retinal nerve fiber layer in primary open angle and capsular glaucoma. Br J Ophthalmol 81:857–861 (1997c).

Hollo G, van den Berg TJTP, Greve EL. Scanning laser Doppler flowmetry in glaucoma. Int Ophthalmol 20:63–70 (1997d).

Hollo G, Szabo A, Vargha P. Scanning laser polarimetry versus frequency-doubling perimetry and conventional threshold perimetry: changes during a 12-month follow-up in preperimetric glaucoma. A pilot study. Acta Ophthalmol Scand 79:403–407 (2001).

Holmer A-K et al. Design, calibration and testing of a laser flare meter. Applied Optics 33:2611–2619 (1994).

Holz FG et al. Simultaneous confocal scanning laser fluorescein and indocyanine green angiography. Am J Ophthalmol 125:227–236 (1998).

Horiguchi M, Ito Y, Miyake Y. Extrafoveal photostress recovery test in glaucoma and idiopathic central serous chorioretinopathy. Br J Ophthalmol 82:1007–1012 (1998).

Horn F, Budde W, Korth M. Contrast-sensitivity testing with scanning-laser ophthalmoscope stimulation in normal, ocular hypertensive, and glaucomatous patients. Ger J Ophthalmol 5:428–434 (1996a).

Horn F et al. Quadrant pattern ERG with SLO stimulation in normals and glaucoma patients. Graefes Arch Clin Exp Ophthalmol 234 (Suppl 1):S174–S179 (1996b).

Horn FK et al. Polarimetric measurement of retinal nerve fiber layer thickness in glaucoma diagnosis. J Glaucoma 8:353–362 (1999).

Hosking S, Flanagan J. Scanning laser tomography: effect of change in keratometry values on retinal distance measures. Ophthal Physiol Opt 18:294–298 (1998).

Hossain P. Scanning laser ophthalmoscopy and fundus fluorescent leucocyte angiography. Br J Ophthalmol 83:1250–1253 (1999).

Hossain P et al. In vivo cell tracking by scanning laser ophthalmoscopy: quantification of leukocyte kinetics. Invest Ophthalmol Vis Sci 39:1879–1887 (1998).

Huang D et al. Optical coherence tomography. Science 254:1178–1181 (1991).

Hudson C et al. Scanning laser tomography Z profile signal width as an objective index of macular retinal thickening. Br J Ophthalmol 82:121–130 (1998).

Hudson HL, Frambach DA, Lopez PF. Relation of the functional and structural fundus changes after submacular surgery for neovascular age-related macular degeneration. Br J Ophthalmol 79:417–423 (1995).

Iester M, De Ferrari R, Zanini M. Topographic analysis to discriminate glaucomatous from normal optic nerve heads with a confocal scanning laser: New optic disk analysis without any observer input. Surv Ophthalmol 44 (Suppl 1):S33–S40 (1999).

Iester M et al. A comparison of healthy, ocular hypertensive, and glaucomatous optic disc topographic parameters. J Glaucoma 6:363–370 (1997).

Iester M et al. Discriminant analysis models for early detection of glaucomatous optic disc changes. Br J Ophthalmol 84:464–468 (2000).

Iida T et al. Evaluation of central serous chorioretinopathy with optical coherence tomography. Am J Ophthalmol 129:16–20 (2000).

Iijima H et al. Optical coherence tomography of orange-red subretinal lesions in eyes with idiopathic polypoidal choroidal vasculopathy. Am J Ophthalmol 129:21–26 (2000).

Ikeda T et al. Examination of patients with cystoid macular edema using a scanning laser ophthalmoscope with infrared light. Am J Ophthalmol 125:710–712 (1998).

Imai M, Iijima H, Hanada N. Optical coherence tomography of tractional macular elevations in eyes with proliferative diabetic retinopathy. Am J Ophthalmol 132:81–84 (2001).

Imai Y, Tanaka K. Direct velocity sensing of flow distribution based on low-coherence interferometry. J Opt Soc Am A 16:2007–2012 (1999).

Imasawa M, Iijima H, Morimoto T. Perimetric sensitivity and retinal thickness in eyes with macular edema resulting from branch retinal vein occlusion. Am J Ophthalmol 131:55–60 (2001).

Ip M et al. Differentiation of degenerative retinoschisis from retinal detachment using optical coherence tomography. Ophthalmology 106:600–605 (1999).

Ishiko S et al. The use of scanning laser ophthalmoscope microperimetry to detect visual impairment caused by macular photocoagulation. Ophthalmic Surg Lasers 29:95–98 (1998).

Ito Y et al. Extrafoveal photostress recovery testing with a scanning laser ophthalmoscope. Jpn J Ophthalmol 41:255–259 (1997).

Jacobson SG et al. Disease expression in X-linked retinitis pigmentosa caused by a putative null mutation in the RPGR gene. Invest Ophthalmol Vis Sci 38:1983–1997 (1997).

Jacobson SG et al. Retinal degenerations with truncation mutations in the cone-rod homeobox (CRX) gene. Invest Ophthalmol Vis Sci 39:2417–2426 (1998).

Jakkola A, Vesti E, Immonen I. The use of confocal scanning laser tomography in the evaluation of retinal elevation in age-related macular degeneration. Ophthalmology 106:274–279 (1999).

Jaschinski-Kruza W. A hand optometer for measuring dark focus. Vision Res 28:1271–1275 (1988).

Jay JL, Mammo RB, Allan D. Effect of age on visual acuity after cataract extraction. Br J Ophthalmol 71:112–115 (1987).

Jonas JB, Hayreh SS. Localized retinal nerve fibre layer defects in chronic experimental high pressure glaucoma in rhesus monkeys. Br J Ophthalmol 83:1291–1295 (1999).

Jones AL et al. The Humphrey optical coherence tomography scanner: quantitative analysis and reproducibility study of the normal human retinal nerve fibre layer. Br J Ophthalmol 85:673–677 (2001).

Junghardt A et al. Reproducibility of the data determined by scanning laser polarimetry. Graefes Arch Clin Exp Ophthalmol 234:628–632 (1996).

Kagemann L et al. Heidelberg retinal flowmetry: factors affecting blood flow measurement. Br J Ophthalmol 82:131–136 (1998).

Kakehashi A et al. Vitreous videography using the scanning laser ophthalmoscope. Jpn J Ophthalmol 39:377–383 (1995).

Kakehashi A et al. Differential diagnosis of macular breaks by microperimetry using the scanning laser ophthalmoscope. Jpn J Ophthalmol 40:116–122 (1996).

Kamal DS et al. Use of sequential Heidelberg retinal tomograph images to identify changes at the optic disc in ocular hypertensive patients at risk of developing glaucoma. Br J Ophthalmol 84:993–998 (2000).

Kamensky VA et al. In-situ observation of IR and UV solid state laser modification of lens and cornea. Proc SPIE Laser-Tissue Interaction IX 3254:390–397 (1998).

Kaneda M et al. Changes of lens protein particles during development and reversal of galactose cataracts. Ophthamic Res 22 (Suppl 1):95–100 (1990).

Kasprzak H, Foerster W, Von Bally G. Holographic measurement of changes of the central corneal curvature due to intraocular pressure differences. Opt Eng 33:198–203 (1994a).

Kasprzak H et al. Analysis of holographic interferograms of the expanded cornea after refractive surgery procedure. Proc SPIE New Techniques and Analysis in Optical Measurements 2340:480–486 (1994b).

Kasprzak H, Foerster W, Von Bally G. Measurement of changes of the central corneal curvature due to intraocular pressure differences using holographic interferometry. Proc SPIE Holography, Interferometry, and Optical Pattern Recognition in Biomedicine III 1889:175–183 (1993a).

Kasprzak H, Foerster W, Von Bally G. Measurement of elastic modulus of the bovine cornea by means of holographic interferometry. Part I. Method and Experiment. Optom Vis Sci 70:535–544 (1993b).

Kasprzak H, Kowalik W, Jaronski J. Interferometric measurements of fine corneal topography. Proc SPIE Optical and Imaging Techniques in Biomedicine 2329:32–39 (1995).

Katsumi O et al. Recording pattern reversal visual evoked response with the scanning laser ophthalmoscope. Acta Ophthalmol 67:243–248 (1989).

Kee C et al. Effect of optic disc size or age on evaluation of optic disc variables. Br J Ophthalmol 81:1046–1049 (1997).

Khoobehi B et al. Repetitive, selective angiography of individual vessels of the retina. Retina 9:87–96 (1989).

Khoobehi B et al. Measurement of circulation time in the retinal vasculature using selective angiography. Ophthalmology 97:1061–1070 (1990c).

Khoobehi B et al. Fluorescent microsphere imaging: a particle-tracking approach to the hemodynamic assessment of the retina and choroid. Ophthalmic Surg Lasers 28:937–947 (1997).

Khoobehi B, Char CA, Peyman GA. Assessment of laser-induced release of drugs from liposomes: an in vitro study. Lasers Surg Med 10:60–65 (1990).

Khoobehi B, Peyman GA. Fluorescent labeling of blood cells for evaluation of retinal and choroidal circulation. Ophthalmic Surg Lasers 30:140–145 (1999).

Khoobehi B, Peyman GA. Fluorescent vesicle system: a new technique for measuring blood flow in the retina. Ophthalmology 101:1716–1726 (1994).

Khoobehi B, Peyman GA, Vo K. Laser-triggered repetitive fluorescein angiography. Ophthalmology 99:72–79 (1992).

Kiel JW, Patel P. Effects of timolol and betaxolol on choridal blood flow in the rabbit. Exp Eye Res 67:501–507 (1998).

Kim J, Yang Y, Sin B, Cho C. Visualization and flow of platelets and leukocytes in vivo in rat retinal and choroidal vessels. Ophthalmic Res 29:374–380 (1997).

Kimura H et al. A new fluorescent imaging procedure in vivo for evaluation of the retinal microcirculation in rats. Curr Eye Res 14:223–228 (1995).

Kirkpatrick JN et al. Fundus imaging in patients with cataract: role for a variable wavelength scanning laser ophthalmoscope. Br J Ophthalmol 79:892–899 (1995).

Kiryu J et al. Enhanced visualization of vitreoretinal interface by laser biomicroscopy. Ophthalmol 100:1040–1043 (1993).

Kiryu J et al. Noninvasive visualization of the choriocapillaris and its dynamic filling. Invest Ophthalmol Vis Sci 35:3724–3731 (1994).

Kiryu J et al. Local response of the primate retinal microcirculation to increased metabolic demand induced by flicker. Invest Ophthalmol Vis Sci 36:1240–1246 (1995).

Knoll HA. Measuring ametropia with a gas laser. Am J Optom Arch Am Acad Optom 43:415–418 (1966).

Koelle JS, Riva CE, Petrig BL, Cranstoun SD. Depth of tissue sampling in the optic nerve head using laser Doppler flowmetry. Lasers Med Sci 8:49–54 (1993).

Kogure S, Chiba T, Tsukahara S. Properties of artifacts on scanning laser polarimetery. Invest Ophthalmol Vis Sci 40 (Suppl):388 (1999a).

Kogure S, Iijima H. Preoperative evaluation by laser interferometry in cataractous eyes with retinitis pigmentosa. Jpn J Ophthalmol 37:282–286 (1993).

Kogure S, Iijima H, Tsukahara S. A new parameter for assessing the thickness of the retinal nerve fiber layer for glaucoma diagnosis. Eur J Ophthalmol 9:93–98 (1999b).

Konno S, Akiba J, Yoshida A. Retinal thickness measurements with optical coherence tomography and the scanning retinal thickness analyzer. Retina 21:57–61 (2001a).

Konno S et al. Retinal blood flow changes in type I diabetes. A long term follow-up study. Invest Ophthalmol Vis Sci 37:1140–1148 (1996).

Konno S et al. Three-dimensional analysis of macular diseases with a scanning retinal thickness analyzer and a coafocal scanning laser ophthalmoscope. Ophthalmic Surg Lasers 32:95–99 (2001b).

Kook MS et al. Study of retinal nerve fibre layer thickness in eyes with high tension glaucoma and hemifield defect. Br J Ophthalmol 85:1167–1170 (2001a).

Kook MS et al. Reproducibility of scanning laser polarimetry (GDx) of peripapillary retinal nerve fiber layer thickness in normal subjects. Graefes Arch Clin Exp Ophthalmol 239:118–121 (2001b).

Kremmer S et al. [Scanning laser topometry and polarimetry before and after cataract surgeries with implantation of intraocular lenses]. Klin Monatsbl Augenheilkd 214:378–385 (1999).

Kremser B et al. Retinal thickness analysis in subjects with different refractive conditions. Ophthalmologica 213:376–379 (1999).

Kubota T et al. Comparative study of retinal nerve fiber layer damage in Japanese patients with normal- and high-tension glaucoma. J Glaucoma 8:363–366 (1999).

Kuck H et al. Diagnosis of occult subretinal neovascularization in age-related macular degeneration by infrared scanning laser videoangiography. Retina 13:36–39 (1993).

Kuckelkorn R et al. Video fluorescein angiography of the anterior eye segment in severe eye burns. Acta Ophthalmol Scand 75:675–680 (1997).

Kulshrestha M et al. Demonstration of the reversibility of optic disc topography by scanning laser ophthalmoscopy. Arch Ophthalmol 117:1664–1665 (1999).

Kunze C et al. Spatial extent of pigment epithelial detachments in age-related macular degeneration. Ophthalmology 106:1830–1840 (1999).

Kutschbach P et al. Retinal capillary density in patients with arterial hypertension: 2-year follow-up. Graefes Arch Clin Exp Ophthalmol 236:410–414 (1998).

Kwon YH et al. Correlation of automated visual field parameters and peripapillary nerve fiber layer thickness as measured by scanning laser polarimetry. J Glaucoma 9:281–288 (2000).

Lang TA, Lindstrom RL. Efficacy of laser interferometry in predicting visual result of YAG laser posterior capsulotomy. J Am Intraocul Implant Soc 11:367–371 (1985).

Larsson LI, Naiji E. Increased permeability of the blood-aqueous barrier after panretinal photocoagulation for proliferative diabetic retinopathy. Acta Ophthalmol Scand 79:414–416 (2001).

Lasa MS, Datiles MB III, Freidlin V. Potential vision tests in patients with cataracts. Ophthalmology 102:1007–1011 (1995).

Lauande-Pimentel R et al. Discrimination between normal and glaucomatous eyes with visual field and scanning laser polarimetry measurements. Br J Ophthalmol 85:586–591 (2001).

Le Gargasson JF et al. Scanning laser ophthalmoscope imaging of fluorescein-labelled blood cells. Graefes Arch Clin Exp Ophthalmol 235:56–58 (1997).

Lee VW, Mok KH. Retinal nerve fiber layer measurement by nerve fiber analyzer in normal subjects and patients with glaucoma. Ophthalmology 106:1006–1008 (1999).

Lee VW, Mok KH. Nerve fibre layer measurement of the Hong Kong Chinese population by scanning laser polarimetry. Eye 14:371–374 (2000).

Lemij HG. The value of polarimetry in the evaluation of the optic nerve in glaucoma. Curr Opin Ophthalmol 12:138–142 (2001).

Lemij HG, Tjon-Fo-Sang. The Nerve Fiber Analyzer. Ophthalmol Clin North Am 11:411–420 (1998).

Lexer F et al. Dynamic coherent focus for transversal resolution enhancement of OCT. Proc SPIE Coherence Domain Optical Methods in Biomedical Science and Clinical Applications II 3251:85–90 (1998).

Libondi T et al. In vivo measurement of the aging rabbit lens using quasielastic light scattering. Curr Eye Res 5:411–419 (1986).

Liem ATA, Keunen JEE, van Norren D. Clinical applications of fundus reflection densitometry. Surv Ophthalmol 41:37–50 (1996).

Lincoff H, Kreissig I. Optical coherence tomography of pneumatic displacement of optic disc pit maculopathy. Br J Ophthalmol 82:367–372 (1998).

Lindblom B. Fluorescein angiograph of the iris in the management of eyes with central retinal vein occlusion. Act Ophthalmol Scand 76:188–191 (1998).

Lindblom B, Bond-Taylor L. Scanning laser ophthalmoscopy as a tool for detecting atrophy of the central retinal nerve fiber layer in Leber's hereditary optic neuropathy. Acta Ophthalmol Scand 76:356–359 (1998).

Littmann H. Zur Bestimmung der wahren Grosse eines Objektes auf dem Hintergrund des lebenden Auges. Klin Monatsbl Augenheilkd 180:286–289 (1982).

Liu C et al. Aggregation in aqueous solutions of bovine lens γ–crystallins: special role of γ_s. Invest Ophthalmol Vis Sci 39:1609–1619 (1998).

Lobo CL et al. Mapping retinal fluorescein leakage with confocal scanning laser fluorometry of the human vitreous. Arch Ophthalmol 117:631–637 (1999).

Loewenstein A et al. Scanning laser ophthalmoscope fundus perimetry after surgery for choroidal neovascularization. Am J Ophthalmol 125:657–665 (1998).

Lotmar W. Apparatus for the measurement of retinal visual acuity by moire fringes. Invest Ophthalmol Vis Sci 19:393–400 (1980).

Lovasik JV, Kergoat H, Kothe AC. The influence of letter size on the focusing response of the eye. J Am Optom Assoc 58:631–639 (1987).

Lovasik JV, Kothe AC. Ocular refraction with body orientation. Aviat Space Environ Med 60:321–328 (1989).

Lusky M, Bosem ME, Weinreb RN. Reproducibility of optic nerve head topography measurements in eyes with undilated pupils. J Glaucoma 2:104–109 (1993).

MacLeod DI, Williams DR, Makous W. A visual nonlinearity fed by single cones. Vision Res 32:347–363 (1992).

Mainster MA et al. Scanning laser ophthalmoscopy. Clinical applications. Ophthalmol 89:852–857 (1982).

Maldonado MJ et al. Optical coherence tomography evaluation of the corneal cap and stromal bed features after laser in situ keratomileusis for high myopia and astigmatism. Ophthalmology 107:81–88 (2000).

Manivannan A et al. Clincal investigation of a true color scanning laser opthalmoscope. Arch Ophthalmol 119:819–824 (2001).

Manivannan A et al. Clinical investigation of an infrared digital scanning lase ophthalmoscope. Br J Ophthalmol 78:84–90 (1994).

Mardin CY et al. Preperimetric glaucoma diagnosis by confocal scanning laser tomography of the optic disc. Br J Ophthalmol 83:299–304 (1999).

Mardin CY et al. Monitoring of morphometric changes of optic discs with morphologic progression of glaucomatous optic atrophy by means of laser scanning tomography. Klin Monatsbl Augenheilkd 217:82–87 (2000a).

Mardin CY et al. Quantification of aqueous melanin granules, intraocular pressure and glaucomatous damage in primary pigment dispersion syndrome. Ophthalmology 107:435–440 (2000b).

Mardin CY, Horn FK. Influence of optic disc size on the sensitivity of the Heidelberg Retina Tomograph. Graefes Arch Clin Exp Ophthalmol 236:641–645 (1998).

Marraffa M et al. Does nerve fiber layer thickness correlate with visual field defects in glaucoma? Ophthalmologica 211:338–340 (1997).

Massin P et al. Optical coherence tomography of idiopathic macular epiretinal membranes before and after surgery. Am J Ophthalmol 130:732–739 (2000).

Matsuda N et al. Visualization of leukocyte dynamics in the choroid with indocyanine green. Invest Ophthalmol Vis Sci 37:2228–2233 (1996).

Matsumoto T et al. Measurement by holographic interferometry of the deformation of the eye accompanying changes in intraocular pressure. Appl Opt 17:358–359 (1978).

Maus TL, McLaren JW, Brubaker RF. A comparison of two methods of measuring aqueous flow in humans: fluorophotometry and flare measurement. Curr Eye Res 12:621–628 (1993).

McCally RL, Farrell RA. Structural implications of small-angle scattering from cornea. Exp Eye Res 34:99–113 (1982).

Melamed S et al. Confocal tomographic angiography of the optic nerve head in patients with glaucoma. Am J Ophthalmol 125:447–456 (1998).

Mendel MJ et al. Eye-tracking laser Doppler velocimeter stabilized in two dimensions: principle, design, and construction. J Opt Soc Am A 10:1663–1669 (1993).

Meyer JH, Guhlmann M, Funk J. Blind spot size depends on the optic disc topography: a study using SLO controlled scotometry and the Heidelberg Retina Tomograph. Br J Ophthalmol 81:355–359 (1997).

Michelson G et al. Simultaneous measurement of ocular micro- and macrocirculation, intraocular pressure, and systemic functions. Ger J Ophthalmol 3:48–53 (1994).

Michelson G et al. Principle, validity, reliability of scanning laser Doppler flowmetry. J Glaucoma 5:99–105 (1996).

Michelson G et al. Visual field defect and perfusion of the juxtapapillary retina and the neuroretinal rim area in primary open-angle glaucoma. Graefes Arch Clin Exp Ophthalmol 236:80–85 (1998a).

Michelson G, Welzenbach Pal I, Harazny J. Automatic full field analysis of perfusion images gained by scanning laser Doppler flowmetry. Br J Ophthalmol 82:1294–1300 (1998b).

Miglior S et al. Scanning laser ophthalmoscopy of the optic disc at the level of the lamina cribrosa. Curr Eye Res 17:453–461 (1998).

Miglior S et al. Clinical ability of Heidelberg retinal tomograph examination to detect glaucomatous visual field changes. Ophthalmology 108:1621–1627 (2001).

Mikelberg FS et al. Ability of the Heidelberg retina tomograph to detect early glaucomatous visual field loss. J Glaucoma 4:242–247 (1995).

Mikelberg FS. Scanning laser ophthalmoscopy of the optic disc in glaucoma with the Heidelberg Retina Tomograph. Ophthalmol Clin North Am 11:435–444 (1998).

Miller ST et al. Predictions of outcomes from cataract surgery in elderly persons. Ophthalmology 95:1125–1129 (1988).

Mistlberger A et al. Heidelberg retina tomography and optical coherence tomography in normal, ocular-hypertensive, and glaucomatous eyes. Ophthalmology 106:2027–2032 (1999).

Miyamoto K et al. In vivo quantification of leukocyte behavior in the retina during endotoxin-induced uveitis. Invest Ophthalmol Vis Sci 37:2708–2715 (1996).

Moller F, Sjolie AK, Bek T. Quantitative assessment of fixational eye movements by scanning laser ophthalmoscopy. Acta Ophthalmol Scand 74:578–583 (1996).

Morgan JE et al. Retinal nerve fiber layer polarimetry: histological and clinical comparison. Br J Ophthalmol 82:684–690 (1998).

Morgan JE, Waldock A. Scanning laser polarimetry of the normal human retinal nerve fiber layer: a quantitative analysis. Am J Ophthalmol 129:76–82 (2000).

Mori M, Araie M. A simple method of determining the time course of timolol's effects on aqueous flow in humans. Arch Ophthalmol 109:1099–1103 (1991).

Moriarty AP et al. Comparison of the anterior chamber inflammatory response to diode and argon laser trabeculoplasty using a laser flare meter. Ophthalmol 100:1263–1267 (1993).

Morrell A, Charman WN. A bichromatic laser optometer. Am J Optom Physiol Opt 64:790–795 (1987).

Morrell A, Whitefoot HD, Charman WN. Ocular chromatic aberration and age. Ophthalmic Physiol Opt 11:385–390 (1991).

Moshfeghi DM et al. Ocular vascular thrombosis following tin ethyl etiopurpurin (SnET2) photodynamic therapy: time dependencies. Ophthalmic Surg Lasers 29:663–668 (1998).

Mulholland DA, Craig JJ, Rankin SJA. Use of scanning laser ophthalmoscopy to monitor papilloedema in idiopathic intracranial hypertension. Br J Ophthalmol 82:1301–1305 (1998).

Mueller AJ et al. Imaging the microvasculature of choroidal melanomas with confocal indocyanine green scanning laser ophthalmoscopy. Arch Ophthalmol 116:31–39 (1998).

Ni M et al. A laboratory evaluation of the Kowa laser flare-cell meter for the study of uveitis. Graefe's Arch Clin Exp Ophthalmol 230:547–551 (1992).

Niessen AGJE et al. Retinal nerve fiber layer assessment by scanning laser polarimetry and standardized photography. Am J Ophthalmol 121:484–493 (1996).

Nishio M et al. Scanning laser ophthalmoscopic findings in a patient with acute zonal occult outer retinopathy. Am J Ophthalmol 125:712–715 (1998).

Nishiwaki H et al. Quantitative evaluation of leukocyte dynamics in retinal microcirculation. Invest Ophthalmol Vis Sci 36:123–130 (1995).

Nishiwaki H et al. Visualization and quantitative analysis of leukocyte dynamics in retinal microcirculation of rats. Invest Ophthalmol Vis Sci 37:1341–1347 (1996).

Nishiwaki H et al. Prednisolone, platelet-activating factor receptor antagonist, or superoxide dismutase reduced leucocyte entrapment induced by interferon alpha in retinal microcirculation. Invest Ophthalmol Vis Sci 38:811–816 (1997).

Nussenblatt RB. Macular alterations secondary to intraocular inflammatory disease. Ophthalmology 93:984–988 (1986).

O'Brart DP et al. Indocyanine green angiography of the peripapillary region in glaucomatous eyes by confocal scanning laser ophthalmoscopy. Am J Ophthalmol 123:657–666 (1997).

Odom JV, Chao GM, Weinstein GW. Preoperative prediction of postoperative visual acuity in patients with cataracts: a quantitative review. Doc Ophthalmol 70:5–17 (1988).

Ogura Y et al. Feasibility of targeted drug delivery to selective areas of the retina. Invest Ophthalmol Vis Sci 32:2351–2356 (1991).

Ogura Y et al. Occlusion of retinal vessels using targeted delivery of a platelet aggregating agent. Br J Ophthalmol 77:233–237 (1993).

Ogura Y, Honda Y. Evaluation of idiopathic epiretinal membranes by a scanning laser ophthalmoscope. Br J Ophthalmol 77:534–535 (1993).

Ohnishi Y et al. Capillary blood flow velocity measurements in cystoid macular edema with the scanning laser ophthalmoscope. Am J Ophthalmol 117:24–29 (1994).

Okada AA et al. Videofunduscopy and videoangiography using the scanning laser ophthalmoscope in Vogt-Koyanagi-Harada syndrome. Br J Ophthalmol 82:1175–1181 (1998).

Okubo H, Gherezghiher T, Koss MC. Long posterior ciliary arterial blood flow and systemic blood pressure. Invest Ophthalmol Vis Sci 31:819–826 (1990).

Ong LS et al. Use of the nerve fibre analyser after occipital coritical infarcts. Clin Experiment Ophthalmol 28:71 (2000).

Orgul S et al. Sources of variability of topometric data with a scanning laser ophthalmoscope. Arch Ophthalmol 114:161–164 (1996).

Orzalesi N et al. Microperimetry of localized retinal nerve fiber layer defects. Vision Res 38:763–771 (1998).

Oshika T. The laser flare-cell meter: its application to clinical studies. In: Khoo CY et al., eds. New frontiers in ophthalmology. New York: Excerpta Medica 641–648 (1991).

Oshika T, Araie M. Time course of changes in aqueous protein concentration and flow rate after oral acetazolamide. Invest Ophthalmol Vis Sci 31:527–534 (1990).

Oshima Y, Emi K. Optical cross-sectional assessment of the macula by retinal thickness analyzer in optic disk pit maculopathy. Am J Ophthalmol 128:106–109 (1999).

Oshima Y, Harino S, Tano Y. Scanning laser ophthalmoscope microperimetric assessment in patients with successful laser treatment for juxtafoveal choroidal neovascularization. Retina 18:109–117 (1998).

Ott D, Eckmiller R, Lades M. The scanning laser ophthalmoscope (SLO) as eye movement measurement system. In: Nasemann JE, Burk ROW, eds. Scanning laser ophthalmoscopy and tomography. Muenchen: Quintessenz, 1990; 14:147–158.

Ozdek S et al. Scanning laser polarimetry in corneal topographic changes after photorefractive keratectomy. Int Ophthalmol 22:113–117 (1999).

Paczka JA et al. Diagnostic capabilities of frequency-doubling technology, scanning laser polarimetry, and nerve fiber layer photographs to distinguish glaucomatous damage. Am J Ophthalmol 131:188–197 (2001).

Papastergiou GI et al. Ocular axial length and choroidal thickness in newly hatched chicks and one-year-old chickens fluctuate in a diurnal pattern that is influenced by visual experience and intraocular pressure. Exp Eye Res 66:195–205 (1998).

Parisi V et al. Visual function correlates with nerve fiber layer thickness in eyes affected with ocular hypertension. Invest Ophthalmol Vis Sci 40:1828–1833 (1999).

Park RJ et al. Effects of cataract extraction with intraocular lens placement on scanning laser polarimetry of the peripapillary nerve fiber layer. Am J Ophthalmol 132:507–511 (2001).

Parnaby-Price A et al. Leukocyte trafficking in experimental autoimmune uveitis in vivo. J Leukoc Biol 64:434–440 (1998).

Peyman GA et al. A fluorescent vesicle system for the measurement of blood velocity in the choroidal vessels. Ophthalmic Surg Lasers 27:459–466 (1996a).

Peyman GA et al. Fluorescent vesicle angiography with sodium fluorescein and indocyanine green. Ophthalmic Surg Lasers 27:279–284 (1996b).

Peyman GA et al. Blood velocity in an experimental iris tumor. Ophthalmic Surg Lasers 29:506–509 (1998).

Phillips DE, McCarter GS, Dwyer WO. Validity of the laser refraction technique for meridional measurement. Am J Optom Physiol Opt 53:447–450 (1976).

Phillips D, Sterling W. Validity of the laser refraction technique for determining cylindrical error. Am J Optom Physiol Opt 52:328–331 (1975).

Pieroth L et al. Evaluation of focal defects of the nerve fiber layer using optical coherence tomography. Ophthalmology 106:570–579 (1999).

Piltz-Seymour JR. Laser Doppler flowmetry of the optic nerve head in glaucoma. Surv Ophthalmol 43 (Suppl 1):S191–S198 (1999).

Poinoosawmy D et al. Variation of nerve fiber layer thickness measurements with age and ethnicity by scanning laser polarimetry. Br J Ophthalmol 81:350–354 (1997).

Poinoosawmy D et al. Longitudinal nerve fibre layer thickness change in normal-pressure glaucoma. Graefes Arch Clin Exp Ophthalmol 238:965–969 (2000).

Poinoosawmy D et al. The ability of the GDx nerve fibre analyzer neural network to diagnose glaucoma. Graefes Arch Clin Exp Ophthalmol 239:122–127 (2001).

Pons et al. Vitreous opacities affect scanning laser polarimetry measurements. Am J Ophthalmol 131:511–513 (2001).

Post RB, Johnson CA, Tsuetaki TK. Comparison of laser and infrared techniques for measurement of the resting focus of accommodation: mean differences and long-term variability. Ophthalmic Physiol Opt 4:327–332 (1984).

Puliafito CA et al. Imaging of macular diseases with optical coherence tomography. Ophthalmology 102:217–229 (1995).

Puliafito CA et al. Optical coherence tomography of ocular diseases. Thorofare, NJ: Slack Inc., 1996.

Quigley HA et al. The size and shape of the optic disc in normal human eyes. Arch Ophthalmol 108:51–57 (1990).

Remky A, Arend O, Toonen F. Infrared imaging of central serous chorioretinopathy: a follow-up study. Act Ophthalmol Scand 76:339–342 (1998).

Remky A, Beausencourt E, Elsner AE. Angioscotometry with the scanning laser ophthalmoscope. Comparison of the effect of different wavelengths. Invest Ophthalmol Vis Sci 37:2350–2355 (1996).

Remky A et al. Infrared imaging of cystoid macular edema. Graefes Arch Clin Exp Ophthalmol 237:897–901 (1999).

Repka MX, Quigley HA. The effect of age on normal human optic nerve fiber number and diameter. Ophthalmology 96:26–32 (1989).

Reyes RDC, Tomita G, Kitazawa Y. Retinal nerve fiber layer thickness within the area of apparently normal visual field in normal-tension glaucoma with hemifield defect. J Glaucoma 7:329–335 (1998).

Richman JE, Kozol N, Crawford RD. Use of interferometry in preschool children. J Am Optom Assoc 60:357–360 (1989).

Richter H, Franzen O, von Sandor R. Quantitative judgments and matching of subjective speed of apparent laser speckle flow induced by refractive defocus. Behav Brain Res 62:81–91 (1994).

Riva CE et al. Blood velocity and volumetric flow rate in human retinal vessels. Invest Ophthalmol Vis Sci 26:1124–1132 (1985).

Riva CE et al. Choroidal blood flow in the foveal region of the human ocular fundus. Invest Ophthalmol Vis Sci 35:4273–4281 (1994a).

Riva CE et al. Local choroidal blood flow in the cat by laser Doppler flowmetry. Invest Ophthalmol Vis Sci 35:608–618 (1994b).

Riva CE et al. Optic nerve and choroidal blood flow in humans by laser Doppler flowmetry. Proc SPIE Lasers in Ophthalmology II 2330:122–133 (1995).

Riva CE, Grunwald JE, Petrig BL. Reactivity of the human retinal circulation to darkness: a laser Doppler velocimetry study. Invest Ophthalmol Vis Sci 24:737–740 (1983).

Riva CE, Petrig BL. Choroidal blood flow by laser Doppler flowmetry. Opt Eng 34:746–752 (1995).

Rivero ME et al. Automated scanning laser ophthalmoscope image montages of retinal diseases. Ophthalmology 106:2296–2300 (1999).

Roberts CW, Brennan KM. A comparison of topical diclofenac with prednisolone for postcataract inflammation. Arch Ophthalmol 113:725–727 (1995).

Roh S et al. Effect of optic nerve head drusen on nerve fiber layer thickness. Ophthalmology 105:878–885 (1998).

Rohrschneider K et al. Factors influencing three-dimensional data in follow-up studies with the laser tomographic scanner. In: Nasemann JE, Burk ROW, eds. Scanning laser ophthalmoscopy and tomography. Muenchen: Quintessenz, 1990; 17:183–192.

Rohrschneider K et al. Fundus-controlled examination of reading in eyes with macular pathology. Ger J Ophthalmol 5:300–307 (1996).

Rohrschneider K et al. Normal values for fundus perimetry with the scanning laser ophthalmoscope. Am J Ophthalmol 126:52–58 (1998).

Rohrschneider K et al. Scanning laser ophthalmoscope fundus perimetry before and after laser photocoagulation for clinically significant diabetic macular edema. Am J Ophthalmol 129:27–32 (2000).

Rosenfield M. Comparison of accommodative adaptation using laser and infra-red optometers. Ophthalmic Physiol Opt 9:431–436 (1989).

Rovati L et al. Diabetic retinopathy assessed by dynamic light scattering and corneal autofluorescence. J Biomed Opt 3:357–363 (1998).

Rovati L, Fankhauser F, Ricka J. Dynamic light scattering spectroscopy of in-vivo human vitreous. Proc SPIE Lasers in Ophthalmology III 2632:73–78 (1996).

Rutgard JJ, Snyder J, Thompson HS. Interferometric acuity testing devices and loss of visual acuity [letter]. Arch Ophthalmol 98:187 (1980).

Saari KM et al. Measurement of protein concentration of aqueous humour in vivo: correlation between laser flare measurements and chemical protein determination. Acta Ophthalmol Scand 75:63–66 (1997).

Sabates NR et al. Scanning laser ophthalmoscope macular perimetry in the evaluation of submacular surgery. Retina 16:296–304 (1996).

Sanchez-Galeana C et al. Using optical imaging summary data to detect glaucoma. Ophthalmology 108:1812–1818 (2001).

Saruhan A et al. Descriptive information of topographic parameters computed at the optic nerve head with the Heidelberg Retina Tomograph. J Glaucoma 7:420–429 (1998).

Sawa M. Clinical application of laser flare-cell meter. Jpn J Ophthalmol 34:346–363 (1990).

Sawa M et al. New quantitative method to determine protein concentration and cell number in aqueous in vivo. Jpn J Ophthalmol 32:132–142 (1988).

Schalnus R, Ohrloff C. Quantification of blood-aqueous barrier function using laser flare measurement and fluorophotometry—a comparative study. Lens Eye Toxic Res 9:309–320 (1992).

Schaudig U et al. Limitations of imaging choroidal tumors in vivo by optical coherence tomography. Graefes Arch Clin Exp Ophthalmol 236:588–592 (1998).

Scheider A, Kaboth A, Neuhauser L. Detection of subretinal neovascular membranes with indocyanine green and an infrared scanning laser ophthalmoscope. Am J Ophthalmol 113:45–51 (1992).

Scheider A, Nasemann JE, Lund O-E. Fluorscein and indocyanine green angiographies of central serous choroidopathy by scanning laser ophthalmoscopy. Am J Ophthalmol 115:50–56 (1993).

Scheider A, Schroedel C. High resolution indocyanine green angiography with a scanning laser ophthalmoscope. Am J Ophthalmol 108:458–459 (1989).

Schmetterer LF et al. Topical measurement of fundus pulsations. Opt Eng 34:711–716 (1995).

Schmetterer L et al. Fundus pulsation measurements in diabetic retinopathy. Graefes Arch Clin Exp Ophthalmol 235:283–287 (1997a).

Schmetterer L et al. Effects of antiglaucoma drugs on ocular hemodynamics in healthy volunteers. Clin Pharmacol Ther 61:583–595 (1997b).

Schmetterer L et al. Noninvasive investigations of the normal ocular circulation in humans. Invest Ophthalmol Vis Sci 39:1210–1220 (1998a).

Schmetterer L et al. Topical fundus pulsation measurements in age-related macular degeneration. Graefes Arch Clin Exp Ophthalmol 236:160–163 (1998b).

Schmetterer L et al. A comparison between laser interferometric measurement of fundus pulsation and pneumotonometric measurement of pulsatile blood flow. 1. Baseline considerations. Eye 14:39–45 (2000).

Schmetterer LF, Wolzt M. Laser interferometric investigations of pulsatile choroidal blood flow: review and new results on the validity of the technique. J Biomed Opt 3:246–252 (1998).

Schneider U et al. Indocyanine green angiographically well-defined choroidal neovascularization: angiographic patterns obtained using the scanning laser ophthalmoscope. Ger J Ophthalmol 4:67–74 (1995).

Schneider U et al. Assessment of visual function in choroidal neovascularization with scanning laser microperimetry and simultaneous indocyanine green angiography. Graefes Arch Clin Exp Ophthalmol 234:612–617 (1996).

Schneider U et al. Detection of choroidal aneurysms with indocyanine green videoangiography. Graefes Arch Clin Exp Ophthalmol 236:193–195 (1998).

Schocket LS et al. The effect of pregnancy on retinal hemodynamics in diabetic versus nondiabetic mothers. Am J Ophthalmol 128:477–484 (1999).

Schoenfeld C-L et al. Prognostic factors in vitreous surgery for proliferative diabetic retinopathy. Ger J Ophthalmol 3:137–143 (1994).

Schuchard RA. Validity and interpretation of Amsler grid reports. Arch Ophthalmol 111:776–780 (1993).

Schuman JS. Optical coherence tomography for imaging and quantification of nerve fiber layer thickness. In: Schuman JS, ed. Imaging in glaucoma. Thorofare, NJ: Slack Inc., 1997; 7:95–130.

Schuman JS et al. Quantification of nerve fiber layer thickness in normal and glaucomatous eyes using optical coherence tomography. Arch Ophthalmol 113:586–596 (1995).

Schuman JS et al. Reproducibility of nerve fiber layer thickness measurements using optical coherence tomography. Ophthalmology 103:1889–1898 (1996).

Schworm HD et al. Investigations on subjective and objective cyclorotatory changes after inferior oblique muscle recession. Invest Ophthalmol Vis Sci 38:405–412 (1997).

Sebag J et al. Anterior optic nerve blood flow decreases in clinical neurogenic optic atrophy. Ophthalmology 93:858–865 (1986).

Sekiguchi N, Williams DR, Packer O. Nonlinear distortion of gratings at the foveal resolution limit. Vision Res 31:815–831 (1991).

Selenow A et al. Prognostic value of laser interferometric visual acuity in amblyopia therapy. Invest Ophthalmol Vis Sci 27:273–277 (1986).

Seong GJ, Lee HK, Hong YJ. Effects of 0.005% latanoprost on optic nerve head and peripapillary retinal blood flow. Ophthalmologica 213:355–359 (1999).

Serguhn S, Gramer E. Is staging of glaucomatous disease possible by in vivo measurement of retinal nerve fiber layer thickness with laser polarimetry? A clinical study. Ophthalmology 93:527–534 (1996).

Shah SM et al. A comparison of the laser flare cell meter and fluorophotometry in assessment of the blood-aqueous barrier. Invest Ophthalmol Vis Sci 34:3124–3130 (1993).

Shah SM, Spalton DJ, Taylor JC. Correlations between laser flare measurements and anterior chamber protein concentrations. Invest Ophthalmol Vis Sci 33:2878–2884 (1992).

Shahidi M et al. Foveal thickening in retinitis pigmentosa patients with cystoid macular edema. Retina 14:243–247 (1994).

Shahidi M et al. A new method for noninvasive optical sectioning of the chorioretinal vasculature. Invest Ophthalmol Vis Sci 39:2733–2743 (1998).

Sharma V, Levi DM, Coletta NJ. Sparse-sampling of gratings in the visual cortex of strabismic amblyopes. Vision Res 39:3526–3536 (1999).

Sharp PF et al. Laser imaging of the retina. Br J Ophthalmol 83:1241–1245 (1999).

Sherman J et al. Presurgical prediction of postsurgical visual acuity in patients with media opacities. J Am Optom Assoc 59:481–488 (1988).

Shiraga F et al. Feeder vessel photocoagulation of subfoveal choroidal neovascularization secondary to age-related macular degeneration. Ophthalmology 105:662–669 (1998).

Shirakashi M et al. Measurement of thickness of retinal nerve fiber layer by scanning laser polarimetry and high-pass resolution perimetry in patients with primary open-angle or normal-tension glaucoma. Act Ophthalmol Scand 75:641–644 (1997).

Shirakashi M et al. Measurement of retinal nerve fiber layer by scanning laser polarimetry and high pass resolution perimetry in normal tension glaucoma with relatively high or low intraocular pressure. Br J Ophthalmol 83:353–357 (1999).

Simon F, Rassow B. Retinal visual acuity with pattern VEP normal subjects and reproducibility. Graefes Arch Clin Exp Ophthalmol 224:160–164 (1986).

Sinai MJ et al. Diffuse and localized nerve fiber layer loss measured with a scanning laser polarimeter: sensitivity and specificity of detecting glaucoma. J Glaucoma 9:154–162 (2000).

Smiddy WE et al. Use of the potential acuity meter and laser interferometer to predict visual acuity after macular hole surgery. Retina 14:305–309 (1994).

Smolek M. Elasticity of the bovine sclera measured with real-time holographic interferometry. Am J Optom Physiol Opt 65:653–660 (1988).

Smolek MK. Holographic interferometry of intact and radially incised human eye-bank corneas. J Cataract Refract Surg 20:277–286 (1994).

Solbach U et al. Imaging of retinal autofluorescence in patients with age-related macular degeneration. Retina 17:385–389 (1997).

Sourdille P, Santiago PY. Optical coherence tomography of macular thickness after cataract surgery. J Cataract Refract Surg 25:256–261 (1999).

Spraul CW et al. Choroidal blood flow in AMD [letter]. Invest Ophthalmol 39:2201–2202 (1998).

Spurny RC et al. Instruments for predicting visual acuity. A clinical comparison. Arch Ophthalmol 104:196–200 (1986).

Steel DHW, Waldock A. Measurement of the retinal nerve fiber layer with scanning laser polarimetry in patients with previous demyelinating optic neuritis. J Neurol Neurosurg Psychiatry 64:505–509 (1998).

Steinert RF, Minkowski JS, Boruchoff SA. Pre-keratoplasty potential acuity evaluation: laser interferometer and potential acuity meter. Ophthalmology 91:1217–1221 (1984).

Stetter M et al. SLO saccade profile measurements and the effects of retinal raster size and distortion. Proc SPIE Lasers in Ophthalmology III. 2632:98–109 (1996).

Stetter M, Obermayer K. Simulation of scanning laser techniques for optical imaging of blood-related intrinsic signals. J Opt Soc Am A 16:58–70 (1999).

Straubhaar M et al. Choroidal laser Doppler flowmetry in healthy subjects. Arch Ophthalmol 118:211–215 (2000).

Strong N. Interferometer assessment of potential visual acuity before YAG capsulotomy: relative performance of three instruments. Graefes Arch Clin Exp Ophthalmol 230:42–46 (1992).

Sullivan P et al. The influence of ocular pulsatility on scanning laser Doppler flowmetry. Am J Ophthalmol 128:81–87 (1999).

Sunness JS, Bressler NM, Maguire MG. Scanning laser ophthalmoscopic analysis of the pattern of visual loss in age-related geographic atrophy of the macula. Am J Ophthalmol 119:143–151 (1995).

Sunness JS et al. Fixation patterns and reading rates in eyes with central scotomas from advanced atrophic age-related macular degeneration and Stargardt disease. Ophthalmology 103:1458–1466 (1996).

Suzuki Y et al. Measurement of blood flow velocity in retinal vessels utilizing laser speckle phenomenon. Jpn J Ophthalmol 35:4–15 (1991).

Swanson EA et al. High-speed optical coherence domain reflectometry. Opt Lett 17:151–153 (1992).

Swanson EA et al. In vivo retinal imaging by optical coherence tomography. Opt Lett 18:1864–1866 (1993).

Swanson WH et al. Interoperator variability in images obtained by laser polarimetry of the nerve fiber layer. J Galucoma 4:414–418 (1995).

Swindale NV et al. Automated analysis of normal and glaucomatous optic nerve head topography images. Invest Ophthalmol Vis Sci 41:1730–1742 (2000).

Tabbut SE, Lindstrom RL. Laser retinometry versus clinical estimation of media: a comparison of efficacy in predicting visual acuity in patients with lens opacities. J Cataract Refract Surg 12:140–145 (1986).

Takamine Y et al. Retinal sensitivity measurement over drusen using scanning laser ophthalmoscope microperimetry. Graefes Arch Clin Exp Ophthalmol 236:285–290 (1998).

Tamaki Y et al. An application of laser speckle phenomenon for noninvasive two-dimensional evaluation of microcirculation in ocular fundus—a preliminary report. Jpn J Ophthalmol 37:178–186 (1993).

Tamaki Y et al. Non-contact, two-dimensional measurement of retinal microcirculation using laser speckle phenomenon. Invest Ophthalmol Vis Sci 35:3825–3834 (1994).

Tamaki Y et al. Non-contact, two-dimensional measurement of tissue circulation in choroid and optic nerve head using laser speckle phenomenon. Exp Eye Res 60:373–383 (1995).

Tamaki Y et al. Real-time measurement of human optic nerve head and choroid circulation, using the laser speckle phenomenon. Jpn J Ophthalmol 41:49–54 (1997a).

Tamaki Y et al. Effect of topical timolol on tissue circulation in the optic nerve head. Jpn J Ophthalmol 41:297–304 (1997b).

Tamaki Y et al. Effect of topical carteolol on tissue circulation in the optic nerve head. Jpn J Ophthalmol 42:27–32 (1998).

Tamaki Y et al. Acute effects of cigarette smoking on tissue circulation in human optic nerve head and choroids-retina. Ophthalmology 106:564–569 (1999a).

Tamaki Y et al. Effect of topical betaxolol on tissue circulation in the human optic nerve head. J Ocul Pharmacol Ther 15:313–321 (1999b).

Tamaki Y et al. Effects of pranidipine, a new calcium antagonist, on circulation in the choroid, retina and optic nerve head. Curr Eye Res 19:241–247 (1999c).

Tanna AP et al. Optical cross-sectional imaging of the macular with the retinal thickness analyzer in X-linked retinoschisis. Arch Ophthalmol 116:1036–1041 (1998).

Tannenbaum DP et al. Relationship between visual field testing and scanning laser polarimetry in patients with a large cup-to-disk ratio. Am J Ophthalmol 132:501–506 (2001).

Tezel TH et al. Correlation between scanning laser ophthalmoscope microperimetry and anatomic abnormalities in patients with subfoveal neovascularization. Ophthalmology 103:1829–1836 (1996).

Theodossiadis PG et al. Optical coherence tomography in the study of the Goldmann-Favre syndrome. Am J Ophthalmol 129:542–544 (2000).

Thibos LN, Bradley A. Use of interferometric visual stimulators in optometry. Ophthal Physiol Opt 12:206–208 (1992).

Thurschwell LM. Presurgical evaluation of patients with cataracts. Optom Clin 1:159–187 (1991).

Thurston GM et al. Quasielastic light scattering study of the living human lens as a function of age. Curr Eye Res 16:197–207 (1997).

Timberlake GT, Van de Velde FJ, Jalkh AE. Clinical use of scanning laser ophthalmoscope retinal function maps in macular disease. Lasers Light Ophthalmol 2:211–222 (1989).

Tjon-Fo-Sang MJ, de Vries J, Lemij HG. Measurement by nerve fiber analyzer of retinal nerve fiber layer thickness in normal subjects and patients with ocular hypertension. Am J Ophthalmol 122:220–227 (1996).

Tjon-Fo-Sang MJ et al. Improved reproducibility of measurements with the Nerve Fiber Analyzer. J Glaucoma 6:203–211 (1997).

Tjon-Fo-Sang MJ, Lemij HG. The sensitivity and specificity of nerve fiber layer measurements in glaucoma as determined with scanning laser polarimetry. Am J Ophthalmol 123:62–69 (1997).

Tjon-Fo-Sang MJ, Lemij HG. Retinal nerve fiber layer measurements in normal black subjects as determined with scanning laser polarimetry. Ophthalmology 105:78–81 (1998).

Tole DM et al. The correlation of the visual field with scanning laser ophthalmoscope measurements in glaucoma. Eye 12:686–690 (1998).

Tomidokoro A et al. In vivo measurement of iridial circulation using laser speckle phenomenon. Invest Ophthalmol Vis Sci 39:364–371 (1998).

Tomidokoro A et al. Effects of topical carteolol and timolol on tissue circulation in the iris and choroid. Curr Eye Res 18:381–390 (1999).

Toonen F et al. Microperimetry in patients with central serous retinopathy. Ger J Ophthalmol 4:311–314 (1995).

Toprak AB, Yilmaz OF. Relation of optic disc topography and age to thickness of retinal nerve fibre layer as measured using scanning laser polarimetry, in normal subjects. Br J Ophthalmol 84:473–478 (2000).

Tornow RP, Stilling R. Variation in sensitivity, absorption and density of the central rod distribution with eccentricity. Acta Anat (Basel) 162:163–168 (1998).

Toth CA et al. Argon laser retinal lesions evaluated in vivo by optical coherence tomography. Am J Ophthalmol 123:188–198 (1997a).

Toth CA et al. A comparison of retinal morphology viewed by optical coherence tomography and by light microscopy. Arch Ophthalmol 115:1425–1428 (1997b).

Trauzettel-Klossinski S, Reinhard J. The veritical field border in hemianopia and its significance for fixation and reading. Invest Ophthal Vis Sci 39:2177–2186 (1998).

Trible JR et al. Accuracy of scanning laser polarimetry in the diagnosis of glaucoma. Arch Ophthalmol 117:1298–1304 (1999).

Trick GL et al. Quantitative evaluation of papilledema in pseudotumor cerebri. Invest Ophthalmol Vis Sci 39:1964–1971 (1998).

Tsai YY, Lin JM. Effect of laser-assisted in situ keratomileusis on the retinal nerve fiber layer. Retina 20:342–345 (2000).

Tsujikawa M et al. Differentiating full thickness macular holes from impending macular holes and macular pseudoholes. Br J Ophthalmol 81:117–122 (1997).

Tsujikawa A et al. In vivo evaluation of leukocyte dynamics in retinal ischemia reperfusion injury. Invest Ophthalmol Vis Sci 39:793–800 (1998).

Tsujikawa A et al. Quantitative analysis of diabetic macular edema after scatter laser photocoagulation with the scanning retinal thickness analyzer. Retina 19:59–64 (1999).

Tuulonen A, Yalvac IS. Pseudodefects of the retinal nerve fiber layer examined using optical coherence tomography. Arch Ophthalmol 118:575–576 (2000).

Uchida H, Brigatti L, Caprioli J. Detection of structural damage from glaucoma with confocal laser image analysis. Invest Ophthalmol Vis Sci 37:2393–2401 (1996a).

Uchida H et al. Relationship of nerve fiber layer defects and parafoveal visual field defects in glaucomatous eyes. Jpn J Ophthalmol 40:548–553 (1996b).

Uchino E et al. Postsurgical evaluation of idiopathic vitreomacular traction syndrome by optical coherence tomography. Am J Ophthalmol 132:122–123 (2001).

Uhlhorn SR et al. Corneal group refractive index measurement using low-coherence interferometry. Proc SPIE Ophthamic Technologies VIII 3246:14–21 (1998).

Van Blokland GJ. Ellipsometry of the human retina in vivo: preservation of polarization. J Opt Soc Am A 2:72–75 (1985).

Van Blokland GJ, Verhelst SC. Corneal polarization in the living human eye explained with a biaxial model. J Opt Soc Am A 4:82–90 (1987).

Van de Velde FJ, Tassignon MJ, Trau R. Scanning laser retinoscopy: a new technique for evaluating optical properties of the cornea after refractive surgery. Proc SPIE Medical Applications of Lasers in Dermatology, Ophthalmology, Dentistry, and Endoscopy. 3192:187–194 (1997).

Van Laethem M et al. Photon correlation spectroscopy of light scattered by eye lenses in in vivo conditions. Biophys J 59:433–444 (1991).

Van Meel GJ et al. Scanning laser densitometry in multiple evanescent white dot syndrome. Retina 13:29–35 (1993).

VanderMeulen DL et al. Laser mediated release of dye from liposomes. Photochem Photobiol 56:325–332 (1992).

Varano M et al. Scanning laser ophthalmoscopy in the early diagnosis of vitreoretinal interface syndrome. Retina 17:300–305 (1997).

Varano M, Scassa C. Scanning laser ophthalmoscope microperimetry. Semin Ophthalmol 13:203–209 (1998).

Varma R, Skaf M, Barron E. Retinal nerve fiber layer thickness in normal human eyes. Ophthalmology 103:2114–2119 (1996).

Vernon SA et al. White light interferometry in amblyopic children—a pilot study. Eye 4:802–805 (1990).

Vetrugno M et al. Retinal nerve fiber layer measurements using scanning laser polarimetry after photorefractive keratectomy. Eur J Ophthalmol 10:137–143 (2000).

Vieira P et al. Tomographic reconstruction of the retina using a confocal scanning laser ophthalmoscope. Physiol Meas 20:1–19 (1999).

Vitale S et al. Screening performance of functional and structural measurements of neural damage in open-angle glaucoma: a case-control study from the Baltimore Eye Surgery. J Glaucoma 9:346–356 (2000).

Von Rueckmann A, Fitzke FW, Bird AC. Fundus autofluorescence in age related macular disease imaged with a laser scanning ophthalmoscope. Invest Ophthalmol Vis Sci 38:478–486 (1997a).

Von Rueckmann A, Fitzke FW, Bird AC. In vivo fundus autofluorescence in macular dystrophies. Arch Ophthalmol 115:609–615 (1997b).

Von Rueckmann A, Fitzke FW, Gregor ZJ. Fundus autofluorescence in patients with macular holes imaged with a laser scanning ophthalmoscope. Br J Ophthalmol 82:346–351 (1998).

Waelti R et al. Rapid and precise in vivo measurement of human corneal thickness with optical low-coherence reflectometry in normal human eyes. J Biomed Opt 3:253–258 (1998).

Waldock A et al. Clinical evaluation of scanning laser polarimetry: I. Intraoperator reproducibility and design of a blood vessel removal algorithm. Br J Ophthalmol 82:252–259 (1998a).

Waldock A et al. Clinical evaluation of scanning laser polarimetry: II. Polar profile shape analysis. Br J Ophthalmol 82:260–266 (1998b).

Wang L, Yamasita R, Hommura S. Corneal endothelial changes and aqueous flare intensity in pseudoexfoliation syndrome. Ophthalmologica 213:387–391 (1999a).

Wang M et al. Detection of shallow detachments in central serous chorioretinopathy. Acta Ophthalmol Scand 77:402–405 (1999b).

Watts P, KaraKucuk S, McAllister J. Measurement of the retinal nerve fiber layer thickness with a nerve fiber analyzer in normal subjects. Lasers Light 7:79–84 (1996).

Weale RA. Sex, age and the birefringence of the human crystalline lens. Exp Eye Res 29:449–461 (1979).

Webb RH. Scanning laser ophthalmoscope. In: Masters BR, ed. Noninvasive diagnostic techniques in ophthalmology. New York: Springer-Verlag, 1990; 22:438–450.

Webb RH, Delori FC. How we see the retina. In: Marshall J, ed. Laser technology in ophthalmology. Amsterdam: Kugler and Ghedini, 1988; 3–14.

Webb RH, Hughes GW, Pomerantzeff. Flying spot TV ophthalmoscope. Appl Opt 19:2991–2997 (1980).

Weinberger D et al. Three-dimensional measurements of topographical changes in macular diseases using confocal laser tomography. Lasers Light 8:39–45 (1997).

Weinreb RN. Laser scanning tomography to diagnose and monitor glaucoma. Curr Opinion Ophthalmol 4;II:3–6 (1993).

Weinreb RN, Dreher AW, Bille JF. Quantitative assessment of the optic nerve head with the laser tomographic scanner. Intl Ophthalmol 13:25–29 (1989).

Weinreb RN et al. Histopathologic validation of Fourier-ellipsometry measurements of retinal nerve fiber layer thickness. Arch Ophthalmol 108:557–560 (1990).

Weinreb RN et al. Effect of repetitive imaging on topographic measurements of the optic nerve head. Arch Ophthalmol 111:636–638 (1993).

Weinreb RN et al. Association between quantitative nerve fiber layer measurement and visual field loss in glaucoma. Am J Ophthalmol 120:732–738 (1995a).

Weinreb RN, Shakiba S, Zangwill L. Scanning laser polarimetry to measure the nerve fiber layer of normal and glaucomatous eyes. Am J Ophthalmol 119:627–636 (1995b).

Weinreb RN et al. Detection of glaucoma with scanning laser polarimetry. Arch Ophthalmol 116:1583–1589 (1998).

Whitefoot HD, Charman WN. A comparison between laser and conventional subjective refraction. Ophthalmic Opt 20:169–173 (1980).

Whitefoot HD, Charman WN. Dynamic retinoscopy and accommodation. Ophthalmic Physiol Opt 12:8–17 (1992).

Williams DR et al. Double-pass and interferometric measures of the optical quality of the eye. J Opt Soc Am A 11:3123–3135 (1994).

Wolf S, Arend O, Reim M. Measurement of retinal hemodynamics with scanning laser ophthalmoscopy: reference values and variation. Surv Ophthalmol 38 (Suppl):S95–S100 (1994).

Wolf S et al. Retinal capillary blood flow measurement with a scanning laser ophthalmoscope. Preliminary results. Ophthalmol 98:996–1000 (1991).

Wolf S et al. Indocyanine green video angiography in patients with age-related maculopathy-related retinal pigment epithelial detachments. Ger J Ophthalmol 3:224–227 (1994).

Wollstein G et al. Identifying early glaucomatous changes. Comparison between expert clinical assessment of optic disc photographs and confocal scanning ophthalmoscopy. Ophthalmology 107:2272–2277 (2000).

Wollstein G, Garway-Heath DF, Hitchings RA. Identification of early glaucoma cases with the scanning laser ophthalmoscope. Ophthalmology 105:1557–1563 (1998).

Woon WH et al. The scanning laser ophthalmoscope. Basic principles and applications. J Ophthalmic Photography 12:17–23 (1990).

Wormington CM, Alaniz RV. Retinal nerve fiber layer thickness in normal vs. glaucomatous eyes of black subjects. Invest Ophthalmol Vis Sci 75 (Suppl): 39 (1998).

Xu L et al. Quantitative nerve fiber layer measurement using scanning laser polarimetry and modulation parameters in the detection of glaucoma. J Glaucoma 7:270–277 (1998).

Yamada N et al. Glaucoma screening using the scanning laser polarimeter. J Glaucoma 9:254–261 (2000).

Yamagishi N et al. Mapping structural damage of the optic disk to visual field defect in glaucoma. Am J Ophthalmol 123:667–676 (1997).

Yamazaki Y et al. Influence of myopic disc shape on the diagnositic precision of the Heidelberg retina tomograph. Jpn J Ophthalmol 43:392–397 (1999).

Yan DB et al. Study of regional deformation of the optic nerve head using scanning laser tomography. Curr Eye Res 17:903–916 (1998).

Yang Y, Kim S, Kim J. Fluorescent dots in fluorescein angiography and fluorescein leukocyte angiography using a scanning laser ophthalmoscope in humans. Ophthalmology 104:1670–1676 (1997a).

Yang Y, Kim S, Kim J. Visualization of retinal and choroidal blood flow with fluorescein leukocyte angiography in rabbits. Graefes Arch Clin Exp Ophthamol 235:27–31 (1997b).

Yokotsuka K, Kishi S, Shimizu K. White dot fovea. Am J Ophthalmol 123:76–83 (1997).

Yoshida A et al. New laser Doppler system for examining optic nerve head circulation. J Biomed Opt 3:396–400 (1998a).

Yoshida A et al. Radiating retinal fields detected by scanning laser ophthalmoscopy using a diode laser in a dark-field mode in idiopathic macular holes. Graefes Arch Clin Exp Ophthalmol 236:445–450 (1998b).

Yu N-T et al. Development of a noninvasive diabetes screening device using the ratio of fluorescence to Rayleigh scattered light. J Biomed Opt 1:280–288 (1996).

Zaczek A, Hallnas K, Zetterstrom C. Aqueous flare intensity in relation to different stages of diabetic retinopathy. Eur J Ophthalmol 9:158–164 (1999).

Zambarakji HJ et al. Reproducibility of volumetric measurements of normal maculae with the Heidelberg retina tomograph. Br J Ophthalmol 82:884–891 (1998).

Zambarakji HJ, Butler TKH, Vernon SA. Assessment of the Heidelberg Retina Tomograph in the detection of sight-threatening diabetic maculopathy. Eye 13:136–144 (1999).

Zangwill L, de Souza Lima M, Weinreb RN. Confocal scanning laser ophthalmoscopy to detect glaucomatous optic neuropathy. In: Schuman JS, ed. Imaging in glaucoma. Thorofare, NJ: Slack Inc., 1997b; 4:45–58.

Zangwill L et al. Reproducibility of retardation measurements with the Nerve Fiber Analyzer II. J Glaucoma 6:384–389 (1997a).

Zangwill L et al. Effect of cataract and pupil size on image quality with confocal scanning laser ophthalmoscopy. Arch Ophthalmol 115:983–990 (1997c).

Zangwill L, Williams JM, Weinreb RN. Quantitative methods for evaluating the retinal nerve fiber layer in glaucoma. Ophthalmol Clin North Am 11:233–241 (1998).

Zangwill LM et al. New technologies for diagnosing and monitoring glaucomatous optic neuropathy. Optometry Vis Sci 76:526–536 (1999).

Zangwill LM et al. Discriminating between normal and glaucomatous eyes using the Heidelberg retina tomograph, GDx nerve fiber analyzer, and optical coherence tomograph. Arch Ophthalmol 119:1985–1993 (2001).

Zeimer R et al. Quantitative detection of glaucomatous damage at the posterior pole by retinal thickness mapping. Ophthalmology 105:224–231 (1998).

Zeimer RC et al. Visualization of the retinal microvasculature by targeted dye delivery. Invest Ophthalmol Vis Sci 31:1459–1465 (1990).

Zeimer RC et al. A new method for rapid mapping of the retinal thickness at the posterior pole. Invest Ophthalmol Vis Sci 37:1994–2001 (1996).

Zhao J et al. Delayed macular choriocapillary circulation in age-related macular degeneration. Int Ophthalmol 19:1–12 (1995).

Chapter 4
Clinical Laser Vision Correction

David Gubman

I. Indications and Contraindications—Patient Candidacy

A. Patient Identification

1. Patients may call to inquire about refractive procedures as a result of direct marketing by television, radio, and print media.

2. Patients may inquire during a clinical office visit for their comprehensive ocular examination or during a follow-up visit where the primary reason for the visit is something other than refractive surgery.

3. Patients who complain about contact lens or spectacle intolerance may ask for alternative treatment options.

4. Doctors may suggest refractive procedures based on examination findings as one of several methods for the treatment of refractive disorders. The advent of the ophthalmic excimer laser has moved refractive procedures into the realm of an accepted treatment modality along with glasses and contact lenses.

B. Patient Expectations

1. The patient can reasonably expect to become dramatically less dependent on traditional optical prosthetic devices such as glasses and contact lenses following refractive procedures. Those originally 100% dependent on optical aids, even to find the bathroom at night, will usually find 85% to 100% freedom from these devices. Published clinical data show 93% of eyes achieving 20/40 or better distance visual acuity following PRK (Farah et al., 1998; McDonald et al., 1989, 1990).

2. Despite these impressive results, the patient's occupation, avocation, and visual demands dictate the degree of freedom from glasses and contact lenses that any given patient may achieve.

3. The patient's personality and psychology also play a role in the level of visual clarity demanded. Some patients are content with 20/30 visual acuity, while others are bothered by even the mildest blur despite 20/20 or 20/15 acuity.

4. Excimer refractive procedures do not treat presbyopia directly. Therefore, patients cannot reasonably expect to discard their optical aids for the rest of their lives. Monovision is an important pre-procedural consideration that warrants exploration with each patient in order to provide the most functional correction over the long term. Although it is not desirable for all or perhaps even the majority of patients, monovision should be considered and possibly tested with disposable contact lenses prior to the procedure.

5. Mild refractive changes requiring spectacle or contact lens prescription adjustment over the years are common (Curtin, 1985). Refractive procedures do not prevent this occurrence.

6. An optimal clinical outcome following a refractive procedure may be experienced as a failure by a patient with unrealistic expectations.

II. Pre-Procedural Examination

A. *Introduction*

1. The initial examination may serve as a pre-procedural evaluation depending on the status of previous contact lens wear.

2. Patients currently in lens wear must discontinue all contact lens wear for 2 weeks for hydrogel and 3 weeks for hard lens wear.

3. Polymethylmethacrylate wearers, especially those displaying even the mildest signs of microcystic edema, will benefit from a temporary refit into a rigid gas permeable material prior to any refractive procedure. This will minimize the chances of corneal distortion upon discontinuation of PMMA lens wear (Rengstorff, 1992).

4. Ultimately, corneal stability and therefore refractive stability at the patient's true baseline is the pre-procedure goal.

B. *Ocular and Systemic History*

1. As with any medical procedure, the history should document the patient's chief complaint and symptoms, especially intolerance to optical aids.

2. Previous ocular trauma, family ocular history including relatives with cataracts and glaucoma, and the age of onset should be reviewed and compared with the **ocular relative versus absolute contraindications** (Table 4–1). Systemic history and current medications should also be reviewed and compared with the **systemic relative versus absolute contraindications** (Table 4–2).

C. *Contact Lens History*

1. The length of time glasses and contact lenses have been worn as well as any complications of these treatments should be recorded.

Table 4–1 Ocular Contraindications for Refractive
Surgery Procedures

Ocular Relative Contraindications	*Ocular Absolute Contraindications*
Unstable refractive error	Cataract
Keratoconjunctivitis sicca	Glaucoma
Blepharitis	Keratoconus
Recurrent or active ocular disease	Amblyopia—monocular function
Irregular astigmatism by topography	
Exposure keratitis/lagophthalmos	
HSV keratitis (active/inactive)	
Previous ocular surgery	

2. Daily or extended wearing times, vision, comfort, and care systems in all lens types worn will describe the patient's contact lens experience and compliance.

D. *Corneal Curvature*

1. Keratometry values with demonstrable stability and repeatability, especially in light of any contact lens wear, are critical prior to any corneal procedure and should be recorded.

2. Mire quality should be recorded and any distortion of the mire reflection described. A simple observation of the mires between blinks is a valuable and noninvasive method of evaluating ocular surface tear–break-up time.

3. A comparison of the corneal toricity and the overall astigmatic refractive error will allow for an accurate interpretation of residual astigmatism, an important factor for a given patient's prognosis.

4. A diagnostic spherical rigid contact lens trial evaluation will confirm the visual significance of any residual astigmatism.

Table 4–2 Systemic Contraindications for Refractive
Surgery Procedures

Systemic Relative Contraindications	*Systemic Absolute Contraindications*
Diabetes mellitus	Pregnant/lactating women
Atopy—severe allergy, eczema, asthma	Rheumatoid arthritis
	Systemic lupus erythematosus
	Collagen vascular disease

5. Corneal topography is an essential tool because of the increased number of data points analyzed and the additional information revealed about the peripheral corneal surface. Furthermore, corneal topography has proven to be the most sensitive clinical instrument in detecting early keratoconus or other peripheral degenerations (Koch & Husain, 1995; Maguire & Bourne, 1989, Maguire & Lowry, 1991, Nesburn et al., 1992; Wilson & Klyce, 1994).

E. *Refractive Error Analysis*

1. The heart of the field of refractive surgery quite obviously centers on the patient's refractive error.

2. Uncorrected visual acuity and best-corrected visual acuity should be documented OD, OS, and OU.

3. The nature and magnitude of the baseline refraction will determine the refractive treatments and procedures available to the patient.

4. Experienced objective retinoscopy followed by subjective refractive refinement to best-corrected acuity defines the starting point for refractive error analysis.

5. Cycloplegia is recommended with 1% cyclopentolate (2 gtts; 5 min apart) because of its rapid onset (20 to 45 min), relatively short duration of action (8 to 24 hr) and most importantly, its efficacy, resulting in minimal residual accommodation (Gettes & Belmont, 1961). One drop of 2.5% phenylephrine is also used for maximal dilation and retinal evaluation. Objective and subjective retinoscopy should then be repeated and the results compared with the dry or non-cyclopleged data to rule out any accommodative component or pseudomyopia.

6. This baseline data should be recorded and the refraction repeated on at least one additional occasion to demonstrate refractive stability. Unstable refractive findings may result from undiagnosed/borderline diabetes, corneal distortion from CL wear, accommodative infacility/hysteresis, or progressive myopic changes, etc. Refractive fluctuation has the potential to cause serious over- or undercorrection and must therefore be detected, diagnosed and treated prior to any permanent refractive procedure.

F. *Binocular Vision*

1. Binocular function often has a significant impact on refractive error and stability.

2. Evaluation for high phoria, intermittent strabismus, and accommodative dysfunction must also be performed prior to refractive surgery in order to ensure an optimal outcome.

3. A patient with undiagnosed accommodative infacility may habitually wear stronger refractive correction than indicated by the true refractive error. Similarly, a patient with convergence insufficiency may be utilizing more accommodative convergence than normal in order to maintain fusion.

4. A sudden change in refractive status has the potential to create diplopia due to previously undetected binocular dysfunction (Mandava et al., 1996).

5. Furthermore, binocular inefficiency in the vergence or accommodative systems can easily be the underlying etiology for visual and refractive fluctuation.

6. Once again, these conditions must therefore be detected, diagnosed, and treated prior to any permanent refractive procedure.

7. Because refractive surgery does not treat presbyopia, ocular dominance should be determined and a monovision result considered.

G. Ocular Health Assessment

1. Anterior segment evaluation should rule out pre-existing disease such as blepharitis, keratoconus, corneal dystrophy, and any notable lens changes or early cataracts. Corneal scarring or vascularization from contact lens wear should also be described.

2. Pupil size, especially in dim illumination, should be measured and compared with the known treatment zone sizes for refractive surgery procedures. Large pupil size is a significant risk factor for visual disturbances such as glare and halos, particularly at night.

3. Intraocular pressure is measured and used as a baseline guide both to rule out risk factors for glaucoma and because the patient may require temporary topical steroid administration following a refractive procedure.

4. Complete dilated funduscopic evaluation is required especially in myopes due to their increased risk for retinal disease. Prophylactic treatment may be indicated for peripheral retinal lesions or lattice holes.

H. **Determine best procedure** based on patient's refractive error and occupation/avocation.

I. **Determine target refraction:** emmetropia vs. monovision. Discuss and demonstrate where appropriate including a trial monovision fitting to evaluate tolerance.

J. **Determine patient motivation and expectations** especially in reference to occupation and avocation.

1. Law enforcement officers and others at risk for ocular trauma are better candidates for excimer than incisional techniques.

2. Medically qualified candidates for a refractive procedure who indicate that 20/20 perfect vision is the only acceptable result should be considered noncandidates on the basis of inappropriate expectation.

3. Freedom from their current dependence on glasses and contact lenses, but allowing the possibility for using a thin pair of glasses about 10% of the time, is a more realistic expectation of the results attained with these procedures.

188 • *Chapter 4: Clinical Laser Vision Correction*

K. Pain

1. Advise patients that all refractive procedures on the eye will involve some ocular discomfort or pain (depending on the degree of epithelial disruption). Pain is a very individual experience, and some will experience significant discomfort while others may go about their normal activities with only a mild scratchy sensation.

2. Prepare all patients by telling them that they may very well experience discomfort or pain for the first 1 to 3 days but that there are methods for treating and managing these symptoms. However, this discomfort is typically not so severe that patients avoid having the second eye treated. Patients usually take off 1 to 2 days of work, and the first day following the procedure is best tolerated by rest, limited activity, and sleep.

III. Photorefractive Keratectomy (PRK)

A. Laser Preparation

1. **Calibration**
   a. Summit—gelatin filter—number of pulses required to ablate and resulting pattern evaluated for calibration.
   b. VISX—PMMA test plastics evaluated on lensometer for refractive effect and ablation quality under magnification.
   c. Fluence adjustments are made to bring instruments to optimal calibration.

2. **Laser programming**
   a. Adjustment is performed via a nomogram based on altitude, humidity, patient age, and laser performance.
   b. Input desired optical correction accounting for vertex distance effectiveness.

B. Pre-Procedure Medications

1. Anesthetic—tetracaine or proparacaine—topical only
2. NSAIDs—diclofenac or ketorolac—assist in alleviating immediate post-procedural pain.
3. Antibiotic—prophylaxis.
4. Miotic—pilocarpine 1%—aids in laser alignment for Summit instrument. Glare reduction may benefit patient fixation during procedure. However, asymmetric pupil constriction can cause decentered ablation and subsequent poor visual outcome due to entrance pupil crossing treated and non-treated cornea. Glare, halos, and irregular astigmatism can complicate the outcome.
5. Sedation—occasional use depending on patient anxiety level: Ativan 0.5 to 2.0 mg or Valium 5.0 to 20 mg 20 min prior to the procedure.

C. *Ocular Preparation*

1. Cover fellow eye—this avoids fixation confusion during the procedure.

2. Position the patient beneath the laser and align the eye with aiming beams.

3. Insert lid speculum.

4. Mark ablation center at either the visual axis or unconstricted pupil center depending on instrument and recommended technique.

5. Use optical zone marker to circumscribe the desired treatment zone.

6. Patient orientation tests are recommended to familiarize the patient with the sounds and sensations experienced during treatment. First, a hydroxymethylcellulose drop is placed on the cornea and the laser is applied for a few pulses. This drop is removed with a spear sponge and several additional pulses are applied to the corneal epithelium that produces a characteristic crackling sound. Both of these tests allow the patient to experience the laser application prior to any treatment effects, and the doctor may observe the patient reaction and reinforce instructions and the importance of fixation during lasing.

7. **Epithelial removal**
   a. **Mechanical debridement.** A blunt or sharp instrument is employed to physically remove the epithelium over the treatment zone. Healthy intact epithelium is strongly adherent and requires a firm technique. Beginning at the edge of the optical zone mark, the epithelium is removed until the entire zone is debrided. Some advocate a circular approach leaving the central epithelium to be removed last. Hydration can affect the rate of ablation, and leaving the epithelium intact centrally until the last possible moment is thought to minimize changes in hydration. Mechanical debridement is the preferred and most common technique used for PRK.
   b. **Trans-epithelial ablation.** This is used more frequently for repeat PRK with regression and haze or for RK enhancements. The appropriate endpoint is more difficult to determine using this technique since the endpoint is defined by the absence of fluorescent glow that occurs during epithelial ablation. The epithelium is composed of several layers under constant mitosis and migration and is therefore not a uniform layer. The technique is performed with room and instrument lights dim so the initial fluorescence may be first observed and then its subsequent absence indicating complete epithelial ablation.
   c. **Chemical epithelial removal.** Alcohol 5% to 25% applied for 10–20 sec has been attempted. Although effective in epithelial removal, this procedure has been shown to alter the hydration of the underlying stroma. It has been associated with increased incidence of post-procedural haze and regression (Machat, 1996).

D. Laser Application

1. Alignment and fixation are reconfirmed and the doctor's hands placed on each side of the patient's head to aid stability.

2. The lasing footpedal is depressed to begin the ablation.

3. Continuous encouragement and reinforcement on fixation are given to the patient during treatment that lasts less than 1 min for most refractive errors.

4. Although immediate and efficient transition from epithelial removal to excimer ablation is desired for hydration reasons, during the laser application centration becomes paramount. Any saccade or drift from fixation should cause an immediate temporary cessation of the procedure until fixation and alignment are reestablished. Such realignment should be achieved several times during the procedure, if necessary, in order to ensure all of the pulses are delivered and well centered in the treatment zone.

E. PRK Immediate Post-Laser Application Management

1. 2 gtt Tobradex.

2. 1 gtt Voltaren.

3. Apply therapeutic bandage hydrogel lens—+0.50 disposable.

4. Remove lid speculum.

5. Patient will notice immediate improvement in vision over pre-procedure uncorrected visual acuity.

IV. Laser in Situ Keratomileusis (LASIK)

A. Introduction

1. Laser in situ keratomileusis (LASIK) is a refractive procedure that utilizes the precision of the excimer laser to sculpt corneal tissue along with the microkeratome's accessibility to the inner stroma and Bowman's membrane.

2. LASIK involves ablation of the stroma of the cornea following the creation of a corneal flap using a microkeratome. The corneal flap is usually one-third of the corneal thickness at approximately 130–160 μm thick. This flap has a nasal hinge to allow proper realignment of the flap and prevent flap loss. The corneal flap is repositioned without the need for sutures.

B. LASIK Technique

1. **Surgical preparation**
   a. The microkeratome should be assembled and tested before use. The manufacturer's recommended laser setup should be followed, and laser calibration via fluence testing implemented as usual.

2. Carefully remove bandage hydrogel lens. Use copious lubricants to achieve lens movement and removal.

3. D/C Tobradex.

4. Use FML 0.1% QID.

5. D/C Voltaren. If discomfort persists, see the patient immediately.

6. Expect the VA to be in the 20/40 to 20/100 range.

7. Although the epithelium is closed, it is not smooth and regular so continued mild scratchiness or foreign body sensation may be present for 2 to 3 days.

8. Postoperative instructions: No swimming for 1 month. Patients may swim in chlorinated pool, an ocean, or a lake or river at 1 month after surgery. Avoid all contact lens use in the treated eye. UV protection is indicated, especially for tanning or skiing activities throughout the healing period. UV can dramatically alter the healing process any time during the 6-month healing period by increasing haze and refractive regression toward myopia.

C. One-Month Visit

1. Uncorrected visual acuity—expect 20/15 to 20/60.

2. Objective and subjective refraction—expect mild hyperopia up to +1.00 D.

3. Corneal evaluation (biomicroscopy): grade corneal haze present—normal, none, significant.

4. Check IOP—watch for steroid responders.

5. Diagnose healing type: normal, inadequate, aggressive. Alter topical medications accordingly:
   a. Normal healing—Type I (Durrie et al., 1995)
      1) Taper FML 0.1% by 1 gtt/month
         TID—second month
         BID—third month
         QD—fourth month; then D/C
      2) RTO in 2 months for 3-month visit
   b. Inadequate healing—Type II (Durrie et al., 1995)
      1) Taper FML 0.1% quickly
         TID—4 days
         BID—3 days
         QD—2 days then D/C
      2) RTO in 2 months for 3-month visit
   c. Aggressive healing—Type III (Durrie et al., 1995)
      1) Increase FML 0.1% to FML Forte QID

      2) Add Voltaren TID

      3) RTO in 1 month for follow-up

6. Expectations—many patients will have excellent functional vision at this visit, especially if they are able to accommodate through the initial hyperopia. Others will need reassurance that they have not yet reached their endpoint refraction and their eye is continuing the healing process. This will occur over the subsequent weeks and months.

7. Night vision. Patients may be more aware of their temporary initial hyperopia or halos and glare at night. This is a temporary refractive situation. Once stabilized, many patients eventually benefit from a mild pair of glasses for driving at night. Because we recommend that everyone should own a pair of sunglasses, one common way to provide for both needs is to use photosensitive lenses, which can serve as sunglasses during the day, and will also allow optimal night driving vision.

D. Three-Month Visit

1. Uncorrected visual acuity—expect 20/15 to 20/40.

2. Objective and subjective refraction—expect mild hyperopia up to +0.50 D.

3. Corneal evaluation (biomicroscopy): grade corneal haze present—normal, none, significant.

4. Check IOP—watch for steroid responders.

5. Perform a dilated fundus examination.

6. Confirm healing type
    a. Inadequate healing—consider extended wear bandage lens to induce healing.
    b. Aggressive healing—adjust and taper topicals as appropriate.

7. Second eye—pre-procedure assessment if first eye is stable and healing normally.

E. Six-Month Visit

1. Uncorrected visual acuity—expect 20/15 to 20/60.

2. Objective and subjective refraction—most patients have reached their endpoint refraction by this visit.

3. Corneal evaluation (biomicroscopy): grade corneal haze present—normal, none, significant.

4. Check IOP.

5. If corneal appearance or refractive result departs significantly from intended, consider secondary enhancement procedures.

F. One-Year Visit

1. Uncorrected visual acuity—expect 20/15 to 20/60.

2. Objective and subjective refraction—most patients have reached their endpoint refraction by this visit.

3. Corneal evaluation (biomicroscopy): grade corneal haze present—normal, none, significant.

4. Check IOP.

5. Return for annual examination including dilation and re-educate on risks and signs and symptoms of retinal detachment.

VII. LASIK Post-Procedural Evaluation and Management

A. One-Day Visit

1. Check for displacement of corneal flap.
    a. If it happens, it will usually occur during the first 48 hours.
    b. If the corneal flap is displaced, then the patient must maintain good hydration of the cornea.

2. Visual acuity
    a. It is normal to have acuity fluctuation.
    b. Evaluate uncorrected visual acuity.

3. Anterior segment examination
    a. The flap edge should be smooth. Flap edge lift can occur (Figure 4–1). A rough edge can be due to dehydration during surgery.
    b. Possible superficial punctate keratitis can be present due to the gentian violet dye.
    c. Possible stromal swelling may occur for 48 hours post-op.
    d. Clear epithelial and stromal interface should be seen.

B. One-Week Visit

1. Evaluate uncorrected visual acuity.

2. Perform refraction and determine the best corrected acuity.

3. Evaluate cornea and flap integrity. Watch for epithelial ingrowth.

4. Perform corneal topography.

5. Topical medications should be discontinued by this visit. Use lubricants for comfort and to prevent dryness.

C. One-Month Visit

1. Determine the uncorrected visual acuity. The best uncorrected acuity is reached at this point.

2. Refraction—the post-op refractive error is fairly accurate at this time. It will stabilize within 3 months.

3. Anterior segment examination—there should be a clear epithelial and stromal interface.

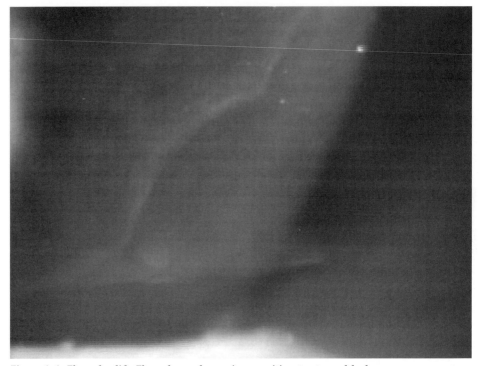

Figure 4–1 Flap edge lift. Flap edge no longer in opposition to stromal bed.

 4. Check flap edge.
    a. It should have healed well.
    b. There may be a ring around the edge secondary to scarring of Bowman's layer from epithelial and underlying stroma interaction.
 5. Corneal topography
    a. This should show central flattening.
    b. Possible induced irregular astigmatism may be seen due to poor realignment of the flap.
 6. Intraocular pressure—use applanation.

D. Three-Month Visit

 1. Visual acuity—acuity should be stabilized at this point.
 2. Manifest refraction
    a. Refractive error should also be stabilized.
    b. Enhancement, when indicated, is usually between 2 to 4 months post-op.
 3. Corneal topography—central flattening should be seen.

4. Anterior segment examination—there may be
   a. interface haze, peripherally greater than centrally, or
   b. increase in the intensity of white ring around flap edge.
5. Intraocular pressure—use applanation.

E. *Six-Month Visit*

1. Visual acuity—acuity should be stabilized at this point.
2. Manifest and cycloplegic refraction
   a. Refractive error should also be stabilized.
   b. Enhancement when indicated is usually between 2 to 4 months post-op.
3. Corneal topography—central flattening should be seen.
4. Anterior segment examination—check flap status and clarity.
5. Intraocular pressure—use applanation.

F. *One-Year Visit*

1. Visual acuity—acuity should be stabilized at this point.
2. Manifest refraction—refractive error should also be stabilized.
3. Corneal topography—central flattening should be seen.
4. Anterior segment examination—check flap status and clarity.
5. Intraocular pressure—use applanation.
6. Return for annual examination including dilation and re-educate on risks and signs and symptoms of retinal detachment.

VIII. Complications of Clinical Laser Vision Correction

A. *Anatomical Factors:* small and deep-set eyes

1. This means it is more difficult to achieve proper suction ring application and to have enough room for the microkeratome to pass.
2. This can be managed with pressure on the lid speculum when applying the suction ring.
3. PRK may be indicated with these patients to avoid intra-procedural flap creation complications.

B. *Intra-Procedural Complications*

1. **LASIK is more invasive** by virtue of the flap formation and has greater potential for complications during the procedure.
2. **Poor position of suction ring**
   a. A scleral ridge forms quickly after suction, making it impossible to reposition suction ring.

  b. Conjunctival tenting will block suction port and prevent adequate pressure.
  c. Prevent by careful alignment of suction ring prior to pressure application and, if necessary, downward pressure on lid speculum for enhanced exposure during microkeratome pass. Also, prevent patient tendency to retract chin toward the chest; keeping the chin up maintains a central eye position within the palpebral aperture.
  d. Manipulation of the suction ring, draping, or lid speculum may lead to loss of suction.
  e. Must postpone operation until original ocular shape is attained.

3. **Hemorrhage from corneal vascularization**
  a. Patients with neovascularization of the cornea secondary to corneal hypoxia from contact lens overwear may have bleeding if the corneal flap involves the vessels.
  b. Management:
    1) Prevent hemorrhage via avoiding neovascular vessels on placement of the suction ring.
    2) Use ALK adjustable ring to create a smaller corneal flap.
    3) Just prior to closing corneal flap, reapply suction to reduce bleeding.
    4) Use 2.5% phenylephrine.
    5) Use local application of air.
    6) Apply a topical steroid.

4. **Incomplete flap—pupil bisection**
  a. Inadequate flap size can occur secondary to the surgeon removing the footswitch too early or an error of adjustable microkeratome stopper.
  b. Inadequate corneal exposure due to the eyelids or drape or speculum may cause blockage of the microkeratome during its application in flap creation.
  c. An incomplete flap results in bisection of the pupil by the flap hinge.
  d. The treatment for an inadequate flap is to abort the procedure and reoperate after three months.
  e. A very experienced and confident surgeon can manage with manual free hand lamellar dissection to complete flap extension.

5. **Thin or buttonhole flap**
  a. This results from either inadequate suction or steep corneal curvature (>45.00 D including high astigmatism).
  b. The buttonhole is created due to central buckling of the cornea during the microkeratome pass.
  c. The midperipheral cornea is thinly cut by the keratome while the central cornea is missed completely. The result is either a thin or buttonhole flap.

6. **Free flap**
  a. This can be a result of improper assembly of the adjustable shaper stop.
  b. A flat cornea has a higher incidence of free flap formation.

    c. A free flap increases the incidence of irregular astigmatism and epithelial ingrowth.

    d. Treatment

        1) Store the free flap in an anti-desiccation chamber with the epithelial side in balanced solution. The stromal side is not hydrated in storage to reduce edema of flap (Machat, 1996).

        2) Replace the flap on the cornea after the ablation is completed.

7. **Perforated flap**

    a. This results from a dull or malfunctioning microkeratome, or inadequate IOP.

    b. It is preventable with good maintenance of the IOP.

    c. Manage by replacing the flap on the cornea to allow for healing. A bandage SCL is used until the epithelium has healed.

    d. Repeat surgery in three months if there is no corneal irregularity.

8. **Corneal perforation—intraocular penetration** (Pallikaris & Siganos, 1997).

    a. This is very rare.

    b. It results from the absence of the depth plate in the microkeratome.

    c. It may result in expulsion of globe contents secondary to elevated ocular pressure produced by the suction ring.

9. **Decentration of laser application**

    a. This is critical in both LASIK and PRK (Doane et al., 1995).

    b. This requires the surgeon to reference initially and to monitor properly throughout treatment (Steinberg & Waring, 1983; Uozato & Guyton, 1987).

    c. Patient fixation should be monitored with treatment interruption and refixation during the procedure when necessary.

C. *Post-Procedural Complications.* Early complications:

    a. **Loss of the bandage hydrogel lens in PRK**—DO NOT REPLACE.

        1) Change Tobradex from solution to ointment—still QID.

        2) Pain may increase depending on epithelial defect size. If necessary, add topical Voltaren QID and oral Mepergan Fortis.

        3) Monitor as usual for epithelial healing.

    b. **Corneal infiltrates**

        1) D/C NSAID (Voltaren)

        2) Use Ciloxan Q2h. Have the patient return daily to monitor for infection.

    c. **Pain and discomfort**

        1) These are generally greater for PRK secondary to large epithelial defect; best managed by bandage hydrogel contact lens and short term NSAIDs; 2- to 3-day duration

2) For LASIK, manage by ensuring the intactness of the flap, and use of topical NSAID and lubrications; 1 to 2 days duration.

d. **Infections**

1) For PRK, the incidence is estimated at 1/1000. This is greater than LASIK due to epithelial debridement (Machat, 1996).

2) For LASIK, there is a low incidence, less than 1/5000, because of minimal disruption of the epithelium (Machat, 1996).

3) There is an increased risk if there is epithelial breakdown.

4) Infection can be minimized by frequent lubrication, prophylactic antibiotic, good hygiene, and an aseptic microkeratome.

e. **Reduced BVA secondary to decentered ablation**

1) Decentration of ablation results in irregular astigmatism.

2) This may require RGP contact lenses for restoration of best-corrected visual acuity.

f. **Night halo and starbursts**

1) Occurrence is partially based on the relationship between pupil size and ablation diameter.

2) The greater the ablation diameter is, the lower the incidence of halos will be.

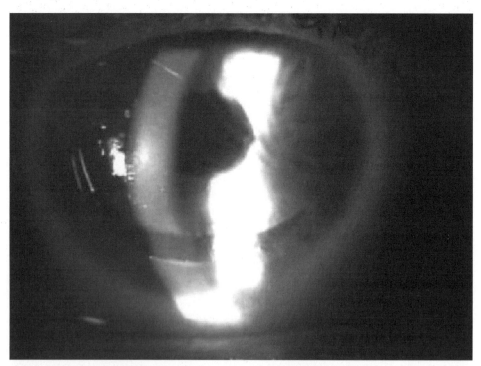

Figure 4–2 Flap displacement. Flap displaced superiorly on patient treated with LASIK to correct refractive error after RK.

3) Patients with large pupil diameters should be detected pre-procedurally; increased treatment zone size should be considered where possible.

g. **Corneal flap displacement** (Buratto & Ferrari, 1997; Perez-Santonja et al., 1997) (Figure 4–2).

1) This is usually seen within the first 12 to 24 hours and consists of flap movement of 1 mm or less.

2) Immediate and frequent lubrication is the appropriate treatment until the flap can be lifted and repositioned.

3) Replacement of the flap as soon as possible not only minimizes the risk of opportunistic infection but also minimizes the severity of flap striae or wrinkling and epithelial ingrowth into the exposed interface (Figure 4–3) (Machat, 1996).

h. **Epithelial ingrowth** (Figures 4–4 and 4–5).

1) The incidence is approximately 2%. This condition occurs when superficial corneal epithelial cells become implanted in the interface (Machat, 1996).

2) Normal epithelial disruption occurs at the flap margins during the microkeratome pass.

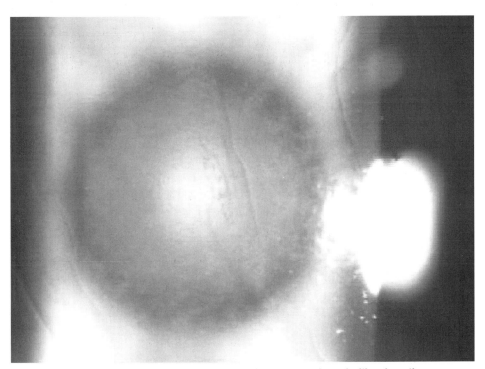

Figure 4–3 Flap wrinkles. Also detectable by retroillumination through dilated pupil.

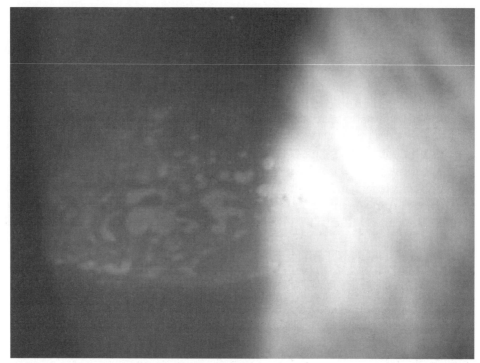

Figure 4–4 Epithelial ingrowth. Peripheral "nests."

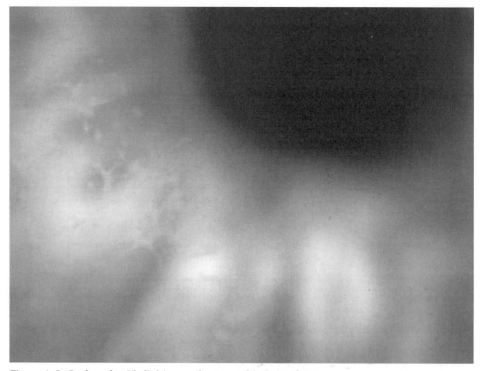

Figure 4–5 Coalesced epithelial ingrowth approaching visual axis.

3) Epithelial ingrowth is generally a peripheral phenomenon occurring more frequently when a frank epithelial defect is present or when poor flap adhesion or flap dislocation occurs.

4) The epithelial ingrowth may migrate and advance toward the central cornea, and/or the epithelial cells may become necrotic leading to a flap melt.

5) This has the potential to significantly affect corneal topography, producing regular or irregular astigmatism and ultimately reducing visual acuity.

6) Peripheral epithelial ingrowth less than 2 mm in diameter without evidence of progression or alteration of topography or refractive error may not require treatment.

7) Aggressive cases require treatment by lifting the flap and mechanically clearing the epithelial cells from the interface surfaces of both the stromal bed and the underside of the flap.

i. **Corneal flap melt or necrosis** (Figure 4–6).

1) This usually develops at the epithelial ingrowth area.

2) Flap necrosis may affect corneal topography and uncorrected or best-corrected vision.

3) There is no relationship between flap melting and flap thickness.

4) This requires similar treatment to epithelial ingrowth but with a poorer prognosis because the corneal flap has sustained damaged (Castillo et al., 1998).

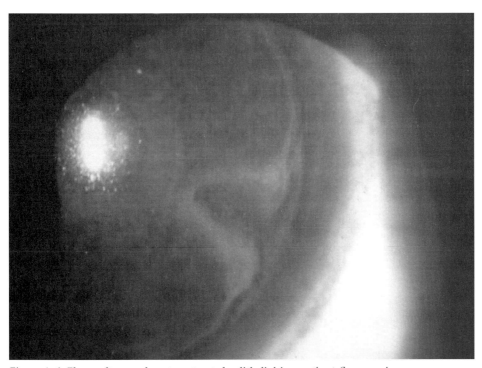

Figure 4–6 Flap melt secondary to untreated eplithelial ingrowth at flap margin.

j. **Haze in stromal bed**
1) For PRK,
   a) Normally trace haze peaks at 3 months and resolves in 6 to 9 months.
   b) Aggressive haze becomes plaque-like and visually significant and is associated with refractive regression toward myopia. The initial treatment is with increased steroids and NSAIDs. Secondary procedures include retreatment and immediate coverage with topical anti-inflammatory agents.
   c) The incidence is estimated at 1% to 5% depending on pre-procedure refractive error (Machat, 1996).
   d) Though commonly utilized, anti-inflammatory use in the treatment of corneal haze remains controversial (Epstein et al., 1994).
2) For LASIK,
   a) The incidence is estimated at 0.1% for PRK-like stromal haze (Machat, 1996).
   b) Non-specific diffuse intralamellar keratitis has recently been described as distinct from previously described haze (Figure 4–7).

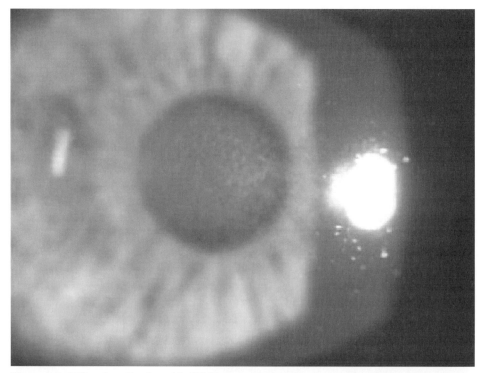

Figure 4–7 Diffuse lamellar keratitis (DLK) central haze following LASIK usually responsive to topical steroid treatment.

c) Early post-procedural granular haze can occur between the corneal flap and stromal bed.

d) The haze is usually diffuse and has a powdery or sifted-sand appearance.

e) Inflammatory reaction is assumed primarily because this keratitis is responsive to a short but aggressive course of topical steroids (Machat, 1998).

k. **Central island formation** (Doane et al., 1995; Maloney, 1990).

1) This is usually detected post-procedurally with associated symptoms of blurred vision, ghost images, and/or monocular diplopia.

2) Topographically this is defined as a central region of at least 2 to 3 mm in diameter showing a 2 D or steeper curvature than the surrounding cornea.

3) Decreased best-corrected visual acuity along with refraction measuring greater myopia than predicted by the corresponding uncorrected visual acuity are typically noted.

4) Less effective ablation centrally may result in local elevation compared to surrounding tissue due to fluid dynamics during treatment of the stromal bed.

5) Treatment consists of lifting the flap and ablating in a similar manner as in PTK for persistent central islands.

l. **Residual refractive error**

1) The final measure of success or failure with any corneal refractive procedure resides in the ability to provide adequate, functional vision with a minimal dependence on optical aids.

2) Inaccurate pre-procedural baseline refraction, perhaps due to the lack of cycloplegia, can result in either primary over- or undercorrection.

3) Variable healing responses can lead to residual refractive errors despite accurate pre-procedural measurements. Normal LASIK recovery shows mild regression within the first weeks following treatment. Biologic variation in this effect will partially determine whether over- or under-correction develops.

4) Management of primary residual refractive error generally involves consideration of surgical enhancement.

5) Persistent irregular astigmatism may require gas permeable contact lens treatment to achieve best potential acuity (see *Additional Reading*). Topographically-linked laser ablation application may become an effective treatment in the near future.

IX. Comparison of LASIK to PRK (Table 4–3).

A. LASIK is a **more invasive procedure due to corneal flap creation**.

B. LASIK has a **greater intraoperative risk of complications**.

C. LASIK involves **quicker visual recovery due to less epithelial disruption**.

D. LASIK results in **less pain/discomfort due to less epithelial disruption**.

E. LASIK involves **less healing variability and less topical steroid use required post-procedure**.

Table 4–3 Comparison of RK, PRK, and LASIK Published Data

Procedure	RK	RK	PRK	LASIK			LASIK
Study	PERK (Waring et al., 1987)	Casebeer (Waring et al., 1996)	FDA (Thompson et al., 1995)	Farah (from journals) (Farah et al., 1998)			Farah (from abstracts) (Farah et al., 1998)
Year	1982–88	1992–93	1997	1987–97			1996–97
# Eyes	435	615	612	1028			11,397
Mean F/U	1 year	1 year	2 yr	6–12 mo			10 days–12 mo
Pre-op Error	–2–8 D		–1–6 D	–1–6 D	–6–12 D	>–12 D	–1–31 D
% Loss 2 or >Lines	3%		7%				0.9%
+/– 1.00 D	60%	89%	78%	93%	74%	42%	83%
UCVA 20/40 OR >	78%	93%	93%	93%	67%	41%	83%
UCVA 20/20 OR >	47%	4%	7%				7%

References

Buratto L, Ferrari M. Indications, techniques, results, limits and complications of laser in situ keratomileusis. Curr Opin Ophthalmol 8:59–66 (1997).

Castillo A et al. Peripheral melt of flap after laser in situ keratomileusis. J Refract Surg 14:61–63 (1998).

Curtin BJ. The myopias: basic science and clinical management. Philadelphia: Harper & Row, 1985.

Doane JF et al. Relation of visual symptoms to topographic ablation zone decentration after excimer laser photorefractive keratectomy. Ophthalmology 102:42–47 (1995).

Durrie DS, Lesher MP, Cavanaugh TB. Classification of variable clinical response after photorefractive keratectomy for myopia. J Refract Surg 11:341–347 (1995).

Epstein D et al. Twenty-four-month follow-up of excimer laser photorefractive keratectomy for myopia. Refractive and visual acuity results. Ophthalmology 101:1558–1563 (1994).

Farah SG et al. Laser in situ keratomileusis: literature review of a developing technique. J Cataract Refract Surg 24:989–1006 (1998).

Gettes BC, Belmont O. Tropicamide: comparative cycloplegic effects. Arch Ophthalmol 66:336–340 (1961).

Koch DD, Husain SE. Corneal topography to detect and characterize corneal pathology. In Gills JP, Sanders DR, Thornton SP, Martin RG, Gayton JL, Holladay JT, Van Der Karr M, eds. Corneal topography: the state of the art. Thorofare, NJ: SLACK Inc, 1995, 159–169.

Machat JJ. Excimer laser refractive surgery: practice and principles. Thorofare, NJ: SLACK Inc, 1996.

Machat JJ. Non-specific diffuse intralamellar keratitis. TLC. Sharing the Vision 4:1–3 (1998).

Maguire LJ, Bourne WM. Corneal topography of early keratoconus. Am J Ophthalmol 108:107–112 (1989).

Maguire LJ, Lowry JC. Identifying progression of subclinical keratoconus by serial topography analysis. Am J Ophthalmol 112:41–45 (1991).

Maloney RK. Corneal topography and optical zone location in photorefractive keratectomy. Refract Corneal Surg 6:363–371 (1990).

Mandava N et al. Ocular deviation following excimer laser photorefractive keratectomy. J Cataract Refract Surg 22:504–505 (1996).

McDonald M et al. Clinical results of central photorefractive keratectomy (PRK) with the 193–nm excimer laser for the treatment of myopia: the blind eye study. Invest Ophthalmol Vis Sci 30 (suppl):216 (1989).

McDonald MB et al. Central photorefractive keratectomy for myopia: the blind eye study. Arch Ophthalmol 108:799–808 (1990).

Nesburn AB et al. Computer assisted corneal topography (CACT) to detect mild keratoconus (KC) in candidates for photorefractive keratectomy. Invest Ophthalmol Vis Sci 33 (suppl): 995 (1992).

Pallikaris IG, Siganos DS. Laser in situ keratomileusis to treat myopia: early experience. J Cataract Refract Surg 23:39–49 (1997).

Perez-Santonja JJ et al. Laser in situ keratomileusis to correct high myopia. J Cataract Refract Surg 23:372–385 (1997).

Rengstorff RH. Corneal rehabilitation. In: Bennett ES, Weissman BA, eds. Clinical contact lens practice. Philadelphia: J.B. Lippincott, 1992, 48:1–10.

Steinberg EB, Waring GO 3rd. Comparison of two methods of marking the visual axis on the cornea during radial keratotomy. Am J Ophthalmol 96:605–608 (1983).

Thompson KP et al. Photorefractive keratectomy with the Summit excimer laser: the phase III U.S. results. In: Salz JJ, McDonnell PJ, McDonald MB, eds. Corneal laser surgery. Philadelphia: Mosby, 1995, 57–63.

Uozato H, Guyton DL. Centering corneal surgical procedures. Am J Ophthalmol 103:264–275 (1987).

Waring GO 3rd, Casebeer JC, Dru RM. One-year results of a prospective multicenter study of the Casebeer system of refractive keratotomy. Casebeer Chiron Study Group. Ophthalmology 103:1337–1347 (1996).

Waring GO 3rd et al. Three-year results of the Prospective Evaluation of Radial Keratotomy (PERK) study. Ophthalmology 94:1339–1354 (1987).

Wilson SE, Klyce SD. Screening for corneal topographic abnormalities before refractive surgery. Ophthalmology 101:147–152 (1994).

Additional Readings

Ackley KD, Caroline P, Davis LJ. Retrospective evaluation of rigid gas permeable contact lenses on radial keratotomy patients. Optom Vis Sci 70(suppl):39 (1993).

Aquavella JV et al. How contact lenses fit into refractive surgery. Rev Ophthalmol 1:36–42 (1994).

Astin CLK. Refractive surgery and contact lenses. In: Hom MM, ed. Manual of contact lens prescribing and fitting. Boston: Butterworth-Heinemann, 1997, 363–380.

Astin CL, Gartry DS, McG-Stecle AD. Contact lens fitting after photorefractive keratectomy. Br J Ophthalmol 80:597–603 (1996).

Koffler BH, Smith VM, Clements LD. Achieving additional myopic correction in undercorrected radial keratotomy eyes using the Lexington RK splint design. CLAO J 25:21–27 (1999).

Lee AM, Kastl PR. Rigid gas permeable contact lens fitting after radial keratotomy. CLAO J 24:33–35 (1998).

Shovlin JP et al. How to fit an irregular cornea. Rev Optom 124(10):88–98 (1987).

Chapter 5
Laser Posterior Capsulotomy

Charles M. Wormington

I. Introduction

A. Posterior Capsule Opacification (PCO)

1. Opacification of the posterior capsule following cataract surgery occurs from 30% to 50% of the time during the first 3 to 5 years after the surgery (Apple et al., 1992; Born & Ryan, 1990; Clark, 2000; Colin & Robinet, 1997; Grusha et al., 1998; Javitt et al., 1992; Koenig et al., 1993; Lyle & Jin, 1996; Mamalis et al., 1996; Martin et al., 1992; Milazzo et al., 1996; Moisseiev et al., 1989; Ninn-Pedersen & Bauer, 1997; Sinskey & Cain, 1978; Sundelin & Sjostrand, 1999; Yamada et al., 1995).

   a. A few studies show a lower rate of opacification, as low as 6.5% at 5 years, which may partly reflect differences in lens design (Born & Ryan, 1990; Frezzotti & Caporossi, 1990). Part of the problem with studies on opacification rates is that definitions of PCO vary from study to study and there is a lack of adjustment for variable follow-up.

   b. A recent meta-analysis found that pooled estimates of the incidence of PCO were 11.8% at 1 year, 20.7% at 3 years, and 28.4% at 5 years after the surgery (Schaumberg et al., 1998). Rates vary from study to study because of differences in surgical techniques, patient characteristics, research designs, and reporting methods.

2. The average time for PCO to occur is 20 to 26 months after the cataract surgery with a range from 4 days to 7.3 years (Colin & Robinet, 1997; Coonan et al., 1985; Nielsen & Naeser, 1993; Ninn-Pedersen & Bauer, 1996; Sinskey & Cain, 1978; Steinert et al., 1991; Wilhelmus & Emery, 1980). For a summary of 22 studies, see the Cataract Management Guideline Panel (1993) review. In those studies, the median time from cataract surgery to laser capsulotomy was 24 months with a range of 1 to 600 months. This wide range probably reflects differences among surgeons in terms of indications and timing of the procedure.

3. Opacification appears to occur more often and sooner in younger patients than in older patients (Apple et al., 1992; Coonan et al., 1985; Frezzotti & Caporossi, 1990; Moisseiev et al., 1989; Ninn-Pedersen & Bauer, 1997).

4. PCO usually results from the migration and proliferation of residual lens epithelial cells (Apple et al., 1992; Green & McDonnell, 1985; Tassin et al., 1979). This process can produce two major types of clinical complication: a fibrosis-type PCO and a pearl-type PCO.

5. The **fibrosis-type PCO** occurs primarily from the fibrous metaplasia of anterior epithelial cells (Apple et al., 1992). They can become fibrocytes that form fibrous membranes that occasionally reduce vision. Contraction of the fibrocytes can produce wrinkling and folds in the posterior capsule, and this can cause distortion of vision, including glare.

6. The **pearl-type PCO** occurs primarily from the migration and proliferation of equatorial epithelial cells (Apple et al., 1992). These result in clusters of cells that resemble pearls. This buildup of cells can then lead to a reduction in vision.

7. Fibrosis tends to occur within about 2 to 6 months after surgery, whereas epithelial pearl formation tends to occur several months to years after surgery (Apple et al., 1992).

8. The incidence of PCO depends on the type of intraocular lens (IOL) (Clark, 2000). In most studies, there appears to be more PCO with polymethylmethacrylate IOLs than with IOLs made of silicone or soft acrylic materials (Hayashi et al., 1998b; Hollick et al., 1999; Olson & Crandall, 1998). However, in one study there was no statistically significant difference (Oshika et al., 1998), and in another it appeared that silicone IOLs induced PCO faster than PMMA lenses (Kim et al., 1999). The polyacrylic IOLs appear to have the least PCO and the lowest laser capsulotomy rates (Hollick et al., 1999). Heparin surface modification of PMMA IOLs may increase the incidence of PCO (Winther-Nielsen et al., 1998).

9. Prevention of PCO is under active investigation and may involve pharmaceutical intervention using a molecular biological approach (Nishi, 1999). In combined glaucoma and cataract surgery cases, the use of mitomycin C apparently decreases the probability of PCO requiring laser capsulotomy (Shin et al., 1998).

10. Using early measurements of PCO, a mathematical model has been developed to predict the time to laser capsulotomy (Clark et al., 1998).

B. Laser Posterior Capsulotomy

1. Before the advent of the Nd:YAG laser, PCO was treated by invasive, surgical procedures involving capsular discission (Lindstrom & Harris, 1980; Simcoe, 1980; Wilhemus & Emery, 1980). These kinds of procedures are still performed if the laser cannot penetrate a very dense membrane on the posterior capsule or if a laser is not available.

2. In the early 1980s, Aron-Rosa in France and Fankhauser in Switzerland applied the Nd:YAG laser as a noninvasive method to open an opacified posterior capsule (Aron-Rosa et al., 1980; Aron-Rosa et al., 1984; Fankhauser et al., 1982).

3. Nd:YAG laser posterior capsulotomy has now replaced the more invasive surgical procedures and is the second most commonly performed ophthalmic surgical procedure that is reimbursed by Medicare (Apple et al., 1992).

II. Laser Instrumentation

A. Nd:YAG Laser System. Almost all laser posterior capsulotomies have been performed with the Nd:YAG laser.

1. An **Nd:YAG laser rod** is the central part of the system. Its subcomponents include
   a. an **active medium** made up of **neodymium (Nd)** ions,
   b. a **crystal rod** whose matrix is composed of **yttrium (Y), aluminum (A), and garnet (G)**, and
   c. a **pump**, which is usually a high intensity **flash lamp** but could be a diode laser.
2. A **high-reflectance mirror** is at one end of the rod.
3. An **output coupler mirror** is at the other end of the rod. This mirror is partially reflective.
4. A **Q-switch** shutter is inserted in the pathway between the two mirrors.
5. A **mode-limiting aperture** can be placed in the pathway, producing a fundamental mode beam, or the aperture can be absent producing a multimode beam.

B. Instrument Parameters

1. The **output** of an Nd:YAG laser is defined by a number of parameters:
   a. The beam is invisible in the **near infra-red** region with a wavelength of **1064 nm**.
   b. The **pulse duration** is from **3 to 7 nsec**.
   c. The beam is usually focused with a **cone angle of 16°**. Thus the beam exits the instrument, converges to a focus point, and then diverges. This feature minimizes the hazard to the cornea, the IOL, and the retina.
   d. The focused **spot size** is from **7 to 20 μm** in diameter.
2. The **cooling system** can be either:
   a. **ambient air** (most clinical instruments use this technique) or
   b. **internal circulating water** (much like a car radiator system).
3. The **electrical requirements** are **110 volts** and **less than 20 amperes**.

C. Delivery Systems

1. An **aiming system** is necessary since the main beam is invisible.
   a. A **helium-neon laser** (HeNe) is usually used in clinical systems, although a diode laser is used in some systems. The pathway of the aiming laser is **coaxial** with the Nd:YAG beam.

b. The **number of beams** in the aiming system can be
1) **single** (rare)—focus is obtained when the smallest, brightest spot is imaged on the target;
2) **dual** (most clinical systems have two aiming beams)—focus is obtained when the two beams merge into one small, bright spot on the target; or
3) **quadruple** (one of the clinical lasers has four aiming beams arranged in a square array)—focus is attained when the four beams merge into one spot.

c. The multiple beam systems can be **stationary or rotating**. A rotating system can add another criterion for focus. In a two-beam system the beams can blink alternately with a frequency that is visible. When the beams are focused and overlap, the blinking frequency is doubled and is above the flicker fusion frequency. Thus, when the aiming system is in focus the blinking disappears.

d. The **focus** of the aiming system with respect to the focus of the Nd:YAG beam can be
1) **parfocal**, in which both beams focus at the same point, or
2) **offset**, in which the Nd:YAG beam focuses behind the aiming beam (i.e., the YAG focus is farther from the laser than the HeNe focus). This offset can be **variable or fixed**. For example, one laser system can be offset from 0 to 200 μm in 50-μm steps. Another laser system is fixed at 200 μm and still another at 167 μm. For a given energy setting, this offset provides for a maximum photomechanical effect on the target. For higher energy levels, the aiming system may have to be moved slightly posterior to the target.

2. **Beam conditioning optics**
   a. An **inverse Galilean telescope** is used to expand the laser beam.
   b. A **final condensing lens** is used to converge the exiting beam.
   c. The laser beam is **coaxial with** the **slit lamp** biomicroscope viewing optics.

D. *Principles of Critical Focus* (Steinert & Puliafito, 1985).
1. Optical breakdown is nonlinear (i.e., an "all or none" phenomenon).
2. It is desirable to work at or close to the threshold energy density at the focus. This localizes the damage to the area close to the focus.
3. Working above threshold can trigger unwanted plasmas in front of the target.
4. Interfaces (e.g., the posterior surface of the IOL) and debris in the pathway can reduce the threshold and trigger unwanted plasmas.
5. A smaller beam cone angle produces a more anterior breakdown.
6. A larger beam cone angle localizes the plasma formation closer to the focus.

E. *Damage Mechanisms.* The damage from the laser is **photodisruptive**.
1. Focal disintegration of tissue occurs when the plasma forms.

2. Mechanical damage to the tissue results from the shock waves generated after plasma formation.

3. The inherent elasticity of the capsular tissue enhances the damage by stretching the tissue.

F. An **erbium:YAG laser** can also be used to perform a laser capsulotomy (D'Amico et al., 1996).

G. The **Nd:YLF laser** has also been evaluated for laser capsulotomy (Geerling, 1998; Hoppeler & Gloor, 1992; Loya et al., 1995). This laser has also been used to produce micrometer-level polishing of a posterior capsule model as a possible alternative to capsulotomy (Hanuch et al., 1997).

H. The **CO_2 Laser** via an endoprobe has been used to explore PCO prevention and also to perform a posterior capsulotomy in sheep and rabbit eyes (Michaeli-Cohen et al., 1998).

III. Posterior Capsulotomy

A. Indications (Cataract Management Guideline Panel, 1993; Magno et al., 1997; McCarty et al., 1999; Nucci et al., 1995; O'Day, et al. 1993; Royal College of Ophthalmologists, 1995).

1. The **primary indication** for a posterior capsulotomy is an **opacified posterior capsule that interferes with the patient's visual needs (i.e., functional impairment)**. The criteria for capsulotomy are similar to those for cataract extraction.

2. **Functional impairment** includes interference with
   a. activities of daily living (e.g., preparing meals, eating, walking, driving, shopping, using the telephone, doing housework),
   b. occupational needs, or
   c. leisure-time activities (e.g., reading, watching TV, stamp collecting, playing baseball).

3. Other factors that need to be taken into consideration are
   a. decreased visual acuity (the most prevalent reported measure was best-corrected vision of 20/50 or worse),
   b. symptoms of glare,
   c. photophobia,
   d. symptoms of loss of contrast sensitivity,
   e. potential risks associated with the capsulotomy versus potential benefits,
   f. the actual extent of posterior capsule opacification,
   g. exclusion of other ocular causes of functional impairment, or
   h. need to diagnose or treat other ocular conditions (e.g., diabetic retinopathy, retinal detachment, tumors).

4. Just as with cataract, there are subjective, objective, and educational **criteria** for capsulotomy:
   a. **Subjective**: impairment of necessary or desirable activities
   b. **Objective**: confirmation of posterior capsular opacification and exclusion of other ocular causes of functional impairment
   c. **Educational**: discussion of the nature of the capsulotomy procedure, as well as the risks and benefits of the procedure, with the patient

5. Justification for the capsulotomy should be **well documented** in the patient's file.

6. Judging the degree of visual impairment in young or nonverbal children can be difficult. Indications of decreased vision in children can include parent-noticed functional impairment, presence of a manifest ocular deviation, as well as retinoscopic and ophthalmoscopic distortion.

7. In addition to cases after cataract surgery, PCO can occur also after clear lens extraction and IOL implantation (Colin & Robinet, 1997; Lee & Lee, 1996; Siganos & Pallikaras, 1998).

8. An uncommon indication is **malignant glaucoma** (Chapter 8).

B. *Contraindications* (Table 5–1).

1. Uncontrolled intraocular pressure (IOP)

2. Inadequate visualization of the target
   a. This can occur if there are corneal or aqueous opacities or haze.
   b. Dense opacities can obstruct view of the target as well as absorb part of the laser beam.

3. Inadequate stability of the eye

4. No potential visual function of eye

Table 5–1 Indications and Contraindications for Laser Posterior Capsulotomy

Indication
    Opacified posterior capsule resulting in functional impairment
Contraindications
    Uncontrolled IOP
    Inadequate target visualization
    Inadequate stability of the eye
    No potential visual function of eye
Relative contraindications
    Active intraocular inflammation
    Corneal edema
    Glass intraocular lens
    Brief time following cataract extraction

C. Relative Contraindications

1. Active intraocular inflammation
   a. Inflammation increases the risk of cystoid macular edema (CME).
   b. Treat and eliminate the inflammation before proceeding with the capsulotomy.

2. Corneal edema

3. Glass IOL

4. Brief time following cataract extraction
   a. Capsulotomy is rarely indicated within 3 months of the procedure. Waiting at least 3 months will allow time for the capsule to stretch, thus requiring fewer laser exposures.
   b. Capsulotomy is uncommon within the first 6 months.
   c. Maintaining the barrier function of the posterior capsule between the anterior and posterior compartments of the eye for as long as possible is desirable.
   d. If your patient has had a no-stitch or one-stitch cataract procedure and a soft silicon IOL has been implanted, capsulotomy needs to be delayed for at least 6 months. Dislocation of the IOL could occur if the laser is used before enough fibrosis has occurred to clamp the IOL in position.

D. Pre-Treatment Examination (Cataract Management Guideline Panel, 1993; Steinert & Puliafito, 1985) (Table 5–2).

1. **Thorough history** that should include the following:
   a. Check for contraindications for capsulotomy or potential medications.
   b. Check for history of retinal detachment.

Table 5–2 Elements of a Pre-Treatment Examination

Thorough history
Subjective refraction
Direct ophthalmoscopy
Retinoscopy
Red-reflex evaluation
Slit-lamp biomicroscope exam
Applanation tonometry
Potential visual acuity assessment
Binocular indirect ophthalmoscopy
Angiography (if necessary)
B-scan ultrasonography (if necessary)
Glare and contrast sensitivity
Informed, written consent

      c. Rule out CME or macular degeneration if the patient has had poor vision since the cataract surgery.

      d. Determine the type of IOL the surgeon placed in your patient's eye.

2. **Subjective refraction**

      a. This must be done to ensure that the patient's reduced vision is not correctable with a simple change in spectacle prescription.

      b. If after the refraction vision is still reduced, use a pinhole to verify that the reduction is nonrefractive.

3. **Direct ophthalmoscopy**—This may be the single most reliable technique for assessing the capsular opacity. Your ability to see in is an indication of the patient's ability to see out.

4. **Retinoscopy**

5. **Red-reflex evaluation** using the slit-lamp biomicroscope and the direct and indirect ophthalmoscopes

6. **Slit-lamp biomicroscope examination**

      a. Cornea—Check the clarity and integrity of the cornea.

      b. Aqueous—Check for cells and flare (i.e., inflammation).

      c. Iris/pupil

          1) Note the position and shape of the pupil and its diameter.

          2) Dilation may result in a slightly decentered pupil, so note any landmarks before dilation.

          3) Alternatively, a marker lesion in the capsule in the center of the undilated pupil may be made.

      d. IOL—Note whether

          1) the IOL is decentered or centered

          2) there are areas of separation between the IOL and the posterior capsule

          3) there are any posterior synechia

      e. Posterior capsule—Retroillumination (Figure 5–1) and side illumination may be used to note

          1) the degree, type, and thickness of the opacification (e.g., Elschnig pearls vs. fibrosis)—it will take more laser energy to photodisrupt a thick membrane compared to a thin one

          2) tension lines or folds in the capsule

          3) empty space between the posterior capsule and the vitreous face

      f. Vitreous

          1) Note whether there is a posterior vitreous detachment.

          2) Note whether there are cells in the vitreous indicating a vitritis.

      g. Retina—Using a +66 D, +78 D, +90 D lens or similar lens, check for:

          1) CME,

          2) age-related macular degeneration (ARMD),

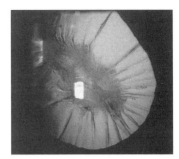

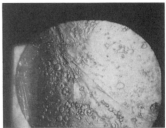

Figure 5–1 Retroillumination of the posterior capsule shows different types of opacification: capsular fibrosis and contracture (top), Elschnig pearl formation (middle), and combined fibrosis and Elschnig pearl formation (bottom). (Reprinted from Sawusch MR, McDonnell PJ. Posterior capsule opacification. Curr Opin Ophthalmol 1:28–33 [1990], with permission from Lippincott Williams & Wilkins.)

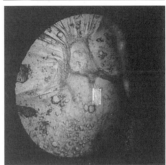

   3) macular lesions, and

   4) optic neuropathy/glaucoma.

7. **Applanation tonometry**

   a. Accurate intraocular pressure readings must be taken to ensure that the IOP is under control and not elevated before the capsulotomy.

   b. The capsulotomy procedure can result in an IOP spike, so the pre-procedure level must be assessed.

8. **Potential visual acuity assessment**

   a. **Clinical interferometer** or **potential acuity meter** assessment may indicate macular function behind the opacified capsule (Faulkner, 1982, 1983; Hanna et al., 1989; Klein et al., 1986; Lang & Lindstrom, 1985; McGraw & Barrett, 1996; Spurny et al., 1986; Strong, 1992). Either technique may give false positives due to macular edema or a number of other factors.

  b. A new **illuminated near card** can also be used to assess potential acuity before laser capsulotomy (Hofeldt, 1996).

  c. Recently, the **scanning laser ophthalmoscope** has been used to predict visual acuity in cataract patients (Cuzzani et al., 1998). It may also be useful for predicting acuity in patients with PCO. Because of the reduced scattering of its red and near-infrared laser beams and the versatility of its projected targets, it may be able to image and test visual function behind opacified capsules as well as behind cataracts.

  d. **Entoptic phenomena** can also be used to predict potential visual acuity. A new method has been devised to elicit striking Purkinje vessel shadows along with a foveal granular pattern (Murillo-Lopez et al., 2000). Perception of the foveal granular pattern using this device had 86% sensitivity and 88% specificity for good vision.

9. **Binocular indirect ophthalmoscopy**—Check especially for
  a. Lattice degeneration
  b. Retinal holes
  c. Retinal detachment
  d. CME
  e. ARMD

10. **Angiography** (if necessary).
  a. This should be performed if it is necessary to diagnose CME.
  b. Fluorescein angiography may also be indicated if the appearance of the capsular opacification does not seem to account for the magnitude of the decreased visual acuity.

11. **B-scan ultrasonography** (if necessary).
  a. If the fundus cannot be evaluated because of the density of the capsular opacification, B-scan may be indicated.
  b. B-scan may also be indicated if the degree of capsular opacification does not appear to account for the level of decreased visual acuity.

12. **Glare sensitivity and contrast sensitivity** (Claesson et al., 1994; Hard et al., 1993; Knighton et al., 1985; Magno et al., 1997; Sunderraj et al., 1992; Tan et al., 1998, 1999; Wilkins et al., 1996).
  a. It may be useful to document glare effects before the capsulotomy. This may be particularly helpful in patients that have fairly good visual acuity but experience problems with glare. The typical patient after capsulotomy shows a greater improvement in visual acuity under glare conditions than under standard non-glare conditions.
  b. Various tests may be used to document glare sensitivity (e.g., the Brightness Acuity Tester, the Straylightmeter, or the Miller-Nadler Glare Tester). The Straylightmeter

may be better for measuring glare associated with PCO than the Brightness Acuity Tester (Tan et al., 1998).

    c. In addition, it may be useful to document contrast sensitivity before capsulotomy. Posterior capsule opacification causes a generalized depression of contrast sensitivity (Tan et al., 1999). A laser posterior capsulotomy results in an improvement of the contrast sensitivity across all spatial frequencies (Claesson et al., 1994; Magno et al., 1997; Tan et al., 1999).

    d. A number of tests may be used to assess contrast sensitivity (Tan et al., 1999). Some tests use gratings (e.g. Mentor B-VAT, Vistech VCTS 6500, and computer graphics systems). Others use various optotypes (e.g., Pelli-Robson chart and computer-generated systems).

13. **Informed, written consent** (mandatory).
    a. The procedure should be explained in clear, understandable terms.
    b. The risks should be explained, including retinal detachment, CME, glaucoma, and IOL damage.
    c. Options available to the patient should be explained.

E. *Pretreatment Regimen* (Table 5–3).

1. One drop of 1% **apraclonidine** (Iopidine) should be instilled (Pollack et al., 1988a,b; Silverstone et al., 1992).
    a. This is an α-agonist that decreases aqueous inflow and hence decreases the IOP.
    b. Without prophylaxis, the occurrence of IOP increase $\geq 10\,mm\,Hg$ after laser capsulotomy averages out to about 28% in 27 studies (see Table 5–9). With 1% apraclonidine given before and after the capsulotomy, the occurrence is reduced to about 3% in seven studies. The occurrence was 0% in two studies using 0.5% apraclonidine and in one study with 0.25% apraclonidine.
    c. A β-blocker (e.g., levobunolol) may be substituted unless contraindicated (Migliori et al., 1987; Rakofsky et al., 1997; Richter et al., 1985a; Silverstone et al., 1988;

Table 5–3 Pretreatment Regimen

1 drop 1% apraclonidine
Dilation (optional)
1 drop 0.5% proparacaine
Advise patient about noises and flashes
Ensure patient's head is stabilized
Ensure patient comfort
Ensure adequate stabilization of eye
Focus and adjust slit lamp oculars

Simsek et al., 1998; Stilma & Boen-Tan, 1986). A topical carbonic anhydrase inhibitor (2% dorzolamide) and an alpha-adrenergic agonist (0.25% clonidine) have also been found to be efficacious (Hartenbaum et al., 1999; Ladas et al., 1997; Loewenstein et al., 1991).

    d. If the patient has glaucoma, additional pressure-lowering agents should be considered in addition to the patient's usual regimen.

2. Dilation is optional.

    a. Dilation may be useful for beginners.

    b. **You should not routinely dilate**, because

       1) there is a risk of displacing a malpositioned IOL (Shah et al., 1986), and

       2) centration of the capsulotomy is easier in an undilated eye and the center of the undilated pupil may not be the center of the dilated pupil.

3. **Proparacaine** should be used if a laser contact lens is employed.

4. **Advise the patient about** the snapping or cracking **noises** and/or the bright **flashes** of light that he or she may experience during the procedure. This will help reassure the patient and will help the patient to maintain steady fixation.

5. **Ensure that the patient's head is stabilized** adequately against the slit-lamp forehead and chin rests. This will help to minimize damage to the IOL and other structures of the eye that may occur due to patient movement.

6. **Ensure patient comfort** during the procedure. This will also help to maintain stability of the eye during the capsulotomy.

7. **Ensure adequate stabilization of the eye**.

    a. Some stabilization can be attained by the use of a laser contact lens.

    b. Use of a retrobulbar anesthetic block may be necessary (e.g., with nystagmus).

    c. In patients with large amplitude nystagmus or in uncooperative children, sedation or general anesthesia may be necessary.

    d. For patients with breathing difficulties, have the patient interrupt breathing just before delivering the laser energy to the patient.

8. **Focus and adjust the oculars on the slit-lamp biomicroscope**—This will help ensure precise laser focus.

F. Capsulotomy Technique (Kolder, 1992; Steinert & Puliafito, 1985) (Table 5–4).

1. **Focusing is absolutely critical.**

    a. Make sure you know whether the aiming beam and the infrared beam are parfocal or how much offset there is. Some Nd:YAG lasers have an adjustable offset and others have a single preset offset. This means that the aiming beams may have to be focused at or behind the capsule.

    b. Placing the Nd:YAG infrared focus on the capsule or in front of the capsule increases the risk of IOL damage.

Table 5–4 Capsulotomy Technique

Focusing is absolutely critical
Use minimum energy necessary (0.6 to 1.5 mJ/pulse)
Use the minimum number of shots
Use a laser contact lens
Use dim, broad side illumination or retroillumination with 25×
  magnification
Synchronize triggering of laser with respiratory and circulatory movement
  of eye
Place your first laser pulse offcenter
Identify any areas of IOL-capsule separation, and begin treatment there
If possible, identify and cut across capsular tension lines
Perform cruciate opening if feasible
Make diameter of capsulotomy appropriate (usually 3 to 4 mm)

c. Placing the infrared focus too far behind the capsule (i.e., toward the posterior pole) will increase the possibility of vitreous damage.
d. Be sure the red HeNe aiming beams are focused on or just behind the capsule. Ensure that you don't inadvertently focus on the IOL posterior or anterior surface. There are a number of Purkinje images due to the multiple optical interfaces in the eye.
e. When using a laser contact lens, make sure the face of the lens is perpendicular to the laser beam. Tilting the lens can result in a lengthening of the plasma and an increase in the threshold for plasma formation (Vogel et al., 1998).

2. **Use the minimum energy necessary (0.6 to 1.5 mJ/pulse).** This will help minimize the amount of tissue volume disrupted, damage to the vitreous, and damage to the IOL. One way to do this is to start out with an energy setting of about 0.5 mJ. If this is below threshold, then increase in increments of 0.1 mJ until threshold is reached. If threshold is not reached by 2.5 mJ, reevaluate your laser output.

3. **Use the minimum number of shots.** This can range from 3 up to possibly 125. This precaution will also help minimize the disrupted tissue volume, damage to the vitreous, and damage to the IOL. Avoid the use of the burst mode.

4. **Use a laser contact lens** (e.g., a central Abraham or a Peyman G 12.12 lens) (Figures 5–2 and 5–3) to
   a. improve visualization of the target (via magnification),
   b. increase the beam convergence (thus minimizing risk to the cornea, IOL, vitreous face, and retina),
   c. decrease the beam spot size and hence increase the power density (localizing the damage closer to the focus),

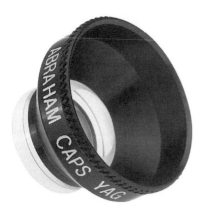

Figure 5–2 Central Abraham button lens for an Nd:YAG posterior capsulotomy. (Courtesy of Ocular Instruments, Inc. Bellevue, WA)

    d. stabilize the eye,

    e. eliminate blinking,

    f. prevent corneal drying, and

    g. provide tamponade if an inadvertent iris hemorrhage occurs.

5. **Use dim, broad, side illumination or retroillumination with 25× magnification.**

6. **Synchronize triggering of the laser with the respiratory and circulatory movement of the patient's eye.**

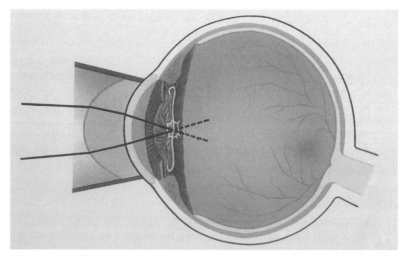

Figure 5–3 Nd:YAG posterior capsulotomy with a contact lens. (Reprinted with permission from Noyori K, Shimizu K, Trokel S. Ophthalmic Laser Therapy. Igaku-Shoin: New York, 1992.)

7. **Place your first laser pulse offcenter.**
   a. If possible, put your first shot either above or below the center of the pupil.
   b. This will allow you to assess the adequacy of the laser power setting and the actual location of the plasma formation without risk to the visual axis.
   c. If the first shot is below threshold for plasma formation, slowly increase the power until you do get a plasma.
   d. If the first shot produces too large a plasma, then the power setting can be reduced.
   e. If the plasma is formed in the wrong location, then the position can be adjusted.

8. **Identify any areas of IOL-capsule separation, and begin treatment there.**
   a. This will decrease the potential for IOL damage.
   b. If the posterior capsule begins to separate from the posterior surface of the IOL during the procedure, wait a moment until maximum separation occurs and then continue.

9. **If possible, identify and cut across capsular tension lines to produce the largest opening per pulse.**
   a. This may involve a relatively linear application of laser pulses.
   b. The capsule edges will separate when the tension is released.
   c. With time, the capsule will usually retract even more and increase the size of the opening.

10. **Perform a cruciate opening if feasible.**
    a. Begin at 12 o'clock **above the center**. If the initial setting or focus is off, the IOL damage won't be in the center along the visual axis, and adjustments could be made.
    b. Progress downward toward 6 o'clock. This in itself may result in an adequate opening.
    c. Cut across from 3 to 9 o'clock, if necessary, to change a slit or oval opening into a circular opening.
    d. Clean up any residual tags.
    e. Avoid large free-floating fragments of capsular material that may disturb the patient's vision.
    f. Continue until the opening is central and of appropriate size (Figure 5–4).

11. **Make the diameter of the capsulotomy opening appropriate** (Goble et al., 1994; Holladay et al., 1985; Shah et al., 1986).
    a. Most clinicians advocate an opening of about **3 to 4 mm** in diameter. In other words, the opening should be **the size of the pupil diameter in ambient light**. Some clinicians advocate limiting the opening to the size of the pupil in darkness.
    b. The point is that the diameter should be sufficient to eliminate visual symptoms and to allow the retina to be fully evaluated or treated, if necessary.

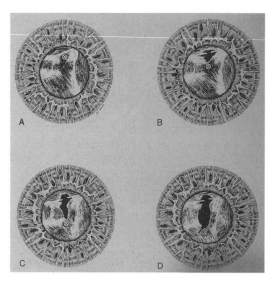

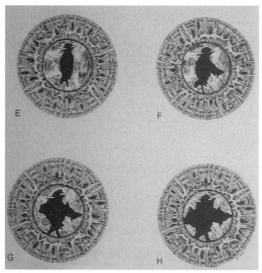

Figure 5–4 A. A cruciate pattern is used to form the capsulotomy by applying the first laser shot superiorly in an area of tension lines. B. The second shot is placed just below the inferior edge of the initial opening. C. The third shot is placed in a similar manner. D. The next shot is placed in an area of tension lines to facilitate widening of the opening. E. The opening is made even wider by placing a shot at the 3 o'clock margin. F. A shot at the 9 o'clock margin extends the opening in that region. G. Finally, a flap at the 7:30 o'clock position is cut and pushed toward the periphery. H. The completed capsulotomy opening will result in a clear pupil when the dilation is reversed. (Reprinted with permission from Steinert RF, Puliafito CA. The Nd-YAG Laser in Ophthalmology. Principles and Clinical Applications of Photodisruption. Philadelphia, PA: WB Saunders, 1985:84–85.)

    c. If the diameter of the capsular opening is smaller than the pupil size
        1) glare may be a problem for the patient,
        2) diffraction may limit the quality of the image formed on the retina, especially if the diameter is less than 2.4 mm, and
        3) evaluation of the retina out to the ora serrata may be precluded in the case of patients with potential retinal problems (e.g., diabetic patients).
    d. If the diameter of the capsular opening is larger than the pupil size
        1) the potential for vitreous prolapse increases,

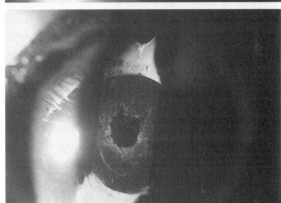

Figure 5–5 Nd:YAG posterior capsulotomy. A. A dense, hazy capsule before the capsulotomy. B. A 3-mm diameter opening in the center of the pupil after capsulotomy. (Reprinted with permission from Noyori K, Shimizu K, Trokel S. Ophthalmic Laser Therapy. Igaku-Shoin: New York, 1992.)

     2) the potential for CME and retinal detachment may increase, and

     3) the potential for IOL dislocation increases.

  e. To make a pupillary-size opening without dilation, first create an opening in the center of the pupil and then have the patient look up, down, to the left, and to the right in order to enlarge the capsular edges posterior to the iris sphincter muscle.

  f. The size and shape of the capsular opening may change with time (Capone et al., 1990; Clayman & Jaffe, 1988; Koch et al., 1989; Thornval & Naeser, 1995). In one study the mean capsulotomy area increased by 32% 6 weeks after the capsulotomy (Capone et al., 1990) (Figure 5–5).

12. **If IOL marking is occurring and/or if the capsule membrane is thick:**

  a. Make an opening in the shape of a Christmas tree from the 12 o'clock to the 4:30 and 7:30 o'clock positions without placing any shots in the central optical zone.

  b. An alternative is to make an opening in the shape of an inverted "U" with a radius of about 1.5 mm and extending about 1 mm below the visual axis (Zeki, 1999).

The resultant flap falls back and down; eventually, it attaches itself to the inferior part of the remaining capsule.

   c. Focus deeper, that is, move further behind the capsule.

   d. Again, avoid the formation of a free-floating capsule fragment.

13. **If Purkinje images from the cornea or IOL are interfering with your visualization of the target area**
   a. adjust the slit-lamp beam or
   b. redirect the patient's gaze slightly to one side.

14. **If bubbles form between the IOL and the capsule**, interrupt the procedure until the bubbles clear enough to allow good visualization of the target area.

G. *Post-Treatment Regimen*

1. Administer one drop of **apraclonidine or a beta-blocker** (e.g., 0.5% Betagan) unless contraindicated.

2. Depending on the level of inflammation, a **steroid** (e.g., prednisolone acetate 1%) may have to be given for a few days. Some clinicians always employ a steroid, and others do not use a steroid unless it is deemed necessary. A **laser flare-cell meter** may be useful in objectively assessing the level of inflammation and for following the progress of therapy.

H. *Follow-Up* (Cataract Management Guideline Panel, 1993; O'Day et al., 1993).

1. **1 to 4 hours**
   a. Check visual acuity and IOP.
   b. Patients with pre-existing glaucoma and especially those with significant visual field loss should be monitored very carefully. Consider maximum medical therapy with these patients.
   c. Instruct the patient:
      1) If headache or eye pain occurs within the first 24 hours, the patient should use an analgesic. If the pain isn't relieved in two hours, you must check the IOP.
      2) Explain the symptoms of retinal detachment and acute glaucoma to the patient.
      3) Give the patient the details concerning access to emergency care.

2. **1 day** (high-risk patients only)

3. **1 week** (certainly within 2 weeks)
   a. Measure IOP.
   b. Check refraction if visual acuity is reduced.
   c. Examine the anterior segment with the slit-lamp biomicroscope and check for adequacy of the capsulotomy and stability of the IOL.

    d. Examine the retina via binocular indirect ophthalmoscopy to check for retinal tears or detachments.

    e. Reinstruct the patient on the symptoms of retinal detachment and glaucoma.

    f. Educate the patient on the need for periodic eye examinations.

    g. Determine an appropriate follow-up schedule for your patient based on risk level and any possible complications.

4. **Routine follow-up**

    a. This should include IOP measurement, slit-lamp biomicroscope examination, and a dilated fundus examination (Table 5–5).

    b. If the patient has experienced a decrease in vision, check for the following:

        1) refractive error shift

        2) CME

        3) retinal detachment

        4) glaucoma

        5) vitreous hemorrhage

Table 5–5 What to Do After the Laser Posterior Capsulotomy

Post-treatment regimen
    1 drop 1% apraclonidine
    Steroid (if necessary)
Follow-up
    1 to 4 hours
        VA
        IOP
        Instruct patient
    1 day (high-risk patients only)
    1 week
        IOP
        Refract (if VA reduced)
        Slit-lamp exam
        BIO
        Reinstruct patient
        Educate patient
        Determine appropriate follow-up schedule
    Routine follow-up
        IOP
        Slit-lamp exam
        Dilated fundus exam

I. Positive Outcomes (Cataract Management Guideline Panel, 1993; Claesson et al., 1994; Magno et al., 1997; Sunderraj et al., 1992).

1. **Improvement of visual acuity.** Snellen visual acuity under standard testing conditions has been shown to improve in 65% to 100% of patients undergoing capsulotomy (Cataract Management Guideline Panel, 1993; Claesson et al., 1994; Knighton et al., 1985; Sunderraj et al., 1992).

2. **Improvement in vision under glare conditions.** Snellen visual acuity under glare conditions has been shown to improve in up to 97% of patients (Claesson et al., 1994; Knighton et al., 1985; Sunderraj et al., 1992; Tan et al., 1998).

3. **Improvement in contrast sensitivity.** In the majority of patients tested, an improvement has been shown in low spatial frequency contrast sensitivity (Claesson et al., 1994; Tan et al., 1999).

4. **Improvement in visual function and health-related quality of life.** The patient's own assessment of improved function is important. Self-assessed as well as interviewer-assessed questionnaires are available (Javitt et al., 1993; Lawrence et al., 1999; Legro, 1991; Mangione et al., 1992).

5. **Improvement in mean opacification density.** Using area densitometry with the Scheimpflug photography system, the mean opacification density value decreased significantly after laser capsulotomy (Hayashi et al., 1998a). This technique may be useful for clinical management as well as for research.

J. Complications (see the following for a review of the literature on complications: Cataract Management Guideline Panel, 1993; Committee on Ophthalmic Procedures Assessment, 1993; Curtis & Javitt, 1994) (Table 5–6).

1. **IOL pits and cracks** (Cataract Management Guideline Panel, 1993; Chehade & Elder, 1997; Dick et al., 1997; Mamalis et al., 1995; Newland et al., 1994) (Table 5–7).
   a. Damage to the patient's IOL occurred with a frequency ranging from 0% to 95%. This usually involved minor pitting of the IOL surface.
   b. Damage to the IOL is usually due to plasma formation on the surface or within the IOL material. Typically, surface cracks and/or pits are formed.
   c. Damage to the IOL can also occur when multiple, subthreshold exposures are made in the same area of the IOL (Sliney et al., 1988). Typically, microfractures or cavities are formed in the bulk of the IOL material. These microlesions increase light scattering and decrease the threshold for plasma formation. Hence, subsequent shots in the same location may result in unintended plasma formation at the IOL.
   d. A few small pits do not affect visual acuity or produce glare problems (Corboy & Novak, 1989; Johnson et al., 1984; Levy & Dodick, 1984; Steinert & Puliafito, 1985).

Table 5–6 Possible Complications
Associated with Laser Posterior
Capsulotomy

IOL pits and cracks
IOP spike
Persistent IOP increase
Cystoid macular edema
Retinal detachment
Inflammation/uveitis
Rupture of the anterior hyaloid face
Vitreous prolapse
Iris hemorrhage
Vitreous hemorrhage
Macular hole
Corneal damage
Corneal graft rejection
Endophthalmitis
Posterior capsule reopacification
Ciliochoroidal effusion
IOL dislocation/entrapment
Aqueous misdirection syndrome
Rubeosis iridis and neovascular glaucoma
Acute hypotonia

e. Larger pits and cracks should be avoided, since they may decrease the visual acuity and cause glare problems (Bath et al., 1987; Gardner et al., 1985; Mamalis et al., 1990; Steinert & Puliafito, 1985).

f. The vulnerability of various types of IOLs to damage from the Nd:YAG laser has been assessed by a number of investigators (Auffarth et al., 1994; Bath et al., 1986a,b; Brancato et al., 1991; Capon et al., 1990; Chehade & Elder, 1997; Johnson & Henderson, 1991; Keates et al., 1987; Kim et al., 1999; Newland et al., 1994; Wilson et al., 1987).

   1) Table 5–8 shows the results on a number of IOLs of the study by Capon and colleagues (Capon et al., 1990).

   2) The results of two other studies show similar results (Bath et al., 1986a,b; Keates et al., 1987).

   3) The flexible silicone and hydrogel IOLs are more subject to laser damage than are the polymethylmethacrylate (PMMA) or the newer acrylic lenses (Bath et al., 1986b; Joo & Kim, 1992; Kim et al., 1999; Newland et al., 1999). Compared to PMMA lenses, the acrylic IOLs have a similar, relatively high resistance to laser damage, but less collateral damage (Newland et al., 1999).

Table 5–7 Occurrence of Damage to the IOL During Nd:YAG Laser Posterior Capsulotomy

Occurrence of IOL Damage (%)	Number of Capsulotomies (n)	Authors
40	30	Terry et al., 1983
29.7	526	Keates et al., 1984
10.3	117	Levy & Dodick, 1984
4	300	Aron-Rosa, 1985
95.4	195	Axt, 1985
10.2	108 (multimode)	Buratto et al., 1985
0	108 (fundamental mode)	
10	210	Chambless, 1985b
81	36	Flohr et al., 1985
39	67	Gardner et al., 1985
11.7	342	Harris et al., 1985
9	158	Levy & Pisacano, 1985
21	94	Liesegang et al., 1985
50	52	Nirankari & Richards, 1985
10	50	Peyman et al., 1985
20	2110	Stark et al., 1985
9.5	367	Wasserman et al., 1985
18.9	595	Bath & Fankhauser, 1986
12	2808	Shah et al., 1986
14	129	Lewis et al., 1987

Table 5–8 Vulnerability of Various Types of IOLs to Damage from the Nd:YAG Laser During Posterior Capsulotomy

Type of IOL	Vulnerability (in descending order)
Compression-molded PMMA with UV absorber	Most vulnerable (lowest damage threshold)
Silicone without UV absorber	
Injection-molded PMMA without UV absorber	
Injection-molded PMMA with UV absorber	
Compression-molded PMMA without UV absorber	
Lathe-cut PMMA with UV absorber	
Polymacon without UV absorber	
Lathe-cut PMMA without UV absorber	Least vulnerable (highest damage threshold)

Data from Capon et al., 1990.

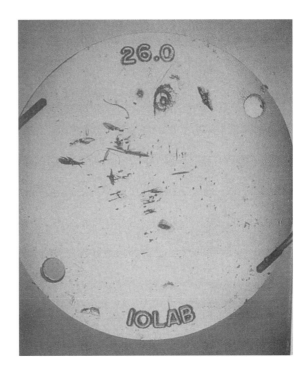

Figure 5–6 Explanted YAG-damaged IOL. (Reprinted from Bath PE, Hoffer KJ, Aron-Rosa, Dang Y. Glare disability secondary to YAG laser intraocular lens damage. J Cataract Refract Surg 13:309–313 [1987], with permission from Elsevier Science.)

    a) Small pits or fracture lines are usually formed in the PMMA lenses.

    b) Lesions that look similar to melted spots can be formed in the silicone lenses.

    c) Be careful not to confuse Nd:YAG laser damage with dark pigment deposits on the IOL (Auffarth et al., 1994). This could lead to further damage in an attempt to remove the "deposits" with the laser.

  4) There appears to be less damage to a foldable IOL with a UV blocker than to a PMMA IOL with a UV blocker (Johnson & Henderson, 1991).

  5) Diffractive IOLs have about the same damage threshold as PMMA IOLs (Brancato et al., 1991). Clinical example (Chambless, 1985b)—Out of a total of 210 patients, 10.4% ended up with pits or cracks. In the first 25 cases, 68% developed pits or cracks. In the remaining 185 cases, only 2.7% were pitted or cracked. This illustrates the effect of practice (Figures 5–6 and 5–7).

2. **IOP spike** (Brown et al., 1985, 1988; Bukelman et al., 1992; Channell & Beckman, 1984; Cullom & Schwartz, 1993; Flohr et al., 1985; Lados et al., 1993; Migliori et al., 1987; Pollack et al., 1988; Richter et al., 1985a,b; Schubert, 1985; Schubert et al., 1985; Shani et al., 1994; Silverstone et al., 1988, 1992; Slomovic & Parrish, 1985a,b; Stark et al., 1985; Stilma & Boen-tan, 1986; van der Feltz van der Sloot et al., 1988).

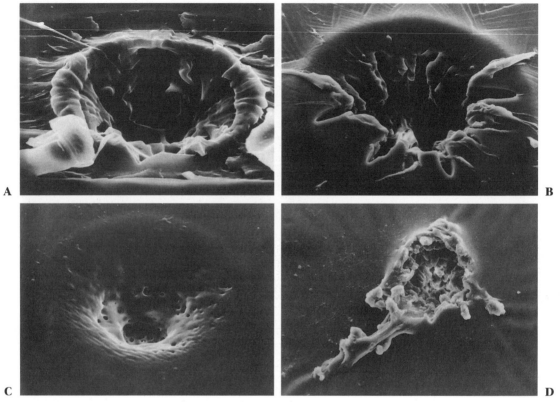

Figure 5–7 Scanning electron microscopy comparison of Nd:YAG laser IOL damage at damage threshold from IOLs. A. Injection-molded PMMA. B. Lathe-cut PMMA. C. Cast-molded PMMA. D. Silicone. (Reprinted from Bath PE, Brown P, Romberger A, Quon D. Quantitative concepts in avoiding intraocular lens damage from the Nd:YAG laser in posterior capsulotomy. J Cataract Refract Surg 12:262–6 (1986), with permission from Elsevier Science.)

    a. IOP increases ≥10 mm Hg or >10 mm Hg have been reported in from 0% to 67% of patients (Table 5–9).

    b. The peak of the IOP increase usually occurs within 4 hours post-treatment, and then it usually declines over the next 24 hours (Gimbel et al., 1990; Richter et al., 1985a,b; Slomovic & Parrish, 1985a). A delayed increase in IOP (e.g., 24 hours later) can occur (Channell & Beckman, 1984; Nesher & Kolker, 1990; Romanowski, 1992).

    c. The IOP spike is due to a reduction in aqueous outflow facility and not to an increase in secretion of aqueous (Wetzel, 1994). The mechanism of the aqueous outflow decrease is unknown. It could be due to capsular debris, acute inflammatory cells, a high molecular weight protein, or a low molecular weight factor from the vitreous (Adams et al., 1996; Deutsch & Goldberg, 1985; Gimbel et al.,

Table 5–9 Occurrence of IOP Increase ≥10 mm Hg After Nd:YAG Posterior Capsulotomy

Placebo (n)	Prophylaxis (n)	Type of Prophylaxis	Authors
59% (37)			Channell & Beckman, 1984
29.3% (393)			Johnson, et al., 1984
29.9% (67)			Leys et al., 1985
66.7% (15)	6.7% (15)	4% pilocarpine	Brown et al., 1985
32.3% (31)			Flohr et al., 1985
36.4% (11)	18.2% (11)	2% pilocarpine	Richter et al., 1985a
	10% (10)	0.5% timolol	
67% (21)			Richter et al., 1985b
28% (32)			Slomovic & Parrish, 1985b
50% (10)	0% (10)	0.5% timolol	Boen-Tan & Stilma, 1986
	0% (10)	0.5% timolol + 250 mg acetazolamide	
22.2% (27)	4.6% (22)	0.5% timolol	Migliori et al., 1987
15% (100)			Schubert, 1987
14% (21)	4% (25)	1% apraclonidine	Brown et al., 1988
17% (30)	3% (33)	1% apraclonidine	Pollack et al., 1988
38% (21)	0% (21)	0.5% levobunolol	Silverstone et al., 1988
27% (33)	0% (30)	0.25% clonidine	Loewenstein et al., 1991
13.8% (65)			Bukelman et al., 1992
25% (164)	2% (163)	1% apraclonidine	Silverstone et al., 1992
27% (22)	4% (53)	1% apraclonidine	Cullom & Schwartz, 1993
30.8% (26)	0% (28)	125 mg acetazolamide	Ladas et al., 1993
4.4% (340)			Shani et al., 1994
	0% (30)	0.5% apraclonidine	Rosenberg et al., 1995
	4% (27)	1% apraclonidine	
57.5% (28)—sulcus fixated IOL			Anand et al., 1996
5% (21)—1 haptic in the bag			
0% (43)—bag-fixated IOL			
	0% (101)	0.5% apraclonidine	Holweger & Marefat, 1997
27.1% (70)	2.9% (70)	125 mg acetazolamide	Ladas et al., 1997
	5.7% (70)	2% dorzolamide	
7.1% (28)	0% (60)	0.5% levobunolol	Rakofsky et al., 1997
	0% (54)	0.5% timolol	
20% (20)	10% (20)	0.5% timolol	Simsek et al., 1998
	0% (20)	0.5% apraclonidine	
	0% (20)	1% apraclonidine	
6.7% (30)	0% (38)	2% dorzolamide	Hartenbaum et al., 1999
	6.8% (133)	1% apraclonidine	Skolnick et al., 2000

1990; Holweger & Marefat, 1997; Kraff et al., 1985; Parker & Clorfeine, 1984; Parker et al., 1984; Richter et al., 1985b; Schubert, 1985; Schubert et al., 1985; Slomovic & Parrish, 1985a). In addition, the Nd:YAG shock wave may contribute to damage to the trabecular meshwork (Channell & Beckman, 1984; Schubert, 1985). After Nd:YAG laser anterior capsulotomy in rabbits, a similar IOP rise has been noted, and fibrin has been identified in the anterior chamber angle (Lin et al., 1994).

d. Risk factors for an IOP increase include the following (Brown et al., 1985; Channell & Beckman, 1984; Hoffer, 1984; Kraff et al., 1985; Migliori et al., 1987; Pollack et al., 1988; Richter et al., 1985a,b; Schubert, 1987; Shah et al., 1986; Slomovic & Parrish, 1985a; Stark et al., 1985):
   1) pre-procedure IOP >20 mm Hg
   2) history of glaucoma
   3) use of high total laser energy
   4) use of cycloplegics
   5) high myopia
   6) aphakia
   7) multiple Nd:YAG laser procedures
   8) large capsular opening
   9) absence of a posterior chamber IOL
   10) vitreous prolapse into the anterior chamber.

e. The increase in IOP following the capsulotomy is significantly higher in sulcus-fixated IOLs than in bag-fixated IOLs (Anand et al., 1996; Gimbel et al., 1990). This may be because bag-fixated IOLs are a better barrier to capsular debris and may dampen the effect of the pressure wave generated by the Nd:YAG laser.

f. The increase in IOP is also significantly higher in aphakes than in pseudophakes (Brown et al., 1985; Hoffer, 1984; Kraff et al., 1985; Migliori et al., 1987; Richter et al., 1985a,b; Slomovic & Parrish, 1985a). This may be because the IOL provides a barrier to capsular debris, and/or it may dampen the Nd:YAG shock wave and prevent damage to the trabecular meshwork. In one case, a marked increase in IOP occurred in an aphake who had experienced recurrent episodes of pupillary block; the patient's IOP went from 22 mm Hg before the laser capsulotomy to 67 mm Hg the next day (Parker et al., 1984). The patient was eventually hospitalized for intravenous treatment.

g. The type of Nd:YAG laser also apparently leads to a different prevalence of IOP spikes. Aron-Rosa (1985) found that a 5 mm Hg or more increase in IOP occurred in 23% of patients treated with a picosecond, mode-locked laser, 31% treated with a nanosecond, fundamental-mode, Q-switched laser, and 48% treated with a nanosecond, multimode, Q-switched laser. When timolol was used prophylactically the prevalences decreased to 2%, 5%, and 8%, respectively.

h. You must carefully monitor and treat patients with preexisting glaucoma, especially those with severe visual field loss. This may include the use of β-blockers, systemic or topical carbonic anhydrase inhibitors, glycerin, or continued use of apraclonidine.

3. **Persistent IOP increase** (Channell & Beckman, 1984; Demer et al., 1986; Fourman & Apisson, 1991; Jahn & Emke, 1996; Kurata et al., 1984; Slomovic & Parrish, 1985a; Stark et al., 1985; Steinert et al., 1991).
   a. This is most common in eyes with a history of glaucoma or with initial IOPs >20 mm Hg.
   b. About 1% of patients have a persistent increase in IOP at 1 week.
   c. 5.9% experience a late-onset increase by 2 to 3 years later (Fourman & Apisson, 1991).
   d. A large IOP increase, especially in a glaucoma patient, can lead to progressive visual field loss (Kurata et al., 1984).

4. **Cystoid macular edema** (Alpar, 1986; Bukelman et al., 1992; Ruiz & Saatci, 1991; Steinert et al., 1991).
   a. There was a 0.0% to 4.4% occurrence of CME (mean: 1.3%) in large-scale studies (n > 100) with at least 6 months of follow-up (Table 5–10). Considering all studies, there was a 0% to 21% occurrence of CME (see Table 5–10). Unfortunately angiographic documentation of the pre-capsulotomy status was not available in most studies. Thus it is difficult to interpret the prevalences.
   b. 80% of the patients recovered within 3 months.
   c. The cause of CME is not completely understood. It appears to be related most often to inflammation, but it may also be associated with tractional, toxic, and/or immunological postoperative complications. Disruption of the anterior hyaloid face may increase the incidence of CME.
   d. Because 80% of patients recover spontaneously, therapy for most cases of postoperative CME is not necessary. However, persistent or severe associated inflammation would require therapy.
   e. If you decide to treat, consider acetazolamide 500 mg po daily (Cox et al., 1988). A number of other forms of therapy with unproven efficacy are also occasionally used.

5. **Retinal detachment (RD)** (Alldredge et al., 1998; Barraquer et al., 1994; Dardenne et al., 1989; Fastenberg et al., 1984; Javitt et al., 1992; Koch et al., 1989; Leff et al., 1987; Lerman et al., 1984; MacEwen & Baines, 1989; Ober et al., 1986; Olsen & Olson, 1995; Powell & Olson, 1995; Ranta & Kivela, 1998; Rickman-Barger et al., 1989; Rosen, 1997; Salvesen et al., 1991; Smith et al., 1995; Steinert et al., 1991; Tasman, 1989; Tielsch et al., 1996; Van Westenbrugge et al., 1992).
   a. There was a **0.0–13% occurrence** in 38 various studies with an overall mean of 1.7% (Table 5–11).

Table 5–10 Occurrence of Cystoid Macular Edema (CME) After Nd:YAG Posterior Capsulotomy

Occurrence of CME (%)	Number of Capsulotomies (n)	Follow-Up Time	Authors
0.04	3253	unknown	Aron-Rosa et al., 1984
0.8	389	>6 mon	Johnson et al., 1984
2.3	526	6 mon	Keates et al., 1984
0	213	6 mon	Axt, 1985
0.9	210	>14.5 mon	Chambless, 1985b
2.3			Durham, 1985
4.4	342	>6 mon	Harris et al., 1985
6.8	74	1 year	Knolle, 1985
1	158	unknown	Levy & Pisacano, 1985
4.3	94	>6 mon	Liesegang et al., 1985
4.3	93	>3 mon	Nirankari & Richards, 1985
2	50	unknown	Peyman et al., 1985
3	67	>1 mon	Slomovic & Parrish, 1985b
1.2	2110	>6 mon	Stark et al., 1985
0.3	367	unknown	Wasserman et al., 1985
0.5	1100	unknown	Winslow & Taylor, 1985
5.7	70 (Microruptor 2)	unknown	Alpar, 1986
21	62 (OPL3)		
2.5	595	6 mon	Bath & Frankhauser, 1986
0.68	2808	unknown	Shah et al., 1986
0	80	>6 mon	Lewis et al., 1987
13	23	1 mon	Wright et al., 1988
0	122	>6 mon	Koch et al., 1989
5.6	54	12 mon	Albert et al., 1990
10	10	>6 mon	Ruiz & Saatci, 1991
1.23	897	>3 mon	Steinert et al., 1991
0.00	65	>2 mon	Bukelman et al., 1992
1.8	51	>3 mon	Lyle & Jin, 1996
0	133	>6 mon	Skolnick et al., 2000

b. The largest study (n = 13,709) reported a probability of RD of **1.6%** during the first 36 months following cataract extraction for patients who underwent capsulotomy (Javitt et al., 1992). Their data indicated that, although infrequent, the **risk of RD increases 3.9-fold** and the risk of retinal break without detachment increases 2.24-fold following capsulotomy. Because of acknowledged limitations of that study, the same group undertook a national case-control study of retinal detachment among Medicare beneficiaries who had undergone extracapsular cataract surgery (Tielsch et al., 1996). In this improved study with 291 cases of retinal detachment and 870 matched controls, the group found that Nd:YAG

Table 5–11 Occurrence of Retinal Detachments Following Nd:YAG Posterior Capsulotomy

RD Occurrence (%)	Number of Capsulotomies (n)	Follow-Up Time	Mean Time Between Capsulotomy and RD	Authors
0.4	210	>14.5 mon	4 mon	Chambless, 1985b
6	48	>14 mon	8.5 mon	Nissen et al., 1998
2.35	383	>12 mon	6.3 mon	Olsen & Olson, 1995
1.6	1000	>12 mon	ca. 10 mon	Dardenne et al., 1989
2.7	74	12 mon		Knolle, 1985
1.35	74	>7 mon	18 mon	Jacobi & Hessemer, 1997
1.5	133	>6 mon		Skolnick et al., 2000
1.0	94	>6 mon	34.4 mon	Liesegang et al., 1985
1.2	342	>6 mon	(3–9 mon)	Harris et al., 1985
0.4	526	>6 mon		Keates et al., 1984
0.5	2110	>6 mon		Stark et al., 1985
1.1	545	>6 mon		Vester et al., 1986
1.4	862	>6 mon	8 mon	Ambler & Constable, 1988
0.5	389	>6 mon	1.6 mon	Johnson et al., 1984
1.2	595	6 mon		Bath & Fankhauser, 1986
0	213	6 mon	N.A.	Axt, 1985
13	45	>3 mon	9.16 mon	Barraquer et al., 1994
2.1	582	>3 mon	(1.25–18 mon)	Ficker et al., 1987
3.6	366	>3 mon	5.79 mon	Rickman-Barger et al., 1989
0.89	897	>3 mon	13.5 mon	Steinert et al., 1991
0.9	51	>3 mon	2 mon	Lyle & Jin, 1996
1.1	93	>3 mon		Nirankari & Richards, 1985
1.2	85	>2 mon	9 mon	Bukelman et al., 1992
0	24	>1 mon	N.A.	Alldredge et al., 1998
0.29	345	>4 d (mean 1.78 years)	2 weeks (only 1 case)	Nielsen & Naeser, 1993
0.82	244	unknown	13.5 mon	Powell & Olson, 1995
2.9	34	unknown	26 mon (only 1 case)	Seward & Doran, 1984
2	50	unknown	unknown	Peyman et al., 1985
3.3	122	unknown		Koch et al., 1989
3.2	95	unknown		Coonan et al., 1985
0.9	1100	unknown	5.3 mon	Winslow & Taylor, 1985
2.0	49	unknown	2.5 mon	Terry et al., 1983
0.17	2808	unknown		Shah et al., 1986
1.6	13709	unknown		Javitt et al., 1992
1.0	198	unknown	16 mon	Van Westenbrugge et al., 1992
1.0	193	unknown	5.7 mon	Salvesen et al., 1991
0.08	3253	unknown	unknown	Aron-Rosa et al., 1984
0.3	367	unknown		Wasserman et al., 1985

posterior capsulotomy was associated with a **3.8-fold excess risk** of pseudopha-kic retinal detachment.

c. In a Swedish study where 24 RDs occurred in 5878 consecutive patients after cataract extraction, the risk of RD was found to increase 4.9-fold after laser cap-sulotomy (Ninn-Pedersen & Bauer, 1996).

d. In a retrospective cohort study of 129 consecutive eyes with pseudophakic retinal detachment, the data suggested that laser capsulotomy increases the risk of RD about **4-fold** (Ranta & Kivela, 1998). This study suggested that atrophic holes, especially superior quadrant holes, may produce RD more easily after laser cap-sulotomy, and if these breaks are identified and treated at the time of capsulo-tomy, detachments might be decreased by a quarter to one third.

e. The risk factors for an RD include:
   1) axial myopia (axial length ≥25 mm)
   2) history of RD in the fellow eye
   3) history of previous RD
   4) lattice degeneration
   5) vitreous prolapse into the anterior chamber
   6) white race
   7) male sex
   8) relative youth
   9) history of ocular trauma after cataract surgery

f. The study with the second highest occurrence of retinal detachment (6%) involved patients that were 40 years of age or older with axial myopia (Nissen et al., 1998). In other words, this whole group of patients was at higher risk for RD. In fact, this is consistent with another study that found that high myopia increased the risk for RD by a factor of about 10 (from 0.5% to 5.4%) (Dardenne et al., 1989).

g. In various studies, the average time interval between capsulotomy and the diag-nosis of RD varied from 1.6 to 34.4 months. The mean of the average time inter-vals in the 17 studies where there was more than one case and the mean was available was 10.4 months. One recent study reported a significantly higher mean of 32 months and a range of 0.4 to 106 months (Ranta & Kivela, 1998). However, this study had a longer follow-up period than most of the others and only involved patients that had no complications during the cataract operation. In one large study of retinal detachments following cataract surgery, it was found that 46% of eyes that developed an RD after a laser capsulotomy developed the RD within 6 months of the laser procedure (Yoshida et al., 1992).

h. Vitreous movement through the capsulotomy opening toward the anterior chamber may contribute to the increased risk of RD, rather than some direct effect of the laser photodisruption (Buratto, 1991; Chambless, 1985a; Krauss et al., 1986). However, damage to the vitreous may also contribute to the increased risk.

1) There is collateral damage, a diffuse depolymerization and decrease in viscosity of the anterior vitreous, near the area of optical breakdown.

2) The capsulotomy may lead to loss of a glycosaminoglycan, hyaluronate, which then leads to vitreous degeneration and posterior vitreous detachment (PVD). The PVD can then lead to RD.

i. The possibility of RD is one of the reasons all patients should have a detailed, dilated fundus examination before and at various intervals after laser capsulotomy. In addition, obviously all patients should be warned of the risks and symptoms of RD.

j. Obviously, if your patient develops an RD, you should refer the patient to a retinologist for treatment. After surgical treatment, the prognosis is usually good.

6. **Inflammation/uveitis** (Altamirano et al., 1992; Cataract Management Guideline Panel, 1993; Lewis et al., 1987) (Table 5–12).

a. There was a 0.0% to 30% occurrence of uveitis. Unfortunately, there was no standard definition of uveitis in these studies.

b. According to one study, up to 83% of patients developed mild inflammation, 16% developed moderate inflammation, and 1.5% developed severe inflammation 24

Table 5–12 Occurrence of Iritis/Uveitis Following Nd:YAG Laser Posterior Capsulotomy

Uveitis Occurrence (no. of capsulotomies)	Authors
0.8% (389)	Johnson et al., 1984
0.4% (526)	Keates et al., 1984
1% (117)	Levy & Dodick, 1984
0% (213)	Axt, 1985
0.4% (216)	Buratto et al., 1985
1.4% (210)	Chambless, 1985b
13% (100)	Gardner et al., 1985
14.6% (342)	Harris et al., 1985
0.6% (158)	Levy & Pisacano, 1985
1% (94)	Liesegang et al., 1985
30% (50)	Peyman et al., 1985
0.6% (2110)	Stark et al., 1985
1% (367)	Wasserman et al., 1985
0.7% (595)	Bath & Fankhauser, 1986
0.1% (2808)	Shah et al., 1986
0.6% (329)	Silverstone et al., 1992
0.8% (133)	Skolnick et al., 2000

hours after the capsulotomy (Lewis et al., 1987). Mild inflammation was present in 6% at one week.

c. A variety of practices are employed.
   1) Some clinicians use steroids on all patients.
   2) Many clinicians only use steroids when necessary.
   3) With less than 30 laser shots of 1 mJ each, treatment with steroids is rarely required.
d. Aqueous flare increased in 34% of patients assessed with the laser flare-cell meter. Only 5% of those with increased flare needed to be treated.
e. Aqueous flare noted clinically occurred in 48% of patients.
f. Anterior chamber particles increased in 48% of patients assessed with the laser flare-cell meter.
g. Anterior chamber inflammation correlates with an increase in IOP following an Nd:YAG capsulotomy.
h. If your patient develops an inflammation:
   1) You may prescribe a steroid (e.g., prednisolone acetate 1%, q 1 to 6h depending on the severity).
   2) Follow up every 1 to 7 days in the acute phase, depending on the severity. At each follow-up visit, evaluate the anterior-chamber reaction and the IOP.
   3) Treat, if necessary, any secondary ocular hypertension.
   4) If the anterior-chamber reaction is improving, then slowly taper the steroid drops (e.g., 1 drop per day every 3 to 7 days). Once all cells have disappeared from the anterior chamber, the steroid can usually be discontinued.
i. If there is a severe inflammatory reaction with excessive pain, consider the possibility of endophthalmitis.

7. **Rupture of the anterior hyaloid face** (Alpar, 1986; Cataract Management Guideline Panel, 1993; Ficker & Steele, 1985; Lewis et al., 1987; Liesegang et al., 1985; Stark et al., 1985; Terry et al., 1983) (Table 5–13).

Table 5–13 Occurrence of Rupture of Anterior Hyaloid Face Following Nd:YAG Laser Posterior Capsulotomy

Anterior Hyaloid Face Rupture Occurrence (no. of capsulotomies)	Authors
12.2% (49)—only occurred in aphakes	Terry et al., 1983
1.9% (213)	Axt, 1985
42% (24)	Ficker & Steele, 1985
48.9% (94)	Liesegang et al., 1985
32% (50)	Peyman et al., 1985
19% (2110)	Stark et al., 1985
11.4% (70)—Microruptor 2	Alpar, 1986
38.7% (62)—OPL3	
18.2% (595)	Bath & Fankhauser, 1986
10% (129)—CL used in all cases	Lewis et al., 1987

   a. This occurs in 1.9% to 49% of patients.
   b. Rupture may increase the risk of vitreous prolapse and cystoid macular edema. The intact posterior capsule may provide a mechanical and chemical barrier separating the chambers. Interrupting the mechanical barrier may allow prolapse of the vitreous with an increase in retinal traction and hence a possible increase in retinal detachments. Interrupting the chemical barrier may allow inflammatory mediators to move from the anterior segment to the posterior segment and thus may increase the likelihood of CME.
   c. It is apparently easier to maintain the integrity of the anterior hyaloid face if the laser capsulotomy is done 6 or more months after the cataract extraction (Alpar, 1986). During this time, the posterior capsule can shrink and tighten, thus increasing the separation of the capsule from the vitreous face.
   d. Use of a laser contact lens may result in less rupture. In addition, use of the lowest possible energy setting and the lowest possible number of laser applications with very accurate focusing should help protect the anterior hyaloid face from disruption.

8. **Vitreous prolapse** (Albert et al., 1990; Harris et al., 1985; Koch et al., 1989; Nirankari & Richards, 1985; Schubert, 1987; Skolnick et al., 2000; Terry et al., 1983).
   a. The occurrence of vitreous prolapse ranges from 0% to 16% in pseudophakes. In aphakes the occurrence ranges from 12.2% to 80%.
   b. Prolapse may increase the risk for CME, RD, corneal edema, IOP rise, and pupillary-block glaucoma.

9. **Iris hemorrhage** (Cataract Management Guideline Panel, 1993; Flohr et al., 1985) (Table 5–14).
   a. The occurrence of iris hemorrhage ranged from 0.2% to 9%.
   b. The occurrence of hyphema ranged from 0.15% to 5%. A layered hyphema is rarely produced.

Table 5–14 Occurrence of Iris Hemorrhage Following Nd:YAG Laser Posterior Capsulotomy

Occurrence of Iris Bleeding (no. of capsulotomies)	*Authors*
5% (3253)	Aron-Rosa et al., 1984
0.6% (526)	Keates et al., 1984
9% (53)	Flohr et al., 1985
3% (100)	Gardner et al., 1985
1.2% (342)	Harris et al., 1985
1% (158)	Levy & Pisacano, 1985
1% (2110)	Stark et al., 1985
0.2% (595)	Bath & Fankhauser, 1986

   c. Hemorrhage can be due to a miss-aim when the laser cuts a blood vessel in the iris.

   d. It may also be caused by the laser shock wave disrupting iris blood vessels in areas of iridocapsular adhesion.

   e. Hemorrhage usually only produces a transient trickle. When using a contact lens, you may apply additional pressure to tamponade the vessel leakage.

   f. If the aqueous becomes too turbid, it may be necessary to interrupt the procedure and complete the capsulotomy at a later time.

10. **Vitreous hemorrhage** (Helbig et al., 1996).

   a. After Nd:YAG laser posterior capsulotomy, vitreous hemorrhage occurred within 6 months in 29% of 21 eyes of diabetic retinopathy patients.

   b. Previous to the capsulotomy, these patients had undergone vitrectomy for diabetic retinopathy. In fact, there was a higher occurrence of capsulotomy in vitrectomized diabetic eyes (60%) than in nondiabetic controls (10%).

11. **Macular hole** (Blacharski & Newsome, 1988; Curtis & Javitt, 1994; Chambless, 1985b; Winslow & Taylor, 1985).

   a. The occurrence of macular holes ranged from 0.2% to 0.4% in those studies that reported holes.

   b. The time interval between capsulotomy and macular hole formation is usually less than 4 weeks.

   c. Vitreous-macular traction bands are probably involved in the formation of the holes.

   d. In patients with a history of a macular hole in the other eye, you should wait until a spontaneous posterior vitreous detachment has occurred. This will decrease the risk.

12. **Corneal damage (stromal scarring and endothelial or epithelial trauma)** (Aron-Rosa et al., 1980; Axt, 1985; Bailey et al., 1988; Canning et al., 1988; Curtis & Javitt, 1994; Ficker & Steele, 1985; Kerr Muir & Sherrard, 1985; Kozobolis et al., 1998; Kraff et al., 1985; Sherrard & Kerr Muir, 1985).

   a. Reported corneal endothelial cell loss/gain in most studies ranged from a gain of 6% to a loss of 7% (Axt, 1985; Kraff et al., 1985; Liesegang et al., 1985; Slomovic et al., 1986; Wasserman et al., 1985). However, in one study, endothelial damage occurred in 56% of eyes (Canning et al., 1988), and in another study, 85% of the eyes had damage to the endothelium upon examination with a specular microscope (Kerr Muir & Sherrard, 1985). In most cases, no evidence of endothelial damage was found after 24 hours (Sherrard & Kerr Muir, 1985), and no persistent damage was detected after 3 months (Canning et al., 1988).

   b. Reported mild transitory corneal edema ranged from 0% to 2% (Table 5–15).

   c. Corneal stromal scarring has also been reported due to miss-aim.

Table 5–15 Occurrence of Corneal Edema Following Nd:YAG Laser Posterior Capsulotomies

Corneal Edema Occurrence (no. of capsulotomies)	Authors
2% (117)	Levy & Dodick, 1984
1% (158)	Levy & Pisacano, 1985
1% (94)	Liesegang et al., 1985
0.3% (2110)	Stark et al., 1985
0% (39)	Slomovic et al., 1986
0.3% (329)	Silverstone et al., 1992

   d. If the laser is mis-aimed, and especially if a laser contact lens is not used, it is possible to damage the corneal epithelium too. Photothermal or photodisruptive damage could occur.

   e. If corneal epithelial damage is sustained, you should treat prophylactically with an antibiotic (e.g., trimethoprim/polymyxin (Polytrim) drops 4 times per day or erythromycin ointment 2 to 3 times per day).

13. **Corneal graft rejection** (Cahane et al., 1992; Crawford et al., 1986; DeBacker et al., 1996; Insler et al., 1990; Meyer & Musch, 1987).

   a. Acute corneal graft rejection has been reported in 4 patients 1 to 11 months following capsulotomy (Cahane et al., 1992; DeBacker et al., 1996). However in other studies, no graft rejections occurred after laser capsulotomy (Crawford et al., 1986; Insler et al., 1990; Meyer & Musch, 1987).

   b. Cahane et al. (1992) suggested that an immunological response resulting in graft rejection may have been triggered by an anterior chamber inflammatory response due to the capsulotomy. However, DeBacker et al. (1996) concluded that the risk of corneal graft rejection did not appear to increase following laser capsulotomy. In their study, 12.5% of the control group experienced graft rejection which was more than the 5% who experienced graft rejection after laser capsulotomy.

14. **Endophthalmitis** (Carlson & Koch, 1988; Koenig et al., 1993; Meisler & Mandelbaum, 1989; Neuteboom & de Vries-Knoppert, 1988; Tetz et al., 1987).

   a. Although very rare, there have been a few case reports of endophthalmitis occurring after capsulotomy.

   b. This may occur by the liberation of previously sequestered microorganisms.

   c. The endophthalmitis can manifest as a chronic inflammation with a white plaque on the IOL or posterior capsule, hypopyon, or granulomatous-appearing keratic precipitates. Treatment may include steroids, intravitreal antibiotics, or surgical intervention.

15. **Posterior capsule reopacification** (Brady et al., 1995; Jones et al., 1995; Kato et al., 1997; Lotery & Sharkey, 1995; McPherson & Govan, 1995).
    a. Massive proliferation of lens epithelial remnants can occur following capsulotomy. Occurrences of up to 0.7% have been reported.
    b. Proliferative disorders of the retina and raised levels of growth factors in the posterior segment may play a role in some cases.
    c. In one study involving 103 eyes, Elschnig pearl formation occurred along the capsulotomy margin in 47.6% of the eyes (Kato et al., 1997). Three-fourths of the eyes developed pearls within the first year after the laser capsulotomy. The pearls caused visual disturbances in 34.7% of the eyes and required a repeat capsulotomy in 36.7% of the eyes with pearls.
    d. Pearl formation from the proliferation and migration of residual lens epithelial cells may involve the use of the posterior surface of the IOL or the anterior hyaloid face as a scaffold. This may occur more often in younger patients (<50).
    e. Many of these cases required further capsulotomy treatments. In fact, in a pediatric population, up to 41% needed a second laser capsulotomy.
    f. Spontaneous disappearance of the pearls after an Nd:YAG capsulotomy has been reported (Caballero et al., 1997). After initial hyperproliferation at the edge of the capsulotomy, the pearls disappeared spontaneously several years after the capsulotomy in six eyes.

16. **Ciliochoroidal effusion** (Schaeffer et al., 1989).
    a. Two cases of ciliochoroidal effusion after laser capsulotomy have been reported. Both patients had a history of glaucoma and a propensity for uveitis.
    b. The effusions were probably secondary to uveitis induced by the laser procedure.

17. **IOL dislocation/entrapment** (Clayman & Jaffe, 1988; Framme et al., 1998; Keates et al., 1984; Kidd et al., 1997; Levy et al., 1990; Melamed et al., 1986; Menapace & Yalon, 1993; Schneiderman et al., 1997; Shah et al., 1986).
    a. The occurrence of IOL dislocation in those papers where one or more cases were reported ranged from 0.1 to 8.4%. In one study with bag-placed Iogel PC-12 lenses, the occurrence of IOL dislocations after capsulotomy dropped from 8.4% when capsulotomy was done within the first 3 months to 0.9% when done from 10 to 14 months and then to 0% when done after 14 months (cited in Menapace, 1996).
    b. Spontaneous enlargement of the capsular opening can result in dislocation of the IOL.
    c. Dilation before capsulotomy followed by an IOP increase can cause entrapment of the IOL.
    d. Silicone IOLs are hydrophobic and can develop adhesions in the capsular bag. This can result in IOL dislocation. Silicone plate haptic IOLs can undergo delayed posterior dislocation through capsular defects up to 6.5 months after laser capsulotomy.

   e. Some bag-placed hydrogel lenses may be too large to withstand capsular bag contraction after implantation with a capsulorhexis. This can result in radial tears in the capsule and displacement of the IOL into the vitreous (Levy et al., 1990). Radial tears and dislocation can also occur with PMMA lenses (Framme et al., 1998).

   f. Caution should also be exercised when considering laser capsulotomy on a previously subluxated lens.

   g. The IOL dislocation can be surgically managed by pars plana vitrectomy and IOL repositioning or exchange.

   h. In one case, asteroid hyalosis made it difficult to diagnose a posterior dislocation following a laser capsulotomy (Kidd et al., 1997).

   i. Nd:YAG posterior capsulotomy produces a backward movement of the IOL (Findl et al., 1999). The range of movement is from 9 μm to 55 μm, and the largest movement occurred with plate-haptic IOLs compared to one-piece PMMA and three-piece foldable IOLs. This small amount of movement will result in a clinically insignificant hyperopic shift.

18. **Aqueous misdirection syndrome** (Mastropasqua et al., 1994).

   a. One case of malignant glaucoma due to aqueous misdirection syndrome has been reported as a complication of Nd:YAG posterior capsulotomy.

   b. There was a persistent rise in IOP in an eye with a flat anterior chamber. This could have been due to the laser effects on the vitreous, diverting the aqueous posteriorly into the anterior vitreous. This could have created a pocket of aqueous, compression of the vitreous, and flattening of the chamber.

19. **Rubeosis iridis and neovascular glaucoma** (Ruiz & Saatci, 1991; Tsopelas et al., 1995).

   a. In patients with diabetic retinopathy and especially those with retinal neovascularization, laser capsulotomy may increase the risk of rubeosis iridis and neovascular glaucoma.

   b. The intact posterior capsule may act as a barrier to prevent growth factors from reaching the anterior segment.

20. **Acute hypotonia** (Walter et al., 1997). One case of episodic acute hypotonia has been reported in which the IOP dropped from 14 to 2 mm Hg following a laser capsulotomy. The patient had a history of recurrent panuveitis and was treated with immunosuppressive and immunomodulating therapy.

21. **Vitreous opacification** (Kumagai et al., 1999). Following Nd:YAG posterior capsulotomy, opacification of the vitreous in contact with the IOL occurred in 1.2% of eyes (n = 728) in one study. The opacification occurred within one month after the capsulotomy and was significantly more prevalent in diabetic eyes compared to non-diabetic eyes. One case spontaneously resorbed, and the others were treated by vitrectomy.

References

Adams EA et al. Effect of neodymium:YAG laser on sodium hyaluronate in vitro as a model for postcapsulotomy intraocular pressure change. J Cataract Refract Surg 22:748–751 (1996).

Albert DW et al. A prospective study of angiographic cystoid macular edema one year after Nd:YAG posterior capsulotomy. Ann Ophthalmol 22:139–143 (1990).

Alldredge CD, Elkins B, Alldredge OC Jr. Retinal detachment following phacoemulsification in highly myopic cataract patients. J Cataract Refract Surg 24:777–780 (1998).

Alpar JJ. Experiences with the neodymium:YAG laser: interruption of anterior hyaloid membrane of the vitreous and cystoid macular edema. Ophthalmic Surg 17:157–165 (1986).

Altamirano D, Mermoud A, Pittet N, et al. Aqueous humor analysis after Nd:YAG capsulotomy with the laser flare-cell meter. J Cataract Refract Surg 18:554–558 (1992).

Ambler JS, Constable IJ. Retinal detachment following Nd:YAG capsulotomy. Aust NZ J Ophthalmol 16:337–341 (1988).

Anand N, Tole DM, Morrell AJ. Effect of intraocular lens fixation on acute intraocular pressure rise after neodymium-YAG laser capsulotomy. Eye 10:509–513 (1996).

Apple DJ et al. Posterior capsule opacification. Surv Ophthalmol 37:73–116 (1992).

Aron-Rosa D. Influence of picosecond and nanosecond YAG laser capsulotomy on intraocular pressure. J Am Intraocul Implant Soc 11:249–252 (1985).

Aron-Rosa D et al. Use of the neodymium-YAG laser to open the posterior capsule after lens implant surgery: a preliminary report. J Am Intraocul Implant Soc 6:352–354 (1980).

Aron-Rosa DS, Aron J-J, Cohn HC. Use of a pulsed picosecond Nd:YAG laser in 6,664 cases. J Am Intraocul Implant Soc 10:35–39 (1984).

Auffarth GU et al. Nd:YAG laser damage to silicone intraocular lenses confused with pigment deposits on clinical examination [letter]. Am J Ophthalmol 118:526–528 (1994).

Axt JC. Nd:YAG laser posterior capsulotomy: a clinical study. Am J Optom Physiol Optics 62:173–187 (1985).

Bailey L, Donzis PB, Kastl PR. Stromal corneal scar following YAG capsulotomy. Ann Ophthalmol 20:188–190 (1988).

Barraquer C, Cavelier C, Mejia LF. Incidence of retinal detachment following clear-lens extraction in myopic patients. Retrospective analysis. Arch Ophthalmol 112:336–339 (1994).

Bath PE et al. Quantitative concepts in avoiding intraocular lens damage from the Nd:YAG laser in posterior capsulotomy. J Cataract Refract Surg 12:262–266 (1986a).

Bath PE et al. Glare disability secondary to YAG laser intraocular lens damage. J Cataract Refract Surg 13:309–313 (1987).

Bath PE, Fankhauser F. Long-term results of Nd:YAG laser posterior capsulotomy with the Swiss laser. J Cataract Refract Surg 12:150–153 (1986).

Bath PE, Romberger AB, Brown P. A comparison of Nd:YAG laser damage thresholds for PMMA and silicone intraocular lenses. Invest Ophthalmol Vis Sci 27:795–798 (1986b).

Blacharski PA, Newsome DA. Bilateral macular holes after Nd:YAG laser posterior capsulotomy [letter]. Am J Ophthalmol 105:417–418 (1988).

Boen-Tan TN, Stilma JS. Prevention of IOP-rise following Nd-YAG laser capsulotomy with pre-operative timolol eye-drops and 1 tablet acetazolamide 250 mg systematically. Doc Ophthalmol 64:59–67 (1986).

Born CP, Ryan DK. Effect of intraocular lens optic design on posterior capsular opacification. J Cataract Refract Surg 16:188–192 (1990).

Brady KM et al. Cataract surgery and intraocular lens implantation in children. Am J Ophthalmol 120:1–9 (1995).

Brancato R et al. Study of laser damage to injection-molded diffractive intraocular lenses. J Cataract Refract Surg 17:639–641 (1991).

Brown RH et al. ALO 2145 reduces the intraocular pressure elevation after anterior segment laser surgery. Ophthalmology 95:378–384 (1988).

Brown SVL et al. Effect of pilocarpine in treatment of intraocular pressure elevation following neodymium:YAG laser posterior capsulotomy. Ophthalmology 92:354–359 (1985).

Bukelman A et al. Cystoid macular oedema following neodymium:YAG laser capsulotomy a prospective study. Eye 6:35–38 (1992).

Buratto L. Cataract surgery in high myopia. Eur J Implant Refract Surg 3:271–278 (1991).

Buratto L, Ricci A, Vitali D. Use of the YAG laser with a seven-micron spot in pseudophakic eyes. Am Intraocular Implant Soc J 11:574–576 (1985).

Caballero A, Salinas M, Marin JM. Spontaneous disappearance of Elschnig pearls after neodymium:YAG laser posterior capsulotomy. J Cataract Refract Surg 23:1590–1594 (1997).

Cahane M et al. Corneal graft rejection after neodymium-yttrium-aluminum-garnet laser posterior capsulotomy. Cornea 11:534–537 (1992).

Canning CR et al. Neodymium:YAG laser iridotomies—short-term comparison with capsulotomies and long-term follow-up. Graefes Arch Clin Exp Ophthalmol 226:49–54 (1988).

Capon MRC et al. Comprehensive study of damage to intraocular lenses by single and multiple nanosecond neodymium:YAG laser pulses. J Cataract Refract Surg 16:603–610 (1990).

Capone A et al. Temporal changes in posterior capsulotomy dimensions following neodymium:YAG laser discission. J Cataract Refract Surg 16:451–456 (1990).

Carlson AN, Koch DD. Endophthalmitis following Nd:YAG laser posterior capsulotomy. Ophthalmic Surg 19:168–170 (1988).

Cataract Management Guideline Panel. Management of functional impairment due to cataract in adults. Appendix O. Literature review: posterior capsular opacification—YAG capsulotomy. Ophthalmology 100 (Supplement):273S–310S (1993).

Chambless WS. Incidence of anterior and posterior segment complications in over 3,000 cases of extracapsular cataract extractions: intact and open capsules. J Am Intraocul Implant Soc 11:146–148 (1985a).

Chambless WS. Neodymium:YAG laser posterior capsulotomy results and complications. J Am Intraocul Implant Soc 11:31–32 (1985b).

Channell MM, Beckman H. Intraocular pressure changes after neodymium-YAG laser posterior capsulotomy. Arch Ophthalmol 102:1024–1026 (1984).

Chehade M, Elder MJ. Intraocular lens materials and styles: a review. Aust N Z J Ophthalmol 25:255–263 (1997).

Claesson M et al. Glare and contrast sensitivity before and after Nd:YAG laser capsulotomy. Acta Ophthalmol 72:27–32 (1994).

Clark DS. Posterior capsule opacification. Curr Opin Ophthalmol 11:56–64 (2000).

Clark DS, Munsell MF, Emery JM. Mathematical model to predict the need for neodymium:YAG capsulotomy based on posterior capsule opacification rate. J Cataract Refract Surg 24:1621–1625 (1998).

Clayman HM, Jaffe NS. Spontaneous enlargement of neodymium:YAG posterior capsulotomy in aphakic and pseudophakic patients. J Cataract Refract Surg 14:667–669 (1988).

Colin J, Robinet A. Clear lensectomy and implantation of a low-power posterior chamber intraocular lens for correction of high myopia: a four-year follow-up. Ophthalmology 104:73–77 (1997).

Committee on Ophthalmic Procedures Assessment. Ophthalmic procedures assessment: Nd:YAG photodisruptors. Ophthalmology 100:1736–1742 (1993).

Coonan P et al. The incidence of retinal detachment following extracapsular cataract extraction. A ten-year study. Ophthalmology 92:1096–1101 (1985).

Corboy JM, Novak EA Jr. Neodymium:YAG laser capsulotomy with a biconvex intraocular lens. J Cataract Refract Surg 15:435–436 (1989).

Cox SN, Hay E, Bird AC. Treatment of chronic macular edema with acetazolamide. Arch Ophthalmol 106:1190–1195 (1988).

Crawford CJ et al. The triple procedure. Analysis of outcome, refraction, and intraocular lens power calculation. Ophthalmology 93:817–824 (1986).

Cullom RD Jr; Schwartz LW. The effect of apraclonidine on the intraocular pressure of glaucoma patients following Nd:YAG laser posterior capsulotomy. Ophthalmic Surg 24:623–626 (1993).

Curtis WJ, Javitt JC. Complications of neodymium: yttrium-aluminum-garnet laser capsulotomy. Current Opinion in Ophthalmology 5:30–34 (1994).

Cuzzani OE et al. Potential Acuity Meter versus scanning laser ophthalmoscope to predict visual acuity in cataract patients. J Cataract Refract Surg 24:263–269 (1998).

D'Amico DJ et al. Initial clinical experience with an erbium:YAG laser for vitreoretinal surgery. Am J Ophthalmol 121:414–425 (1996).

Dardenne M-U et al. Retrospective study of retinal detachment following neodymium:YAG laser posterior capsulotomy. J Cataract Refract Surg 15:676–680 (1989).

DeBacker CM et al. Effect of neodymium:YAG laser posterior capsulotomy on corneal grafts. Cornea 15:15–17 (1996).

Demer JL et al. Persistent elevation in intraocular pressure after Nd:YAG laser treatment. Ophthalmic Surg 17:465–466 (1986).

Deutsch TA, Goldberg MF. Neodymium:YAG laser capsulotomy. Int Ophthalmol Clin 25:87–100 (1985).

Dick B, Schwenn O, Eisenmann D. Reflections on Nd:YAG capsulotomy in lens opacity after multifocal lens implantation. Klin Monatsbl Augenheilkd 211:363–368 (1997).

Fankhauser F, Lortscher H, van der Zypen E. Clinical studies on high and low power laser radiation upon some structures of the anterior and posterior segments of the eye. Experiences in the treatment of some pathological conditions of the anterior and posterior segments of the human eye by means of a Nd:YAG laser, driven at various power levels. Int Ophthalmol 5:15–32 (1982).

Fastenberg DM, Schwartz PL, Lin HZ. Retinal detachment following neodymium-YAG laser capsulotomy. Am J Ophthalmol 97:288–291 (1984).

Faulkner HW. The laser interferometer in predicting efficacy of secondary posterior capsulotomy. Am Intra-Ocular Implant Soc J 8:136–140 (1982).

Faulkner HW. Predicting acuities in capsulotomy patients: interferometers and potential acuity meter. Am Intra-Ocular Implant Soc J 9:434–437 (1983).

Ficker LA et al. Retinal detachment following Nd:YAG posterior capsulotomy. Eye 1:86–89 (1987).

Ficker LA, Steele ADM. Complications of Nd:YAG laser posterior capsulotomy. Trans Ophthalmol Soc UK 104:529–532 (1985).

Findl O et al. Changes in intraocular lens position after neodymium:YAG capsulotomy. J Cataract Refract Surg 25:659–662 (1999).

Flohr MJ, Robin AL, Kelley JS. Early complications following Q-switched neodymium:YAG laser posterior capsulotomy. Ophthalmology 92:360–363 (1985).

Fourman S, Apisson J. Late-onset elevation in intraocular pressure after Q-switched neodymium:YAG laser posterior capsulotomy. Arch Ophthalmol 109:511–513 (1991).

Framme C et al. Delayed intraocular lens dislocation after neodymium:YAG capsulotomy. J Cataract Refract Surg 24:1541–1543 (1998).

Frezzotti R, Caporossi A. Pathogenesis of posterior capsular opacification. Part I. Epidemiological and clinico-statistical data. J Cataract Refract Surg 16:347–352 (1990).

Gardner KM, Straatsma BR, Pettit TH. Neodymium:YAG laser posterior capsulotomy: the first 100 cases at UCLA. Ophthalmic Surg 16:24–28 (1985).

Geerling G et al. Initial clinical experience with the picosecond Nd:YLF laser for intraocular therapeutic applications. Br J Ophthalmol 82:504–509 (1998).

Gimbel HV et al. Effect of sulcus vs capsular fixation on YAG-induced pressure rises following posterior capsulotomy. Arch Ophthalmol 108:1126–1129 (1990).

Goble RR et al. The role of light scatter in the degradation of visual performance before and after Nd:YAG capsulotomy. Eye 8:530–534 (1994).

Green WR, McDonnell PJ. Opacification of the posterior capsule. Trans Ophthalmol Soc UK 104:727–739 (1985).

Grusha YO, Masket S, Miller KM. Phacoemulsification and lens implantation after pars plana vitrectomy. Ophthalmology 105:287–294 (1998).

Hanna IT et al. The role of white light interferometry in predicting visual acuity following posterior capsulotomy. Eye 3:468–471 (1989).

Hanuch OE et al. Posterior capsule polishing with the neodymium:YLF picosecond laser: model eye study. J Cataract Refract Surg 23:1561–1571 (1997).

Hard A-L, Beckman C, Sjostrand J. Glare measurements before and after cataract surgery. Acta Ophthalmol 71:471–476 (1993).

Harris WS, Herman WK, Fagadau WR. Management of the posterior capsule before and after the YAG laser. Trans Ophthalmol Soc U K 104:533–535 (1985).

Hartenbaum D et al. A randomized study of dorzolamide in the prevention of elevated intraocular pressure after anterior segment laser surgery. J Glaucoma 8:273–275 (1999).

Hayashi K et al. In vivo quantitative measurement of posterior capsule opacification after extracapsular cataract surgery. Am J Ophthalmol 125:837–843 (1998a).

Hayashi H et al. Quantitative comparison of posterior capsule opacification after polymethylmethacrylate, silicone, and soft acrylic intraocular lens implantation. Arch Ophthalmol 116:1579–1582 (1998b).

Helbig H et al. Cataract surgery and YAG-laser capsulotomy following vitrectomy for diabetic retinopathy. Ger J Ophthalmol 5:408–414 (1996).

Hofeldt AJ. Illuminated near card assessment of potential visual acuity. J Cataract Refract Surg 22:367–371 (1996).

Hoffer KJ. YAG and IOP [letter]. Ophthalmic Surg 15:610 (1984).

Holladay JT, Bishop JE, Lewis JW. The optimal size of a posterior capsulotomy. Am Intra-Ocular Implant Soc J 11:18–20 (1985).

Hollick EJ et al. The effect of polymethylmethacrylate, silicone, and polyacrylic intraocular lenses on posterior capsular opacification 3 years after cataract surgery. Ophthalmology 106:49–55 (1999).

Holweger RR, Marefat B. Intraocular pressure change after neodymium:YAG capsulotomy. J Cataract Refract Surg 23:115–121 (1997).

Hoppeler T, Gloor B. Preliminary clinical results with the ISL laser. Proc SPIE Ophthalmic Technologies II 1644:96–99 (1992).

Insler MS, Kern MD, Kaufman HE. Results of neodymium:YAG laser posterior capsulotomy following penetrating keratoplasty. J Cataract Refract Surg 16:369–371 (1990).

Jacobi FK, Hessemer V. Pseudophakic retinal detachment in high axial myopia. J Cataract Refract Surg 23:1095–1102 (1997).

Jahn CE, Emke M. Long-term elevation of intraocular pressure after neodymium:YAG laser posterior capsulotomy. Ophthalmologica 210:85–89 (1996).

Javitt JC et al. National outcomes of cataract extraction. Increased risk of retinal complications associated with Nd:YAG laser capsulotomy. The Cataract Patient Outcomes Research Team. Ophthalmology 99:1487–1498 (1992).

Javitt JC et al. Outcomes of cataract surgery. Improvement in visual acuity and subjective visual function after surgery in the first, second, and both eyes. Arch Ophthalmol 111:686–691 (1993).

Johnson S, Kratz R, Olson P. Clinical experience with the Nd:YAG laser. Am Intra-Ocular Implant Soc J 10:452–460 (1984).

Johnson SH, Henderson C. Neodymium:YAG laser damage to UV-absorbing poly(methyl methacrylate) and UV-absorbing MMA-HEMA-EGDMA polymer intraocular lens materials. J Cataract Refract Surg 17:604–607 (1991).

Jones NP, McLeod D, Boulton ME. Massive proliferation of lens epithelial remnants after Nd-YAG laser capsulotomy. Br J Ophthalmol 79:261–263 (1995).

Joo C-K, Kim J-H. Effect of neodymium:YAG laser photodisruption on intra-ocular lenses in vitro. J Cataract Refract Surg 18:562–566 (1992).

Kato K et al. Elschnig pearl formation along the posterior capsulotomy margin after neodymium:YAG capsulotomy. J Cataract Refract Surg 23:1556–1560 (1997).

Keates RH et al. Long-term follow-up of Nd:YAG laser posterior capsulotomy. Am Intra-Ocular Implant Soc J 10:164–168 (1984).

Keates RH, Sall KN, Kreter JK. Effect of the Nd:YAG laser on polymethylmethacrylate, HEMA copolymer, and silicone intra-ocular materials. J Cataract Refract Surg 13:401–409 (1987).

Kerr Muir MG, Sherrard ES. Damage to the corneal endothelium during Nd/YAG photodisruption. Br J Ophthalmol 69:77–85 (1985).

Kidd GR, Cohen KL, Eifrig DE. Asteroid hyalosis and vision loss after posterior capsulotomy. J Cataract Refract Surg 23:1595–1596 (1997).

Kim MJ, Lee HY, Joo CK. Posterior capsule opacification in eyes with a silicone or poly(methyl methacrylate) intraocular lens. J Cataract Refract Surg 25:251–255 (1999).

Klein TB et al. Visual acuity prediction before neodymium-YAG laser posterior capsulotomy. Ophthalmology 93:808–810 (1986).

Knighton RW, Slomovic AR, Parrish RK II. Glare measurements before and after neodymium-YAG laser posterior capsulotomy. Am J Ophthalmol 100:708–713 (1985).

Knolle GE Jr. Knife versus neodymium:YAG laser posterior capsulotomy: a one-year follow-up. Am Intra-Ocular Implant Soc J 11:448–455 (1985).

Koch DD et al. Axial myopia increases the risk of retinal complications after neodymium-YAG laser posterior capsulotomy. Arch Ophthalmol 107:986–990 (1989).

Koenig SB et al. Pseudophakia for traumatic cataracts in children. Ophthalmology 100:1218–1224 (1993).

Kolder HE. Chapter 15—YAG laser capsulotomy. In Weingart TA, Sneed SR, eds. Laser surgery in ophthalmology: Practical applications. Norwalk, CT: Appleton and Lange, 1992.

Kozobolis VP et al. Endothelial corneal damage after neodymium:YAG laser treatment: pupillary membranectomies, iridotomies, capsulotomies. Ophthalmic Surg Lasers 29:793–802 (1998).

Kraff MC, Sanders DR, Lieberman HL. Intraocular pressure and the corneal endothelium after neodymium-YAG laser posterior capsulotomy. Relative effects of aphakia and pseudophakia. Arch Ophthalmol 103:511–514 (1985).

Krauss JM et al. Vitreous changes after neodymium-YAG laser photodisruption. Arch Ophthalmol 104:592–597 (1986).

Kumagai K et al. Vitreous opacification after neodymium:YAG posterior capsulotomy. J Cataract Refract Surg 25:981–984 (1999).

Kurata F et al. Progressive glaucomatous visual field loss after neodymium-YAG laser capsulotomy. Am J Ophthalmol 98:632–634 (1984).

Ladas ID et al. Prophylactic use of acetazolamide to prevent intraocular pressure elevation following Nd-YAG laser posterior capsulotomy. Br J Ophthalmol 77:136–138 (1993).

Ladas ID et al. Topical 2.0% dorzolamide vs oral acetazolamide for prevention of intraocular pressure rise after neodymium:YAG laser posterior capsulotomy. Arch Ophthalmol 115:1241–1244 (1997).

Lang TA, Lindstrom RL. Efficacy of laser interferometry in predicting visual result of YAG laser posterior capsulotomy. Am Intra-Ocular Implant Soc J 11:367–371 (1985).

Lawrence DJ et al. Measuring the effectiveness of cataract surgery: the reliability and validity of a visual function outcomes instrument. Br J Ophthalmol 83:66–70 (1999).

Lee KH, Lee JH. Long-term results of clear lens extraction for severe myopia. J Cataract Refract Surg 22:1411–1415 (1996).

Leff SR, Welch JC, Tasman W. Rhegmatogenous retinal detachment after YAG laser posterior capsulotomy. Ophthalmology 94:1222–1225 (1987).

Legro MW. Quality of life and cataracts: a review of patient-centered studies of cataract surgery outcomes. Ophthalmic Surg 22:431–443 (1991).

Lerman S, Thrasher B, Moran M. Vitreous changes after neodymium:YAG laser irradiation of the posterior lens capsule or mid-vitreous. Am J Ophthalmol 97:470–475 (1984).

Levy JH, Dodick JM. Initial clinical results with YAG laser capsulectomy with a monomode, Q-switched unit (LASAG). Am Intra-Ocular Implant Soc J 10:341–342 (1984).

Levy JH, Pisacano AM. Comparison of techniques and clinical results of YAG laser capsulotomy with two Q-switched units. Am Intra-Ocular Implant Soc J 11:131–133 (1985).

Levy JH, Pisacano AM, Anello RD. Displacement of bag-placed hydrogel lenses into the vitreous following neodymium:YAG laser capsulotomy. J Cataract Refract Surg 16:563–566 (1990).

Lewis H et al. A prospective study of cystoid macular edema after neodymium:YAG laser posterior capsulotomy. Ophthalmology 94:478–482 (1987).

Leys MJJ, Pameijer JH, de Jong PTVM. Intermediate-term changes in intraocular pressure after neodymium-YAG laser posterior capsulotomy. Am J Ophthalmol 100:332–333 (1985).

Liesegang TJ, Bourne WM, Ilstrup DM. Secondary surgical and neodymium-YAG laser discissions. Am J Ophthalmol 100:510–519 (1985).

Lin TY et al. Immunohistological visualization of fibrin in anterior chamber angle after YAG laser capsulotomy. Jpn J Ophthalmol 38:144–147 (1994).

Lindstrom RL, Harris WS. Management of the posterior capsule following posterior chamber lens implantation. Am Intra-Ocular Implant Soc J 6:255–258 (1980).

Loewenstein A et al. Prevention of the rise in intraocular pressure following neodymium-YAG posterior capsulotomy using topical clonidine. Acta Ophthalmol (Copenh) 69:462–465 (1991).

Lotery AJ, Sharkey JA. Proliferation of lens epithelial remnants after Nd-YAG laser capsulotomy [letter]. Br J Ophthalmol 79:964 (1995).

Loya N et al. Effects of the picosecond neodymium:YLF laser on poly(methyl methacrylate) intraocular lenses during experimental posterior capsulotomy. J Cataract Refract Surg 21:586–590 (1995).

Lyle WA, Jin GJC. Phacoemulsification with intraocular lens implantation in high myopia. J Cataract Refract Surg 22:238–242 (1996).

MacEwen CJ, Baines PS. Retinal detachment following YAG laser capsulotomy. Eye 3:759–763 (1989).

Magno BV et al. Evaluation of visual function following neodymium:YAG laser posterior capsulotomy. Ophthalmology 104:1287–1293 (1997).

Mamalis N, Craig MT, Price FW. Spectrum of Nd:YAG laser-induced intraocular lens damage in explanted lenses. J Cataract Refract Surg 16:495–500 (1990).

Mamalis N et al. Effect of intraocular lens size on posterior capsule opacification after phacoemulsification. J Cataract Refract Surg 21:99–102 (1995).

Mamalis N et al. Neodymium:YAG capsulotomy rates after phacoemulsification with silicone posterior chamber intraocular lenses. J Cataract Refract Surg 22:1296–1302 (1996).

Mangione CM et al. Development of the "Activities of Daily Vision Scale." A measure of visual functional status. Med Care 30:1111–1126 (1992).

Martin RG et al. Effect of posterior chamber intraocular lens design and surgical placement on postoperative outcome. J Cataract Refract Surg 18:333–341 (1992).

Mastropasqua L et al. Aqueous misdirection syndrome: A complication of neodymium:YAG posterior capsulotomy. J Cataract Refract Surg 20:563–565 (1994).

McCarty CA, Keefe JE, Taylor HR. The need for cataract surgery: projections based on lens opacity, visual acuity, and personal concern. Br J Ophthalmol 83:62–65 (1999).

McGraw PV, Barrett BT. Assessing retinal/neural function in the presence of ocular media opacities. Graefes Arch Clin Exp Ophthalmol 234:280–283 (1996).

McPherson RJE, Govan JAA. Posterior capsule reopacification after neodymium:YAG laser capsulotomy. J Cataract Refract Surg 21:351–352 (1995).

Meisler DM, Mandelbaum S. Propionibacterium-associated endophthalmitis after extracapsular cataract extraction. Review of reported cases. Ophthalmology 96:54–61 (1989).

Melamed S, Barraquer E, Epstein DL. Neodymium:YAG laser iridotomy as a possible contribution to lens dislocation. Ann Ophthalmol 18:281–282 (1986).

Menapace R. Posterior capsule opacification and capsulotomy rates with taco-style hydrogel intraocular lenses. J Cataract Refract Surg 22 (Suppl 2):1318–1330 (1996).

Menapace R, Yalon M. Exchange of IOGEL hydrogel one-piece foldable intraocular lens for bag-fixated J-loop poly(methyl methacrylate) intraocular lens. J Cataract Refract Surg 19:425–430 (1993).

Meyer RF, Musch DC. Assessment of success and complications of triple procedure injury. Am J Ophthalmol 104:233–240 (1987).

Michaeli-Cohen A et al. Prevention of posterior capsule opacification with the CO_2 laser. Ophthalmic Surg Lasers 29:985–990 (1998).

Migliori ME, Beckman H, Channell MM. Intraocular pressure changes after neodymium–YAG laser capsulotomy in eyes pretreated with timolol. Arch Ophthalmol 105:473–475 (1987).

Milazzo S et al. Long-term follow-up of three-piece, looped, silicone intraocular lenses. J Cataract Refract Surg 22 (Suppl 2): 1259–1262 (1996).

Moisseiev J et al. Long-term study of the prevalence of capsular opacification following extracapsular cataract extraction. J Cataract Refract Surg 15:531–533 (1989).

Murillo-Lopez F, Maumenee AE, Guyton DL. Perception of Purkinje vessel shadows and foveal granular pattern as a measure of potential visual acuity. J Cataract Refract Surg 26:260–265 (2000).

Nesher R, Kolker AE. Delayed increased intraocular pressure after Nd:YAG laser posterior capsulotomy in a patient treated with apraclonidine. Am J Ophthalmol 110:94–95 (1990).

Neuteboom GHG, de Vries-Knoppert WAEJ. Endophthalmitis after Nd:YAG laser capsulotomy. Doc Ophthalmol 70:175–178 (1988).

Newland TJ et al. Neodymium:YAG laser damage on silicone intraocular lenses. A comparison of lesions on explanted lenses and experimentally produced lesions. J Cataract Refract Surg 20:527–533 (1994).

Newland TJ et al. Experimental neodymium:Yag laser damage to acrylic, poly (methlyl methacrylate), and silicone intraocular lens materials. Cataract Refract Surg 25:72–76 (1999).

Nielsen NE, Naeser K. Epidemiology of retinal detachment following extracapsular cataract extraction: a follow-up study with an analysis of risk factors. J Cataract Refract Surg 19:675–680 (1993).

Ninn-Pedersen K, Bauer B. Cataract patients in a defined Swedish population, 1986 to 1990. V. Postoperative retinal detachments. Arch Ophthalmol 114:382–386 (1996).

Ninn-Pedersen K, Bauer B. Cataract patients in a defined Swedish population, 1986 to 1990. VI. YAG laser capsulotomies in relation to preoperative and surgical conditions. Acta Ophthalmol Scand 75:551–557 (1997).

Nirankari VS, Richards RD. Complications associated with the use of the neodymium:YAG laser. Ophthalmology 92:1371–1375 (1985).

Nishi O. Posterior capsule opacification. Part 1: experimental investigations. J Cataract Refract Surg 25:106–117 (1999).

Nissen KR et al. Retinal detachment after cataract extraction in myopic eyes. J Cataract Refract Surg 24:772–776 (1998).

Nucci P, Biglan AW, Rehkopf P. Neodymium:YAG capsulotomy in children. In Tasman W. Jaeger EA, eds. Duane's clinical ophthalmology, volume 6, rev. ed. Philadelphia, PA: Lippincott-Raven Publishers, 1995.

Ober RR et al. Rhegmatogenous retinal detachment after neodymium-YAG laser capsulotomy in phakic and pseudophakic eyes. Am J Ophthalmol 101:81–89 (1986).

O'Day DM, Cataract Management Guideline Panel of the Agency for Health Care Policy and Research. Management of cataract in adults. Quick reference guide for clinicians. Arch Ophthalmol 111:453–459 (1993).

Olsen GM, Olson RJ. Prospective study of cataract surgery, capsulotomy, and retinal detachment. J Cataract Refract Surg 21:136–139 (1995).

Olson RJ, Crandall AS. Silicone versus polymethylmethacrylate intraocular lenses with regard to capsular opacification. Ophthalmic Surg Lasers 29:55–58 (1998).

Oshika T et al. Three year prospective, randomized evaluation of intraocular lens implantation through 3.2 and 5.5 mm incisions. J Cataract Refract Surg 24:509–514 (1998).

Parker WT, Clorfeine GS. YAG capsulotomy and IOP rise [letter]. Ophthalmic Surg 15:787 (1984).

Parker WT, Clorfeine GS, Stocklin RD. Marked intraocular pressure rise following Nd:YAG laser capsulotomy. Ophthalmic Surg 15:103–104 (1984).

Peyman GA et al. Early clinical experience with a new generation Q-switched neodymium:YAG laser. Am Intra-Ocular Implant Soc J 11:292–294 (1985).

Pollack IP et al. Prevention of the rise in intraocular pressure following neodymium-YAG posterior capsulotomy using topical 1% apraclonidine. Arch Ophthalmol 106:754–757 (1988).

Powell SK, Olson RJ. Incidence of retinal detachment after cataract surgery and neodymium:YAG laser capsulotomy. J Cataract Refract Surg 21:132–135 (1995).

Rakofsky S et al. Levobunolol 0.5% and timolol 0.5% to prevent intraocular pressure elevation after neodymium:YAG laser posterior capsulotomy. J Cataract Refract Surg 23:1075–1080 (1997).

Ranta P, Kivela T. Retinal detachment in pseudophakic eyes with and without Nd:YAG laser posterior capsulotomy. Ophthalmology 105:2127–2133 (1998).

Richter CU et al. Prevention of intraocular pressure elevation following neodymium-YAG laser posterior capsulotomy. Arch Ophthalmol 103:912–915 (1985a).

Richter CU et al. Intraocular pressure elevation following Nd:YAG laser posterior capsulotomy. Ophthalmology 92:636–640 (1985b).

Rickman-Barger L et al. Retinal detachment after neodymium:YAG laser posterior capsulotomy. Am J Ophthalmol 107:531–536 (1989).

Romanowski A. Prophylactic use of apraclonidine for intraocular pressure increase after Nd:YAG capsulotomies [letter]. Am J Ophthalmol 114:377–378 (1992).

Rosen B. Retinal detachment after laser capsulotomy [letter]. J Cataract Refract Surg 23:7–8 (1997).

Rosenberg LF et al. Apraclonidine and anterior segment laser surgery. Comparison of 0.5% versus 1.0% apraclonidine for prevention of postoperative intraocular pressure rise. Ophthalmology 102:1312–1318 (1995).

Royal College of Ophthalmologists. Guidelines for cataract surgery. London: Royal College of Ophthalmologists, 1995.

Ruiz RS, Saatci OA. Posterior chamber intraocular lens implantation in eyes with inactive and active proliferative diabetic retinopathy. Am J Ophthalmol 111:158–162 (1991).

Salvesen S, Eide N, Syrdalen P. Retinal detachment after YAG-laser capsulotomy. Acta Ophthalmol 69:61–64 (1991).

Schaeffer AR, Ryll DL, O'Donnell FE. Ciliochoroidal effusions after neodymium YAG posterior capsulotomy: association with pre-existing glaucoma and uveitis. J Cataract Refract Surg 15:567–569 (1989).

Schaumberg DA et al. A systematic overview of the incidence of posterior capsule opacification. Ophthalmology 105:1213–1221 (1998).

Schneiderman TE et al. Surgical management of posteriorly dislocated silicone plate haptic intraocular lenses. Am J Ophthalmol 123:629–635 (1997).

Schubert HD. A history of intraocular pressure rise with reference to the Nd:YAG laser. Surv Ophthalmol 30:168–172 (1985).

Schubert HD. Vitreoretinal changes associated with rise in intraocular pressure after Nd:YAG capsulotomy. Ophthalmic Surg 18:19–22 (1987).

Schubert HD et al. The role of the vitreous in the intraocular pressure rise after neodymium-YAG laser capsulotomy. Arch Ophthalmol 103:1538–1542 (1985).

Seward HC, Doran RML. Posterior capsulotomy and retinal detachment following extracapsular lens surgery. Br J Ophthalmol 68:379–382 (1984).

Shah GR et al. Three thousand YAG lasers in posterior capsulotomies: an analysis of complications and comparison to polishing and surgical discission. Ophthalmic Surg 17:473–477 (1986).

Shani L et al. Intraocular pressure after neodymium:YAG laser treatments in the anterior segment. J Cataract Refract Surg 20:455–458 (1994).

Sherrard ES, Ker Muir MG. Damage to the corneal endothelium by Q-switched Nd:YAG laser posterior capsulotomy. Trans Ophthalmol Soc UK 104:524–528 (1985).

Shin DH et al. Decrease of capsular opacification with adjunctive mitomycin C in combined glaucoma and cataract surgery. Ophthalmology 105:1222–1226 (1998).

Siganos DS, Pallikaris IG. Clear lensectomy and intraocular lens implantation for hyperopia from +7 to +14 diopters. J Refract Surg 14:105–113 (1998).

Silverstone DE et al. Prophylactic treatment of intraocular pressure elevations after neodymium:YAG laser posterior capsulotomies and extracapsular cataract extractions with levobunolol. Ophthalmology 95:713–718 (1988).

Silverstone DE et al. Prophylactic use of apraclonidine for intraocular pressure increase after Nd:YAG capsulotomies. Am J Ophthalmol 113:401–405 (1992).

Simcoe CW. Capsular discission behind posterior chamber lens. Contact Intra-Ocul Lens Med J 6:60–61 (1980).

Simsek S et al. The effect of 0.25% apraclonidine in preventing intraocular pressure elevation after Nd:YAG laser posterior capsulotomy. Eur J Ophthalmol 8:167–172 (1998).

Sinskey RM, Cain W Jr. The posterior capsule and phacoemulsification. Am Intra-Ocular Implant Soc J 4:206–207 (1978).

Skolnick KA et al. Neodymium:YAG laser posterior capsulotomies performed by residents at a Veterans Administration hospital. J Cataract Refract Surg 26:597–601 (2000).

Sliney DH et al. Intraocular lens damage from Nd:YAG laser pulses focused in the vitreous. Part II: mode-locked lasers. J Cataract Refract Surg 14:530–532 (1988).

Slomovic AR et al. Neodymium-YAG laser posterior capsulotomy. Central corneal endothelial cell density. Arch Ophthalmol 104:536–538 (1986).

Slomovic AR, Parrish RK II. Acute elevations of intraocular pressure following Nd:YAG laser posterior capsulotomy. Ophthalmology 92:973–976 (1985a).

Slomovic AR, Parrish RK II. Neodymium:YAG laser posterior capsulotomy: visual acuity outcome and intraocular pressure elevation. Can J Ophthalmol 20:101–104 (1985b).

Smith RT et al. The barrier function in neodymium-YAG laser capsulotomy. Arch Ophthalmol 113:645–652 (1995).

Spurny RC et al. Instruments for predicting visual acuity. A clinical comparison. Arch Ophthalmol 104:196–200 (1986).

Stark WJ et al. Neodymium:YAG lasers: an FDA report. Ophthalmology 92:209–12 (1985).

Steinert RF et al. Cystoid macular edema, retinal detachment, and glaucoma after Nd:YAG laser posterior capsulotomy. Am J Ophthalmol 112:373–380 (1991).

Steinert RF, Puliafito CA. The Nd-YAG laser in ophthalmology: Principles and clinical applications of photodisruption. Philadelphia, PA: WB Saunders Co, 1985.

Stilma JS, Boen-Tan TN. Timolol and intra-ocular pressure elevation following neodymium:YAG laser surgery. Doc Ophthalmol 61:233–239 (1986).

Strong N. Interferometer assessment of potential visual acuity before YAG capsulotomy: relative performance of three instruments. Graefe's Arch Clin Exp Ophthalmol 230:42–46 (1992).

Sundelin K, Sjostrand J. Posterior capsule opacification 5 years after extracapsular cataract extraction. J Cataract Refract Surg 25:246–250 (1999).

Sunderraj P et al. Glare testing in pseudophakes with posterior capsule opacification. Eye 6:411–413 (1992).

Tan JCH, Spalton DJ, Arden GB. Comparison of methods to assess visual impairment from glare and light scattering with posterior capsule opacification. J Cataract Refract Surg 24:1626–1631 (1998).

Tan JCH, Spalton DJ, Arden GB. The effect of neodymium:YAG capsulotomy on contrast sensitivity and the evaluation of methods for its assessment. Ophthalmology 106:703–709 (1999).

Tasman W. Pseudophakic retinal detachment after YAG laser capsulotomy. Aust NZ J Ophthalmol 17:277–279 (1989).

Tassin J, Malaise E, Courtois Y. Human lens cells have an in vitro proliferative capacity inversely proportional to the donor age. Exp Cell Res 123:388–392 (1979).

Terry AC et al. Neodymium-YAG laser for posterior capsulotomy. Am J Ophthalmol 96:716–720 (1983).

Tetz MR et al. A newly described complication of Nd:YAG laser capsulotomy: Exacerbation of an intraocular infection. Case report. Arch Ophthalmol 105:1324–1325 (1987).

Thornval P, Naeser K. Refraction and anterior chamber depth before and after neodymium:YAG laser treatment for posterior capsule opacification in pseudophakic eyes: a prospective study. J Cataract Refract Surg 21:457–460 (1995).

Tielsch JM et al. Risk factors for retinal detachment after cataract surgery. A population-based case-control study. Ophthalmology 103:1537–1545 (1996).

Tsopelas N et al. Extracapsular cataract extraction in diabetic eyes. The role of YAG laser capsulotomy. Doc Ophthalmol 91:17–24 (1995).

Van der Feltz van der Sloot D et al. Prevention of IOP-rise following Nd-YAG laser capsulotomy with topical timolol and indomethacin. Doc Ophthalmol 70:209–214 (1988).

Van Westenbrugge JA et al. Incidence of retinal detachment following Nd:YAG capsulotomy after cataract surgery. J Cataract Refract Surg 18:352–355 (1992).

Vester CAGM et al. Retinal detachment following neodymium:YAG laser capsulotomy. Fortschr Ophthalmol 83:441–443 (1986).

Vogel A et al. Influence of optical aberrations on laser-induced plasma formation in water and their consequences for intraocular photodisruption. Proc SPIE Ophthalmic Technologies VIII 3246:120–131 (1998).

Walter P et al. Episodic acute hypotonia after Nd:YAG laser capsulotomy—retinal function and choroidal swelling. Vision Res 37:2937–2942 (1997).

Wasserman EL, Axt JC, Sheets JH. Neodymium:YAG laser posterior capsulotomy. Am Intra-Ocular Implant Soc J 11:245–248 (1985).

Wetzel W. Ocular aqueous humor dynamics after photodisruptive laser surgery procedures. Ophthalmic Surg 25:298–302 (1994).

Wilhelmus KA, Emery JM. Posterior capsule opacification following phacoemulsification. Ophthalmic Surg 11:264–267 (1980).

Wilkins M, McPherson R, Fergusson V. Visual recovery under glare conditions following laser capsulotomy. Eye 10:117–120 (1996).

Wilson SE, Brubaker RF. Neodymium:YAG laser damage threshold. A comparison of injection-molded and lathe-cut polymethylmethacrylate intraocular lenses. Ophthalmology 94:7–11 (1987).

Winslow RL, Taylor BC. Retinal complications following YAG laser capsulotomy. Ophthalmology 92:785–789 (1985).

Winther-Nielsen A et al. Posterior capsule opacification and neodymium:YAG capsulotomy with heparin-surface-modified intraocular lenses. J Cataract Refract Surg 24:940–944 (1998).

Wright PL et al. Angiographic cystoid macular edema after posterior chamber lens implantation. Arch Ophthalmol 106:740–744 (1988).

Yamada K et al. Effect of intraocular lens design on posteior capsule opacification after continuous curvilinear capsulorhexis. J Cataract Refract Surg 21:697–700 (1995).

Yoshida A et al. Retinal detachment after cataract surgery. Predisposing factors. Ophthalmology 99:453–459 (1992).

Zeki SM. Inverted "U" strategy for short pulsed laser posterior capsulotomy. Acta Ophthalmol Scand 77:575–577 (1999).

Chapter 6
Laser Iridotomy

Charles M. Wormington

I. Introduction and Definitions

A. Pupillary Block

1. This condition occurs when the flow of aqueous from the posterior to the anterior chamber is restricted as it moves between the posterior surface of the iris and the anterior surface of the lens (Mapstone, 1968; Ritch & Lowe, 1996a,b; Shaffer, 1973).

2. The pupillary block can be **absolute** (e.g., if posterior synechiae completely bind down the iris to the lens) or **relative**, where there is a functional or partial restriction in flow.

3. This block may increase the pressure in the posterior chamber enough to push the iris forward, causing it to come into contact with the trabecular meshwork and obstruct aqueous outflow. This would then increase the intraocular pressure (IOP) significantly, resulting in **angle-closure glaucoma**.

4. Relative pupillary block is the underlying mechanism in about 90% of patients with angle-closure glaucoma (Ritch & Lowe, 1996b). The other 10% have angle-closure glaucoma due either to another mechanism or to a combination of mechanisms that could include pupillary block.

B. Iridotomy

1. Iridotomy refers to the creation of a hole in the iris.

2. The most common term for the laser procedure to form this hole is **laser iridotomy**. Less commonly, this procedure is known as *laser iridectomy*.

3. There is also an incisional technique called *surgical iridectomy* that does not involve the use of a laser.

4. An iridotomy by any technique allows aqueous to bypass the pupillary margin and flow from the posterior chamber to the anterior chamber. By equalizing the pressure in the two chambers, it allows the iris to fall back away from the trabecular mesh-

work, reestablishing aqueous outflow. The IOP then decreases, breaking the angle-closure attack.

5. A laser iridotomy has become the procedure of choice in cases of angle-closure glaucoma with a pupillary block component, and it is recommended for eyes with occludable angles.

II. Indications (Table 6–1).

A. The main indication for a laser iridotomy is any form of **angle-closure glaucoma** that has **pupillary block** as a component. These forms include the following:

1. **Acute angle-closure glaucoma**
   a. This should be considered an ophthalmic emergency.
   b. After medical treatment has broken the acute attack and after any active inflammation has been reduced or eliminated, a laser iridotomy should be performed (Ritch & Liebmann, 1996).
   c. If the attack is not broken by a brief period of medical therapy and if the media are clear enough, a laser iridotomy may be performed. If the media are not clear enough, the argon laser may be used to perform a peripheral iridoplasty.
   d. If the eye has an intumescent lens and the cornea is clear enough, a laser iridotomy may be accomplished prior to medical therapy (Ritch & Liebmann, 1996).

Table 6–1 Indications for Laser Iridotomy

Angle-closure glaucoma with pupillary block
    Acute angle-closure glaucoma
    Chronic angle-closure glaucoma
    Pseudophakic or aphakic pupillary block
    Malignant glaucoma
    Nanophthalmos
    Pigment dispersion syndrome and pigmentary glaucoma
    Incomplete incisional surgical iridectomy
    Before argon laser trabeculoplasty in eyes with narrow angles
    Phacomorphic glaucoma
    Uveitic glaucoma
    Combined mechanism glaucoma
Eyes with occludable angles
    Fellow eyes of patients with acute or chronic angle-closure glaucoma
    Eyes with spontaneous apposition of the iris to the trabecular meshwork
    Eyes with small peripheral anterior synechiae
    Eyes with central anterior chamber depths of less than 2.0 to 2.5 mm
    Eyes of patients with pigment dispersion syndrome

2. **Chronic angle-closure glaucoma**
   a. If pupillary block is causing chronic angle-closure glaucoma, a laser iridotomy could stop the development of peripheral anterior synechiae and subsequent angle closure.
   b. An iridotomy may result in a decrease in the IOP (Gieser & Wilensky, 1984). If prior damage had occurred to the trabecular meshwork, the elevated IOP may continue to be a problem and require either medical therapy or filtration surgery.

3. **Pseudophakic or aphakic pupillary block**
   a. An iridotomy may be successful in treating pseudophakic or aphakic pupillary block (Anderson et al., 1975; Cinotti et al., 1986; Forman et al., 1987).
   b. Lack of success with the iridotomy may suggest the possibility of malignant glaucoma (Epstein et al., 1984).

4. **Malignant glaucoma**
   a. After any type of surgery for angle-closure glaucoma, it is possible for the anterior chamber to become shallow or flattened and for the IOP to become elevated. Aqueous humor flow can be forced backward into the vitreous by ciliary body apposition to the lens and/or vitreous. This condition has been called *malignant glaucoma* or *ciliary block glaucoma* (Ritch & Lowe, 1996a; Shaffer, 1973).
   b. Its resistance to treatment makes it a very serious complication of surgery for angle-closure.
   c. An iridotomy is useful in differentiating malignant glaucoma from pupillary block (Liebmann & Ritch, 1996).
   d. Although laser iridotomy is usually unsuccessful in the treatment of malignant glaucoma, prophylactic iridotomy is suggested for the fellow eye (Ritch & Liebmann, 1996; Simmons et al., 1995).

5. **Nanophthalmos** (Campo & Reiss, 1995; Kocak et al., 1997; Ritch & Liebmann, 1996; Singh et al., 1987).
   a. A nanophthalmic eye is an eye with an axial diameter of less than 20 mm or a cycloplegic refraction of greater than +7.50 D.
   b. Anterior chamber crowding places these eyes at risk for the development of angle-closure glaucoma.
   c. In addition to medical treatment, iridotomy should be attempted. If it is ineffective, then laser iridoplasty should be tried. Prophylactic laser iridotomy and/or iridoplasty may also be useful in the contralateral eye.

6. **Pigment dispersion syndrome and pigmentary glaucoma**
   a. Laser iridotomy has been suggested as a treatment for pigment dispersion syndrome where there is reverse pupillary block (Karickhoff, 1992; Potash et al., 1994b).
   b. Reverse pupillary block can be assessed via slit-lamp biomicroscopy by noticing posterior bowing of the peripheral iris.

c. In cases of reverse pupillary block, laser iridotomy may allow the iris to come forward to a planar configuration, and thus reduce pigment dispersion due to zonular rubbing of the iris (Karickhoff, 1992; Lagreze & Funk, 1995). High-resolution ultrasound biomicroscopy has dramatically demonstrated the iris concavity change and the decrease in iridolenticular contact following laser iridotomy (Breingan et al., 1999; Carassa et al., 1998; Caronia et al., 1996; Lagreze & Funk, 1995; Lagreze et al., 1996; Potash et al., 1994b; Figure 6–1). It has also demonstrated that iridotomy eliminates the increased concavity of the iris that occurs in some patients upon accommodation (Carassa et al., 1998; Pavlin et al., 1996).

d. Because many patients with pigmentary glaucoma are myopes and thus more prone to retinal detachment, Moster & George-Lomax (1998) have suggested using the consensual light reflex to constrict the pupil during the iridotomy instead of using pilocarpine.

e. Laser iridotomy is not successful in all patients with pigment dispersion syndrome (Jampel, 1992). And it may not eliminate pigment liberation during vigorous exercise (Haynes et al., 1995).

7. **Incomplete incisional surgical iridectomy**

   a. Occasionally during a surgical iridectomy, the iris pigment epithelium is left intact and only the iris stroma is removed.

   b. Laser iridotomy can be used to remove the pigment epithelium, leaving a patent iridotomy (Tessler et al., 1975).

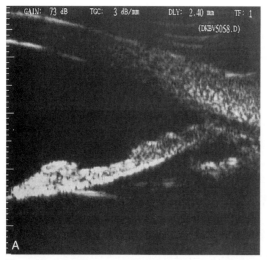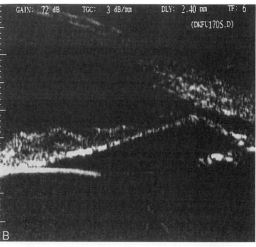

Figure 6–1 A. Ultrasound biomicroscope scan before a laser iridotomy. Note the iris concavity and contact between the central iris and the anterior lens capsule. B. Scan after a laser iridotomy. Note relaxation of the iris concavity and the decreased area of iris contact with the anterior lens capsule. (Reprinted from Potash SD, Tello C, Liebmann J, Ritch R. Ultrasound biomicroscopy in pigment dispersion syndrome. Ophthalmology 101:332–339 (1994b), with permission from Lippincott Williams & Wilkins.)

c. One condition where Nd:YAG iridotomy is not very successful is in reopening failed surgical iridotomies in silicone-oil-filled aphakic eyes (Reddy & Aylward, 1995).

8. **Before argon laser trabeculoplasty in eyes with narrow angles** (Ritch & Liebmann, 1996).
   a. In order to perform an argon laser trabeculoplasty, you must be able to see the angle structures. Narrow angles may occlude those structures.
   b. If relative pupillary block is causing the narrow angle, laser iridotomy may relieve the block and allow visualization of the angle.

9. **Phacomorphic glaucoma** (Potash et al., 1994a; Tomey & Al-Rajhi, 1992).
   a. Angle-closure glaucoma can be precipitated by anterior chamber angle crowding due to the swelling of the lens. The intumescence of the lens could be due to a rapidly maturing cataract or a cataract associated with trauma or inflammation.
   b. Laser iridotomy should be performed to relieve pupillary block prior to cataract surgery (Figure 6–2).

10. **Uveitic glaucoma** (American Academy of Ophthalmology, 1994).
    a. Inflammatory adhesions may develop between the iris and lens resulting in iris bombé and angle closure.
    b. Any pupillary block from this process may be broken by a laser iridotomy.
    c. Unfortunately, continued inflammation may result in closure of the iridotomy and may require reopening.

11. **Combined mechanism glaucoma** (Schuman, 1997). The angle-closure component in combined mechanism glaucoma can be eliminated with laser iridotomy.

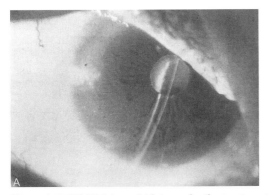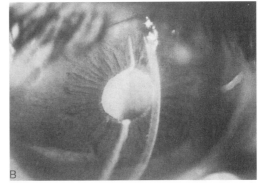

Figure 6–2 Nd:YAG laser iridotomy for the treatment of phacomorphic glaucoma. A. Note the markedly shallow anterior chamber before treatment. B. The same eye after treatment showing significant deepening of the chamber. (Reprinted with permission from Tomey KF, Al-Rajhi AA. Neodymium:YAG laser iridotomy in the initial management of phacomorphic glaucoma. Ophthalmology 99:660–665 (1992).)

B. Eyes with **occludable angles** may be an indication for **prophylactic laser iridotomy** (American Academy of Ophthalmology, 1994; Liebmann & Ritch, 1996; Ritch, 1996; Ritch & Liebmann, 1996; Schuman, 1997; Tomey et al., 1987; Werner, 1995; Wilensky, 1996). This may involve anatomically narrow angles and normal IOPs with no detectable glaucomatous damage. In one large study of patients judged to be at risk for angle-closure based on gonioscopy and a slit-lamp biomicroscope exam, it was found that this group had about a 30% risk of experiencing angle closure within 6 years (Wilensky et al., 1993). In eyes of patients with homocystinuria who have lens subluxation or dislocation, a prophylactic peripheral iridotomy may not be successful in preventing lens dislocation into the anterior chamber (Harrison et al., 1998). Eyes that may be considered for prophylactic laser iridotomy include the following:

1. **Fellow eyes of patients with acute or chronic angle-closure glaucoma** (Ritch, 1996; Wilensky, 1996). If an iridotomy is not performed, 50% to 75% of these fellow eyes experience angle closure within 5 years (Lowe, 1962; Snow, 1977). If a laser iridotomy is temporarily deferred, 50% of subspecialty-trained glaucoma specialists will use pilocarpine and 33% will observe with close follow-up (Davidorf et al., 1996).

2. **Eyes with spontaneous apposition of the iris to the trabecular meshwork.**

3. **Eyes with small peripheral anterior synechiae.** These are often seen at 12 o'clock, and they suggest previous spontaneous appositional angle closure (Ritch, 1996). If anterior synechia are present in more than 50% of the periphery, laser iridotomy may not successfully control the pressure (Kim & Jung, 1997).

4. **Eyes with central anterior chamber depths of less than 2.0 to 2.5 mm** (Werner, 1995). Another study suggested performing prophylactic laser iridotomy on eyes with anterior chamber depths less than 2.70 mm (Lin et al., 1997), whereas using anterior chamber depth has been questioned by others (American Academy of Ophthalmology, 1994; Higginbotham, 1995; Wilensky et al., 1993).

5. **Eyes of patients with pigment dispersion syndrome.** In a study involving 21 patients with pigment dispersion syndrome in both eyes, one eye of each patient was treated with Nd:YAG laser iridotomy and the patients were followed for 2 years (Gandolfi & Vecchi, 1996). During the follow-up period, a significant elevation of intraocular pressure occurred in 53% of untreated eyes and only 5% of treated eyes.

III. Contraindications (Belcher, 1984; Belcher & Schuman, 1992; Liebmann & Ritch, 1996; Ritch & Liebmann, 1996; Schuman, 1997) (Table 6–2).

A. Absolute Contraindication—If there is **no pupillary block**, then a laser iridotomy will not break an angle-closure attack. This includes angle-closure glaucomas that result from anterior mechanisms of closure (e.g., iridocorneal endothelial syndrome or neovascular glaucoma).

Table 6–2 Contraindications for Laser Iridotomy

Absolute
  No pupillary block
Relative
    Inadequate visualization of target
    Very flat or shallow anterior chamber
    Completely sealed anterior chamber angle
    Angle closure due to primary synechial closure of
      the angle
    Poor patient cooperation

B. *Relative Contraindications*

1. **Inadequate visualization of the target**
   a. Corneal opacification or edema may make it difficult or impossible to adequately see the target iris site. This may include dense arcus senilis and posterior crocodile shagreen.
   b. A hyphema or dense cells and flare in the anterior chamber may obscure the target site also.

2. **Very flat or shallow anterior chamber**—A completely flat chamber may make it extremely difficult or impossible to perform a laser iridotomy without producing corneal lesions.

3. **Completely sealed anterior chamber angle**

4. **Angle closure due to primary synechial closure of the anterior chamber angle**

5. **Poor patient cooperation**—If the patient has trouble maintaining fixation, retrobulbar anesthesia may be tried.

IV. Instrumentation

A. *Argon Laser*

1. In the mid-1970s, the argon laser began to be used to create iridotomies.

2. By 1980, it had replaced surgical iridectomy as the procedure of choice for pupillary-block glaucoma.

3. This laser employs a photothermal mechanism to create iridotomies.

B. *Nd:YAG Laser*

1. During the 1980s, the Nd:YAG laser was introduced as another effective instrument to produce iridotomies.

2. This is the **most commonly used laser** today for the creation of iridotomies. It uses a photodisruptive mechanism of action.

3. Many clinicians use the argon laser to thin the iris at the iridotomy site and then use the Nd:YAG laser to penetrate the iris.

4. Even though almost all studies used the Q-switched Nd:YAG laser, the mode-locked Nd:YAG laser has also been used to create iridotomies (Kumar et al., 1990).

C. Nd:YLF Laser

1. The Nd:YLF laser has also been used to perform peripheral iridotomies (Balacco-Gabrieli et al., 1995; Frangie et al., 1992; Geerling et al., 1998; Hoppeler & Gloor, 1992; Oram et al., 1995; Pecorella et al., 1997).

2. This laser, like the Nd:YAG laser, uses plasma-mediated photodisruption to remove tissue.

3. With the Nd:YLF laser, there is a much smaller amount of energy per pulse than in the Nd:YAG system. This may limit collateral damage.

4. Under computer control, this laser can create an iridotomy with a predetermined size, shape, and depth.

D. Semiconductor Diode Laser

1. Numerous diode laser systems are available with outputs in the red and near-infrared region.

2. The near-IR diode laser has been used to create successful iridotomies (Emoto et al., 1992; Hawkins et al., 1994; Jacobson et al., 1990; Schuman et al., 1990). Due to its higher transmittance, it has been suggested that the diode laser may be a better laser than the argon laser for iridotomy in patients with hazy corneas (Chew et al., 2000).

3. These lasers use a photothermal mechanism of damage.

E. Diode Laser-Pumped, Frequency-Doubled Nd:YAG Laser

1. This is a CW laser with an output in the green at 532 nm.

2. The iridotomy produced with this type of laser is very similar to that produced by the argon laser (Abreu et al., 1997).

3. This laser employs a photothermal mechanism of damage and generates thermal damage zones comparable in size to those an argon laser produces.

F. Krypton Laser

1. This is a CW laser with an output in the green (531 nm), yellow (568 nm), and red (647 nm).

2. The red output is the strongest and has been used to create iridotomies (Yassur et al., 1986). It uses the photothermal mechanism of damage.

G. *Dye Laser*

1. The CW dye laser used in one study was tuned to 600 nm (Wishart et al., 1986). Another study did not cite the laser wavelength (Hitchings, 1984). Single pulses have been used to create iridotomies (Bass et al., 1979).

2. A photothermal mechanism vaporized the tissue.

H. *Er:YAG Laser* (Brazitikos et al., 1998).

1. An Er:YAG laser (2.94 μm) with the capability of a high repetition rate (2 Hz to 200 Hz) has recently become available.

2. Iridotomies were performed on pig eyes with an endoprobe (Brazitikos et al., 1998).

3. In addition, iridotomies were performed on patients with an endoprobe (D'Amico et al., 1996).

I. *Laser Contact Lenses*

1. **Abraham iridotomy lens** (Figures 6–3 and 6–4).
   a. This is the most commonly used laser contact lens for iridotomies.
   b. This lens has a peripheral, +66 D, planoconvex button-lens (Abraham, 1981).
   c. Because the diameter of the laser beam on the iris is reduced by about a factor of 2, the energy density on the iris is increased by about a factor of 4.
   d. This configuration also reduces the energy density at the corneal level by about a factor of 4.

2. **Wise iridotomy-sphincterotomy lens**
   a. This lens has a peripheral, +103 D, optical button that magnifies the iris image 2.65× (Wise et al., 1986).
   b. Compared to a plano contact lens, this lens increases the energy density at the iris by a factor of 7.79. This is 2.92 times greater than the energy density when using the Abraham lens.
   c. Compared to a plano contact lens, this lens reduces the retinal energy density to 1.2% of what it would be with the plano lens and 8.7% of what it would be with the Abraham lens.
   d. Unfortunately, the field of view is small, the lens is sensitive to decentration, and there is some distortion due to the high magnification.

3. **Lasag CGI lens** (Riquin et al., 1983) (Figure 6–5).

4. **Shirmer** peripheral iridotomy laser lens (Schirmer, 1983).
   a. This lens has two optical buttons, one for iridotomy and one for peripheral iris and angle.
   b. The lens increases the energy density by a factor of 4.5.

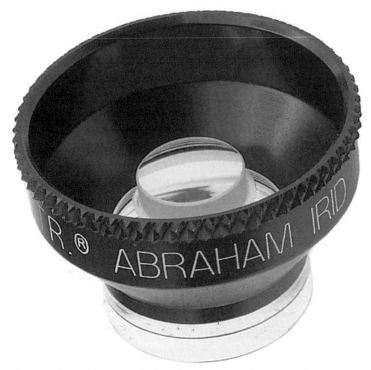

Figure 6–3 An Abraham iridotomy contact lens. (Courtesy of Ocular Instruments, Bellevue, WA.)

5. The **advantages of laser contact lenses** include the following:
   a. The lens **provides magnification of the iris with good depth of field** (compared to the loss of depth of field using the biomicroscope magnification control to increase magnification).
   b. The lens **concentrates the laser energy on the iris**, thus increasing the energy density and minimizing the total energy necessary to achieve a patent iridotomy.
   c. The lens **acts as a speculum** keeping the lids out of the way and making it easier to gain access to the upper iris.
   d. The lens **acts as a heat sink** minimizing corneal damage.
   e. The lens **provides a moderate amount of control over ocular movement** thus stabilizing the target.
   f. The lens **minimizes the energy density on the retina** by increasing the divergence of the beam posterior to the focus point.

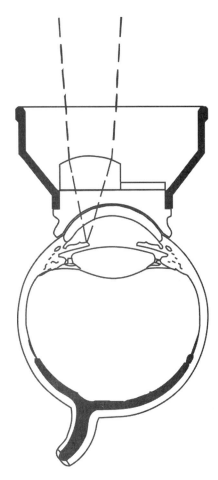

Figure 6–4 Schematic of Abraham iridotomy lens use. (Courtesy of Ocular Instruments, Bellevue, WA.)

V. Pretreatment Procedures (American Academy of Ophthalmology, 1994; Belcher & Schuman, 1992; Liebmann & Ritch, 1996; Ritch & Liebmann, 1996; Schuman, 1997).

A. *Preoperative Ophthalmic Examination* (Table 6–3)

1. **Thorough history** which should include the following:
   a. Check for contraindications for iridotomy or potential medications.
   b. Check for history of retinal detachment.
   c. Rule out cystoid macular edema or macular degeneration if the patient has had poor vision.

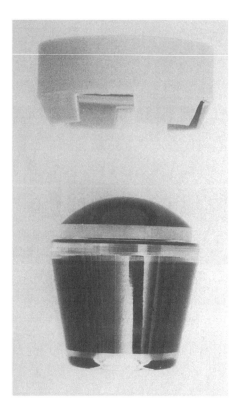

Figure 6–5 A Lasag CGI lens. (Reprinted with permission from Riquin D, Fankhauser F, Loertscher H. Contact lenses for use with high power lasers. Two new contact glasses for microsurgery at the iris, in the pupillary and the retropupillary space. Int Ophthalmol 6:191–200 (1983).)

    d. Check for a history of diplopia or glare problems.

    e. Assess level and location of any current pain.

    f. Ask about previous episodes of sharp pain in or around the eye or halos associated with headache.

    g. Ask about any current or previous episodes of blurry vision.

2. **Visual acuity testing**

3. **Subjective refraction.** Check for hyperopia greater than +7.5 D (i.e., nanophthalmos).

4. **Applanation tonometry**

    a. Accurate IOP readings must be taken to ensure that the IOP is reduced and under control after the iridotomy.

    b. The iridotomy procedure can result in an IOP spike so the pre-procedure level must be assessed.

5. **Slit-lamp biomicroscope examination**

    a. Cornea

Table 6–3 Preoperative Ophthalmic Exam

Thorough history
Visual acuity testing
Subjective refraction
Applanation tonometry
Slit-lamp biomicroscope examination
Gonioscopy
Binocular indirect ophthalmoscopy
Automated threshold perimetry
Informed written consent
Special methods for measurement of anterior
    chamber depth

1) Check the clarity of the cornea, especially in the area of the target site.
2) Evaluate the integrity of the cornea, including a check for corneal guttata.
3) Check for Krukenberg's spindle (keratic precipitates).

b. Aqueous
    1) Check for cells and flare (i.e., inflammation).
    2) Check for shallow anterior chamber.
c. Iris: check for the following:
    1) largest areas of separation of the iris from the corneal endothelium
    2) iris crypts in the target area
    3) areas of increased pigmentation if the patient has a light iris and you are using an argon laser
    4) posterior synechiae
    5) any preexisting iris atrophy
    6) any preexisting pupillary distortion
    7) a partially dilated pupil
    8) iris neovascularization
d. Crystalline lens
    1) Check for an intumescent lens.
    2) Check for a luxated or subluxated lens.
    3) Check for pseudophakia or aphakia.
e. Retina—Using a +78 D, +90 D, or similar lens, assess the following:
    1) optic nerve head
    2) nerve fiber layer
    3) macula (e.g., for CME)

f. Van Herick test to assess the depth of the peripheral anterior chamber (narrow, occludable angles are suggested by chamber depths that are one-fourth of the corneal thickness or less) (Van Herick et al., 1969).

6. **Gonioscopy** (of both eyes)
   a. This test is **essential** to the diagnosis of angle-closure glaucoma and for assessing whether pupil block is present. Gonioscopy should be performed in a darkened room with minimal slit-lamp illumination to prevent stimulation of the pupillary light reflex (Liebmann & Ritch, 1996). Pay particular attention to the superior angle, which is usually the narrowest.
   b. Determine the most posterior structure visible in all quadrants.
   c. Describe the width of the anterior chamber angle (e.g., closed, slit, narrow, moderate, wide).
   d. Describe the position of insertion of the iris root (e.g., below the scleral spur, from the scleral spur, above the scleral spur).
   e. Grade the level of any pigment buildup in the angle. Pigment in angle-closure attacks is usually blotchy and distributed over the trabecular meshwork. It accumulates more in the inferior angle, but in cases of appositional closure limited to the superior angle, it may accumulate more in the superior angle (Desjardins & Parrish, 1985).
   f. Using indentation gonioscopy, check to see if the angle closure is due to apposition of the iris to the trabecular meshwork or if there are anterior synechiae (Forbes, 1966; Gorin, 1971).
   g. Check for plateau iris syndrome.
   h. Evaluate the state of the trabecular meshwork.
   i. Check for angle neovascularization.

7. **Binocular indirect ophthalmoscopy** (if possible)
   a. Check the optic nerve head for glaucomatous damage.
   b. Check the nerve fiber layer for glaucomatous dropout.
   c. Check for CME.
   d. Check for choroidal and retinal detachments.

8. **Automated threshold perimetry**
   a. Assess the level and location of glaucomatous damage, if any.
   b. Check for any preexisting visual field defects other than glaucomatous lesions.

9. **Informed, written consent** (mandatory)
   a. The procedure should be explained in clear, understandable terms.
   b. The risks should be explained.
   c. Any other options available to the patient should also be explained.

10. **Special methods for measurement of anterior chamber depth**
    a. Laser Doppler interferometry/partial coherence interferometry (Drexler et al., 1997; Fercher et al., 1993).

b. Optical coherence tomography (Huang et al., 1991; Izatt et al., 1994)

c. Pachymetry (Lowe, 1966)

d. Scheimpflug photography (Richards et al., 1988)

e. Ultrasound biomicroscopy. The ultrasound biomicroscope may be useful in making the diagnosis of pupillary block glaucoma or in confirming it (Aslanides et al., 1995; Carassa et al., 1998; Pavlin et al., 1992; Tello et al., 1994).

f. Slit-lamp biomicroscope (Chan et al., 1981; Jacobs, 1979; Lowe, 1966; Smith, 1979)

B. Pretreatment Regimen (American Academy of Ophthalmology, 1994; Belcher & Schuman, 1992; Liebmann & Ritch, 1996; Ritch & Liebmann, 1996; Schuman, 1997) (Table 6–4).

1. **Ensure correct diagnosis.**

2. If possible, **break the angle-closure attack with medications**.

   a. This will lower the IOP, decrease the level of inflammation, and increase patient comfort.

   b. If significant inflammation persists after breaking the angle-closure attack, consider treating with topical steroids for 1 to 2 days before performing the iridotomy.

   c. If there is significant damage due to glaucoma, consider using a beta blocker, carbonic anhydrase inhibitor, and/or an oral osmotic agent.

3. **If necessary, perform laser peripheral iridoplasty** to break the angle-closure attack (see *Laser Iridoplasty* in Chapter 8). Medications may not break the attack or may actually worsen it. Alternatively, corneal edema secondary to angle-closure glaucoma may preclude iridotomy, but this can often be resolved via laser iridoplasty.

Table 6–4 Pretreatment Regimen

Ensure correct diagnosis
Break angle-closure attack with medications
Ensure adequate clarity of the cornea
0.5% or 1% apraclonidine (1 hr before)
2% to 4% pilocarpine (30 to 60 min before)
0.5% proparacaine (just before contact lens
    placement)
Advise patient about noises and/or bright flashes
Ensure patient's head is stabilized
Ensure patient comfort
Ensure laser operator comfort
Ensure adequate stabilization of the eye
Focus and adjust oculars on slit-lamp biomicroscope
Ensure alignment of laser beam

4. **Ensure adequate clarity of the cornea.**
   a. Getting the pressure under better control with medications will be of assistance.
   b. Topically applied glycerin may be useful in reducing corneal edema.

5. One drop of 1% **apraclonidine** (Iopidine) should be instilled 1 to 1.5 hr before the procedure. A recent study concluded that administration of 0.5% apraclonidine is as effective as 1% apraclonidine (Rosenberg et al., 1995).
   a. This will help prevent any IOP spike following the iridotomy.
   b. The vasoconstriction due to the apraclonidine may be useful in enhancing hemostasis following Nd:YAG laser iridotomy.
   c. A beta-blocker (e.g., levobunolol), osmotic agent, or carbonic anhydrase inhibitor may be substituted unless contraindicated. One of these other drugs should be used if the patient is already taking apraclonidine for glaucoma treatment.
   d. If the patient has glaucoma, additional pressure-lowering agents should be considered.

6. If the pupil is not in a state of maximal miosis from previous glaucoma medications, use **2% to 4% pilocarpine** or an equivalent drug 30 to 60 min prior to the procedure to produce strong miosis. In addition to the usual delivery of pilocarpine as ophthalmic drops, pilocarpine can also be delivered effectively as a spray (Doe & Campagna, 1998).
   a. This will stretch the iris, making it thinner, and thus decrease the amount of laser energy necessary to penetrate the iris.
   b. This will also help minimize iris movement during the procedure.

7. Instill one or two drops of 0.5% **proparacaine** to anesthetize the cornea before placement of the laser contact lens.

8. **Advise the patient about the noises and/or the bright flashes of light** that he or she may experience during the procedure. This will help reassure the patient and will help the patient to maintain steady fixation.

9. **Ensure the patient's head is stabilized** adequately against the slit-lamp forehead- and chin-rests. This will help to minimize damage to the cornea and lens that may occur due to patient movement.

10. **Ensure patient comfort during the procedure.** This will also help to maintain stability of the eye during the iridotomy.

11. **Ensure laser operator comfort**. To increase comfort and to decrease fine tremor movement of the hand, the operator should use an elbow support.

12. **Ensure adequate stabilization of the eye.**
    a. Some stabilization is attained by the use of a laser contact lens.
    b. Very rarely, use of a retrobulbar block may be necessary (e.g., with severe nystagmus).

   c. For patients with breathing difficulties, have the patient interrupt breathing just before delivering the laser energy to the patient.

13. **Focus and adjust the oculars on the slit-lamp biomicroscope**—This will help ensure precise laser focus.

14. **Ensure alignment of the laser beam.** Loss of power and/or precise focus can occur if the laser is not aligned properly.

VI. Site Selection (American Academy of Ophthalmology, 1994; Belcher, 1984; Belcher & Schuman, 1992; Hill, 1999; Ritch & Liebmann, 1996; Schuman, 1997).

A. **Select either the 11-o'clock or the 1-o'clock position on the iris.**

 1. This location usually allows the upper lid to cover the iridotomy hole and thus minimizes diplopia and glare difficulties.

 2. The 12-o'clock position is avoided because
    a. bubbles generated during the procedure can move to this area and obscure the target site, and
    b. a hemorrhage at this site can be visually disturbing to the patient (i.e., blood can trickle down over the pupil).

 3. When a continuous wave laser is used, the superior and nasal location is preferred because it lessens the risk of macular damage.

B. **If possible, focus on an iris crypt**, especially when using the argon or diode lasers.

 1. The iris is thinner in the base of the crypt.

 2. This minimizes the amount of laser energy necessary and thus helps protect other ocular structures.

C. **Choose an area of increased pigmentation** (e.g., a nevus) when using the argon or diode lasers on a light blue iris. This will facilitate absorption of the laser beam and thus reduce the amount of laser energy needed.

D. **Choose a site as close to the limbus as possible.**

 1. This usually involves an area about two-thirds to three-quarters of the way from the pupil to the limbus (Figure 6–6).

 2. This will help place the iridotomy under the upper lid and thus avoid diplopia or glare problems.

 3. This also minimizes any damage to the lens capsule and the iris sphincter muscle.

 4. In addition, the iris is thinner and the blood vessels are more widely spaced in the periphery.

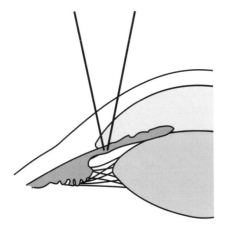

Figure 6–6 Diagram of appropriate position for placement of a laser iridotomy.

5. The main limitation on distance toward the limbus is the increased risk for corneal endothelial lesions as you approach the limbus.
6. Avoid any area of dense corneal arcus senilis.
    a. The arcus can obscure the target site.
    b. The arcus can also absorb part of the laser beam and thus require higher laser energy with subsequent increases in risk.

E. **Choose a site where the white collagen beams are slightly separated** in lightly pigmented irides.

F. **Reevaluate the target site after beginning the procedure**. If difficulty is encountered at the onset, consider shifting to a new site.

VII. Argon Laser Iridotomy Procedures (Table 6–5).

A. *Types of Argon Laser Thermal Delivery* (Ritch & Liebmann, 1996; Shields, 1992).
1. **Contraction burn**
    a. These burns usually use a large spot size (500 μm), a long duration (0.5 sec), and low power (200 to 400 mW).
    b. The power should be adjusted according to the level of iris pigmentation (e.g., 300 mW in light irides and 200 mW in dark irides).
    c. The power should be reduced if pigment is released or if bubbles are forming.
    d. By thermally contracting iris tissue, these burns will move adjacent iris tissue toward the burn area and compact the stroma under the burn. This enhances absorption of the laser energy in lightly colored irides.

Table 6–5 Basic Parameters for Argon Laser Thermal Delivery

Type of Burn	Spot Size (μm)	Duration (sec)	Power (mW)
Contraction	500	0.5	200–400
Stretch	200	0.2	200
Penetration	50	0.01–0.02	600–1500
		0.1–0.2	
Cleanup	50	0.01–0.02	400–600
		0.1–0.2	200–600

   e. These burns can also be used to generate a "hump" for subsequent penetrating burns.

   f. This type of burn can also be used for iridoplasty or pupilloplasty.

2. **Stretch burn**

   a. These burns usually use a smaller spot size (200 μm), a shorter duration (0.2 sec), and low power (200 mW).

   b. These burns are less effective than contraction burns at contracting iris tissue.

3. **Penetrating burn**

   a. These burns (previously called *punch burns*) usually use a smaller spot size (50 μm), a very short duration (0.01 to 0.02 sec), and higher power (600 to 1500 mW) (Ritch & Liebmann, 1996; Kolker, 1984; Shields, 1992; Yamamoto et al., 1982, 1985). This has been called a *chipping* technique.

   b. Longer duration (0.1 to 0.2 sec) burns have also been used (Pollack, 1979; Robin & Pollack, 1984). Bubbles can form, especially with the long-duration burns. Continue to apply burns through the bubble, focusing on the base of the bubble.

   c. The shorter duration helps prevent charring of the iris tissue, lessens complications, and reduces the total energy used.

   d. These burn parameters are useful for vaporizing tissue and hence penetrating the iris.

   e. A variation on these parameters has been suggested involving higher power (1500 to 2500 mW) burns (Ritch & Palmberg, 1982).

4. **Cleanup burn** (Ritch & Liebmann, 1996; Shields, 1992).

   a. These burns can use a low-power (400 to 600 mW) penetrating burn (50 μm spot size, 0.01 to 0.02 sec duration), or a longer, low-power burn (50 μm spot size, 0.1 to 0.2 sec duration, and 200 to 600 mW of power).

   b. After penetrating the iris stroma, they can be used to remove the pigment epithelium with minimal risk to the anterior lens capsule.

B. *Argon Laser Iridotomy Techniques* (Figure 6–7).

1. **Linear incision** (Wise, 1985, 1987).
   a. This technique involves multiple laser burns placed in a line approximately 500 μm long two-thirds of the way from the pupil margin to the limbus. The burns are made parallel to the limbus, thus cutting across the radial fibers of the iris.
   b. Penetrating burns of small spot size (50 μm), short duration (0.02 sec), and high power (800 to 1500 mW) are used. If this doesn't provide adequate effect in light blue irides, the duration can be increased to 0.05 or even 0.10 sec at 1500 mW.
   c. As the radial iris fibers are cut, they separate and place the deeper fibers under greater tension. This aids in the efficiency of the procedure and results in fairly round holes.
   d. Individual strands that are left bridging the gap should be cut at the base on either side rather than towards the middle.
   e. After penetrating the stroma, the iris tension lines may pull open the pigment epithelium. If not, low power and short duration burns are used to cleave the pigment epithelium.
   f. This method requires about 150 to 300 laser shots, except for lightly pigmented irides that require up to 500 shots.

2. **Penetrating burns on a contraction burn bed** (Ritch & Liebmann, 1996; Stetz et al., 1983).
   a. In this technique, two to four contraction burns are placed in a line parallel to the limbus. They should partially overlap. These burns compact the stroma and enhance the absorption of the laser energy.

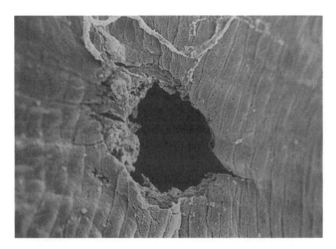

Figure 6–7 Scanning electron micrograph of a posterior view of an argon laser iridotomy. Note the segmented disturbance of the posterior iris pigment epithelium. (Reprinted with permission from Hawkins TA, Stewart WC, McMillan TA, Gwynn DR. Analysis of diode, argon, and Nd:YAG peripheral iridectomy in cadaver eyes. Doc Ophthalmol 87:367–376 (1994).)

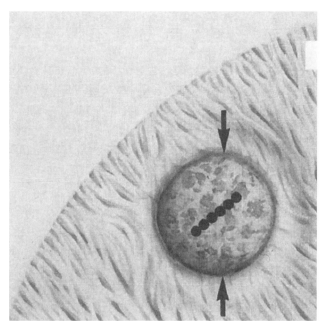

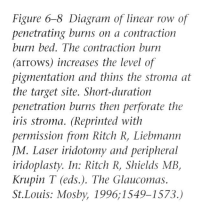

Figure 6–8 Diagram of linear row of penetrating burns on a contraction burn bed. The contraction burn (arrows) increases the level of pigmentation and thins the stroma at the target site. Short-duration penetration burns then perforate the iris stroma. (Reprinted with permission from Ritch R, Liebmann JM. Laser iridotomy and peripheral iridoplasty. In: Ritch R, Shields MB, Krupin T (eds.). The Glaucomas. St.Louis: Mosby, 1996;1549–1573.)

    b. Penetrating burns are then placed inside the thinned area of the contraction burns. These penetrating burns can be fully superimposed on each other or placed in a linear incision configuration (Figure 6–8).

    c. This has been useful in lightly pigmented irides, especially when there are no crypts in the target area.

3. **Iris hump method** (Abraham, 1976, 1981; Belcher, 1984; Hoskins & Migliazzo, 1984; Ritch & Liebmann, 1996).

    a. This is a two-step technique.

    b. The first step is to use a contraction burn to form two iris humps on either side of the burn.

    c. The second step is to place a long duration (1.0 sec or less) penetrating burn at the peak of one of the humps (Abraham, 1981). Alternatively, a high power (1500 mW), long-duration (0.5 sec or less) penetrating burn is used (Hoskins & Migliazzo, 1984).

    d. Unfortunately, this method often resulted in pain and did not become widely used.

4. **Drumhead technique** (Belcher, 1984; Podos et al., 1979; Pollack, 1979; Ritch & Liebmann, 1996).

a. In this method, three to eight burns are positioned in a circle around the target site. The burns involve a large spot size (200 μm), long duration (0.1 to 0.2 sec), and low power (200 mW).
b. The thin, taut area in the center of the circle of burns is then perforated with penetrating burns applied in a "chipping" technique.
c. This method is not used much currently.
d. A **modified drumhead technique** has been found useful in light brown irides. An iris crypt is stretched open by placing two contraction burns on either side of the crypt. The exposed area is then perforated with penetrating burns.

C. Iris Color. Which technique is used depends on a number of factors, including the iris color.

1. **Medium brown irides**
   a. This color of iris is usually the easiest to penetrate.
   b. One approach is with long duration (0.1 to 0.2 sec) penetration burns to perforate the stroma and then cleanup burns to penetrate the pigment epithelium (Belcher & Schuman, 1992; Shields, 1992). This may take on the order of 1 to 30 laser shots.
   c. Another approach is the modified drumhead technique (Ritch & Liebmann, 1996).

2. **Dark brown irides**
   a. Because of the thick, dense stroma, these irises are harder to penetrate.
   b. One approach here is to use the short duration (0.01 to 0.02 sec) penetration (*chipping*) burns to perforate the stroma and then cleanup burns for the pigment epithelium (Belcher & Schuman, 1992; Kolker, 1984; Ritch & Palmberg, 1982; Yamamoto et al., 1982, 1985). This may take on the order of 50 to 300 laser shots.
   c. Another approach is the linear incision technique (Ritch & Liebmann, 1996).
   d. The shorter duration burns are used to prevent charring. Once charring occurs it can interfere with subsequent burns.

3. **Blue irides**
   a. Because the lightly pigmented iris absorbs less laser energy, the blue iris can be difficult to penetrate.
   b. One approach is to use long duration (even up to 0.5 sec) penetration burns for the stroma and cleanup burns for the pigment epithelium, just like the technique with medium brown irides (Belcher & Schuman, 1992; Kolker, 1984).
   c. Another approach is to use penetrating burns on a contraction burn bed (Stetz et al., 1983) or to modify this technique by adding a linear incision (Ritch & Liebmann, 1996).
   d. The iris hump method has also been advocated (Hoskins & Migliazzo, 1984).

VIII. Neodymium:YAG Laser Iridotomy Procedures (Figure 6–9).

A. Advantages of the Nd:YAG Laser over the argon laser (McAllister et al., 1984; Robin & Pollack, 1984; Schuman, 1997).

1. The Nd:YAG laser requires **less laser energy** to achieve a patent iridotomy.

2. The Nd:YAG laser also requires **fewer pulses** and hence **less time** to create iris penetration.

3. There is **less central corneal cell loss** with the Nd:YAG laser.

4. There is a **decreased occurrence of focal lenticular opacity formation**.

5. There is a significantly **reduced** occurrence of subsequent **iridotomy closure** with the Nd:YAG laser.

6. The Nd:YAG laser photodisruption mechanism is much **less dependent on iris pigmentation**.

B. Nd:YAG Laser Parameters for Iridotomies (Del Priore et al., 1988; Drake, 1987; Klapper, 1984; McAllister et al., 1984; Moster et al., 1986; Naveh et al., 1987; Ritch & Liebmann, 1996; Robin et al., 1986; Robin & Pollack, 1984, 1986; Schuman, 1997; Schwartz et al., 1986; Wise, 1987).

1. **Energy level**
   a. The energy levels range from 1 to 15 mJ per pulse, but are usually 4 to 6 mJ.
   b. The appropriate energy depends on a number of factors, including the specific fixed laser parameters (e.g., spot size and pulse duration), the type of laser contact lens used, the pattern of energy delivery, and the clarity of the media.

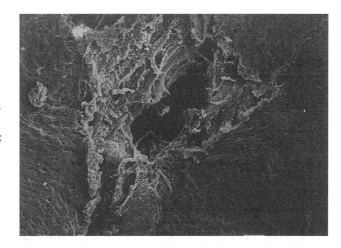

Figure 6–9 Scanning electron micrograph of a posterior view of an Nd:YAG laser iridotomy. Note the irregular opening. (Reprinted with permission from Hawkins TA, Stewart WC, McMillan TA, Gwynn DR. Analysis of diode, argon, and Nd:YAG peripheral iridectomy in cadaver eyes. Doc Ophthalmol 87:367–376 (1994).)

c. It is usually best to begin with lower energy (e.g., 1.5 to 3 mJ) and then assess the effect. If the effect is inadequate, the energy can be increased to 4 to 6 mJ, which will often be satisfactory.

2. **Pulses per burst**
   a. The number of pulses per burst ranges from one to four.
   b. One pulse per burst allows better control over the energy delivery. If the second or third pulse in a burst of four penetrates the iris, there is an increased risk of anterior lens capsule injury. The risk to the corneal endothelium also increases.
   c. Bursts of five or six pulses have led to lens damage (Welch et al., 1986).

3. **Total number of pulses**
   a. In most studies the *mean* number of pulses to achieve a patent iridotomy has ranged from two to six.
   b. The range of pulses has been from 1 to 30 pulses.

IX. Argon Pretreatment Followed by Neodymium: YAG Treatment (Goins et al., 1990; Ho & Fan, 1992; Kumar et al., 1990; Lim et al., 1996; Naveh-Floman & Blumenthal, 1985; Schuman, 1997; Zborwski-Gutman et al., 1988).

A. **The argon laser can be used to thin the iris and coagulate blood vessels.** The Nd:YAG laser is then used to complete the penetration of the stroma and pigment epithelium.

B. **The use of argon pretreatment followed by the Nd:YAG treatment has a number of advantages.** Such pretreatment

1. significantly reduces the incidence of hemorrhage following the Nd:YAG laser treatment because the argon coagulates and seals the blood vessels;
2. reduces the pigment dispersion that can occur with the Nd:YAG laser alone;
3. reduces the likelihood of retinal injury from the argon laser;
4. reduces the incidence of focal lenticular damage compared to argon treatment alone; and
5. apparently reduces the incidence of iridotomy closure compared to argon laser alone.

C. Some eyes are difficult or impossible to penetrate with the argon laser alone.

X. General Procedure (Table 6–6)

A. Perform Preoperative Ophthalmic Examination.

B. Administer Pretreatment Regimen.

C. Use Fairly High Magnification (e.g., 25×) on the Slit Lamp.

Table 6–6 General Procedure for Laser Iridotomy

Perform preoperative ophthalmic examination
Administer pretreatment regimen
Use fairly high magnification (e.g., 25×) on the slit lamp
Use a laser contact lens
Aim laser beam away from the macula
Focusing is absolutely critical
Choose initial laser parameters based on color of iris and media clarity
Adjust laser parameters as appropriate
Use the minimum energy necessary
Use the minimum number of shots
Make the diameter of the iridotomy opening appropriate
Be sure the iridotomy is patent
Treat tissue around circumference of iris to enlarge opening
Administer post-treatment regimen
Conduct follow-up examinations

D. *Use a Laser Contact Lens.*

1. Be sure that the beam is kept perpendicular always to the front surface of any laser contact lens. The more deviation there is, the more the loss of power at the target site.

2. Aim the laser beam at the center of the button.

3. Focus the laser beam precisely on the iris.

E. *Aim the Laser Beam Away from the Macula* (Figure 6–10).

F. *Focusing Is Absolutely Critical.*

1. Make sure you know whether the aiming beam and the infrared beam on the Nd:YAG laser are parfocal or how much offset there is. Some Nd:YAG lasers have an adjustable offset and others have a single preset offset.

2. Placing the Nd:YAG or argon focus in front of the iris increases the risk of corneal endothelial damage.

3. Placing the focus deep in the iris or behind the iris increases the risk of anterior lens capsule damage.

G. *Choose Initial Laser Parameters* (based on color of iris and media clarity).

H. *Adjust Laser Parameters as Appropriate.*

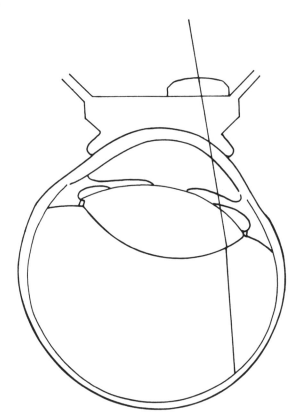

Figure 6–10 When enlarging an iridotomy, the Abraham lens and the laser beam should be angled away from the macula. (Reprinted with permission from Berger BB. Foveal photocoagulation from laser iridotomy. Ophthalmology 91:1029–1033 (1984).)

I. Use the Minimum Energy Necessary.

1. Start out with a low level of energy or power.

2. Assess the effect of this initial energy setting.

3. Increase the energy if needed or consider moving to another location.

J. Use the Minimum Number of Shots.

K. Make the Diameter of the Iridotomy Opening Appropriate.

1. An opening of **at least 150 to 200 μm** has been recommended (Brainard et al., 1982; Fleck, 1990; Fleck et al., 1992).

2. Acute angle-closure glaucoma has been shown to occur in some cases where the iridotomy had diameters in the range of 50 to 150 μm (Brainard et al., 1982; Gray et al., 1989; Mandelkorn et al., 1981; Wishart & Hitchings, 1986).

L. Be Sure the Iridotomy Is Patent.

1. The best way to assure patency is to **directly visualize the anterior lens capsule** through the iridotomy.

2. Another helpful indication of patency is when a gush of pigment from the iris pigment epithelium flows into the anterior chamber through the iridotomy.

3. Deepening of the anterior chamber is not a clear indication of patency.
   a. Pupillary block can be relieved during the procedure if the pupil is distorted.
   b. With time, the pupil can regain its normal shape and the pupillary block can return.

4. Iridotomy transillumination is also not a good indication of patency, especially when using the Nd:YAG laser.
   a. It is possible for the photodisruptive effect to remove the iris pigment epithelium and still leave a thin layer of impermeable stroma.
   b. Because the pigment epithelium is gone, there is a good red reflex, but the pupillary block remains.

M. To Enlarge the Iridotomy, Treat the Tissue Around the Circumference of the Iridotomy Rather Than Any Strands That Bridge the Gap. Use one pulse per burst. This will minimize damage to the crystalline lens.

N. Administer Post-Treatment Regimen.

O. Conduct Follow-up Examinations.

XI. Post-Treatment Regimen (American Academy of Ophthalmology, 1994; Liebmann & Ritch, 1996; Schuman, 1997) (Table 6–7).

A. **Instill another drop of 1% apraclonidine** to blunt any IOP spike.

B. **Begin topical steroids** (e.g., 1% prednisolone acetate, four times daily for 3 to 5 days) and then taper.

Table 6–7 Post-Treatment Regimen

1% apraclonidine
Topical steroids
Continue preoperative glaucoma medications
Avoid miotics
Postoperative Examinations
   Applanation tonometry
   Gonioscopy
   Slit-lamp biomicroscopy
   Dilation of patient if iridotomy is patent
   Automated threshold perimetry

C. **Continue preoperative anti-glaucoma medications** initially until the eye stabilizes and is reassessed.

D. **Avoid miotics,** if possible, to prevent posterior synechiae from forming. Some clinicians use miotics for a few weeks in case of iridotomy closure.

XII. Follow-up (American Academy of Ophthalmology, 1994; Schuman, 1997).

A. *Schedule*

1. 1 to 3 hr

2. 1 day (if necessary due to marked IOP elevation or intraoperative problems)

3. 1 week

4. 2 to 4 weeks

5. 3 months

6. Every 3 to 6 months

B. *Examinations Should Include*

1. **Applanation tonometry**

2. **Gonioscopy**
   a. Check the angle and the extent of opening. Be sure to assess all four quadrants.
   b. Check for peripheral anterior synechiae and areas of synechial closure.
   c. Check the contour of the iris. If the relative pupillary block has been relieved, then the iris should be rather flat instead of convex.
   d. Rule out plateau iris syndrome.

3. **Slit-lamp biomicroscopy**. Check for the following:
   a. iridotomy patency (is the lens capsule definitely visible through the iridotomy opening?)
   b. inflammation
   c. posterior synechiae
   d. pupillary distortion
   e. clarity of the lens
   f. corneal damage

4. **Dilation of the patient if the iridotomy is patent**
   a. A dilated fundus examination can be performed, especially if it had not been possible preoperatively.
      1) Check for laser-related posterior pole pathology.
      2) Evaluate the optic nerve head and nerve fiber layer.

b. Posterior synechiae formation is thereby prevented.

c. The patency of the iridotomy can be confirmed by this mydriatic provocative test.

d. Prescription of mydriatics for home use by patients is not recommended since the iridotomy could close during the first 6 weeks. Instead, dilation should be accomplished in the office on follow-up visits.

5. **Automated threshold perimetry** (especially if not possible preoperatively)

XIII. Complications: Prevention and Management (Table 6–8).

A. IOP Spikes

1. The IOP spikes more than 10 mm Hg in the first 3 hr in about 25% of patients following either argon or Nd:YAG laser iridotomy (Table 6–9).

   a. Out of the 10 studies examined, the pressure spiked following argon laser iridotomy on the average in 25.1% of the patients (range = 10% to 43%).

   b. In 11 other studies, the pressure spiked following Nd:YAG laser iridotomy on the average in 23.5% of the patients (range = 7% to 42%).

2. Usually the IOP elevations peak within 3 hr following the laser iridotomy and return to preoperative levels by 24 hr.

3. The IOP elevations are usually relatively mild but can rise up to 40 mm Hg above the preoperative baseline (Moster et al., 1986). In one case report, the pressure remained high and required a filtering operation (Henry et al., 1986).

4. Unfortunately, there does not appear to be any preoperative or immediate postoperative parameter that can accurately predict which eye will have an IOP spike after the iridotomy (Krupin et al., 1985; Lewis et al., 1998; Robin, 1989; Robin & Pollack, 1984, 1986; Robin et al., 1987). However, there may be a direct relationship between the preoperative outflow facility and the maximum postoperative IOP spike (Wetzel, 1994).

5. The IOP spike may be due to an influx of tissue debris and inflammatory cells into the trabecular meshwork after the laser treatment (Greenidge et al., 1984; Pollack, 1979; Schwartz et al., 1978). Similar IOP spikes occur in rabbits, and it was found that transient accumulation of blood plasma with fibrin occurs in the tissue of the anterior chamber angle after argon laser iridotomy (Tawara & Inomata, 1987). The blood plasma and fibrin apparently come from damage to iris blood vessels and the consequent breaks in the blood-aqueous barrier in the iris and iris processes (Tawara & Inomata, 1987).

Table 6–8 Complications of Laser Iridotomy

IOP spikes
Transient iritis
Closure of the iridotomy site
Pupillary distortion
Corneal damage
   Focal corneal opacities
   Corneal epithelial defects
   Corneal decompensation
   Focal corneal edema
   Linear cracks in Descemet's membrane
   Focal denudement of the corneal endothelium
   Cellular pleomorphism
   Decreased endothelial cell count
   Increased endothelial cell size
Lenticular damage
   Focal opacification
   Rupture of lens capsule
   Zonular rupture
   Lens dislocation
Posterior synechiae formation
Precipitation of angle-closure attack
Iris hemorrhage
Retinal damage
   Retinal photothermal and/or photochemical
     damage
   Retinal and choroidal detachment
Cystoid macular edema
Hypopyon
Pigmented pupillary pseudomembranes
Failure to perforate the iris
Phacoanaphylactic endophthalmitis
Malignant glaucoma
Diplopia and glare
Blurry vision
Monocular blurring
Iris atrophy and enlargement of the iridotomy
Loss of central visual acuity
Reactions to medications used pre- and
     postoperatively

Table 6–9 Occurrence of IOP Elevations Greater Than 10 mm Hg Following Laser Iridotomy

Occurrence of IOP Elevation >10 mm Hg (n)	Type of Laser	Occurrence of IOP Elevation >10 mm Hg for Prophylaxis (n)	Prophylaxis	Authors
35% (20)	Ar			Robin & Pollack, 1984
22% (50)	Ar			Krupin et al., 1985
12% (43)	Ar	6% (32)	0.25% timolol	Liu & Hung, 1987
43% (14)	Ar	0% (14)	1% apraclonidine	Robin et al., 1987
27% (45)	Ar			Taniguchi et al., 1987
21% (19)	Ar	0% (17)	1% apraclonidine	Brown et al., 1988
	Ar	0% (28)	1% apraclonidine	Robin, 1989
	Ar	27% (26)	0.5% timolol	Robin, 1989
36% (11)	Ar	0% (11)	1% apraclonidine	Fernandez-Bahamonde & Alcaraz-Michelli, 1990
10% (31)	Ar	11% (92)	125 mg acetazolamide & 1% carteolol	Chang & Hung, 1991
27% (11)	Ar	0% (18)	1% apraclonidine	Hong et al., 1991
18% (129)	Ar	2% (115)	1% apraclonidine	Krupin et al., 1992
30% (20)	Nd:YAG			Robin & Pollack, 1984
27% (33)	Nd:YAG			Robin & Pollack, 1986
30% (182)	Nd:YAG			Schwartz et al., 1986
23% (48)	Nd:YAG			Wishart & Hitchings, 1986
42% (40)	Nd:YAG			Naveh et al., 1987
27% (45)	Nd:YAG			Taniguchi et al., 1987
10% (100)	Nd:YAG			Wand et al., 1988
25% (12)	Nd:YAG			Goins et al., 1990
21% (212)	Nd:YAG			Shani et al., 1994
17% (29)	Nd:YAG	3.4% (29)	0.5% apraclonidine	Kitazawa et al., 1989
	Nd:YAG	6% (35)	0.5% apraclonidine @ 1 hr	Rosenberg et al., 1995
	Nd:YAG	11% (27)	1% apraclonidine @ 1 hr	Rosenberg et al., 1995
7% (29)	Nd:YAG	1% (137)	125 mg acetazolamide & 1% carteolol	Chang & Hung, 1991
62.5% (8)	Nd:YAG	16.7% (6)	2% dorzolamide	Hartenbaum et al., 1999
	Nd:YAG	0.7% (289)	0.5% or 1% apraclonidine	Lewis et al., 1998
	A few Ar then Nd:YAG			
42% (12)	Ar then Nd:YAG			Goins et al., 1990

Table continued on following page

Table 6–9 Occurrence of IOP Elevations Greater Than 10 mm Hg Following Laser Iridotomy *Continued*

Occurrence of IOP Elevation >10 mm Hg (n)	Type of Laser	Occurrence of IOP Elevation >10 mm Hg for Prophylaxis (n)	Prophylaxis	Authors
25% (20)	Ar then Nd:YAG			Ho & Fan, 1992
17% (18)	Nd:YLF			Oram et al., 1995
20% (40)	Diode			Emoto et al., 1992
66% (52)	Dye			Wishart & Hitchings, 1986

≥10 mm Hg: Shani et al., 1994

6. The **use of 1% or even 0.5% apraclonidine to blunt the pressure spike is highly effective** (see Table 6–9). In most studies, no patients had an IOP rise more than 10 mm Hg above the preoperative baseline. In the largest study, only two eyes (0.7%) out of 289 experienced an IOP rise of more than 10 mm Hg (Lewis et al., 1998). In this study, 278 of the iridotomies were done with the Nd:YAG laser alone and 11 were done with a combination of argon and Nd:YAG lasers. This study also suggested that routine IOP monitoring after laser iridotomy may not be required even though it is the current standard of practice.

7. Timolol does blunt the IOP spike but not nearly as well as apraclonidine (Liu & Hung, 1987; Robin, 1989). Pilocarpine has also been used (Schrems et al., 1984), and a combination of carteolol and acetazolamide has been tried (Chang & Hung, 1991). Dorzolamide has also been employed (Hartenbaum et al., 1999).

8. Obviously, those patients with significant glaucomatous damage preoperatively should be monitored closely following laser iridotomy.

B. Transient Iritis

1. Most studies indicate that essentially 100% of patients experience a low-grade transient inflammation of the anterior segment following laser iridotomy (Goins et al., 1990; Harrad et al., 1985; Mishima et al., 1985; Robin & Pollack, 1984, 1986; Yassur et al., 1979).

2. There is apparently less clinically significant uveitis following Nd:YAG laser iridotomy than after argon laser iridotomy (Cohen et al., 1984; Schwartz et al., 1986; Shin, 1984; Drake, 1987).

3. "Cells" in the anterior chamber following iridotomy may include aggregates of fibrin or protein in addition to real inflammatory cells (Liu et al., 1993).

4. The inflammation caused by laser iridotomies is due to iris trauma leading to the release of tissue and pigment debris, the release of inflammatory mediators like the eicosanoids, and subsequent breakdown of the blood-aqueous barrier (Gailitis et al., 1986; Joo & Kim, 1992; Sanders et al., 1983; Schrems et al., 1984; Sugiyama et al., 1990; Tawara & Inomata, 1987; Unger et al., 1977; Unger & Bass, 1977; Weinreb et al., 1985).

5. The inflammation usually resolves within 48 hr with topical steroid treatment. However, the iritis can persist for months (Choplin & Bene, 1983; Moster et al., 1986).

C. *Closure of the Iridotomy Site*

1. **Argon laser iridotomies tend to close in 16% to 34% of patients** (Table 6–10). These iridotomies can induce pigment proliferation and progressive scarring of iris tissue (Del Priore et al., 1988; Schwartz et al., 1978).

2. **Nd:YAG iridotomies rarely close** (see Table 6–10). Even 3 to 5 years after the iridotomy, there appeared to be no proliferation of the iris pigment epithelium or fibrous scar formation (Tetsumoto et al., 1992). A rare case of repeated closure has been reported (Melamed & Wagoner, 1988).

3. Iridotomies made by argon laser pretreatment followed by Nd:YAG laser treatment also rarely close (see Table 6–10).

4. If the iridotomy opening decreases in size so that its minimum diameter is less than 75 µm, it should be enlarged (Robin & Pollack, 1984). Based on more recent studies, other clinicians suggest that the opening diameter be at least 150 to 200 µm (Fleck, 1990; Fleck et al., 1992).

5. If closure occurs, it usually happens within the first 6 weeks (Del Priore et al., 1988; Pollack, 1979). As a rule-of-thumb, iridotomies that are patent at 6 weeks postop will remain open for at least a year (Quigley, 1981).

6. Closure can occur due to occlusion by
   a. settling of circulating debris into the opening,
   b. landsliding of iris pigment epithelium from the area around the opening,
   c. proliferation of iris pigment epithelium,
   d. swollen iris stromal tissue surrounding the opening, or
   e. posterior synechiae surrounding the opening (Brainard et al., 1982; Mandelkorn et al., 1981; Pollack, 1979; Robin & Pollack, 1986).

7. Risk factors for closure include rubeosis and any pre-existing active inflammatory process (Klapper, 1984; Lim et al., 1996; Quigley, 1981; Robin & Pollack, 1986).

Table 6–10 Occurrence of Iridotomy Closure by Laser Type

Occurrence of Closure	Number of Iridotomies (n)	Type of Laser	Follow-up Time	Authors
22%	45	Ar	≥2 mon	Podos et al., 1979
34%	77	Ar	1 mon	Pollack, 1979
30%	20	Ar	1 mon	Robin & Pollack, 1984
16%	38	Ar	≥8 mon	Moster et al., 1986
18%	28	Ar	1 mon	Robin et al., 1987
21%	43	Ar	≥20 mon	Del Priore et al., 1988
20%	25	Ar	1–8 mon	McAllister et al., 1984
12%	68	red Kr	≥6 mon	Yassur et al., 1986
4%	25	Nd:YAG	1–8 mon	McAllister et al., 1984
0%	20	Nd:YAG	≥3 mon	Klapper, 1984
0%	20	Nd:YAG	1 mon	Robin & Pollack, 1984
0%	38	Nd:YAG	≥8 mon	Moster et al., 1986
6%	33	Nd:YAG	≥1 mon	Robin & Pollack, 1986
8%	51	Nd:YAG	unknown	Drake, 1987
10%	40	Nd:YAG	≥4 mon	Naveh et al., 1987
0%	53	Nd:YAG	≥10 mon	Canning et al., 1988
0%	43	Nd:YAG	≥20 mon	Del Priore et al., 1988
0%	36	Nd:YAG	8.6 mon (mean)	Bertoni et al., 1988
0%	16	Ar then Nd:YAG	≥4 mon	Zborwski-Gutman et al., 1988
9%	11	Ar then Nd:YAG	1 wk–8 mon	Lim et al., 1996
5%	20	Ar then Nd:YAG	≥6 mon	Ho & Fan, 1992
0%	18	Nd:YLF	1–6 mon	Oram et al., 1995

8. To minimize late closure
   a. make the opening at least 200 μm,
   b. use the Nd:YAG laser, and
   c. do not perform iridotomies on patients with active inflammation.
9. The simplest way to treat late closure is to reopen the iridotomy with the Nd:YAG laser. The argon laser could also be used, but there is less reclosure with the Nd:YAG laser.

D. Pupillary Distortion

1. Pupillary distortion appears to occur slightly more often in argon laser iridotomies than in Nd:YAG iridotomies (Table 6–11). However, many studies did not specifically mention the occurrence of pupillary distortion and so are not listed in the table.

Table 6–11 Occurrence of Pupillary Distortion Following Laser Iridotomies

Occurrence of Pupillary Distortion	Number of Iridotomies (n)	Type of Laser	Authors
2.2%	45	Ar	Podos et al., 1979
10.5%	38	Ar	Moster et al., 1986
42%	53	Ar-Kr	Yassur et al., 1979
7.9%	38	Nd:YAG	Moster et al., 1986
3%	182	Nd:YAG	Schwartz et al., 1986
70%	40	Diode	Emoto et al., 1992

2. When distortion occurs, the pupil is usually dragged toward the iridotomy opening.

3. Usually the pupil regains its normal shape after several weeks (Belcher, 1984; Yassur et al., 1979).

E. Corneal Damage

1. Corneal changes can occur following laser iridotomies. These lesions include the following:

   a. **Focal corneal opacities**

      1) The mean occurrences of focal corneal opacities following argon and Nd:YAG laser iridotomies are essentially the same (Table 6–12). However, the sequential use of Ar and then Nd:YAG lasers resulted in a much lower mean percentage of opacities.

         a) The mean occurrence of opacities after use of the argon laser in 8 studies is 24% with a range of 8% to 57%.

         b) The mean occurrence of opacities after use of the Nd:YAG laser in 13 studies is 22% with a range of 0% to 69%.

         c) The mean occurrence of opacities after sequential use of the argon and then Nd:YAG lasers in 2 studies is 9% with a range of 8% to 10%.

      2) The argon laser can produce epithelial burns by photothermal absorption and endothelial burns by thermal conduction from the iris surface.

      3) Following argon laser iridotomies, focal corneal opacities involved a discrete whitening of the endothelium, Descemet's membrane, and posterior stroma (Del Priore et al., 1988).

      4) The Nd:YAG laser can produce endothelial damage via the plasma-generated shock wave.

      5) Following Nd:YAG iridotomies, the focal corneal opacities involved stretch deformations or linear fractures of Descemet's membrane and posterior stroma (Del Priore et al., 1988).

Table 6–12 Occurrence of Corneal Opacities Following Laser Iridotomy

Occurrence of Corneal Opacities	Number of Iridotomies (n)	Type of Laser	Authors
9%	45	Ar	Podos et al., 1979
25%	20	Ar	Robin & Pollack, 1984
19%	52	Ar	Harrad et al., 1985
57%	101	Ar (long-burn)	Mishima et al., 1985
26%	197	Ar (short-burn)	Mishima et al., 1985
21%	28	Ar	Robin et al., 1987
26%	43	Ar	Del Priore et al., 1988
8%	25	Ar	McAllister et al., 1984
3%	68	red Kr	Yassur et al., 1986
0%	20	Nd:YAG	Klapper, 1984
8%	25	Nd:YAG	McAllister et al., 1984
35%	20	Nd:YAG	Robin & Pollack, 1984
25%	44	Nd:YAG	Robin et al., 1986
18%	33	Nd:YAG	Robin & Pollack, 1986
4%	182	Nd:YAG	Schwartz et al., 1986
2.5%	40	Nd:YAG	Naveh et al., 1987
2%	45	Nd:YAG	Taniguchi et al., 1987
69%	26	Nd:YAG	Canning et al., 1988
30%	43	Nd:YAG	Del Priore et al., 1988
33%	12	Nd:YAG	Goins et al., 1990
0%	38	Nd:YAG	Bertoni et al., 1988
58%	52	Nd:YAG	Fleck et al., 1991
10%	20	Ar then Nd:YAG	Ho & Fan, 1992
8%	12	Ar then Nd:YAG	Goins et al., 1990
5%	40	Diode	Emoto et al., 1992
0%	18	Nd:YLF	Oram et al., 1995

6) Because these focal opacities are in the periphery, they do not interfere with the patient's vision. Many of them are transient and heal within a few days. However, intraoperatively they may absorb part of the laser beam and thus make the procedure more difficult and put the cornea at even more risk for damage. Another target site may need to be chosen.

b. **Corneal epithelial defects**

1) Epithelial damage can occur with the argon laser due to photothermal absorption and subsequent coagulation (Figure 6–11).

2) Mishima et al. (1985) found that with longer duration burns the occurrence of corneal epithelial defects was 44%; whereas with short duration burns the occurrence was reduced to 2%.

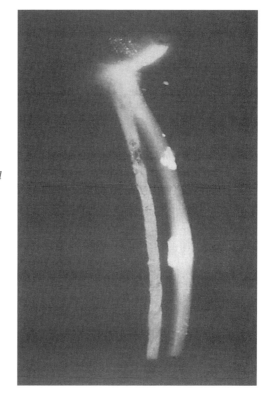

Figure 6–11 Corneal epithelial lesion following a high power argon laser iridotomy. Note the focal thermal coagulation of the epithelium and superficial stroma. (Reprinted with permission from Ritch R, Liebmann JM. Laser iridotomy and peripheral iridoplasty. In: Ritch R, Shields MB, Krupin T (eds.). The Glaucomas. St.Louis: Mosby, 1996; 76:1549–1573.)

    3) No epithelial defects were noted in many studies (Klapper, 1984; Goins et al., 1990).

    4) Some of the epithelial defects may be induced by laser contact lens abrasion, especially in patients with epithelial basement membrane dystrophy (Goins et al., 1990).

    5) Just like endothelial opacities, these opacities are in the periphery and hence do not interfere with the patient's vision. But they also absorb part of the laser energy and hence increase the difficulty of the procedure and the risk to the cornea. They also may require the choice of another target site.

  c. **Corneal decompensation** (Jeng et al., 1991; Kalnins & Mandelkorn, 1989; Pollack, 1984; Schwartz et al., 1988; Wilhemus, 1992; Zabel et al., 1991; Zadok et al., 1993).

    1) Rarely, corneal decompensation occurs following argon laser iridotomy. This damage can evolve over months or years as a foreign body sensation, progressive corneal edema, and bullous keratopathy.

      2) Possible risk factors include the following:
         a) diabetes
         b) corneal guttata
         c) prior angle closure occurrences with pressure elevation and inflammation
         d) high laser energy (Jeng et al., 1991; Schwartz et al., 1989; Wilhelmus, 1992)
      3) Check for patients with preexisting corneal problems that may predispose the patient to corneal decompensation.
      4) Treatment may require hypertonic saline, a bandage contact lens, or even penetrating keratoplasty.
  d. **Focal corneal edema**
      1) The argon laser can produce transient focal corneal edema, especially when higher powers and/or longer durations are used (Kalnins & Mandelkorn, 1989; Pollack, 1984).
      2) The Nd:YAG laser can also produce transient focal edema that resolves within a week (Fleck et al., 1991, 1997; Naveh et al., 1987).
  e. **Linear cracks in Descemet's membrane** (Drake, 1987).
  f. **Focal denudement of the corneal endothelium** (Drake, 1987; Kerr Muir & Sherrard, 1985; Power & Cullom, 1992).
  g. **Cellular pleomorphism** (Kerr Muir & Sherrard, 1985).
  h. **Decreased endothelial cell count**
      1) Small decreases in endothelial cell count of up to 8% have been noted following *argon* laser iridotomies (Hong et al., 1983; Robin & Pollack, 1984). However, when followed for up to 1 year, usually no statistically significant cell loss has been noted (Hirst et al., 1982; Panek et al., 1988; Smith & Whitted, 1984; Thoming et al., 1987).
      2) Decreased counts following *Nd:YAG* iridotomies have ranged from 0% to 16% with most being statistically insignificant (Kozobolis et al., 1998; Marraffa et al., 1995; Panek et al., 1991; Robin & Pollack, 1984; Schrems et al., 1986; Schwenn et al., 1995; Wishart et al., 1986). As expected, there is a greater loss of cells when the iridotomy is more peripheral and when the angle is narrower (Marraffa et al., 1995).
  i. **Increased endothelial cell size**
      1) Hong et al. (1983) reported a significant increase in endothelial cell size by 3 months following an argon laser iridotomy.
      2) This increase in cell size was significantly correlated with the amount of laser energy employed.
2. Damage to the cornea can occur by
  a. heat conduction from an argon laser-treated iris site,
  b. direct absorption of laser energy by the cornea, or
  c. mechanical shock waves from the plasma at an Nd:YAG-treated iris site.

3. To minimize the occurrence of corneal damage
    a. use the minimum energy necessary (i.e., lower power and/or shorter duration) (Hong et al., 1983; Meyer et al., 1984),
    b. use a laser contact lens (Meyer et al., 1984; Power & Collum, 1992),
    c. focus very carefully,
    d. choose a target site with adequate clearance between the cornea and iris,
    e. avoid areas of prominent corneal arcus, and
    f. move to a new site if an opacity begins to form early in the treatment.

F. Lenticular Damage

1. **Focal opacification**
    a. Lenticular opacities are much more frequent following argon laser iridotomies (up to 54% occurrence) than after Nd:YAG iridotomies (typically 0% occurrence) (Table 6–13). Very few, if any, opacities form following argon laser pretreatment and then Nd:YAG laser iridotomies (0% to 5%).
    b. These opacities are usually small and nonprogressive.
    c. The argon laser can produce photothermal coagulation of the capsule and lens tissues.
    d. The Nd:YAG laser can cause photodisruptive damage. Scanning electron microscopy of human lenses following Nd:YAG iridotomies showed craters in the superficial anterior lens capsule and superficial cortex (Welch et al., 1986). These depressions had a smooth-contoured surface.
    e. An opacity of the anterior capsule has been noted under the site of an Nd:YAG laser iridotomy prior to implantation of a phakic IOL (Zadok & Chayet, 1999).

2. **Rupture of lens capsule** (Berger et al., 1989; Fernandez-Bahamonde, 1991; Margo et al., 1992; Montgomery & Dutton, 1987; Wollensak et al., 1997)
    a. The anterior lens capsule may be perforated.
    b. In one case, capsular rupture of an intumescent cataract led to one-half of the anterior chamber being filled with liquid cortex (Fernandez-Bahamonde, 1991). This was followed by an emergency cataract extraction (Figure 6–12).
    c. In another case, a subcapsular perforation rosette of the posterior pole of the lens was found along with a ring of pigment located inside the lens (Wollensak et al., 1997). The anterior capsule was perforated directly behind the Nd:YAG laser iridotomy site. The rosette disappeared in about 4 weeks, and the patient's vision returned to normal. The patient had pigment dispersion syndrome, and the case was probably related to a concave iris placing the iris in close proximity to the lens.

3. **Zonular rupture** (Berger et al., 1989).

4. **Lens dislocation**—one case of lens dislocation may have been precipitated by an Nd:YAG iridotomy (Melamed et al., 1986).

Table 6–13 Occurrence of Lenticular Opacities Following Laser Iridotomies Using Different Types of Lasers

Occurrence of Opacities	Number of Iridotomies (n)	Type of Laser	Authors
4%	45	Ar	Podos et al., 1979
35%	20	Ar	Robin & Pollack, 1984
40%	52	Ar	Harrad et al., 1985
54%	101	Ar (long-burn)	Mishima et al., 1985
6%	197	Ar (short-burn)	Mishima et al., 1985
18%	28	Ar	Robin et al., 1987
53%	43	Ar	Del Priore et al., 1988
4%	25	Ar	McAllister et al., 1984
47%	53	Ar, Kr	Yassur et al., 1979
31%	68	red Kr	Yassur et al., 1986
0%	25	Nd:YAG	McAllister et al., 1984
0%	20	Nd:YAG	Klapper, 1984
0%	20	Nd:YAG	Robin & Pollack, 1984
0%	33	Nd:YAG	Robin & Pollack, 1986
0%	182	Nd:YAG	Schwartz et al., 1986
2.5%	40	Nd:YAG	Naveh et al., 1987
0%	45	Nd:YAG	Taniguchi et al., 1987
0%	43	Nd:YAG	Del Priore et al., 1988
8%	12	Nd:YAG	Goins et al., 1990
0%	38	Nd:YAG	Bertoni et al., 1988
4%	52	Nd:YAG	Fleck et al., 1991
0%	16	Ar then Nd:YAG	Zborwski-Gutman et al., 1988
0%	12	Ar then Nd:YAG	Goins et al., 1990
5%	20	Ar then Nd:YAG	Ho & Fan, 1992
5%	40	Diode	Emoto et al., 1992
0%	18	Nd:YLF	Oram et al., 1995

5. To minimize lenticular damage
   a. Use the minimum laser energy necessary.
   b. Use single-pulse bursts.
   c. Focus precisely.
   d. Avoid enlargement of an already patent iridotomy.
   e. Use the Nd:YAG instead of the argon laser.
   f. Perform the procedure peripherally where there is the greatest separation between the iris and the anterior lens capsule.

G. Posterior Synechiae Formation

1. Similar occurrences of posterior synechiae formation have been reported for both argon and the Nd:YAG laser iridotomies (Table 6–14). One problem in the reporting

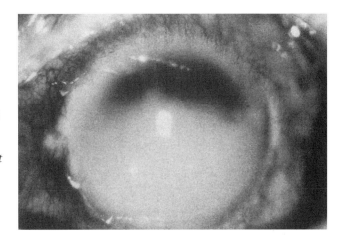

Figure 6–12 Rupture of the lens capsule followed by leakage of liquid cortex into the anterior chamber. An Nd:YAG laser iridotomy had been attempted. (Reprinted with permission from Fernandez-Bahamonde JL. Iatrogenic lens rupture after a neodymium: yttrium aluminum garnet laser iridotomy attempt. Ann Ophthalmol 23:346–348 (1991).)

has been that a number of studies did not specifically comment on the presence or absence of posterior synechiae and thus were not included in the table.

2. There is a strong positive correlation between the postoperative use of miotics and the formation of posterior synechiae (Lederer & Price, 1989; McGalliard & Wishart, 1990; Figure 6–13).

3. Posterior synechiae usually respond to intense pupil dilation (Pollack & Patz, 1976).

4. To minimize the occurrence of posterior synechiae
   a. Use the minimum amount of laser energy necessary.
   b. Use topical steroid therapy postoperatively.
   c. Discontinue the use of miotics in the immediate postoperative period (2 to 4 weeks) if the patient does not have significant combined-mechanism glaucoma.
   d. Dilate the pupil frequently in the immediate postoperative period if the patient has a patent iridotomy and does not have plateau iris syndrome.

Table 6–14 Occurrence of Posterior Synechiae Following Laser Iridotomy

Occurrence of Posterior Synechiae	Number of Iridotomies (n)	Type of Laser	Authors
14%		Ar	Abraham & Miller, 1975
4%	45	Ar	Podos et al., 1979
5%	38	Ar	Moster et al., 1986
37%	83 Ar/3 Nd:YAG	mostly Ar	Lederer & Price, 1989
3%	38	Nd:YAG	Moster et al., 1986
7%	182	Nd:YAG	Schwartz et al., 1986
21%	81	Nd:YAG	McGalliard & Wishart, 1990
6%	52	Nd:YAG	Fleck et al., 1991

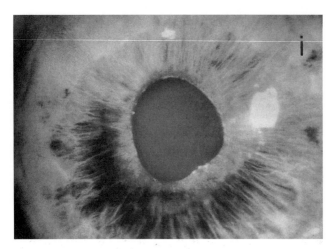

Figure 6–13 Extensive posterior synechiae following an Nd:YAG laser iridotomy. This patient had been on long-term treatment with pilocarpine. The iridotomy (i) is at about 2 o'clock. (Reprinted with permission from McGalliard JN, Wishart PK. The effect of Nd:YAG iridotomy on intraocular pressure in hypertensive eyes with shallow anterior chambers. Eye 4:823–829 (1990).)

H. Precipitation of Angle-Closure Glaucoma Attack

1. There have been a few cases of acute angle-closure glaucoma following laser iridotomy even with a patent opening (Brainard et al., 1982; Brazier, 1989; Fleck et al., 1997; Gray et al., 1989; Mandelkorn et al., 1981; Morsman, 1991; Pollack & Patz, 1976; Wishart & Hitchings, 1986).

2. Failure of the laser iridotomy in these cases could be due to the following:
   a. plateau iris syndrome
   b. non-patent opening
   c. pigment "avalanche" occluding a patent opening
   d. posterior synechiae surrounding the iridotomy opening
   e. patent iridotomy too small for adequate aqueous flow

3. Patients should be instructed to return immediately if they experience intense pain, redness, or a decrease in vision.

I. Iris Hemorrhage

1. **Iris hemorrhage during or following an argon laser iridotomy is very rare** because of the photothermal coagulation of the blood vessels (Table 6–15).
   a. There are a few case reports of small hemorrhages with the argon laser (Beckman & Sugar, 1973; Perkins & Brown, 1973; Snyder et al., 1975).
   b. Using the argon laser, the risk factors for hemorrhage include patients with rubeosis iridis and uveitis and patients on anticoagulative medications, like heparin (Beckman & Sugar, 1973; Quigley, 1981; Perkins & Brown, 1973; Snyder et al., 1975).
   c. There has been one report of hemorrhage and hyphema in a patient with no apparent predisposing condition (Hodes et al., 1982).

Table 6–15 Occurrence of Iris Hemorrhage During Laser Iridotomy

Occurrence of Iris Hemorrhage	Number of Iridotomies (n)	Type of Laser	Authors
0%	20	Ar	Robin & Pollack, 1984
0%	38	Ar	Moster et al., 1986
0%	43	Ar	Del Priore et al., 1988
0%	25	Ar	McAllister et al., 1984
28%	25	Nd:YAG	McAllister et al., 1984
15%	20	Nd:YAG	Klapper, 1984
45%	20	Nd:YAG	Robin & Pollack, 1984
34%	38	Nd:YAG	Moster et al., 1986
52%	44	Nd:YAG	Robin et al., 1986
36%	33	Nd:YAG	Robin & Pollack, 1986
20%	182	Nd:YAG	Schwartz et al., 1986
20%	40	Nd:YAG	Naveh et al., 1987
36%	45	Nd:YAG	Taniguchi et al., 1987
44%	43	Nd:YAG	Del Priore et al., 1988
100%	100	Nd:YAG	Wand et al., 1988
67%	12	Nd:YAG	Goins et al., 1990
58%	52	Nd:YAG	Fleck et al., 1991
39%	54	Nd:YAG	Fleck et al., 1997
0%	16	Ar then Nd:YAG	Zborwski-Gutman et al., 1988
17%	12	Ar then Nd:YAG	Goins et al., 1990
27%	52	Mode-locked Nd:YAG	Kumar et al., 1990
44%	52	Ar then mode-locked Nd:YAG	Kumar et al., 1990
56%	18	Nd:YLF	Oram et al., 1995

    d. There is also one report of delayed hyphema after an argon laser iridotomy possibly due to macrophage activity and necrosis postoperatively (Rubin et al., 1984).

2. **Iris hemorrhage during Nd:YAG iridotomies is very common** because the photodisruptive mechanism does not provide coagulation of the blood vessels (see Table 6–15 and Figure 6–14). Out of 14 studies examined, the average occurrence of hemorrhage was 42% (range = 15% to 100%).

    a. Hyphema following Nd:YAG iridotomies has a mean occurrence of 1.6% in 11 studies (Table 6–16). Most of them are small and easily resolve.

    b. There is one case report of a serious 40% hyphema and secondary iris traction that occurred in a patient that experienced repeated closures and reopenings of an iridotomy and subsequent iridectomy (Gilbert et al., 1984).

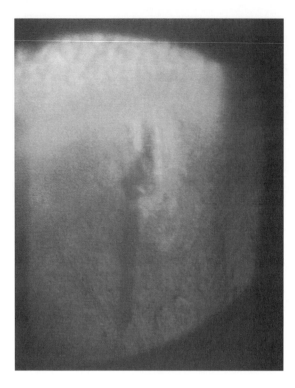

Figure 6–14 Iris hemorrhage 15 min after an Nd:YAG laser iridotomy. This self-limited type of hemorrhage is usually gone by the following day. (Reprinted from Drake MV. Neodymium:YAG laser iridotomy. Surv Ophthalmol 32:171–177 (1987), with permission from Elsevier Science.)

3. Iris hemorrhage occurrence appears to be low (mean = 8%; range = 0% to 17%) during iridotomies where the argon laser is used for pretreatment and the Q-switched Nd:YAG laser is used for completion. The occurrence of hyphema also appears to be very low (mean = 2%; range = 0% to 10%).

4. In one study, the mode-locked Nd:YAG laser was used either with or without argon laser pretreatment (Kumar et al., 1990). The results are shown in Table 6–15.

5. **To minimize and manage iris hemorrhage:**
    a. Use the argon laser for the iridotomy or as pretreatment, especially in patients with uveitis or rubeosis iridis or who are on anticoagulant drugs.
    b. Avoid iris blood vessels when aiming the laser.
    c. Apply increased pressure on the globe using the laser contact lens to tamponade any hemorrhage that occurs.
    d. If the hemorrhage does not stop with applied pressure, consider using the argon laser to coagulate the vessel.

6. There is one reported case of an **intralenticular hemorrhage** following an Nd:YAG laser iridotomy (Montgomery & Dutton, 1987). This probably involved a small rupture of the anterior lens capsule, entry of blood, and subsequent sealing of the capsule.

Table 6–16 Occurrence of Hyphema Following Laser Iridotomy

Occurrence of Hyphema	Number of Iridotomies (n)	Type of Laser	Authors
0%	20	Ar	Robin & Pollack, 1984
0%	38	Ar	Moster et al., 1986
0%	43	Ar	Del Priore et al., 1988
0%	13	Ar	Lim et al., 1996
0%	25	Ar	McAllister et al., 1984
0%	25	Nd:YAG	McAllister et al., 1984
0%	20	Nd:YAG	Klapper, 1984
5%	20	Nd:YAG	Robin & Pollack, 1984
3%	38	Nd:YAG	Moster et al., 1986
0%	33	Nd:YAG	Robin & Pollack, 1986
2%	48	Nd:YAG	Wishart & Hitchings, 1986
2.5%	40	Nd:YAG	Naveh et al., 1987
2.6%	38	Nd:YAG	Bertoni et al., 1988
0%	43	Nd:YAG	Del Priore et al., 1988
2%	100	Nd:YAG	Wand et al., 1988
0%	12	Nd:YAG	Goins et al., 1990
0%	16	Ar then Nd:YAG	Zborwski-Gutman et al., 1988
0%	11	Ar then Nd:YAG	Lim et al., 1996
0%	12	Ar then Nd:YAG	Goins et al., 1990
10%	20	Ar then Nd:YAG	Ho & Fan, 1992
10%	52	Dye	Wishart & Hitchings, 1986

J. Retinal Damage

1. **Retinal photothermal and /or photochemical damage** (Anderson et al., 1989; Berger, 1984; Bongard & Pederson, 1985; Karmon & Savir, 1986; Pollack & Patz, 1976)

   a. The most significant risk of retinal damage comes from the argon laser. This laser is capable of both photothermal and photochemical damage.

      1) Most studies detected no retinal damage following laser iridotomies.

      2) In one study, 96% of patients undergoing argon laser iridotomy sustained focal peripheral retinal damage detected by static perimetry and fluorescein angiography (Karmon & Savir, 1986). No ophthalmoscopically visible damage was detected and the patients were asymptomatic. In this study a laser contact lens was not used, and the energy levels were higher than usual.

      3) There is also one case report of ophthalmoscopically visible foveal damage following an argon laser iridotomy (Berger, 1984). This patient was symptomatic since the visual acuity was reduced permanently to 20/400.

    4) One further report noted a small decrease in contrast sensitivity at high spatial frequencies and a small increase at low spatial frequencies (Anderson et al., 1989). These changes may not have been laser-related.

  b. Laser contact lenses, like the Abraham iridotomy lens, significantly reduce the potential for retinal damage during a laser iridotomy (Bongard & Pederson, 1985; Wise et al., 1986).

  c. The most dangerous part of the procedure occurs just after penetration, when the opening is being enlarged (Quigley, 1981). Part or all of the laser beam can be transmitted through the opening.

  d. To avoid a macular lesion
    1) use the minimum laser energy necessary,
    2) use a laser contact lens, and
    3) tilt the contact lens and angle the laser beam away from the macula during the procedure.

2. **Retinal and choroidal detachment**
  a. One case involving a large choroidal detachment along with a total serous retinal detachment has been reported three weeks following argon laser iridotomy (Corriveau et al., 1986).

  b. Similarly, one patient developed bilateral nonrhegmatogenous retinal detachment and choroidal detachment two weeks following Nd:YAG laser iridotomies to both eyes (Karjalainen et al., 1986).

  c. Both cases may have been due to the relatively high cumulative energy levels employed. In the argon laser case, a total of 442 burns (over 35,000 mJ) were delivered to the eye during two separate procedures. In the Nd:YAG laser case, a total of 61 shots (220 mJ) were delivered to the right eye and 6 shots (22 mJ) were delivered to the left eye.

K. Cystoid Macular Edema

1. One case of cystoid macular edema occurring about 3 months after an argon laser iridotomy has been reported (Choplin & Bene, 1983). The edema resolved within 3 weeks.

2. This incident was most likely due to vitreous inflammation secondary to postlaser chronic iritis.

L. Hypopyon

1. Hypopyon formation following laser iridotomy is very rare (Cohen et al., 1984; Margo et al., 1992; Shin, 1984).

2. Rubeosis iridis was a predisposing factor in one of the cases.

M. Pigmented Pupillary Pseudomembranes

1. At least four cases of pigmented pupillary pseudomembranes have been reported following argon laser iridotomy (Lotufo et al., 1993; Geyer et al., 1991; Goldberger et al., 1989). They involve the formation of a confluent pigment mass that can occlude the pupil.

2. These incidents were probably due to laser-induced inflammation and long-term miotic treatment.

3. It is possible that these cases represented extension of posterior synechiae into the area of the pupil.

4. To minimize the occurrence of these pseudomembranes, dilate the patient periodically if miotic treatment is continued postoperatively. Use of the Nd:YAG laser for the iridotomy may also decrease the incidence.

N. Failure to Perforate the Iris (Belcher, 1984; Belcher & Schuman, 1992; Bertoni et al., 1988; Fleck et al., 1997; Oh & Rosenquist, 1994; McAllister et al., 1984).

1. Most attempts at iris iridotomy are successful, but light blue and dark brown irides can be difficult, especially with the argon laser. Other causes of failure include omission of pilocarpine, inadequate visualization of the target, inadequate laser power setting, inexperience of the operator, and poor cooperation of the patient.

2. If the iridotomy at one site is too difficult to complete, consider
   a. moving to another target site,
   b. using an Nd:YAG laser instead of the argon laser or in combination with it,
   c. scheduling another treatment at a later time, and
   d. performing incisional surgical iridectomy if laser iridotomy is not feasible.

O. Phacoanaphylactic Endophthalmitis

1. One case of lens-induced endophthalmitis following an Nd:YAG laser iridotomy was reported (Margo et al., 1992).

2. This occurred in a blind eye with a mature cataract and involved capsular rupture following two Nd:YAG iridotomies in the same eye.

P. Malignant Glaucoma

1. A number of cases of malignant glaucoma after laser iridotomy have been reported (Abe et al., 1994; Aminlari & Sassani, 1993; Blondeau, 1983; Brooks et al., 1989; Cashwell & Martin, 1992; Levene, 1988; Robinson et al., 1990; Small & Maslin, 1995; Takeuchi & Okubo, 1986).

2. Whether laser iridotomy causes malignant glaucoma is still controversial (Fourman, 1992; Geyer et al., 1990; Hodes, 1992; Loewenstein & Lazar, 1994). A number of risk factors for the development of malignant glaucoma are associated with patients who

undergo laser iridotomies. They include narrow angles, use of miotics, trauma, and transient inflammation. Risk factors such as these were present in essentially all the reported cases.

3. Malignant glaucoma can be precipitated even when there is a patent iridotomy (Blondeau, 1983; Brooks et al., 1989; Cashwell & Martin, 1992; Robinson et al., 1990; Small & Maslin, 1995). In fact, the patent iridotomy rules out the possibility of pupillary block glaucoma.

Q. Diplopia and Glare

1. A few cases of monocular diplopia and glare problems following argon iridotomy have been reported (Harrad et al., 1985; Kublin & Simmons, 1987). Generally, they occurred in patients with large iridotomies (e.g., 0.5 mm and 1.0 mm diameter).

2. If postoperative progressive enlargement of the iridotomy opening occurs, the risk of diplopia and glare may increase (Quigley, 1981; Sachs & Schwartz, 1984).

3. See *Monocular Blurring* for a related complication.

4. **To minimize the occurrence of diplopia and glare, ensure that the iridotomy is totally covered by the upper lid.**

5. To treat patients who experience diplopia and glare postoperatively
   a. prescribe tinted soft contact lenses (Kublin & Simmons, 1987),
   b. design a prism ballast contact lens with an opaque tint applied over the iridotomy site (Fresco & Trope, 1992), or
   c. prescribe lightly tinted spectacle lenses (Murphy & Trope, 1991).

R. Blurry Vision (Liebmann & Ritch, 1996; Quigley, 1981; Ritch & Liebmann, 1996)

1. Transient blurry vision can occur immediately after a laser iridotomy.

2. This problem can be due to residual gonioscopic solution, photoreceptor bleaching by the visible argon laser light, anterior segment inflammation, hyphema, residual pilocarpine effect, or pigment dispersion.

S. Monocular Blurring

1. This complication involves the perception of monocular blurring or a thin, colored (e.g., dark bluish or silver) line directly in front of the eye with the laser peripheral iridotomy (Murphy & Trope, 1991; Weintraub & Berke, 1992).
   a. In these cases, the iridotomy was partially covered by the lid.
   b. Usually, the line moves with lid movement.

2. This symptom occurs in up to 2% of patients following Nd:YAG laser iridotomies (Murphy & Trope, 1991).

3. The cause of the symptom is probably a diffractive effect compounded with chromatic and or spherical aberration (Murphy & Trope, 1991). Another contributing

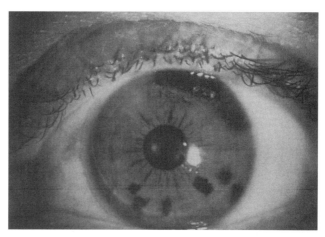

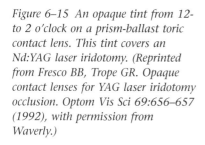

Figure 6–15 An opaque tint from 12- to 2 o'clock on a prism-ballast toric contact lens. This tint covers an Nd:YAG laser iridotomy. (Reprinted from Fresco BB, Trope GR. Opaque contact lenses for YAG laser iridotomy occlusion. Optom Vis Sci 69:656–657 (1992), with permission from Waverly.)

factor may be the base-up prism effect of the upper lid tear meniscus (Weintraub & Berke, 1992).

4. Prevention of this symptom involves placement of the iridotomy so that the lid
   a. completely covers the iridotomy site (best option), or
   b. completely exposes the iridotomy site, if complete coverage is not possible.
5. Resolution of the symptom may be accomplished by
   a. prescription of lightly tinted spectacle lenses (Murphy & Trope, 1991),
   b. design of a prism ballast contact lens with an opaque tint applied over the iridotomy site (Fresco & Trope, 1992; Figure 6–15), or
   c. prescription of tinted soft contact lenses (Kublin & Simmons, 1987).

T. Iris Atrophy and Enlargement of the Iridotomy

1. It is possible for an iridotomy to increase in size with time.
2. Sachs and Schwartz (1984) noted an enlargement in 33% of the eyes they followed for 5 months or more.
3. Quigley (1981) also noticed a number of cases of enlargement with time.

U. Loss of Central Visual Acuity

1. In addition to the case of foveal burn from the argon laser mentioned under *Retinal Damage,* one case of dramatic loss of central vision occurred following another argon laser iridotomy (Balkan et al., 1982).
2. Preoperatively, this patient had a pale disc with almost total cupping. The postlaser drop in vision from 20/25 to light perception probably represented "snuffing."

V. Reactions to Medications Used Pre- or Postoperatively. These include allergy, response to toxicity, or side effects of the medications.

References

Abe H et al. Bilateral malignant glaucoma after laser iridotomy: report of a case. Glaucoma 16:57–61 (1994).

Abraham RK. Procedure for outpatient argon laser iridectomies for angle-closure glaucoma. Int Ophthalmol Clin 16:1–14 (1976).

Abraham RK. Protocol for single-session argon laser iridectomy for angle-closure glaucoma. Int Ophthalmol Clin 21:145–165 (1981).

Abraham RK, Miller GC. Outpatient argon laser iridectomy for angle closure glaucoma: A two year study. Trans Am Acad Ophthalmol Otolaryngol 79:529–538 (1975).

Abreu MM, Sierra RA, Netland PA. Diode laser-pumped, frequency-doubled neodymium:YAG laser peripheral iridotomy. Ophthalmic Surg Lasers 28:305–310 (1997).

American Academy of Ophthalmology. Laser peripheral iridotomy for pupillary-block glaucoma. Ophthalmology 101:1749–1758 (1994).

Aminlari A, Sassani JW. Simultaneous bilateral malignant glaucoma following laser iridotomy. Graefe's Arch Clin Exp Ophthalmol 231:12–14 (1993).

Anderson DR, Forster RK, Lewis ML. Laser iridotomy for aphakic pupillary block. Arch Ophthalmol 93:343–346 (1975).

Anderson DR, Knighton RW, Feuer WJ. Evaluation of phototoxic retinal damage after argon laser iridotomy. Am J Ophthalmology 107:398–402 (1989).

Aslanides IM et al. High frequency ultrasound imaging in pupillary block glaucoma. Br J Ophthalmol 79:972–976 (1995).

Balacco-Gabrieli C et al. Peripheral iridotomy performed with Nd:YLF laser (1053 nm). Ann Ophthalmol 27:256–259 (1995).

Balkan RJ et al. Loss of central visual acuity after laser peripheral iridectomy. Ann Ophthalmol 14:721–723 (1982).

Bass MS et al. Single treatment laser iridotomy. Br J Ophthalmol 63:29–30 (1979).

Beckman H, Sugar HS. Laser iridectomy therapy of glaucoma. Arch Ophthalmol 90:453–455 (1973).

Belcher CD III. Laser iridectomy. In Belcher CD III, Thomas JV, Simmons RJ, eds. Photocoagulation in glaucoma and anterior segment disease. Baltimore, MD: Williams & Wilkins, 1984; 6:87–110.

Belcher CD III, Schuman JS. Laser iridectomy—1992. Seminars in Ophthalmology 7:156–162 (1992).

Berger BB. Foveal photocoagulation from laser iridotomy. Ophthalmology 91:1029–1033 (1984).

Berger CM, Lee DA, Christensen RE. Anterior lens capsule perforation and zonular rupture after Nd:YAG laser iridotomy. Am J Ophthalmol 107:674–675 (1989).

Bertoni G et al. Angle re-opening after Nd:YAG laser iridotomy. In Marshall J, ed. Laser technology in ophthalmology. Amsterdam: Kugler & Ghedini, 1988; 53–55.

Blondeau P. Late flat anterior chamber following a laser iridotomy. J Ocul Ther Surg 2:68–70 (1983).

Bongard B, Pederson JE. Retinal burns from experimental laser iridotomy. Ophthalmic Surg 16:42–44 (1985).

Brainard JO, Landers JH, Shock JP. Recurrent angle closure glaucoma following a patent 75–micron laser iridotomy: a case report. Ophthalmic Surg 13:1030–1032 (1982).

Brazier DJ. Neodymium-YAG laser iridotomy. J R Soc Med 79:658–660 (1986).

Brazitikos PD et al. Experimental ocular surgery with a high-repetition-rate erbium:YAG laser. Invest Ophthalmol Vis Sci 39:1667–1675 (1998).

Breingan PJ et al. Iridolenticular contact decreases following laser iridotomy for pigment dispersion syndrome. Arch Ophthalmol 117:325–328 (1999).

Brooks AMV, Harper CA, Gillies WE. Occurrence of malignant glaucoma after laser iridotomy. Br J Ophthalmol 73:617–620 (1989).

Brown RH et al. ALO 2145 reduces the intraocular pressure elevation after anterior segment laser surgery. Ophthalmology 95:378–384 (1988).

Campo RV, Reiss GR. Glaucoma associated with retinal disorders and retinal surgery. In Tasman W, Jaeger EA, eds. Duane's clinical ophthalmology, volume 3. Philadelphia, PA: Lippincott-Raven, 1995; 54E:1–22.

Canning CR et al. Neodymium:YAG laser iridotomies—short-term comparison with capsulotomies and long-term follow-up. Graefe's Arch Clin Exp Ophthalmol 226:49–54 (1988).

Carassa RG et al. Nd:YAG laser iridotomy in pigment dispersion syndrome: an ultrasound biomicroscopic study. Br J Ophthalmol 82:150–153 (1998).

Caronia RM et al. Increase in iris-lens contact after laser iridotomy for pupillary block angle-closure. Am J Ophthalmol 122:53–57 (1996).

Cashwell LF, Martin TJ. Malignant glaucoma after laser iridotomy. Ophthalmology 99:651–659 (1992).

Chan RY, Smith JA, Richardson KT. Anterior segment configuration correlated with Shaffer's grading of anterior chamber angle. Arch Ophthalmol 99:104–107 (1981).

Chang S-W, Hung P-T. Effect of carteolol on intraocular pressure elevation following laser iridotomy. J Clin Laser Med Surg 9:259–263 (1991).

Chew PTK et al. Corneal transmissibility of diode versus argon lasers and their photothermal effects on the cornea and iris. Clin Exp Ophthalmol 28:53–57 (2000).

Choplin NT, Bene CH. Cystoid macular edema following laser iridotomy. Ann Ophthalmol 15:172–173 (1983).

Cinotti DJ et al. Neodymium:YAG laser therapy for pseudophakic pupillary block. J Cataract Refract Surg 12:174–179 (1986).

Cohen JS, Bibler L, Tucker D. Hypopyon following laser iridotomy. Ophthalmic Surg 15:604–606 (1984).

Corriveau LA, Nasr Y, Fanous S. Choroidal and retinal detachment following argon laser iridotomy. Can J Ophthalmol 21:107–108 (1986).

D'Amico DJ et al. Multicenter clinical experience using an erbium:YAG laser for vitreoretinal surgery. Ophthalmology 103:1575–1585 (1996).

Davidorf JM, Baker ND, Derick R. Treatment of the fellow eye in acute angle-closure glaucoma: a case report and survey of members of the American Glaucoma Society. J Glaucoma 5:228–232 (1996).

Del Priore LV, Robin AL, Pollack IP. Neodymium:YAG and argon laser iridotomy. Long-term follow-up in a prospective, randomized clinical trial. Ophthalmology 95:1207–1211 (1988).

Desjardins D, Parrish RK II. Inversion of anterior chamber pigment as a possible prognostic sign in narrow angles [letter]. Am J Ophthalmol 100:480–481 (1985).

Doe EA, Campagna JA. Pilocarpine spray: an alternative delivery method. J Ocul Pharmacol Ther 14:1–4 (1998).

Drake MV. Neodymium:YAG laser iridotomy. Surv Ophthalmol 32:171–177 (1987).

Drexler W et al. Submicrometer precision biometry of the anterior segment of the human eye. Invest Ophthalmol Vis Sci 38:1304–1313 (1997).

Emoto I, Okisaka S, Nakajima A. Diode laser iridotomy in rabbit and human eyes. Am J Ophthalmol 113:321–327 (1992).

Epstein DL, Steinert RF, Puliafito CA. Neodymium-YAG laser therapy to the anterior hyaloid in aphakic malignant (ciliovitreal block) glaucoma. Am J Ophthalmol 98:137–143 (1984).

Fercher AF, Li HC, Hitzenberger CK. Slit lamp laser Doppler interferometer. Lasers Surg Med 13:447–452 (1993).

Fernandez-Bahamonde JL. Iatrogenic lens rupture after a neodymium: yttrium aluminum garnet laser iridotomy attempt. Ann Ophthalmol 23:346–348 (1991).

Fernandez-Bahamonde JL, Alcaraz-Michelli V. The combined use of apraclonidine and pilocarpine during laser iridotomy in a Hispanic population. Ann Ophthalmol 22:446–449 (1990).

Fleck BW. How large must an iridotomy be? Br J Ophthalmol 74:583–588 (1990).

Fleck BW et al. A randomized, prospective comparison of Nd:YAG laser iridotomy and operative peripheral iridectomy in fellow eye. Eye 5:315–321 (1991).

Fleck BW, Fairley E, Wright E. A photometric study of the effect of pupil dilatation on Nd:YAG laser iridotomy area. Br J Ophthalmol 76:678–680 (1992).

Fleck BW, Wright E, Fairley EA. A randomised prospective comparison of operative peripheral iridectomy and Nd:YAG laser iridotomy treatment of acute angle closure glaucoma: 3 year visual acuity and intraocular pressure control outcome. Br J Ophthalmol 81:884–888 (1997).

Forbes M. Gonioscopy with corneal indentation. Arch Ophthalmol 76:488–92 (1966).

Forman JS et al. Pupillary block following posterior chamber lens implantation. Ophthalmic Laser Therapy 2:85–97 (1987).

Fourman S. "Malignant" glaucoma post laser iridotomy [letter]. Ophthalmology 99:1751–1752 (1992).

Frangie JP, Park SB, Aquavella JV. Peripheral iridotomy using Nd:YLF laser. Ophthalmic Surg 23:220–221 (1992).

Fresco BB, Trope GR. Opaque contact lenses for YAG laser iridotomy occlusion. Optom Vis Sci 69:656–657 (1992).

Gailitis R et al. Prostaglandin release following Nd:YAG iridotomy in rabbits. Ophthalmic Surg 17:467–469 (1986).

Gandolfi SA, Vecchi M. Effect of a YAG laser iridotomy on intraocular pressure in pigment dispersion syndrome. Ophthalmology 103:1693–1695 (1996).

Geerling G et al. Initial clinical experience with the picosecond Nd:YLF laser for intraocular therapeutic applications. Br J Ophthalmol 82:504–509 (1998).

Geyer O et al. Pigmented pupillary pseudomembranes as a complication of argon laser iridotomy. Ophthalmic Surg 22:162–164 (1991).

Geyer O, Rothkoff L, Lazar M. Malignant glaucoma after laser iridectomy [letter]. Br J Ophthalmol 74:576 (1990).

Gieser DK, Wilensky JT. Laser iridectomy in the management of chronic angle-closure glaucoma. Am J Ophthalmol 98:446–450 (1984).

Gilbert CM, Robin AL, Pollack IP. Hyphema complicating neodymium:YAG iridotomy [letter]. Ophthalmology 91:1123 (1984).

Goins K, Schmeisser E, Smith T. Argon laser pretreatment in Nd:YAG iridotomy. Ophthalmic Surg 21:497–500 (1990).

Goldberger S et al. Pigmented pupillary pseudomembranes as a complication of argon laser iridotomy. Ophthalmology 96 (Suppl):126 (1989).

Gorin G. Re-evaluation of gonioscopic findings in angle-closure glaucoma. Am J Ophthalmol 71:894–897 (1971).

Gray RH, Hoare Nairne J, Aycliffe WHR. Efficacy of Nd:YAG laser iridotomies in acute angle closure glaucoma. Br J Ophthalmol 73:182–185 (1989).

Greenidge KC et al. Acute intraocular pressure elevation after argon laser trabeculoplasty and iridectomy: a clinicopathologic study. Ophthalmic Surg 15:105–110 (1984).

Harrad RA, Stannard KP, Shilling JS. Argon laser iridotomy. Br J Ophthalmol 69:368–372 (1985).

Harrison DA et al. Management of ophthalmic complications of homocystinuria. Ophthalmology 105:1886–1890 (1998).

Hartenbaum D et al. A randomized study of dorzolamide in the prevention of elevated intraocular pressure after anterior segment laser surgery. J Glaucoma 8:273–275 (1999).

Hawkins TA et al. Analysis of diode, argon, and Nd:YAG peripheral iridectomy in cadaver eyes. Doc Ophthalmol 87:367–376 (1994).

Haynes WL et al. Incomplete elimination of exercise-induced pigment dispersion by laser iridotomy in pigment dispersion syndrome. Ophthalmic Surg Lasers 26:484–486 (1995).

Henry JC et al. Increased intraocular pressure following neodymium-YAG laser iridectomy [letter]. Arch Ophthalmol 104:178 (1986).

Higginbotham EJ. Laser iridotomy [letter]. Ophthalmology 102:859 (1995).

Hill RA. Nonincisional glaucoma surgery. In Sassani JW, ed. Ophthalmic fundamentals: glaucoma. Thorofare, NJ: SLACK, 1999; 12:193–202.

Hirst LW et al. Corneal endothelial changes after argon-laser iridotomy and panretinal photocoagulation. Am J Ophthalmol 93:473–481 (1982).

Hitchings RA. Combined dye and argon laser treatment for narrow angle glaucoma. Trans Ophthalmol Soc UK 104:52–54 (1984).

Ho T, Fan R. Sequential argon-YAG laser iridotomies in dark irides. Br J Ophthalmol 76:329–331 (1992).

Hodes BL. Malignant glaucoma after laser iridotomy [letter]. Ophthalmology 99:1641–1642 (1992).

Hodes BL, Bentivegna JF, Weyer NJ. Hyphema complicating laser iridotomy. Arch Ophthalmol 100:924–925 (1982).

Hong C et al. Effect of apraclonidine on acute intraocular pressure rise after argon laser iridotomy. Korean J Ophthalmol 5:37–41 (1991).

Hong C, Kitazawa Y, Tanishima T. Influence of argon laser treatment of glaucoma on corneal endothelium. Jpn J Ophthalmol 27:567–574 (1983).

Hoppeler T, Gloor B. Preliminary clinical results with the ISL laser. Proc SPIE Ophthalmic Technologies II 1644:96–99 (1992).

Hoskins HD, Migliazzo CV. Laser iridectomy—a technique for blue irises. Ophthalmic Surg 15:488–490 (1984).

Huang D et al. Micron-resolution ranging of cornea anterior chamber by optical reflectometry. Lasers Surg Med 11:419–425 (1991).

Izatt JA et al. Micrometer-scale resolution imaging of the anterior eye in vivo with optical coherence tomography. Arch Ophthalmol 112:1584–1589 (1994).

Jacobs IH. Anterior chamber depth measurement using the slit-lamp microscope. Am J Ophthalmol 88:236–238 (1979).

Jacobson JJ et al. Diode laser peripheral iridectomy. Int Ophthalmol Clin 30:120–122 (1990).

Jampel HD. Lack of effect of peripheral laser iridotomy in pigment dispersion syndrome [letter]. Arch Ophthalmol 111:1606 (1992).

Jeng S, Lee J-S, Huang SCM. Corneal decompensation after argon laser iridectomy—a delayed complication. Ophthalmic Surg 22:565–569 (1991).

Joo C-K, Kim J-H. Prostaglandin E in rabbit aqueous humor after Nd-YAG laser photodisruption of iris and the effect of topical indomethacin pretreatment. Invest Ophthalmol Vis Sci 33:1685–1689 (1992).

Kalnins LY, Mandelkorn RM. Corneal decompensation after argon laser iridectomy [letter]. Arch Ophthalmol 107:792 (1989).

Karickhoff JR. Pigmentary dispersion syndrome and pigmentary glaucoma: a new mechanism concept, a new treatment, and a new technique. Ophthalmic Surg 23:269–277 (1992).

Karjalainen K, Laatikainen L, Raitta C. Bilateral nonrhegmatogenous retinal detachment following neodymium-YAG laser iridotomies [letter]. Arch Ophthalmol 104:1134 (1986).

Karmon G, Savir H. Retinal damage after argon laser iridotomy. Am J Ophthalmol 101:554–560 (1986).

Kerr Muir MG, Sherrard ES. Damage to the corneal endothelim during Nd/YAG photodisruption. Br J Ophthalmol 69:77–85 (1985).

Kim YY, Jung HR. Dilated, miotic-resistant pupil and laser iridotomy in primary angle-closure glaucoma. Ophthalmologica 211:205–208 (1997).

Kitazawa Y, Taniguchi T, Sugiyama K. Use of apraclonidine to reduce acute intraocular pressure rise following Q-switched Nd:YAG laser iridotomy. Ophthalmic Surg 20:49–52 (1989).

Klapper RM. Q-switched neodymium:YAG laser iridotomy. Ophthalmology 91:1017–1021 (1984).

Kocak I et al. Treatment of glaucoma in young nanophthalmic patients. Int Ophthalmol 20:107–111 (1997).

Kolker AE. Techniques of argon laser iridectomy. Trans Am Ophthalmol Soc 82:302–306 (1984).

Kozobolis VP et al. Endothelial corneal damage after neodymium:YAG laser treatment: pupillary membranectomies, iridotomies, capsulotomies. Ophthalmic Surg Lasers 29:793–802 (1998).

Krupin T et al. Acute intraocular pressure response to argon laser iridotomy. Ophthalmology 92:922–926 (1985).

Krupin T, Stank T, Feitl ME. Apraclonidine pretreatment decreases the acute intraocular pressure rise after laser trabeculoplasty or iridotomy. J Glaucoma 1:79–86 (1992).

Kublin J, Simmons RJ. Use of tinted soft contact lenses to eliminate monocular diplopia secondary to laser iridectomies. Ophthalmic Laser Therapy 2:111–113 (1987).

Kumar H, Sood NN, Kalra VK. Evaluation of argon pretreatment for mode-locked Nd:YAG laser peripheral iridotomy in angle-closure glaucoma. Glaucoma 12:122–126 (1990).

Lagreze WD, Funk J. Iridotomy in the treatment of pigmentary glaucoma: documentation with high resolution ultrasound. Ger J Ophthalmol 4:162–166 (1995).

Lagreze WD, Mathieu M, Funk J. The role of YAG-laser iridotomy in pigment dispersion syndrome. Ger J Ophthalmol 5:435–438 (1996).

Lederer CM, Price PK. Posterior synechiae after laser iridectomy. Ann Ophthalmol 21:61–64 (1989).

Levene R. Malignant glaucoma: proposed definition and classification. In Shields MB, Pollack IP, Kolker AE, eds. Perspectives in glaucoma: Transactions of First Scientific Meeting of The American Glaucoma Society. Thorofare, NJ: Slack, 1988; 27:243–250.

Lewis R et al. The rarity of clinically significant rise in intraocular pressure after laser peripheral iridotomy with apraclonidine. Ophthalmology 105:2256–2259 (1998).

Liebmann JM, Ritch R. Laser iridotomy. Ophthalmic Surg Lasers 27:209–227 (1996).

Lim L, Seah SKL, Lim ASM. Comparison of argon laser iridotomy and sequential argon laser and Nd:YAG laser iridotomy in dark irides. Ophthalmic Surg Lasers 27:285–288 (1996).

Lin YW, Wang TH, Hung PT. Biometric study of acute primary angle-closure glaucoma. J Formos Med Assoc 96:908–912 (1997).

Liu CJL et al. Flow cytometric study of anterior chamber aqueous humor after neodymium: yttrium aluminum garnet laser iridotomy. Ann Ophthalmol 25:174–179 (1993).

Liu PF, Hung PT. Effect of timolol on intraocular pressure elevation following argon laser iridotomy. J Ocular Pharm 3:249–255 (1987).

Loewenstein A, Lazar M. Does YAG laser iridotomy cause malignant glaucoma? Ophthalmic Surg 25:554 (1994).

Lotufo DG et al. Pigmented pupillary pseudomembranes with visual loss after argon laser treatment. Glaucoma 15:164–169 (1993).

Lowe RF. Acute angle-closure glaucoma. The second eye: an analysis of 200 cases. Br J Ophthalmol 46:641–650 (1962).

Lowe RF. New instruments for measuring anterior chamber depth and corneal thickness. Am J Ophthalmol 62:7–11 (1966).

Mandelkorn RM et al. Short exposure times in argon laser iridotomy. Ophthalmic Surg 12:805–809 (1981).

Mapstone R. Mechanics of pupil block. Br J Ophthalmol 52:19–25 (1968).

Margo CE et al. Lens-induced endophthalmitis after Nd:YAG laser iridotomy. Am J Ophthalmol 113:97–98 (1992).

Marraffa M et al. Ultrasound biomicroscopy and corneal endothelium in Nd:YAG-laser iridotomy. Ophthalmic Surg Lasers 26:519–523 (1995).

McAllister JA et al. Laser peripheral iridectomy comparing Q-switched neodymium YAG with argon. Trans Ophthalmol Soc UK 104:67–69 (1984).

McGalliard JN, Wishart PK. The effect of Nd:YAG iridotomy on intraocular pressure in hypertensive eyes with shallow anterior chambers. Eye 4:823–829 (1990).

Melamed S, Barraquer E, Epstein DL. Neodymium: YAG laser iridotomy as a possible contribution to lens dislocation. Ann Ophthalmol 18:281–282 (1986).

Melamed S, Wagoner MD. Recurrent closure of neodymium:YAG laser iridotomies requiring multiple treatments in pseudophakic pupillary block. Ann Ophthalmol 20:105–108 (1988).

Meyer KT, Pettit TH, Straatsma BR. Corneal endothelial damage with neodymium:YAG laser. Ophthalmology 91:1022–1028 (1984).

Mishima S, Kitasawa Y, Shirato S. Laser therapy for glaucoma. Aust NZ J Ophthalmol 13:225–235 (1985).

Montgomery DMI, Dutton GN. Intralenticular hemorrhage complicating pulsed laser iridotomy [letter]. Br J Ophthalmol 71:484 (1987).

Morsman CDG. Acute glaucoma in the presence of patent neodymium:YAG laser iridotomies. Acta Ophthalmologica 69:68–70 (1991).

Moster MR et al. Laser iridectomy. A controlled study comparing argon and neodymium:YAG. Ophthalmology 93:20–24 (1986).

Moster MR, George-Lomax KM. The use of the consensual light reflex as an aid to performing laser peripheral iridectomy in patients with pigment dispersion syndrome and pigmentary glaucoma. J Glaucoma 7:93–94 (1998).

Murphy PH, Trope GE. Monocular blurring. A complication of YAG laser iridotomy. Ophthalmology 98:1539–1542 (1991).

Naveh N, Zborowsky-Gutman L, Blumenthal M. Neodymium-YAG laser iridotomy in angle closure glaucoma: preliminary study. Br J Ophthalmol 71:257–261 (1987).

Naveh-Floman N, Blumenthal M. A modified technique for serial use of argon and neodymium-YAG lasers in laser iridotomy. Am J Ophthalmol 100:485–486 (1985).

Oh YG, Rosenquist RC. Laser treatment in glaucoma. In Higginbotham EJ, Lee DA, eds. Management of difficult glaucoma: a clinician's guide. Oxford, UK: Blackwell Scientific Publications, 1994; 29:299–315.

Oram O et al. Picosecond neodymium:yttrium lithium fluoride (Nd:YLF) laser peripheral iridotomy. Am J Ophthalmol 119:408–414 (1995).

Panek WC, Lee DA, Christensen RE. Effects of argon laser iridotomy on the corneal endothelium. Am J Ophthalmol 105:395–397 (1988).

Panek WC, Lee DA, Christensen RE. The effects of Nd:YAG laser iridotomy on the corneal endothelium. Am J Ophthalmol 111:505–507 (1991).

Pavlin CJ et al. Accommodation and iridotomy in the pigment dispersion syndrome. Ophthalmic Surg Lasers 27:113–120 (1996).

Pavlin CJ, Harasiewicz K, Foster FS. Ultrasound biomicroscopy of anterior segment structures in normal and glaucomatous eyes. Am J Ophthalmol 113:381–389 (1992).

Pecorella I et al. Histological & iridographic comparison of the collateral damage produced by in vivo experimental iridotomies with Nd:YLF-1053 nm & Nd:YAG-1064 nm lasers. Annals Ophthalmol 29:219–224 (1997).

Perkins ES, Brown NAP. Iridotomy with a ruby laser. Br J Ophthalmol 57:487–498 (1973).

Podos SM et al. Continuous wave argon laser iridectomy in angle-closure glaucoma. Am J Ophthalmol 88:836–842 (1979).

Pollack IP. Use of argon laser energy to produce iridotomies. Trans Am Ophthalmol Soc 77:674–706 (1979).

Pollack IP. Current concepts in laser iridotomy. Int Ophthalmol Clin 24:153–180 (1984).

Pollack IP, Patz A. Argon laser iridotomy: an experimental and clinical study. Ophthalmic Surg 7:22–30 (1976).

Potash SD et al. Ultrasound biomicroscopy in pigment dispersion syndrome. Ophthalmology 101:332–339 (1994b).

Potash SD, Liebmann J, Ritch R. Laser iridotomy and peripheral iridoplasty. In Benson WE, Coscas G, Katz LJ, eds. Current techniques in ophthalmic laser surgery. Philadelphia, PA: Current Medicine 15:155–166 (1994a).

Power WJ, Collum LMT. Electron microscopic appearances of human corneal endothelium following Nd:YAG laser iridotomy. Ophthalmic Surg 23:347–350 (1992).

Quigley HA. Long-term follow-up of laser iridotomy. Ophthalmology 88:218–224 (1981).

Reddy MA, Aylward GW. The efficacy of neodymium:YAG laser iridotomy in the treatment of closed peripheral iridotomies in silicone-oil-filled aphakic eyes. Eye 9:757–759 (1995).

Richards DW, Russel SR, Anderson DR. A method for improved biometry of the anterior chamber with a Scheimpflug technique. Invest Ophthalmol Vis Sci 29:1826–1836 (1988).

Riquin D, Fankhauser F, Loertscher H. Contact lenses for use with high power lasers. Two new contact glasses for microsurgery at the iris, in the pupillary and the retropupillary space. Int Ophthalmol 6:191–200 (1983).

Ritch R. Definitive signs and gonioscopic visualization of appositional angle closure are indications for prophylactic laser iridectomy. Surv Ophthalmol 41:33–36 (1996).

Ritch R, Liebmann JM. Laser iridotomy and peripheral iridoplasty. In Ritch R, Shields MB, Krupin T. The glaucomas. St.Louis, MO: Mosby, 1996; 76:1549–1573.

Ritch R, Lowe RF. Angle-closure glaucoma: clinical types. In Ritch R, Shields MB, Krupin T. The glaucomas. St.Louis, MO: Mosby, 1996a; 38:821–840.

Ritch R, Lowe RF. Angle-closure glaucoma: mechanisms and epidemiology. In Ritch R, Shields MB, Krupin T. The glaucomas. St.Louis, MO: Mosby, 1996b; 37:801–809.

Ritch R, Palmberg P. Argon laser iridectomy in densely pigmented irides. Am J Ophthalmol 93:800–801 (1982).

Robin AL. The role of apraclonidine hydrochloride in laser therapy for glaucoma. Trans Am Ophthalmol Soc 87:729–761 (1989).

Robin AL et al. Q-switched neodymium-YAG laser iridotomy. Arch Ophthalmol 104:526–530 (1986).

Robin AL, Pollack IP. A comparison of neodymium:YAG and argon laser iridotomies. Ophthalmology 91:1011–1016 (1984).

Robin AL, Pollack IP. Q-switched neodymium-YAG laser iridotomy in patients in whom the argon laser fails. Arch Ophthalmol 104:531–535 (1986).

Robin AL, Pollack IP, deFaller JM. Effects of topical ALO 2145 (p-aminoclonidine hydrochloride) on the acute intraocular pressure rise after argon laser iridotomy. Arch Ophthalmol 105:1208–1211 (1987).

Robinson A et al. The onset of malignant glaucoma after prophylactic laser iridotomy. Am J Ophthalmol 110:95–96 (1990).

Rosenberg LF et al. Apraclonidine and anterior segment laser surgery. Comparison of 0.5% versus 1.0% apraclonidine for prevention of postoperative intraocular pressure rise. Ophthalmology 102:1312–1318 (1995).

Rubin L, Arnett J, Ritch R. Delayed hyphema after argon laser iridectomy. Ophthalmic Surg 15:852–853 (1984).

Sachs SW, Schwartz B. Enlargement of laser iridotomies over time. Br J Ophthalmol 68:570–573 (1984).

Sanders DR et al. Studies on the blood-aqueous barrier after argon laser photocoagulation of the iris. Ophthalmology 90:169–174 (1983).

Schirmer KE. Argon laser surgery of the iris, optimized by contact lenses. Arch Ophthalmol 101:1130–1132 (1983).

Schrems W, Belcher CD III, Tomlinson CP. Changes in the human central corneal endothelium after neodymium:YAG laser surgery. Ophthalmic Laser Ther 1:143–152 (1986).

Schrems W, Eichelbroenner O, Krieglstein GK. The immediate IOP response of Nd-YAG-laser iridotomy and its prophylactic treatability. Acta Ophthalmologica 62:673–680 (1984).

Schrems W et al. The effect of yag laser iridotomy on the blood aqueous barrier in the rabbit. Graefes Arch Clin Exp Ophthalmol 221:179–181 (1984).

Schuman JS. Laser peripheral iridectomy. In Epstein DL, Allingham RR, Schuman JS, eds. Chandler and Grant's glaucoma. Baltimore, MD: Williams & Wilkins, 1997; 56:472–483.

Schuman JS, Puliafiton CA, Jacobson JJ. Semiconductor diode laser peripheral iridotomy. Arch Ophthalmol 108:1207–1208 (1990).

Schwartz AL, Martin NF, Weber PA. Corneal decompensation after argon laser iridectomy. Arch Ophthalmol 106:1572–1574 (1988).

Schwartz LW et al. Argon laser iridotomy in the treatment of patients with primary angle-closure or pupillary block glaucoma: a clinicopathologic study. Ophthalmology 85:294–309 (1978).

Schwartz LW et al. Neodymium-YAG laser iridectomies in glaucoma associated with closed or occludable angles. Am J Ophthalmol 102:41–44 (1986).

Schwenn O et al. Prophylactic Nd:YAG-laser iridotomy versus surgical iridectomy: a randomized, prospective study. Ger J Ophthalmol 4:374–379 (1995).

Shaffer RN. A suggested anatomic classification to define the pupillary block glaucomas. Invest Ophthalmol 12:540–542 (1973).

Shani L et al. Intraocular pressure after neodymium:YAG laser treatments in the anterior segment. J Cataract Refract Surg 20:455–458 (1994).

Shields MB. Textbook of glaucoma, 3rd ed. Baltimore: Williams and Wilkins, 1992.

Shin DH. Another hypopyon following laser iridotomy [letter]. Ophthalmic Surg 15:968 (1984).

Simmons RJ, Belcher CD III, Dallow RL. Primary angle-closure glaucoma. In Tasman W, Jaeger EA, eds. Duane's clinical ophthalmology, Volume 3. Philadelphia, PA: Lippincott-Raven, 1995; 53:1–32.

Singh OS, Belcher CD, Simmons RJ. Nanophthalmic eyes and neodymium-YAG laser iridectomies [letter]. Arch Ophthalmol 105:455–456 (1987).

Small KM, Maslin KF. Malignant glaucoma following laser iridotomy. Aust NZ J Ophthalmol 23:339–341 (1995).

Smith J, Whitted P. Corneal endothelial changes after argon laser iridotomy. Am J Ophthalmol 98:153–156 (1984).

Smith RJH. A new method of estimating the depth of the anterior chamber. Br J Ophthalmol 63:215–220 (1979).

Snow JT. Value of prophylactic peripheral iridectomy on the second eye in angle-closure glaucoma. Trans Ophthalmol Soc UK 97:189–191 (1977).

Snyder WB, Vaiser A, Hutton WL. Laser iridectomy. Trans Am Acad Ophthalmol Otolaryngol 79:OP381–386 (1975).

Stetz D, Smith H Jr, Ritch R. A simplified technique for laser iridectomy in blue irides. Am J Ophthalmol 96:249–251 (1983).

Sugiyama K et al. Biphasic intraocular pressure response to Q-switched Nd:YAG laser irradiation of the iris and the apparent mediatory role of prostaglandins. Exp Eye Res 51:531–536 (1990).

Takeuchi H, Okubo K. A case of malignant glaucoma following laser iridotomy. Jpn J Clin Ophthalmol 40:399–402 (1986).

Taniguchi T et al. Intraocular pressure rise following Q-switched neodymium:YAG laser iridotomy. Ophthalmic Laser Therapy 2:99–104 (1987).

Tawara A, Inomata H. Histological study on transient ocular hypertension after laser iridotomy in rabbits. Graefes Arch Clin Exp Ophthalmol 225:114–122 (1987).

Tello C et al. Measurement of ultrasound biomicroscopy images: intraobserver and interobserver reliability. Invest Ophthalmol Vis Sci 35:3549–3552 (1994).

Tessler HH et al. Argon laser iridotomy in incomplete peripheral iridectomy. Am J Ophthalmol 79:1051–1052 (1975).

Tetsumoto K, Kuechle M, Naumann GOH. Late histopathological findings of neodymium:YAG laser iridotomies in humans. Arch Ophthalmol 110:1119–1123 (1992).

Thoming C, Van Buskirk EM, Samples JR. The corneal endothelium after laser therapy for glaucoma. Am J Ophthalmol 103:518–522 (1987).

Tomey KF, Al-Rajhi AA. Neodymium:YAG laser iridotomy in the initial management of phacomorphic glaucoma. Ophthalmology 99:660–665 (1992).

Tomey KF, Traverso CE, Shammas IV. Neodymium-YAG laser iridotomy in the treatment and prevention of angle closure glaucoma. Arch Ophthalmol 105:476–481 (1987).

Unger WG, Bass MS. Prostaglandin and nerve-mediated response of the rabbit eye to argon laser irradiation of the iris. Ophthalmologica 175:153–158 (1977).

Unger WG, Brown NAP, Edwards J. Response of the human eye to laser irradiation of the iris. Br J Ophthalmol 61:148–153 (1977).

Van Herick W, Shaffer RN, Schwartz A. Estimation of width of angle of anterior chamber. Am J Ophthalmol 68:626–629 (1969).

Wand M, Clark JA, Hill DA. Nd:YAG laser iridectomies: 100 consecutive cases. Ophthalmic Surg 19:399–402 (1988).

Weinreb RN, Weaver D, Mitchell MD. Prostanoids in rabbit aqueous humor. Effect of laser photocoagulation of the iris. Invest Ophthalmol Vis Sci 26:1087–1092 (1985).

Weintraub J, Berke SJ. Blurring after iridotomy [letter]. Ophthalmology 99:479–480 (1992).

Welch DB et al. Lens injury following iridotomy with a Q-switched neodymium-YAG laser. Arch Ophthalmol 104:123–125 (1986).

Werner E. Laser iridotomy [letter]. Ophthalmology 102:859 (1995).

Wetzel W. Ocular aqueous humor dynamics after photodisruptive laser surgery procedures. Ophthalmic Surg 25:298–302 (1994).

Wilensky JT. Narrow angles accompanied by slit-lamp and gonioscopic evidence of risk are indications for prophylactic laser iridectomy. Surv Ophthalmol 41:31–32 (1996).

Wilensky JT et al. Follow-up of angle-closure glaucoma suspects. Am J Ophthalmol 115:338–346 (1993).

Wilhelmus KR. Corneal edema following argon laser iridotomy. Ophthalmic Surg 23:533–537 (1992).

Wise JB. Iris sphincterotomy, iridotomy, and synechiotomy by linear incision with the argon laser. Ophthalmology 92:641–645 (1985).

Wise JB. Low-energy linear-incision neodymium:YAG laser iridotomy versus linear-incision argon laser iridotomy. Ophthalmology 94:1531–1537 (1987).

Wise JB, Munnerlyn CR, Erickson PJ. A high-efficiency laser iridotomy-sphincterotomy lens. Am J Ophthalmol 101:546–553 (1986).

Wishart PK et al. Corneal endothelial changes following short pulsed laser iridotomy and surgical iridectomy. Trans Ophthalmol Soc UK 105:541–548 (1986).

Wishart PK, Hitchings RA. Neodymium YAG and dye laser iridotomy—a comparative study. Trans Ophthalmol Soc UK 105:521–540 (1986).

Wollensak G, Eberwein P, Funk J. Perforation rosette of the lens after Nd:YAG laser iridotomy. Am J Ophthalmol 123:555–557 (1997).

Yamamoto T, Shirato S, Kitazawa Y. Argon laser iridotomy in angle-closure glaucoma: a comparison of two methods. Jpn J Ophthalmol 26:387–396 (1982).

Yamamoto T, Shirato S, Kitazawa Y. Treatment of primary angle-closure glaucoma by argon laser iridotomy: a long-term follow-up. Jpn J Ophthalmol 29:1–12 (1985).

Yassur Y et al. Laser iridotomy in closed-angle glaucoma. Arch Ophthalmol 97:1920–1921 (1979).

Yassur Y et al. Iridotomy with red krypton laser. Br J Ophthalmol 70:295–297 (1986).

Zabel RW, MacDonald IM, Mintsioulis G. Corneal endothelial decompensation after argon laser iridotomy. Can J Ophthalmol 26:367–373 (1991).

Zadok D, Chayet A. Lens opacity after neodymium:YAG laser iridectomy for phakic intraocular lens implantation. J Cataract Refract Surg 25:592–593 (1999).

Zadok J et al. Aron and neodymium: yttrium aluminum garnet laser iridotomy in the treatment of pupillary-block and narrow-angle glaucoma: a retrospective clinical investigation of 252 eyes. Glaucoma 15:18–23 (1993).

Zborwski-Gutman L et al. Sequential use of argon and Nd:YAG lasers to produce an iridotomy—a pilot study. Metabolic, Pediatric and Systemic Ophthalmology 11:58–60 (1988).

Chapter 7
Laser Trabeculoplasty

Charles M. Wormington

I. Introduction

A. In the 1970s, a number of clinicians began to use lasers to treat open-angle glaucoma.

1. The initial attempts involved using laser energy to form holes from the anterior chamber, through the trabecular meshwork, and into Schlemm's canal (Krasnov, 1973; Worthen & Wickham, 1974). This procedure was variously labeled *trabeculopuncture* (Witschel & Rassow, 1976), *trabeculotomy* (Ticho et al., 1978), *laseropuncture* (Krasnov, 1973), or *goniopuncture* (Krasnov, 1974).

2. These puncture holes eventually closed within weeks to months due to fibrous scarring (Epstein et al., 1985; Melamed et al., 1987; Ticho et al., 1978; Witschel & Rassow, 1976).

3. Enthusiasm for this procedure was also dampened when another group of investigators noted that glaucoma could be created in monkeys by high-energy argon laser exposures to the trabecular meshwork (Gaasterland & Kupfer, 1974).

B. The turning point came in 1979 when Wise and Witter (1979) reported promising results by using low-energy argon laser exposures to the trabecular meshwork.

1. Their procedure involved making about 100 laser burns scattered evenly over the 360° of the angle.

2. The laser parameters were 0.1 sec duration, 50-μm spot size, and about 1000 mW of power.

C. The technique of Wise and Witter (1979) became known as *laser trabeculoplasty* (LTP). In modified form, it rapidly gained widespread acceptance as a major form of treatment for open-angle glaucoma.

II. Role in Open-Angle Glaucoma Therapy

A. The three most common methods of open-angle glaucoma management are medical treatment (topical and/or oral), laser trabeculoplasty, and surgery (usually trabeculectomy). The usual hierarchy of treatment has been medical first, then laser, and finally, if necessary, surgery (American Academy of Ophthalmology, 1996b; Migdal, 1992).

B. A number of new suggestions for the role of ALT have surfaced in the last few years (Savitt & Wilensky, 1992; Schwartz, 1993; Van Buskirk, 1991).

1. Early on, ALT was limited to patients who had end-stage glaucoma, patients who had refused or failed filtering surgery, or patients who were poor surgical risks (Schwartz, 1993).

2. Today, most clinicians perform ALT before filtering surgery if the patient is on maximum medical therapy and the glaucoma is not controlled. What is considered maximum medical therapy is in a state of flux.
   a. Previously, most clinicians considered three topical drugs and one oral drug as maximum therapy.
   b. Now many clinicians will opt for ALT after a series of topical drugs have been tried, sparing the patient the side effects of carbonic anhydrase inhibitors (CAIs).
   c. Other clinicians will go to ALT after trying a β-blocker or epinephrine but before trying a miotic drug.

3. The possibility of using ALT before medical or surgical management has been considered by a number of groups (Glaucoma Laser Trial Research Group [GLTRG], 1989, 1990, 1995a,b; Jampel, 1998; Migdal et al., 1994; Migdal & Hitchings, 1984, 1986; Odberg & Sandvik, 1999; Rosenthal et al., 1984; Schwartz, 1993; Sharma & Gupta, 1997; Thomas et al., 1984; Tuulonon, 1984). A survey of American Glaucoma Society members found that 42.9% never use ALT as initial therapy and 43.7% rarely use it as the initial treatment (Schwartz, 1993).

C. *The Glaucoma Laser Trial* was a controlled, randomized, multi-center, clinical trial of the safety and efficacy of argon laser trabeculoplasty (ALT) as initial therapy of newly diagnosed primary open-angle glaucoma (GLTRG, 1989, 1990, 1995a). Initially, for each patient in the study, one eye was treated with ALT and the other eye was treated with timolol only.

1. During the first 2 years of follow-up, laser-treated eyes had lower mean intraocular pressures (IOPs) than medically treated eyes.

2. After 2 years of follow-up, 44% of the laser-treated eyes were controlled by ALT alone. Of the medically treated eyes, 30% were controlled by timolol alone.

3. Of the laser-treated eyes, 89% were controlled by ALT, or ALT plus medication. Of the medically treated eyes, 66% were controlled with timolol or timolol plus other medications.

4. With respect to visual fields through 3.5 years of follow-up, the laser-treated group had slightly more improvement and slightly less loss than the medically treated group.

5. Initial ALT allows about a 2-year delay in drug treatment in the majority of patients. This could be a significant consideration for elderly patients.

D. *The Glaucoma Laser Trial Follow-up Study* involved extended follow-up for 203 of the original 271 patients in the Glaucoma Laser Trial (GLTRG, 1995b). For patients in the Glaucoma Laser Trial, the median duration of follow-up was 3.5 years with a maximum of 5.5 years. For patients in the combined Glaucoma Laser Trial and Glaucoma Laser Trail Follow-up Study, the median duration of follow-up was 7 years with a maximum of 9 years.

1. Throughout follow-up in the combined Glaucoma Laser Trial and Glaucoma Laser Trial Follow-up Study, there was a reduction in the mean IOPs for both the laser-treated eyes and the medically treated eyes. The IOP in laser-treated eyes was reduced by 7 to 10 mm Hg, and the IOP in medically treated eyes was 6 to 9 mm Hg. Laser-treated eyes had 1.2 mm Hg more reduction than medically treated eyes ($P < 0.001$).

2. Averaged over all the combined study times, laser-treated eyes showed a 0.6 dB greater improvement in visual field than medically treated eyes.

3. Overall, laser-treated eyes were similar to or better than the medically treated eyes. This finding led to the conclusion that initially treating with argon laser trabeculoplasty is at least as efficacious as initially treating with timolol.

E. *The Moorfields Primary Therapy Trial* was a randomized prospective study that compared laser, medical, and surgical treatment as initial therapies (Migdal et al., 1994). The patients were followed for a minimum of 5 years.

1. The surgery-treated group ended up with the lowest mean IOP and no statistically significant visual field loss.

2. After 5 years of follow-up, the laser-treated group had a higher mean IOP and significantly more visual field loss. The visual field loss could be accounted for by the differences in IOP values noted after 6 months of follow-up.

3. The medically treated group had the same mean IOP as the laser group, but even more visual field loss.

4. At 5 years of follow-up, the percentages of success for the surgery, laser, and medicine groups were 98%, 68%, and 83%, respectively.

F. *The Advanced Glaucoma Intervention Study (AGIS)* was a ongoing, long-term follow-up, multicenter investigation to compare the sequence of the therapies (Schwartz, 1993; The AGIS Investigators, 1998).

1. AGIS was begun in 1988 to look at the clinical course and outcomes of sequential surgical therapy after the failure of medical therapy. The patients entered into the study had open-angle glaucoma without previous invasive or laser trabecular ocular surgery. There were 249 white patients, 332 black patients, and 10 patients of other races recruited into the study.

2. Eyes were randomly assigned to either a trabeculectomy-argon laser trabeculoplasty (ALT)-trabeculectomy sequence (TAT) or to an ALT-trabeculectomy-trabeculectomy (ATT) sequence. The sequences indicated the order in which interventions were offered after failure of the first and then second interventions.

3. The initial report found a difference in the 7-year results for black and white patients (AGIS Investigators, 1998). A subsequent report found similar results (AGIS Investigators, 2001). The data supported the use of the TAT sequence for white patients without life-threatening health problems and the ATT sequence for black patients. This new recommendation for white patients is different from current standard management.

G. *The Early Manifest Glaucoma Trial* will evaluate the effectiveness of IOP reduction in early, previously untreated open-angle glaucoma (Leske et al., 1999). The patients were randomized to treatment or no initial treatment coupled with close follow-up. Treatment included laser trabeculoplasty and topical betaxolol twice daily. The patients will be followed for at least 4 years.

H. Factors to consider when determining which form of treatment should be attempted first include:

1. Age of the patient

2. Severity of the glaucoma

3. IOP at time of diagnosis

4. Presence of systemic diseases or other health problems

5. Patient's visual requirements

6. Patient's access to medical care

7. Likelihood of patient's compliance with prescribed medications (Savitt & Wilensky, 1992).

III. Indications and Patient Selection (Table 7–1).

A. Laser trabeculoplasty is indicated in most patients with open-angle glaucoma in whom the IOP is not low enough to prevent progressive optic nerve damage and visual field deterioration (Werner, 1993).

B. The type of glaucoma is an important consideration (American Academy of Ophthalmology, 1996a). LTP is more effective in certain types of glaucoma than others (Reiss et al., 1991; Thomas, 1984; Weinreb & Tsai, 1996; Werner, 1993).

Table 7–1 Indications for Laser Trabeculoplasty Based on Expected Initial Success Rates in Descending Order

Good (>67% initial success)
   Combined-mechanism glaucoma
   Exfoliation syndrome glaucoma
   Angle-closure glaucoma
   Pigmentary glaucoma
   Glaucoma after failed filtering surgery
   Primary open-angle glaucoma
Fair (33% to 67% initial success)
   Low-tension glaucoma
   Aphakia or pseudophakia
   Neovascular glaucoma
   Iridocorneal endothelial (ICE) syndrome glaucoma
   Trabeculodysgenesis
   Angle-recession glaucoma
   Uveitic glaucoma
   Sturge-Weber glaucoma
Poor (<33% initial success)
   Congenital glaucoma
   Juvenile glaucoma
   Steroid-induced glaucoma
   Essential atrophy glaucoma
   Marfan syndrome glaucoma
   Glaucoma with elevated episcleral venous pressure

C. See Table 7–1 for a list of the indications for ALT. This table is based on the initial success rates obtained from the literature (see also Tables 7–9 to 7–12).

IV. Contraindications (Table 7–2).

A. There are a number of conditions that make ALT difficult or impossible. They include:

1. **Inadequate visualization of the trabecular meshwork**
   a. This could be due to **corneal edema** or **opacities**. Not only would the edema obscure the target, but it would absorb a significant amount of the laser beam and could lead to significant corneal damage. One way to minimize edema is to avoid procedures that involve corneal manipulation for at least 1 day prior to treatment.
   b. Extensive **peripheral anterior synechiae**, extensive **iris processes**, or **hazy media** can also obscure the bulk of the angle. **Inflammation** can contribute to a hazy view of the angle and can also be complicated by additional laser-induced

Table 7–2 Contraindications for Laser Trabeculoplasty

Inadequate visualization of target
   Corneal edema or opacities
   Extensive peripheral anterior synechiae
   Extensive iris processes
   Hazy media
   Narrow angle
Uncooperative patient
Relative contraindications
   Congenital glaucoma
   Juvenile glaucoma
   Steroid-induced glaucoma
   Essential atrophy glaucoma
   Marfan syndrome glaucoma
   Glaucoma with elevated episcleral venous pressure
   Patients less than 35 years old

inflammation. Treating an angle largely closed by peripheral anterior synechiae can lead to a significant IOP elevation after the procedure. Laser iridoplasty can be used to try to break the synechiae.

  c. Inability to view the angle can also be caused by a **narrow angle**. In this case, consider laser iridotomy and/or iridoplasty to allow an adequate view of the target sites.

2. **Uncooperative patients**
  a. The patient should be able to sit still for the procedure.
  b. There should also be adequate control over eye movements.
  c. A psychiatric or physical illness may affect the patient's ability to cooperate.

B. A number of **relative contraindications** include conditions in which ALT is relatively ineffective (Reiss et al., 1991; Weinreb & Tsai, 1996; Wilensky, 1994). Some of these conditions include:

1. **Congenital glaucoma**

2. **Juvenile glaucoma**

3. **Steroid-induced glaucoma**

4. **Essential atrophy glaucoma**

5. **Marfan syndrome glaucoma**

6. **Glaucoma with elevated episcleral venous pressure**

7. **Patients less than 35 years old**

V. Instrumentation

A. *Argon Laser* (see Figure 2–3).

1. In 1973, the application of the argon laser to treat the trabecular meshwork was first reported (Krasnov, 1973; Worthen & Wickham, 1973).

2. Since the 1970s, the argon laser has been the principal laser used for laser trabeculoplasty.

3. The argon laser is usually used in the blue-green (488 and 514 nm) mode. By limiting the output to the green line (just 514 nm), there is no significant difference in the pressure-lowering effect or in complications (Smith, 1984).

B. *Krypton Laser*

1. The krypton red (647 nm) and krypton yellow (568 nm) lines have also been used for laser trabeculoplasty (Makabe, 1986; Reiss et al., 1991; Spurny & Lederer, 1984).

2. The short-term pressure-lowering effect of either krypton wavelength is comparable to that of the argon laser.

C. *Nd:YAG Lasers.* Table 7–3 shows the short-term effectiveness of laser trabeculoplasty with Nd:YAG lasers.

1. **Continuous wave (CW) mode** (200 to 400 msec pulse duration)
   a. The CW mode uses a photothermal damage mechanism.
   b. The pressure-lowering effect of this mode is comparable to that of the argon laser (Kwasniewska et al., 1993).

2. **Free-running mode** (10 to 20 msec pulse duration)
   a. This mode uses a photothermal damage mechanism.
   b. The pressure-lowering effect of this mode is also comparable to that of the argon laser (Belgrado et al., 1988; Fankhauser, 1983; Martenet & Schwarzenbach, 1986; Mermoud et al., 1992a,b).
   c. Nd:YAG near-infrared radiation penetrates deeper into tissue than the argon laser radiation (Van der Zypen et al., 1987). The Nd:YAG laser effect extends to the juxtacanalicular meshwork, whereas the argon laser effect is limited to the first two or three trabecular meshwork layers. Otherwise, similar tissue reactions are produced by the two thermal lasers.
   d. There is apparently less inflammation after the Nd:YAG laser treatment than after ALT (Mermoud et al., 1992a,b).

3. **Q-switched mode** (ca. 10 nsec pulse duration)
   a. The Nd:YAG used in the Q-switched mode uses a photodisruptive damage mechanism and is called **Nd:YAG laser trabeculopuncture** (YLT).
   b. The pressure-lowering effect of this mode in open-angle glaucoma is comparable to that of the argon laser (del Priore et al., 1988).

Table 7–3 Nd:YAG Laser Trabeculoplasty Short-Term Effectiveness

Laser Type	Type of Glaucoma	Number of ALTs (n)	IOP Before (mm Hg)	Decrease in IOP	Amount of Angle Treated	Success	Follow-up (mean)	Authors
Nd:YAG CW 1064 nm	Mixture	106	29.0	25%	180	97% 93% 83% 79% 71.5%	1 mon 3 mon 6 mon 1 yr 2 yr	Kwasniewska et al., 1993
Nd:YAG Q-switched 1064 nm	Mixture	79	28.9	25% (1 mon)	36	76% 46%	1 mon 1 yr	del Priore et al., 1988
Nd:YAG 1064 nm	Angle recession	7 4 (after ALT)	31 26	52% 38%	180 or 90	91% 79.5%	1 yr 1.5 yr	Fukuchi et al., 1993
Nd:YAG Q-switched 1064 nm	Angle recession	12	34.3	22%	30	42%	1 yr	Melamed et al., 1992
Nd:YAG Q-switched 1064 nm	Juvenile glaucoma	8	25.6	24%	focal (4 holes) confluent (60°)	75%	6 mon	Melamed et al., 1987
Nd:YAG Q-switched 1064 nm	Adult open-angle glaucoma	6 (5)*	31.7 (C) 30.8* (C)	4% (C) 19%* (C)	360 (4–6 sites)	N/A	2–11 mon	Epstein et al., 1985
Nd:YAG Q-switched 1064 nm	Juvenile open-angle glaucoma	3	35 (C)	35% (C)	360 (4–6 sites)	50%	2–11 mon	Epstein et al., 1985
Nd:YAG Q-switched 1064 nm	Mixture	25	30	30%	36 (10 spots)	68%	5 mon	Robin & Pollack, 1985

Nd:YAG Q-switched 1064 nm	Juvenile glaucoma	8	26	27%	3–8.5 hours	62.5%	4–24 mon	Yumita et al., 1984
Nd:YAG free-running	Mixture	23	21.5	28% (1 mon)	180	N/A	22.9 mon	Belgrado et al., 1988
Nd:YAG free-running	N/A	42	N/A	N/A	360	48%	N/A	Fankhauser, 1983
Nd:YAG free-running	Mixture (17 POAG, 5 EXG)	22	24.4 (from graph)	24.5% (3 mon)	180	82%	6 mon	Mermoud et al., 1992a,b
Nd:YAG free-running	EXG	5	29.2	25%	180	N/A	1–4.5 mon	Martenet & Schwarzenbach, 1986
Nd:YAG free-running	POAG	14	24.3	16%	180	N/A	1–4.5 mon	Martenet & Schwarzenbach, 1986

*5 of the 6 OAG patients (without the patient that had an emergency filtering operation due to a 22 mm Hg increase in IOP over baseline)

c. The pressure-lowering effect of this mode in angle-recession glaucoma has been reported to be significantly better than that of ALT (Fukuchi et al., 1993) or comparable to that of ALT (Melamed et al., 1992).

d. The pressure-lowering effect of this mode in juvenile glaucoma is significantly better than that of ALT and might be used in case of failed ALT (Epstein et al., 1985; Kwasniewska & Fankhauser, 1988; Melamed et al., 1987; Yumita et al., 1984).

e. The mechanism of this effect is unknown, but it may include: uveoscleral outflow increase from a small cyclodialysis cleft, micropuncture into Schlemm's canal, an inflammatory effect, or a mechanism similar to that proposed for ALT (del Priore et al., 1988; Melamed, 1987).

f. Closure of a trabeculopuncture site may involve one or a combination of three different mechanisms:

    1) growth of an impermeable sheet of endothelial cells over the trabecular meshwork

    2) fibrosis due to a healing process triggered by factors released during tissue breakdown

    3) fibrosis following hemorrhage and blood reflux from Schlemm's canal (probably not a major factor)

g. **Low energy, Q-switched Nd:YAG laser trabeculoplasty** has been explored as a means to get around the obstruction caused by scarring in trabeculopuncture (Follmann et al., 1994; Fukuchi et al., 1993; Hollo, 1996). During 1 to 18 months of follow-up in the most recent study, there was no statistically significant difference in the amount of IOP decrease between eyes treated with the argon laser and those treated with the low-energy, Q-switched Nd:YAG laser (Hollo, 1996). Histologically, the Nd:YAG laser exposures caused severe focal damage in the uveoscleral meshwork but no damage in the juxtacanalicular tissue (Hollo, 1996).

h. **Selective laser trabeculoplasty (SLT). A Q-switched, frequency-doubled (532 nm) Nd:YAG laser** has been used to selectively target pigmented trabecular meshwork cells in tissue culture (Latina et al., 1998; Latina & Park, 1995) (Figure 7–1). This could avoid the collateral thermal damage seen in ALT. This technique may allow exploration of the role and function of trabecular meshwork cells. Clinical results suggest that this technique is safe and effective for reducing the IOP in patients with open-angle glaucoma (Damji et al., 1999; Gracner, 2001; Kajiya et al., 2000; Latina et al., 1998). The ability of SLT to reduce IOP is equivalent to that of ALT (Damji et al., 1999; Lanzetta et al., 1999; Pirnazar et al., 1998; Tabak et al., 1998). SLT may also be useful in treating patients that have already been treated with ALT (Damji et al., 1999). Diurnal IOP variations appear to be decreased after frequency-doubled Nd:YAG laser trabeculoplasty (Guzey et al., 1999).

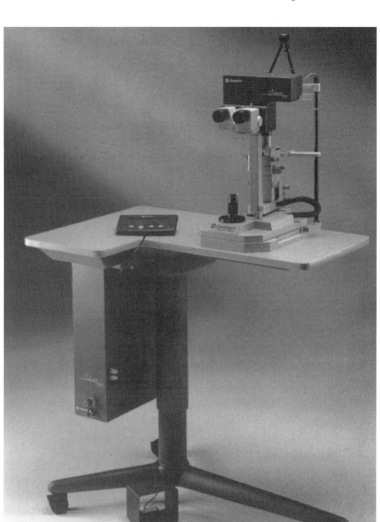

Figure 7–1 Coherent Selectra 7000 for selective laser trabeculoplasty. This is a Q-switched, frequency-doubled (532 nm) Nd:YAG laser. (Courtesy of Coherent Medical, Santa Clara, CA.)

D. Diode Lasers

1. The effective output of diode lasers is in the near-infrared (780 to 850 nm). Because there is less absorption by melanin of the near-infrared radiation compared to the visible argon lines, the burns from a diode laser are deeper (Farrar et al., 1999; McHugh et al., 1990).

Table 7–4 Short-Term IOP Effect with Diode Laser Trabeculoplasty

Type of Glaucoma	Number of ALTs (n)	IOP Before (mm Hg)	Decrease in IOP	Amount of Angle Treated	Success	Follow-up (mean)	Authors
Mixture	50	23	17%	180		3 mon	Brooks & Gillies, 1993
	20	28.3	33%	180		6 mon	McHugh et al., 1990
	11	21.6	2.4%	180		3 mon	Englert et al., 1997
	22	21.2	22%	180		3 mon	Chung et al., 1998
	17	26.8	27%	180		2 mon	Moriarty et al., 1993b

2. The pressure-lowering effect of the diode laser (Table 7–4) is comparable to that of the argon laser (Brancato et al., 1991; Brooks & Gillies, 1993; Chung et al., 1998; Moriarty et al., 1993b). Even with follow-up out to 5 years, there was no statistically significant difference in IOP or in Kaplan-Meier survival curves (Chung et al., 1998). Only one study suggested that there was a difference in efficacy between the two types of lasers, but in that study the power output of the diode laser was not measured and the sample size was small (Englert et al., 1997).

3. However, the diode laser reportedly causes less inflammation, less pain, and less peripheral anterior synechiae formation (Moriarty et al., 1993a,b). In a study by Chung et al. (1998), there was no difference between the diode and the argon lasers with respect to these three parameters. Notably, Moriarty et al. (1993a) used a laser flare meter to assess the amount of inflammation and Chung et al. (1998) used slit-lamp biomicroscope clinical assessment. Englert et al. (1997) found no apparent difference in inflammation by slit-lamp examination, although there was more patient discomfort with the argon laser.

4. There is also less blanching and almost no or very mild tissue alteration on gross inspection (Brooks & Gillies, 1993; Chung et al., 1998; McHugh et al., 1992; McMillan et al., 1994). This characteristic also makes it more difficult to determine the last application location when rotating the contact lens (Chung et al., 1998).

5. At the scanning electron microscope level, the tissue effects of the diode and argon lasers are comparable at similar levels of energy per area (McMillan et al., 1994). At typical clinical energy levels, the diode laser produces a smaller area of superficial coalescence and the argon laser causes a deeper disruption of more trabecular meshwork tissue (McMillan et al., 1994).

E. Copper Vapor Laser

1. The copper vapor laser emits significant power at two wavelengths: 511 nm (green) and 578 nm (yellow).

2. Trabeculoplasty has been performed with the laser (Nesterov et al., 1996).

F. Contact Lenses

1. The **advantages of laser contact lenses** include:
   a. The lens mirrors **provide access to the angle structures** so the laser can be directed to the trabecular meshwork.
   b. The lens may **provide magnification of the trabecular meshwork area with good depth of field** (compared to the loss of depth of field using the biomicroscope magnification control to increase magnification).
   c. The lens may **concentrate the laser energy on the trabecular area**, thus increasing the energy density and minimizing the total energy necessary to achieve effective trabeculoplasty.
   d. The lens **acts as a speculum** keeping the lids out of the way.
   e. The lens **acts as a heat sink** minimizing corneal damage.
   f. The lens **provides a moderate amount of control over ocular movement** thus stabilizing the target.
   g. The lens **minimizes the energy density on the retina** by increasing the divergence of the beam posterior to the focus point.

2. A **disadvantage** of the mirror lenses is the oblique, off-axis beam pathway (Rol et al., 1986). This pathway introduces a number of **aberrations** like spherical aberrations, coma, and astigmatism.

3. **Goldmann-type three-mirror lens**
   a. This lens was the first to be used for laser trabeculoplasty (Wise & Witter, 1979) and has been used in the majority of the later studies.
   b. Except for the special antireflection coating on the front surface, this is the standard Goldmann-type three-mirror lens.
   c. The mirror used for laser trabeculoplasty is inclined at an angle of 59° and allows a view of the angle. The other mirrors are angled for viewing the fundus from the equator to the ora (67°) and from the equator to the posterior pole (73°).
   d. One disadvantage of this lens is that it must be rotated three times (270°) to view all four quadrants of the anterior chamber angle. Another disadvantage is that tipping the lens leads to a change in the beam shape and effective diameter at the treatment site.
   e. Besides the standard lens and the standard lens with a flange, a variety of styles are available, including infant, pediatric, and small.

4. **Ritch trabeculoplasty laser lens**
   a. Because the superior angle is often narrower than the inferior angle, the Ritch trabeculoplasty lens was developed (Ritch, 1985).
   b. This lens has an antireflective coating and four mirrors. Two of the mirrors are inclined at 59° to treat the inferior angle, and the other two mirrors are inclined

at an angle of 64° to treat the superior half of the angle. The 59° mirrors have a rounded top, and the 64° mirrors have a flat top.

   c. To provide 1.4× magnification of the treatment site, one of the 59° mirrors and one of the 64° mirrors have a +17-diopter plano-convex button lens aligned over each. This button reduces the size of the laser spot from 50 μm to 35 μm and, hence, increases the laser energy by a factor of about 2. The focal point of the lenses is at the trabecular meshwork.

5. **Thorpe four-mirror gonioscopy lens**
   - a. The Thorpe lens has four mirrors inclined at 62° (Thorpe, 1966). This is a compromise position set halfway between the mirror angles optimized for treating the inferior angle (59°) and the superior angle (64°).
   - b. Having all the mirrors set at the same angle eliminates the need to rotate the lens to treat the entire anterior chamber angle.

6. **Trokel single-mirror YAG laser lens**
   - a. This lens is designed for use with the Nd:YAG laser and has a single mirror inclined at 68° (Dieckert et al., 1984).
   - b. The anterior surface of the lens has a convex curvature providing magnification and a 10° prismatic offset. The offset is to prevent beam clipping due to the large 16° cone angle of the Nd:YAG laser converging beam.

7. **Single-mirror gonioscopy lens**
   - a. This lens has a single mirror inclined at an angle of 62° (Dieckert et al., 1984). The mirror takes up one-third of the diameter of the lens.
   - b. This lens has the same disadvantage that the Goldmann-type lens has: one must rotate the lens 270° in order to see or treat the entire anterior chamber angle.

8. **Lasag CGA lens**
   - a. This is a mirrored contact lens with a spherical front surface (Rol et al., 1986; Roussel & Fankhauser, 1983).
   - b. Because of its curved front surface, this lens can be tipped without significantly affecting the diameter of the focused laser beam. This is especially important when using high-power lasers like the Nd:YAG laser for trabeculoplasty.

VI. Pretreatment Procedures

A. Preoperative Ophthalmic Examination (Richter, 1997; Schuman, 1997; Thomas, 1984) (Table 7–5).

1. **Thorough history** which should include:
   - a. Check for contraindications for trabeculoplasty or potential medications.
   - b. Rule out cystoid macular edema or macular degeneration if the patient has had poor vision.

Table 7–5 Preoperative Ophthalmic Examination

Thorough history
Visual acuity testing
Subjective refraction
Applanation tonometry
Slit-lamp biomicroscope examination
Gonioscopy
Binocular indirect ophthalmoscopy
Automated threshold perimetry
Fundus stereophotography
Informed, written consent

   c. Assess the systemic as well as ocular history. Check for conditions that can cause secondary glaucoma.

   d. Check for a history of trauma.

   e. Check for a history of glaucoma filtering surgery.

   f. Check for history of uveitis.

2. **Visual acuity testing**

3. **Subjective refraction**

4. **Applanation tonometry**

   a. Accurate IOP readings must be taken to ensure that the IOP is reduced and under control after the trabeculoplasty.

   b. The trabeculoplasty procedure can result in an IOP spike, so the pre-procedure level must be assessed.

   c. Check the IOP at different times of the day to estimate peak IOP in diurnal curve.

5. **Slit-lamp biomicroscope examination**

   a. Cornea

      1) Check the clarity of the cornea.

      2) Evaluate the integrity of the cornea, including a check for corneal guttata.

      3) Check for Krukenberg's spindle (keratic precipitates) and pigment on the endothelium.

      4) Check for a fine, hammered-metal appearance of the corneal endothelium (as in, for example, the iridocorneal endothelial (ICE) syndrome).

   b. Aqueous

      1) Check for cells and flare (i.e., inflammation).

      2) Check for shallow anterior chamber.

    c. Iris—check for:
       1) Any preexisting iris atrophy (as in, for example, essential iris atrophy, Chandler's syndrome, and ICE syndrome)
       2) Iris neovascularization
       3) Exfoliation material on the anterior iris surface and reduction of pupillary ruff
       4) Prior iridotomy
    d. Crystalline lens
       1) Check for exfoliation material on the anterior lens surface.
       2) Check for a luxated or subluxated lens.
       3) Check for pseudophakia or aphakia.
    e. Retina: Using a +66 D, +78 D, +90 D, or similar lens, assess the following:
       1) Optic nerve head
       2) Nerve fiber layer
       3) Macula (e.g., for CME)
    f. Van Herick test to assess the depth of the peripheral anterior chamber (narrow, occludable angles are suggested by chamber depths that are one-fourth of the corneal thickness or less)

6. **Gonioscopy** (of both eyes)
    a. This test is essential to the diagnosis of the type of glaucoma and for assessing whether pupil block is present.
    b. Determine the most posterior structure visible and note it in the patient's record.
    c. Describe the width of the anterior chamber angle (e.g., closed, slit, narrow, moderate, wide).
    d. Describe the position of insertion of the iris root (e.g., below the scleral spur, from the scleral spur, above the scleral spur).
    e. Grade the level of any pigment buildup in the angle.
    f. Check for peripheral anterior synechiae. In the ICE syndrome, the synechiae often extend beyond Schwalbe's line. If there is angle closure, use indentation gonioscopy to check to see if the angle closure is due to apposition of the iris to the trabecular meshwork or if there are anterior synechiae.
    g. Check for plateau iris syndrome.
    h. Evaluate the state of the trabecular meshwork.
    i. Check for angle neovascularization.
    j. Check for angle recession.

7. **Binocular indirect ophthalmoscopy**
    a. Check the optic nerve head for glaucomatous damage.
    b. Check the nerve fiber layer for glaucomatous dropout.
    c. Check for CME.
    d. Check for choroidal and retinal detachments.

8. **Automated threshold perimetry**
   a. Assess the level and location of glaucomatous damage, if any.
   b. Check for any preexisting visual field defects other than glaucomatous lesions.
9. **Fundus stereophotography**
10. **Informed, written consent** (mandatory)
    a. The procedure should be explained in clear, understandable terms.
    b. The risks should be explained.
    c. Any other options available to the patient should also be explained.

B. *Pretreatment Regimen* (Richter, 1997; Schuman, 1997; Thomas, 1984) (Table 7–6).

1. **Ensure correct diagnosis.** As noted before, knowing the type of glaucoma is important for determining whether laser trabeculoplasty is appropriate for the patient. If pupillary block is a component of the patient's glaucoma, laser iridotomy should be done before the trabeculoplasty.

2. **Continue the patient's pre-ALT glaucoma medications.**

3. **Ensure adequate clarity of the cornea.** If the cornea is edematous due to high IOP.
   a. Getting the pressure under better control with medications will be of assistance.
   b. Topically applied glycerin may be useful in reducing the corneal edema.

4. **One drop of 1% apraclonidine (Iopidine) should be instilled 1 hour before the procedure.**

Table 7–6 Pretreatment Regimen

Ensure correct diagnosis
Continue the patient's pre-ALT glaucoma
    medications
Ensure adequate clarity of the cornea
Instill one drop of 1% apraclonidine 1 hour before
    procedure
Instill two drops of 0.5% proparacaine
Advise the patient about the noises and/or the bright
    flashes of light
Ensure the patient's head is stabilized
Ensure patient comfort during the procedure
Ensure laser operator comfort
Ensure adequate stabilization of the eye
Focus and adjust the oculars on the slit-lamp
    biomicroscope
Ensure alignment of the laser beam

a. This will help prevent any IOP spike following the trabeculoplasty.

b. A beta-blocker (e.g., levobunolol), osmotic agent, or brimonidine may be substituted unless contraindicated (see Table 7–15).

5. Instill one or two drops of 0.5% **proparacaine** to anesthetize the cornea before placement of the laser contact lens.

6. **Advise the patient about the noises and/or the bright flashes of light** that he or she may experience during the procedure. This will help reassure the patient and will help the patient to maintain steady fixation.

7. **Ensure the patient's head is stabilized** adequately against the slit-lamp forehead- and chin-rests. This will help to minimize damage to the cornea and lens that may occur due to patient movement.

8. **Ensure patient comfort during the procedure.** This will also help to maintain stability of the eye during the iridotomy.

9. **Ensure laser operator comfort.** To increase comfort and to decrease fine tremor movement of the hand, the operator should use an elbow support.

10. **Ensure adequate stabilization of the eye.**
    a. Some stabilization is attained by the use of a laser contact lens.
    b. Very rarely, use of a retrobulbar block may be necessary (e.g., with severe nystagmus).
    c. For patients with breathing difficulties, have the patient interrupt breathing just before delivering the laser energy to the patient.

11. **Focus and adjust the oculars on the slit-lamp biomicroscope.** This will help ensure precise laser focus (Blumenthal & Serpetopoulos, 1998).

12. **Ensure alignment of the laser beam.** Loss of power and/or precise focus can occur if the laser is not aligned properly.

VII. Treatment Procedures

A. *Use of the Gonioprism* (Thomas, 1984).

1. After insertion of the goniolens, **assess the patient's ability to follow the fixation light**. If unable to follow the fixation light, the patient is instructed to look straight ahead and, when necessary, make slight changes in direction. It will obviously be more difficult to achieve adequate control with the latter technique.

2. **Use 25× magnification on the slit-lamp biomicroscope.**
   a. In order to appropriately visualize the angle structures, the minimum magnification is 16×.
   b. Using greater than 25× magnification reduces the depth of field to an unsatisfactory level.

3. Prior to treatment, **examine the entire 360° of the angle**.
   a. Start with the superior mirror of the goniolens and examine the inferior angle. The inferior angle usually is wider, has the most pigment, and is thus the easiest part of the angle to visualize.
   b. In each of the quadrants identify the four angle structures: (1) ciliary body, (2) scleral spur, (3) trabecular meshwork (both pigmented and nonpigmented), and (4) Schwalbe's line. This is important in order to avoid inadvertent treatment of the ciliary body or the cornea and to target the most effective portion of the angle.
   c. Identify any areas of peripheral anterior synechiae or blood vessels. These structures need to be avoided during laser application.
   d. The most important structure to identify is scleral spur. This can act as your point of reference for determining the position of the trabecular meshwork. You should be able to trace scleral spur and meshwork around the entire 360° of the angle.

4. If necessary, **use the focal line technique to identify Schwalbe's line** (see Figure 7–1).
   a. With relatively narrow angles, pigment deposited above Schwalbe's line (Sampaolesi's line) can be mistaken for trabecular meshwork.
   b. Move the slit lamp out of clickstop about 5° to 10° to the side, narrow the slit beam to an optic section, and focus on the angle.
   c. With the optic section, identify the two corneal reflections, one from the front and one from the back of the cornea. Follow these reflections posteriorly until the two reflections come together. This point identifies the position of Schwalbe's line.

5. **If it is difficult to identify structures in a portion of the angle due to lack of pigment, rotate back to an area where the scleral spur can be identified.** Where there is a lack of pigment over the trabecular meshwork, it is important to differentiate the ciliary body from the meshwork. Inadvertent treatment of the ciliary body can lead to acute pain, formation of peripheral anterior synechiae, more severe iritis, and IOP elevation (Lichter, 1982).

6. **If it is difficult to visualize the angle when the patient is in primary gaze, move the fixation light in the direction of the mirror.** This will change the patient's gaze into the same direction as the mirror. For example, when examining the inferior angle with the superior mirror, move the fixation light up. This will allow you to see around the edge of the iris further down into the angle.

7. **If the patient's angle is too narrow to visualize and treat the meshwork, consider using laser iridoplasty (gonioplasty) to flatten the peripheral iris** (Lieberman et al., 1983).

8. **If combined-mechanism glaucoma is present or if the angle is capable of closing, consider performing a laser iridotomy about a week before trabeculoplasty.**

B. Argon Laser Parameters

1. **Spot size**
   a. **Use a 50-µm spot size.** Essentially every study since Wise and Witter (1979) has used the 50-µm spot size.
   b. Decreasing the spot size to 25 µm did not provide a significant advantage over the 50-µm spot size (Schwartz et al., 1983).
   c. Increasing the spot size to 150 µm or 350 µm results in good IOP reduction, although it is harder to focus the 350 µm spots (Sherwood et al., 1987).
   d. Wise (1984) found that improperly focused lasers produced oversized spots up to 160 µm in diameter when nominally set for 50 µm. The diameter of the spot should be checked before using the laser, and the eyepieces should be focused by the operator before use.

2. **Duration**
   a. **Use 0.1 sec duration.** Almost all studies have used 0.1 sec durations.
   b. Increasing the duration to 0.2 sec does not lead to a statistically significant difference in effect when treating to the same endpoint with up to 2 years of follow-up (Blondeau et al., 1987; Hugkulstone, 1990, 1993).
   c. Increasing the duration to 0.2 sec leads to more discomfort immediately after the procedure (Hugkulstone, 1990).
   d. Decreasing the duration to 0.01 or 0.02 sec did not offer any advantage in one study (Wickham & Worthen, 1979), whereas decreasing the duration to 0.02 sec or 0.05 sec appeared to improve the results in another study (de Heer & Peperkamp, 1979).
   e. Increasing the duration beyond 0.2 sec may put the patient at more risk (Blondeau et al., 1987; Gaasterland & Kupfer, 1974; Quigley & Hahman, 1983).

3. **Power/energy level**
   a. **Start with a power level of about 500 mW.** Assess the tissue response after the first laser application.
   b. **Increase the power level in 100-mW steps until the desired tissue endpoint is reached.**
   c. Because of variation in pigmentation of the meshwork around the circumference of the angle, the power level may need to be adjusted throughout the procedure. The more meshwork pigment there is, the less power will be needed to achieve the same endpoint.
   d. The power levels cited in the literature range from 100 to 1750 mW, but most fall within the range of 500 to 1200 mW. The average power level when titrating the tissue response is about 800 mW.
   e. Maximal success occurs with laser powers greater than 500 mW and energy levels greater than 3.0 J (Rouhiainen & Terasvirta, 1986).

f. Energy levels below 10 J appear to give a more predictable IOP effect and cause less tissue disruption and less formation of peripheral anterior synechiae (Wickham & Worthen, 1979).

g. The laser energy level did not show any significant correlation with the effectiveness of the ALT with up to a 5 year follow-up (Bergea, 1986b; Tuulonen et al., 1985; Rouhiainen et al., 1995). In fact in one study, the patients were randomized into groups for treatment with 500, 600, 700, or 800 mW without titration to a given tissue response endpoint (Rouhiainen et al., 1995). In this study, neither the visible tissue response nor the laser power level affected the IOP-reducing effect or the success rate. Another clinician has advocated using a standard laser power of 900 mW for all patients (Wilensky, 1985).

h. Laser power levels higher than 800 mW are associated with a higher incidence of peripheral anterior synechiae formation (Rouhiainen et al., 1988) and a higher incidence and magnitude of post-treatment IOP elevation (Rosenblatt & Luntz, 1987; Rouhiainen et al., 1987).

i. In some studies, there was no correlation between average laser power and peripheral anterior synechiae formation (GLTRG, 1989; Thomas et al., 1982a).

4. **Wavelength**

   a. See *Instrumentation*.

   b. While almost all studies of argon laser trabeculoplasty have used the blue-green mode of the laser, Smith (1984) found that limiting the laser to the green line gave comparable results.

C. *Laser Burn Application*

1. **Placement of burns** (Figure 7–2)

   a. The burns should be placed anteriorly in the trabecular meshwork at or near the junction of the pigmented and nonpigmented meshwork (Mattox & Schuman, 1992; Thomas, 1984; Weinreb & Tsai, 1996). If there is very little or no pigment over the trabecular meshwork, the burns can be placed in the middle of the meshwork area (Thomas, 1984). This can usually be identified as the area that is slightly grayish or at least differing in texture and whiteness from the more anterior non-filtering meshwork and the more posterior scleral spur.

   b. There appears to be no statistically significant difference in IOP-lowering effect between placing burns in the anterior or posterior portion of the meshwork (Higgins, 1985; Schwartz et al., 1983; Traverso et al., 1984). Only one study dissented from this view, indicating success in 66.5% of patients with ALT to the trabecular pigment band or its posterior aspect versus 33.7% of patients with ALT to the anterior portion of the band (Eguchi et al., 1985).

   c. Treatment of either the superior or inferior half of the angle does not affect significantly the duration of the ALT effect (Grayson et al., 1994).

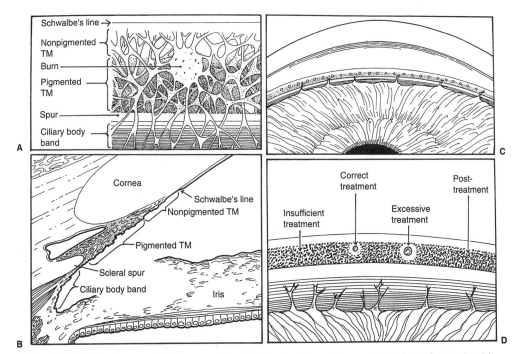

Figure 7–2 A. The laser applications are placed at the junction of the anterior 1/3 and posterior 2/3 of the trabecular meshwork. B. Damage to the filtering portion of the trabecular meshwork, the more posterior portion, is minimized, with access to Schlemm's canal. C. The laser spots are placed 100–150 μm apart (about 3 spot diameters) so that 50 spots span 180° of angle. D. The desired endpoint is a blanch or small bubble. Excessive power will generate large bubbles or bubbles that burst. (Reprinted with permission from Schuman JS. Laser trabeculoplasty. In Epstein DL, Allingham RR, Schuman JS, eds. Chandler and Grant's Glaucoma. Baltimore, MD: William & Wilkins, 1997; 52:456–463.)

    d. Treatment of the anterior trabecular meshwork results in a lower incidence of acute IOP elevation immediately post-ALT (Schwartz et al., 1983) and a lower incidence of peripheral anterior synechiae (GLTRG, 1989; Hoskins et al., 1983; Rouhiainen et al., 1988; Traverso et al., 1984).

2. **Number and spacing of burns/extent of angle treated** (see Figure 7–2)
    a. *Treat 180° of angle with 40 to 50 evenly spaced burns* (GLTRG, 1989, 1990; Grayson et al., 1993; Mattox & Schuman, 1992; Richter, 1997; Thomas, 1984). *If the IOP reduction is not sufficient or if the IOP creeps back up in time, treat the other half of the angle.* In a survey of American Glaucoma Society Members, 19.4% always treat 180° initially and another 37.1% usually treat 180° (Schwartz, 1993). In other words, 56.5% of glaucomatologists usually or always treat 180° initially.

b. The alternative is to *treat 360° of angle with approximately 100 evenly spaced burns*. In the survey of glaucomatologists, 12.8% always treat 360° and another 22.4% usually treat 360° in one sitting (Schwartz, 1993). Thus, 35.2% of the glaucomatologists polled would usually or always treat 360°. In addition, 51.5% place 96 to 105 burns and 39.7% place 80 to 95 burns.

c. The initial paper describing laser trabeculoplasty treated 360° with 100 burns (Wise & Witter, 1979).

d. Treating 180° versus 360° of the angle results in a comparable IOP-lowering effect (Heijl, 1984; Horns et al., 1983; Lustgarten et al., 1984; Schwartz et al., 1983; Thomas et al., 1982a; Weinreb et al., 1983a). One study of aphakic and pseudophakic eyes showed no correlation between ALT success and the use of 180° versus 360° treatment (Schwartz et al., 1997).

e. Treating 180° of the angle with 50 burns results in a lower magnitude and/or incidence of IOP spikes post-ALT (Eguchi et al., 1985; Heijl, 1984; Hoskins et al., 1983; Krupin et al., 1992; Thomas et al., 1982a; Weinreb et al., 1983b), less long-lasting inflammation (Eguchi et al., 1985), and may result in less peripheral anterior synechiae (Eguchi et al., 1985; Hoskins et al., 1983; Weinreb et al., 1983a) compared to treating 360° with 100 burns.

f. Treating 180° of meshwork first and then waiting for the initial treatment effect to decrease before treating the remaining 180° delays filtering surgery longer than treating 360° initially (Grayson et al., 1993).

g. In one study, applying 25 burns over 90° of the angle did not reduce the IOP as much as 50 burns over 180°, 50 burns over 360°, or 100 burns over 360° (Schwartz et al., 1983). Whereas, in another study, applying 25 burns over 90° resulted in an IOP reduction (23%) comparable to that in most studies with 100 burns over 360° (Wilensky & Weinreb, 1983b).

h. There was no statistically significant difference in long-term success of ALT when comparing 65 burns to 100 burns in two groups of patients (Fink et al., 1988).

i. The difference in intraocular pressure reduction at 9 to 12 months was not statistically significant when applying 35 burns to 120° versus applying 50 burns to 180° (Frenkel et al., 1997). Doing only a third of the angle at first would allow the possibility of two retreatments.

j. One retrospective study claimed a better success rate and a larger reduction in IOP in a group treated 360° compared to a group treated 180° (Honrubia et al., 1992). However, the IOP reduction in the 180° group was anomalous (13%). It was less than half of the IOP reductions obtained in 14 other studies that also treated 180° (range: 21% to 44%) (see Tables 7–4 and 7–6). Also, the two treatment groups differed in that the 360° group had a higher percentage of exfoliation glaucoma patients and a higher pre-treatment mean IOP than the 180° group. And both of these differences could lead to a larger effect and higher success rate in the 360° group.

k. Another study found a positive correlation between the IOP reduction and the amount of angle treated (Higgins, 1985). The number of eyes done at each angle extent was not noted nor was the statistical significance mentioned. There seemed to be a similar amount of IOP reduction with less than 70 spots. There was a significantly higher IOP reduction with more than 70 spots, but the reduction was similar with >70, >80, >90, and >100 spots.

3. **Endpoint** (see Figure 7–2)
   a. The desired endpoint is a blanching of the trabecular meshwork (Lustgarten et al., 1984; Thomas, 1984; Weinreb & Tsai, 1996).
   b. Many clinicians qualify the endpoint by requiring either blanching *or* very small bubble formation (Mattox & Schuman, 1992; Shields, 1992; Thomas, 1984) and others do not even require a visible tissue response (Rouhiainen et al., 1995; Wilensky, 1985).

D. *General Procedure* (Table 7–7) (Mattox & Schuman, 1992; Richter, 1997; Schuman, 1997; Shields, 1992; Thomas, 1984; Weinreb & Tsai, 1996).

1. **Perform preoperative ophthalmic examination.**
2. **Check the laser for proper functioning and focusing.**
3. **Administer pretreatment regimen.**
4. **Use a laser contact lens.**

Table 7–7 General Procedure

Perform preoperative ophthalmic examination
Check laser for proper functioning and focusing
Administer pretreatment regimen
Use a laser contact lens
Aim at junction between posterior pigmented and
   anterior nonpigmented meshwork
Choose initial laser parameters
   50-μm spot size
   0.1 sec duration
   500 mW power
Adjust laser power until blanching of meshwork
   occurs
Treat 180° of the angle using 40 to 50 burns
Administer post-treatment regimen
Conduct follow-up examinations
Treat the remaining 180° later, if necessary

    a. Be sure the beam is kept perpendicular always to the front surface of any laser contact lens. The more deviation there is, the more the loss of power at the target site.

    b. Aim the laser beam at the center of the button and/or mirror.

5. **Focus** the laser beam precisely on the anterior trabecular meshwork **at the junction between the posterior pigmented and the anterior nonpigmented meshwork**.

6. **Choose initial laser parameters** (usually 50-μm spot size, 0.1-sec duration, and 500 mW).

7. **After an initial burn application, adjust the laser power until blanching of the meshwork occurs.**

8. **Treat 180° of the angle using about 40 to 50 burns**, continuously adjusting the laser power to generate the same endpoint tissue reaction.

    a. Begin treatment at 6 o'clock and evenly space the burns over the 180° area.

    b. Always treat the same quadrants initially if possible (e.g., the nasal 180°). This procedure avoids confusion if retreatment is necessary. Inadvertent treatment of the same 180° area on a subsequent visit may further damage the meshwork and lead to a pressure elevation.

    c. When rotating the contact lens to treat the next portion of the trabecular meshwork, rotate it so that the previously treated section is still visible. Thus the treatment can begin again adjacent to the last treated spot.

9. **Administer post-treatment regimen.**

10. **Conduct follow-up examinations.**

11. **Treat the remaining 180°, if necessary** at a later time.

VIII. Post-Treatment Regimen (Mattox & Schuman, 1992; Shields, 1992; Weinreb & Tsai, 1996).

A. **Instill another drop of 1% apraclonidine** to blunt any IOP spike.

B. **Begin topical steroids** (e.g., 1% prednisolone acetate, four times daily for 4 to 5 days) **as needed** and then taper.

1. Fluoromethalone can also be effective in attenuating the inflammation after ALT (Shin et al., 1996). This corticosteroid has a relatively low risk of inducing IOP elevation compared to dexamethasone (Kass et al., 1986).

2. An alternative would be topical nonsteroidal anti-inflammatory drugs which are also effective (Herbort et al., 1993; Huk et al., 1991). Although diclofenac may be useful in treating inflammation post-ALT (Diestelhorst et al., 1995; Herbort et al., 1993), indomethacin and flurbiprofen may (Goethals et al., 1994) or may not be effective (Hotchkiss et al., 1984).

3. Steroids and nonsteroidal anti-inflammatory drugs apparently do not affect the outcome of the ALT in terms of IOP-lowering effect or success rate (Herbort et al., 1993; Pappas et al., 1985; Ruderman et al., 1983; Shin et al., 1996; Thomas et al., 1982b; Ustundag & Diestelhorst, 1997; Weinreb et al., 1984).

C. **Continue pretreatment glaucoma medications** initially until the eye stabilizes and is reassessed. If there is a significant IOP reduction a few months post-treatment, one medication may be withdrawn at a time, starting with any oral carbonic anhydrase inhibitor.

IX. Follow-up

A. Schedule

1. 1 to 3 hours
2. 1 day (if necessary due to marked IOP elevation or intraoperative problems)
   a. A recent study suggested that a 1-day IOP check is not necessary for most patients (Mittra et al., 1995). In fact, the 1-day IOP measurement was not associated significantly with the type of glaucoma, laser parameters, extent of angle treated, pre-ALT IOP, 1-hour IOP, or whether it was an initial ALT or a repeat ALT.
   b. However, if the patient has a marked IOP elevation immediately post-ALT or advanced glaucomatous damage, a 1-day follow-up is appropriate.
3. 2 to 3 weeks (Mittra et al., 1995)
4. 4 to 6 weeks (Schuman, 1997)
5. 3 months
6. every 3 months thereafter

B. Examinations should include (Table 7–8)

1. **Visual acuity**
2. **Applanation tonometry**

Table 7–8 Follow-up Ophthalmic Examinations

Visual acuity
Applanation tonometry
Gonioscopy
Slit-lamp biomicroscopy
Dilated fundus examination (periodically)
Automated threshold perimetry (periodically)

   a. If the immediate post-treatment IOP spikes more than 10 mm Hg over the pre-ALT IOP or the IOP is more than 30 mm Hg, then consider 500 mg of oral acetazolamide.

   b. If the patient is already on acetazolamide, consider oral glycerin, 1 gm/kg of body weight.

   c. If the patient has advanced glaucomatous damage and significant visual field loss, consider assessing the IOP after 1 to 3 hours post-ALT.

3. **Gonioscopy**
   a. Check the angle and the extent of opening.
   b. Check for areas of peripheral anterior synechiae.
   c. Check for inflammatory precipitates on the trabecular meshwork.

4. **Slit-lamp biomicroscopy.** Check for:
   a. inflammation
   b. corneal burns

5. **Dilated fundus examination** (periodically)
   a. Evaluate the optic nerve head and nerve fiber layer.
   b. Check for cystoid macular edema.
   c. Stereo fundus photography should be performed periodically to check for progression.

6. **Automated threshold perimetry.** This should be done periodically to monitor for progression.

X. Results of Treatment

A. *Short-Term Control* (Tables 7–9 and 7–10)

1. ALT reduces IOP in the vast majority of patients.

2. The full IOP-lowering effect is achieved by about the sixth post-treatment week (Forbes & Bansal, 1981; Schwartz et al., 1981; Thomas et al., 1982a; Wilensky & Jampol, 1981). Some reports indicate that the full effect may take 3 or 4 weeks (Pavan et al., 1992; Wilensky & Jampol, 1981), 2 months (Schwartz et al., 1985), or 6 to 9 months (Fink et al., 1988) to become manifest.

3. Another benefit of ALT appears to be a decrease in the daily IOP variation, a flattening of the IOP diurnal curve (Greenidge et al., 1983). Both the IOP fluctuations and the mean peak IOP fell 25% following ALT.

B. *Long-Term Control* (Table 7–11)

1. In many patients, ALT can control IOP for years and even eliminate the need for filtering surgery in some.

Text continued on page 348

Table 7-9 Short-Term (i.e., <2 Years) Effectiveness of ALT

Type of Glaucoma	Number of ALTs (n)	IOP Before (mm Hg)	Decrease in IOP	Amount of Angle Treated	Success	Follow-up (mean)	Authors
POAG	141	27.4	36% (12 mon)	360°	77.3%	12 mon	Goldberg, 1985
	37	25.73	31% (1 mon)	360	N/A	12 mon	Heijl, 1984
		25.36	26% (1 mon)	180		12 mon	
	28	22.4	26% (2 mon)	180	64%	14.75 mon	Higginbotham & Richardson, 1986
	121	27	26% (9 mon)	360 & 180	82%	9 mon	Gilbert et al., 1986
	52	21.2	22% (12 mon)	360	65%	12 mon	Tuulonen & Airaksinen, 1983
	74	25.8	24% (15.3 mon)	360	80%	15.3 mon	Lieberman et al., 1983
	9	23.4	27% (6 mon)	360	57% ("20 mm Hg)	12 mon	Levy & Bonney, 1982
	28	29	41% (3 mon)	360	79%	18 mon	Pollack et al., 1983
	237	23	30% (5 mon)	360 180/180	85%	5 mon	Thomas et al., 1982a
	26	30.2	33%	360		7.6 mon	Thomas et al., 1984
	16	23.4	21%	180	94%	2.5 mon	Elsas & Harstad, 1983
	186	21.7	19%	360	58%	9 mon	Traverso et al., 1986
	15	33.6	44%	180	73%	6 mon	Migdal & Hitchings, 1984
	58	N/A	N/A	360	84%	10.5 mon	Forbes & Bansal, 1981
	62	25.1	26%	180	84%	1–12 mon	Martenet & Schwarzenbach, 1986
	112	27.1	32% (1 yr)	360	79%	12 mon	Grinich et al., 1987
	237	26.45	18% (11 yr)	360	78%	12 mon	Lotti et al., 1995
	159	23.61	29% (5 yr)	360	81%	12 mon	Moulin et al., 1991
	143	N/A	N/A	180 180/180	76%	12 mon	Atmaca & Karel, 1993
	21	25.6	30%	360	81%	12 mon	Tuulonen, 1984

Table continued on following page

53	N/A	N/A	Mixture	78%	18 mon	Tuulonen et al., 1985
684	N/A	N/A	360	60%	1.84 yr	Lund, 1988
416		N/A	180	95%	1.5 mon	
84	N/A		360 180	94% 86%	1 yr 1 mon	Brooks & Gillies, 1984
43	31.7	28% (4–6 weeks)	360	65%	12 mon	Rosenthal et al., 1984
61	22.3	20% (9–12 mon)	180 (50 burns)			Frenkel et al., 1997
61	22.8	17% (9–12 mon)	120 (35 burns)			
50	23	22% (3 mon)	180	N/A	3 mon	Brooks & Gillies, 1993
66	26.9	30%	360	82%	10.5 mon	Forbes & Bansal, 1981
380	25.9	31%	360 180	81%	9 mon	Horns et al., 1983
21	25.0	25% (2 mon)	180	N/A	2 mon	Moriarty et al., 1993b
31	26	38% (1 mon)	360	87%	12 mon	Pollack & Robin, 1982
35	24.4	39% (2 mon)	360	97%	12 mon	Schwartz et al., 1981
22	27.5	26% (11 mon)	360	100%	11 mon	Wilensky & Jampol, 1981
52	27.6	26% (1 mon)	360	65%	20.6 mon	Wilensky & Weinreb, 1983a
150	28.37	43% (6 mon)	360	85%	6 mon	Wise, 1981
59	27.3	33% (3 mon)	360	82%	6 mon	Zborowski et al., 1984
30	27.4	36% (3 mon)	360	87%	3–12 mon	Pohjanpelto, 1981
30	30.3	33%	360	83%	7.5 mon	Thomas et al., 1984
19	29.4	32%	360	89%	12 mon	Tuulonen et al., 1989
109	N/A	N/A	360 180/180	68%	12 mon	Spaeth & Baez, 1992
118	29.1	30% (3 yr)	360	88%	12 mon	Ticho & Nesher, 1989
60	35.2	56% (2.8 yr)	360 180/180	73%	12 mon	Elsas & Johnsen, 1991
93	26.1	29% (1 mon)	360	77%	12 mon	Shingleton et al., 1993
49	N/A	N/A	superior 180	70%	12 mon	Grayson et al., 1994
53	N/A	N/A	inferior 180	66%	12 mon	Grayson et al., 1994
11	24.4	30%	180		3 mon	Englert et al., 1997

Mixture

Table 7-9 Short-Term (i.e., <2 Years) Effectiveness of ALT *Continued*

Type of Glaucoma	Number of ALTs (n)	IOP Before (mm Hg)	Decrease in IOP	Amount of Angle Treated	Success	Follow-up (mean)	Authors
	28	21.5	31% (1 yr)	180	~83%	12 mon	Chung et al., 1998
	20	36.3	N/A	180	65%	12 mon	Elsas, 1987
	26	35.9		360	88%	12 mon	
	82	26.8	30%	360	87%	≥12 mon	Scrivanti et al., 1988
	60	28	35%		82%	≥12 mon	
	100	28	36%	50–60 burns	82%	4–30 mon	Mohan et al., 1988
EXG	22	29.9	37% (1 yr)	360	73%	12 mon	Grinich et al., 1987
	54	32	53% (12 mon)	360	91%	12 mon	Goldberg, 1985
	40	27.77 29.03	41% (1 mon) 35%	360 180	N/A	12 mon	Heijl, 1984
	26	25.5	38% (2 mon)	180	59%	14.75 mon	Higginbotham & Richardson, 1986
	35	28.5	42%	360	89%	3–12 mon	Pohjanpelto, 1981
	34	28.5	44% (5 mon)	360 180/180	97%	5 mon	Thomas et al., 1982a
	79	24.1	37%	360	68%	12 mon	Tuulonen & Airaksinen, 1983
	7	34.7	31%	360	71%	15.3 mon	Lieberman et al., 1983
	2	27.5	27%	360	N/A	6 mon	Thomas et al., 1984
	34	27.4	34%	180	94%	4.1 mon	Elsas & Harstad, 1983
	4	33	52%	360	100%	19 mon	Robin & Pollack, 1983
	19	28.7	31%	180	N/A	1–5 mon	Logan et al., 1983
	26	27.5	33%	360	84%	9 mon	Traverso et al., 1986
	4	N/A	N/A	360	100%	10.5 mon	Forbes & Bansal, 1981
	2	31.5	51% (1–2 mon)	360	100%	1–2 mon	Lichter, 1982
	42	27.0	36% (12 mon)	360	100% 94%	12 mon 18 mon	Tuulonen, 1984

Group	n	IOP	%	Degrees	%	Time	Reference
	14	N/A	N/A	360 180/180	50%	1 yr	Spaeth & Baez, 1992
	48	30.2	42%	360 180	87.5%	8 mon	Horns et al., 1983
	36	27.1	37%	180	94%	1–12 mon	Martenet & Schwarzenbach, 1986
	100	N/A	N/A	Mixture	72%	1.7 yr	Tuulonen et al., 1985
	42	27.0	36%	360	100% 94%	12 mon 18 mon	Tuulonen, 1984
	227 412	N/A	N/A	360 180	97% 86%	1.5 mon 1 yr	Lund, 1988
	25	N/A	N/A	360 180	88%	1 mon	Brooks & Gillies, 1984
PIG	6	25.0	40% (13.5 mon)	360 180/180	100%	13.5 mon	Thomas et al., 1982a
	2	25.0	48%	180	100%	4 mon	Elsas & Harstad, 1983
	11	32	31%	360	73%	7 mon	Robin & Pollack, 1983
	20	22	30%	360	81%	10.5 mon	Traverso et al., 1986
	16	27.8	12%	360	44%	15.3 mon	Lieberman et al., 1983
	6	23.3	36%	360 180	100%	7 mon	Horns et al., 1983
	4	23.75	31% (1–2 mon)	360	50%	1–2 mon	Lichter, 1982
	13	25.0	43%	360 180/180	62%	12.8 mon	Lunde, 1983
	19	N/A	N/A	360 180	79% 91%	1.5 mon 12 mon	Lund, 1988
	32	27.8	N/A	360 180	80%	12 mon	Ritch et al., 1993
	10	N/A	N/A	180 180/180	60%	1 yr	Brooks et al., 1988

POAG = Primary open-angle glaucoma
EXG = Exfoliation syndrome glaucoma
PIG = Pigmentary glaucoma

Table 7–10 Mean Values of Short-Term Effectiveness of ALT for Different Types of Glaucoma

Type of Glaucoma	IOP Reduction (range)	Mean Success (range)	Mean Follow-up (range)
Combined-mechanism G	24% (22–26%)	85% (70–100%)	ca. 12 mon
EXG	39% (27–53%)	82% (50–100%)	11.8 mon (8–15.3 mon)
Angle-closure G	42% (32–52%)	79% (50–100%)	10.3 mon (7–12 mon)
PIG	34% (12–48%)	77% (44–100%)	11.3 mon (7–15.3 mon)
After filtering surgery	28% (14–38%)	77% (67–89%)	9.6 mon (3.8–20 mon)
POAG	28% (19–44%)	76% (57–94%)	12.3 mon (9–18 mon)
LTG	29% (16–40%)	67% (46–86%)	27.6 mon (12–48 mon)
Neovascular G	29%	45% (40–50%)	N/A
ICE syndrome G	4% (−14–22%)	41.5% (33–50%)	3.75 mon (2–5.5 mon)
Trabeculodysgenesis	56% ↑	40%	4.3 mon
ARG	26% (2–45%)	39% (0–75%)	11.6 mon (4.6–18 mon)
Uveitic G	14% (−7–33%)	33.5% (0–75%)	8.75 mon (3–17 mon)
Sturge-Weber G	31% (17–45%)	33% (0–100%)	N/A
Congenital G	17% (9.6–24%)	25% (0–50%)	8.5 mon (5–12 mon)
Juvenile G	5.6% (−7.2–16%)	23% (0–40%)	ca.10.9 mon (1.5–24 mon)
Steroid-induced G	N/A	0%	3.2 mon
Essential atrophy G	5%	0%	1–2 mon
Marfan syndrome G	72% ↑	0%	N/A
Elevated episcleral venous pressure G	N/A	0%	10.5 mon
Phakia	31% (26–35%)	87% (81–100%)	>9 mon (5–≥12 mon)
Pseudophakia	31.5% (30–33%)	63% (33–80%)	21.2 mon (12–36 mon)
Aphakia	25% (10–50%)	63% (17–100%)	8.8 mon (1–18 mon)
Mixture	33% (22–56%)	82% (65–100%)	11.3 mon (7.5–12 mon)
Repeat treatment	21.4% (7–36%)	50% (21–73%)	12 mon (all 12 mon)

2. However, on the average, the IOP-lowering effect of ALT wears off progressively over time (see later discussion). With up to 10 years of follow-up, the annual failure rate is about 7% to 10% per year (Grinich et al., 1987; Lund, 1988; Moulin et al., 1991; Moulin & Haut, 1993; Shingleton et al., 1987; Spaeth & Baez, 1992).

3. After ALT, some patients are able to reduce the number of antiglaucoma medications (Forbes & Bansal, 1981; Horns et al., 1983; Pollack & Robin, 1982; Pollack et al., 1983; Sharpe & Simmons, 1985; Thomas et al., 1982a).

   a. In one study, 64% of patients were able to stop carbonic anhydrase inhibitors, 57% could stop the miotic, and 18% stopped all medications (Pollack et al., 1983). In a prior study, some of the same authors found that 67% of patients could stop carbonic anhydrase inhibitors, 75% the miotic, and 33% required no medications (Pollack & Robin, 1982).

Text continued on page 356

Table 7–11 Long-Term (i.e., ≥2 Years) Effectiveness of ALT for Different Types of Glaucoma

Type of Glaucoma	Number of ALTs	IOP Before (mm Hg)	Decrease in IOP	Amount of Angle Treated	Success	Follow-up (mean)	Authors
POAG	45	36.24	29% (0.75 mon)	60	80%	5 years	Brooks et al., 1988
	66	23.2	25% (4–6 mon)	180	(no filtration)		Threlkeld et al., 1996b
			23% (16–18 mon)		91%	1 year	
					78%	3 years	
					(no filtration, 3rd laser, or IOP ≥ 22)		
					81%	1 year	
					64%	3 years	
	269	27	33% (3 mon)	180/180	44%	2 yr	GLTRG, 1990
	112	27.1	32% (1 yr)	360	79%	1 yr	Grinich et al., 1987
					69%	2 yr	
					59%	3 yr	
	237	26.45	18% (11 yr)	360	78%	1 yr	Lotti et al., 1995
					71%	3 yr	
					61%	5 yr	
					40%	10.5 yr	
	55 or 57 (unclear in paper)	34.9	48% (2 yr)	180/180	86% (laser alone or laser + pilo)	7–36 mon	Migdal & Hitchings, 1986
					44% (laser alone)		
	55	35	40% (6 mon)	180/180	68% (laser alone or laser + pilo)	5 yr	Migdal et al., 1994
	159	23.61	29% (5 yr)	360	81%	1 yr	Moulin et al., 1991
					70%	2 yr	Moulin & Haut, 1993
					59%	3 yr	
					52%	4 yr	

Table continued on following page

Table 7–11 Long-Term (i.e., ≥2 Years) Effectiveness of ALT for Different Types of Glaucoma *Continued*

Type of Glaucoma	Number of ALTs	IOP Before (mm Hg)	Decrease in IOP	Amount of Angle Treated	Success	Follow-up (mean)	Authors
	61	27.4	20% (24 mon)	360 (100 burns)	48% 17% 11% 71%	5 yr 8 yr 10 yr 1.9 yr	Fink et al., 1988
	21	26.1	19% (24 mon)	360 (65 burns)	43% 79% 50%	3.5 yr 2.1 yr 3.5 yr	
	195	25.2	28% (6 mon)	360 180	50%	5.5 yr	Eendebak et al., 1990
	61	26	33% (6 mon)	180	74%	4.4 yr	Amon et al., 1990
	143	N/A	N/A	180 180/180	76% 61.5% 50%	1 yr 2 yr 3 yr	Atmaca & Karel, 1993
	10	24.0	32% (5 yr)	360	70% (50%–complete)	5 yr	Tuulonen et al., 1987
	15	22.7	29% (2 yr)	180/180	100%	2 yr	Blondeau et al., 1987
	15 (<40 yo)	32	16% (2 yr)	360	40%	2 yr	Safran et al., 1984
	29 (>40 yo)	30	40% (2 yr)	360	93%	2 yr	
	11	N/A	N/A	180/180	73%	2 yr	Bergea et al., 1994
	49	25.9	N/A	360	45%	2 yr	Bergea, 1986b
	43	N/A	N/A	360	39%	3.65 yr	Searle et al., 1990
	50	N/A	N/A	360	54%	10 yr	Ticho & Nesher, 1989
	60	N/A	N/A	360	57% 31%	4 yr 10 yr	Shingleton et al., 1987 Shingleton et al., 1993
	64	N/A	N/A	180	57%	2 yr	Eguchi et al., 1985
	66	N/A	N/A	360	79%	2 yr	Schwartz & Kopelman, 1983

Group	N						Reference
	52	N/A	N/A	360	46%	5 yr	Schwartz et al., 1985
	24	23.8	30%	360 (150-μm spot size)	79%	2.9 yr	Sherwood et al., 1987
	684	N/A	N/A	360	95%	1.5 mon	Lund, 1988
	416			180	94%	1 yr	
	149				82%	2 yr	
	47				72%	3 yr	
	110				82%	4 yr	
	23	N/A	N/A	180	39%	3 yr	Ustundag & Diestelhorst, 1997
POAG (Indians only)	36	25.48	29% (2 yr)			2 yr	Sharma & Gupta, 1997
	103	28.6		360	73%	1 year	Ghosh et al., 1996
					49%	2 years	
					26%	3 years	
					9%	4 years	
COAG	93	27.6	32% (1 mon)	180	80%	1 yr	Odberg & Sandvik, 1999
					67%	5 yr	
					67%	8 yr	
OAG	108	N/A	N/A	360	50% IOP criteria / 29% visual field criteria	2 yr	Balacco Gabrieli et al., 1993
Mixture	45	N/A	N/A	360 (100 burns)	54%	4 years	Grayson et al., 1993
				360 (50 burns)	62%	4 years	
				180 (50 burns)	76%	4 years	
	109	N/A	N/A	360 180/180	68%	1 yr	Spaeth & Baez, 1992
					58%	2 yr	
					51%	3 yr	
					44%	4 yr	

Table continued on following page

Table 7-11 Long-Term (i.e., ≥2 Years) Effectiveness of ALT for Different Types of Glaucoma *Continued*

Type of Glaucoma	Number of ALTs	IOP Before (mm Hg)	Decrease in IOP	Amount of Angle Treated	Success	Follow-up (mean)	Authors
					35%	5 yr	
					28%	6 yr	
					26%	7 yr	
					26%	8 yr	
	123	25.8	21% (5.4 yr)	360	55%	5.4 yr	Honrubia et al., 1992
	73	24.8	13% (4.7 yr)	180	36%	4.7 yr	
	36	24.0	N/A	360 (100 burns)	39%	3.25 yr	Eguchi et al., 1985
	84	24.6		180 (50 burns) P	67%	1.4 yr	
	37	24.2		180 (50 burns) A	34%	0.7 yr	
	118	29.1	30% (3 yr)	360	88%	1 yr	Ticho & Nesher, 1989
					77%	2 yr	
					70%	3 yr	
					55%	6 yr	
					57%	10 yr	
	60	35.2	56% (2.8 yr)	360	73%	1 yr	Elsas & Johnsen, 1991
				180/180	66%	2 yr	
					57%	3 yr	
					50%	4 yr	
	110	29.6	42% (6 yr)	360	61%	5 yr	Wise, 1987
					56%	6 yr	
	27	27.3	29% (0.7 mon)	180	64%	2 yr	Odberg, 1990
	85	N/A	N/A	180	52%	5 yr	Rouhiainen et al., 1995
	81	24.8	32% (1 yr)	360	77%	2 yr	Schwartz et al., 1985
					46%	5 yr	

85	N/A	N/A	360 270 180/180 180 90 × 4	46%	2.5 yr	Sharpe & Simmons, 1985
93	26.1	29% (1 mon)	360	77% 49% 32%	1 yr 5 yr 10 yr	Shingleton et al., 1993
24	28.2	33% (3 yr)	180	75%	3 yr	Dreyer & Gorla, 1993
49	N/A	N/A	superior 180	70% 64%	1 yr 2 yr	Grayson et al., 1994
53	N/A	N/A	inferior 180	66% 57%	1 yr 2 yr	Grayson et al., 1994
109	26	31%	360 270 180 90	85%	2 yr	Higgins, 1985
100 (dark brown eyes)	28	36% (in successful eyes)	180	82%	.3–2.5 yr	Mohan et al., 1988
63	25.1	30% (3 mon) 33% (1 year)	360 180 × 1 180 × 2	50% 34%	1.92 yr 3 yr	Schwartz et al., 1997
39	24.7	N/A	180	46%	3 yr	Ustundag & Diestelhorst, 1997
28	21.5	18% (3 mon) 31% (1 yr)	180	58%	5 yr	Chung et al., 1998

Table continued on following page

Table 7-11 Long-Term (i.e., ≥2 Years) Effectiveness of ALT for Different Types of Glaucoma Continued

Type of Glaucoma	Number of ALTs	IOP Before (mm Hg)	Decrease in IOP	Amount of Angle Treated	Success	Follow-up (mean)	Authors
EXG	29	25.8	35% (4–6 mon) 35% (16–18 mon)	180	(no filtration) 92% 78% (no filtration, 3rd laser, or IOP ≥ 22) 86% 60%	1 yr 3 yr 1 yr 3 yr	Threlkeld et al., 1996b
	22	29.9	37% (1 yr)	360	73% 54% 54%	1 yr 2 yr 3 yr	Grinich et al., 1987
	29	N/A	N/A	180/180	59%	2 yr	Bergea et al., 1994
	79	30.6	N/A	360	76%	2 yr	Bergea, 1986b
	22	26.4	37% (5 yr)	360	50%	5 yr	Tuulonen et al., 1987
	18	N/A	N/A	360 180	6%	9.5 yr	Gillies et al., 1994
	20	N/A	N/A	360 180	94%	2 yr	Eguchi et al., 1985
	9	N/A	N/A	360	89%	2 yr	Schwartz & Kopelman, 1983
	11	N/A	N/A	360	55%	5 yr	Schwartz et al., 1985
	12	N/A	N/A	360	75%	10 yr	Ticho & Nesher, 1989
	14	N/A	N/A	360 180/180	50% 43% 36%	1 yr 5 yr 8 yr	Spaeth & Baez, 1992
	227 412 64	N/A	N/A	360 180	97% 86% 53%	1.5 mon 1 yr 2 yr	Lund, 1988

Group	n			Degrees	Success	Follow-up	Reference
	19	N/A	N/A	180	37%	3 yr	Ustundag & Diestelhorst, 1997
	26				50%	4 yr	
	6	N/A	N/A	180	83%	3 yr	
	75	30.1	31% (1 mon)	180	80%	1 yr	Odberg & Sandvik, 1999
					53%	5 yr	
					36%	8 yr	
PIG	9	29.0	14% (3 mon)	360	89%	5.5 yr	Lehto, 1992
	19	N/A	N/A	360	79%	1.5 mon	Lund, 1988
	12			180	91%	1 yr	
	8				50%	2 yr	
	4				25%	3 yr	
	32	27.8	N/A	360	80%	1 yr	Ritch et al., 1993
				180	62%	2 yr	
					45%	6 yr	
	4	N/A	N/A	360	50%	2 yr	Schwartz & Kopelman, 1983
	2	N/A	N/A	360	50%	10 yr	Ticho & Nesher, 1989
	2	23.5	40%	360	100%	2 yr	Goldberg, 1985
				180/180			
				180			
	10	N/A	N/A	180	60%	1 yr	Brooks et al., 1988
				180/180	30%	4 yr	
	10	N/A	N/A	180	40%	3 yr	Ustundag & Diestelhorst, 1997
	2	N/A	N/A	360	50%	5 yr	Schwartz et al., 1985

POAG = Primary open-angle glaucoma
EXG = Exfoliation syndrome glaucoma
PIG = Pigmentary glaucoma

   b. In another study, 26% of patients with POAG and 41% of patients with exfoliation syndrome glaucoma were able to taper their medications (Thomas et al., 1982a).

   c. In still another study, 28% of phakic POAG patients, 26.5% of aphakic POAG, and 39% of exfoliation syndrome glaucoma patients were able to reduce medications (Horns et al., 1983).

   d. Sharpe and Simmons (1985) found that 24% of patients in their study could taper medications after ALT.

   e. Tuulonen and colleagues (1989) reported that 53% of their patients who had ALT as their first form of therapy required no medications post-ALT.

C. Patient Factors

1. Age

   a. ALT is more effective in older compared to younger patients (Eguchi et al., 1985; Forbes & Bansal, 1981; Grinich et al., 1987; Moulin et al., 1991; Safran et al., 1984; Schwartz & Kopelman, 1983; Schwartz et al., 1981; Shingleton et al., 1987; Thomas et al., 1982a; Ticho & Nesher, 1989; Wilensky & Jampol, 1981; Wise, 1981, 1987; Wise & Witter, 1979; Zborowski et al., 1984).

   b. In marked contrast, ALT apparently has a greater chance of long-term success in younger patients with pigmentary glaucoma (Lunde, 1983; Ritch et al., 1993).

   c. There are also reports that age does not have a relationship with the IOP changes after ALT (Odberg & Sandvik, 1999; Schwartz et al., 1997; Threlkeld et al., 1996b; Traverso et al., 1986; Tuulonen et al., 1985). However, in some of the studies there was a relative lack of young subjects.

   d. In low-tension glaucoma, age apparently does not affect the success rate of ALT (Schwartz et al., 1984).

2. Race

   a. A number of reports suggest that ALT is equally effective in treating black and white patients (Forbes & Bansal, 1981; Krupin et al., 1986; Schwartz et al., 1981, 1984, 1997; Thomas et al., 1982a; Wilensky & Jampol, 1981; Wise, 1981; Zborowski et al., 1984).

   b. Long-term success of ALT in open-angle glaucoma may be better in white as compared to black patients (Schwartz et al., 1985).

3. Gender

Gender apparently does not affect the success rate of ALT (Odberg & Sandvik, 1999; Schwartz et al., 1984; Schwartz et al., 1997; Shingleton et al., 1987; Thomas et al., 1982a; Threlkeld et al., 1996b; Tuulonen et al., 1985; Zborowski et al., 1984). One study indicated that males had a greater percent decrease in IOP even though gender had no significant effect on success rate (Threlkeld et al., 1996b).

4. **Angle pigmentation**
   a. There are a number of studies that suggest that the degree of trabecular mesh-work pigmentation does not affect the outcome of ALT (Bergea, 1984; Forbes & Bansal, 1981; Grinich et al., 1987; Threlkeld et al., 1996b; Tuulonen et al., 1985; Wilensky & Jampol, 1981).
   b. However, there are also reports that the ALT success rate is higher in patients with higher degrees of pigmentation (Bergea, 1986b; Brooks & Gillies, 1984; Higgins, 1985; Odberg & Sandvik, 1999; Rouhiainen et al., 1995; Traverso et al., 1986).
      1) In one report, there was a greater IOP-lowering effect in patients that had 4+ angle pigmentation compared to those with lower levels (Traverso et al., 1986). However, there was no correlation with degree of pigment in the lower levels.
      2) Brooks & Gillies (1984) found that the IOP reduction was greatest in those patients with moderate angle pigment compared to light and heavy pigment.
      3) Bergea (1986b) speculated that the higher success rates in patients with greater degrees of pigment may be due to the higher incidence of exfoliation syndrome glaucoma in the more successful group.
      4) Higgins (1985) found that there was a positive correlation of IOP reduction with degree of pigment in the angle. Threlkeld et al. (1996b) also found that patients with higher pigment grades had greater percent decreases in their IOP.

5. **Pretreatment IOP**
   a. Patients with initially high IOPs tend to have a larger decrease in IOP following ALT than those patients with initially lower IOPs (Bergea, 1984; Brooks & Gillies, 1984; Grinich et al., 1987; Higgins, 1985; Horns et al., 1983; Klein et al., 1985; Lieberman et al., 1983; Rosenthal et al., 1984; Thomas et al., 1982a, 1984; Threlkeld et al., 1996b; Traverso, et al., 1986; Watson et al., 1984; Zborowski et al., 1984). In other words, the higher the pretreatment IOP, the greater the decrease in posttreatment IOP. In one study, the same correlation occurred except for patients with pretreatment IOPs above 35 mm Hg where the post-treatment IOP change decreased (Forbes & Bansal, 1981). A small sample size (six patients) may have contributed to this anomaly.
   b. However, even though a higher pretreatment IOP may lead to a larger IOP decrease right after ALT, the long-term success may be lower (Elsas & Johnsen, 1991; Forbes & Bansal, 1981; Odberg & Sandvik, 1999; Rosenthal et al., 1984; Schwartz & Kopelman, 1983; Tuulonen et al., 1985). This could be due to the fact that patients with high pre-ALT IOPs may need an even larger IOP decrease than is normally attainable.
   c. There are also reports that the pretreatment IOP level does not correlate with success rate (Bergea, 1986b; Shingleton et al., 1987; Threlkeld et al., 1996b).

6. **Prior filtering operation**

ALT appears to be effective in patients who have uncontrolled IOP after filtration surgery (Amon et al., 1990; Elsas & Harstad, 1983; Fellman et al., 1984; Goldmann & Mellin, 1987; Robin, 1991; Robin & Pollack, 1983; Thomas et al., 1982a).

7. **Prior penetrating keratoplasty**

ALT also appears to be effective in patients who have had corneal transplants (Van Meter et al., 1988).

D. *Type of Glaucoma* (Table 7–12; see also Tables 7–9 to 7–11).

1. Reported variations in success rates in the tables may be due to differences in:
   a. ALT technique (e.g., power, number of burns, placement of burns)
   b. Patient selection (including the types of glaucoma and how many eyes of each patient were included)
   c. Criteria for success which could include:
      1) IOP value (e.g., "21 mm Hg or "20 mm Hg)
      2) Degree of change in IOP (e.g., ≥2 mm Hg or ≥5 mm Hg)
      3) Avoidance of surgery
      4) "Clinical control"
      5) Lack of visual field loss
      6) Reduction of level of medication
      7) Avoidance of repeat ALT
      8) Lack of progressive optic nerve damage
   d. Number of patients lost to follow-up
   e. Use of Kaplan-Meier life-table analysis of survival or another method
   f. Interpretation of "maximum tolerated therapy"
   g. Level of laser operator experience

2. **Combined-mechanism glaucoma** (see Tables 7–10 and 7–12).
   a. Success rates in combined-mechanism glaucoma patients with follow-up of approximately 1 year ranged from 70% to 100% with a mean of 85% (two studies).
   b. The mean IOP reduction was 24% in two studies.

3. **Exfoliation syndrome glaucoma (EXG)** (see Tables 7–9 to 7–11).
   a. Success rates in EXG patients with follow-up of 8 to 15.3 months ranged from 50% to 100% with a mean of 82% (13 studies). The mean IOP reduction was 39% in 18 studies.
   b. Mean success rate in EXG patients with a mean follow-up of 2 years was 71% in six studies with a range of 54% to 94%.
   c. Mean success rate in EXG patients with a mean follow-up of 5 years was 49% in 3 studies with a range of 43% to 55%.
   d. Mean success rate in EXG patients with a mean follow-up of 10 years was 40.5% in 2 studies with a range of 6% to 75%.

Text continued on page 365

Table 7–12 Effectiveness of ALT with Secondary Glaucomas

Type of Glaucoma	Number of ALTs	IOP Before (mm Hg)	Decrease in IOP	Amount of Angle Treated	Success	Follow-up (mean)	Authors
Uveitic G	14	29.2	7% ↑	360	29%	5.4 mon	Spaeth et al., 1983
	8	41	27%	360	37.5%	8 mon	Robin & Pollack, 1983
	3	39.0	3% ↑	360	33%	3 mon	Goldberg, 1985
				180/180			
				180			
	6	25.7	17%	360	33%	8.25 mon	Horns et al., 1983
				180			
	3	N/A	N/A	360	0%	15.3 mon	Lieberman et al., 1983
	4	35.5	33%	360	75%	4.3 mon	Thomas et al., 1982a
				180/180			
	11	33	15%	360	27%	17 mon	Goldmann & Mellin, 1987
	6	N/A	N/A	180	17%	5 yr	Brooks et al., 1988
				180/180			
Juvenile G	3	36	7.2% ↑	360	0%	6 weeks	Thomas et al., 1982a
				180/180			
	1	N/A	N/A	360	0%	10.5 mon	Forbes & Bansal, 1981
	6	N/A	N/A	360	33%	1 yr +	Wilensky & Weinreb, 1983a
	10	27.7	8%	360	40%	6.45 mon	Horns et al., 1983
				180			
	15 (<40 yr)	32	16%	360	40%	2 yr	Safran et al., 1984
Congenital G	3	34.3	9.6%	360	0%	5 mon	Thomas et al., 1982a
				180/180			
	4	37	24%	360	50%	12 mon	Robin & Pollack, 1983
ARG	2	34.5	45%	360	N/A	6.5 mon	Thomas et al., 1984
	4	40	27.5%	360	0%	14 mon	Robin & Pollack et al., 1983
	1	N/A	N/A	360	0%	10.5 mon	Forbes & Bansal, 1981

Table continued on following page

359

Table 7-12 Effectiveness of ALT with Secondary Glaucomas Continued

Type of Glaucoma	Number of ALTs	IOP Before (mm Hg)	Decrease in IOP	Amount of Angle Treated	Success	Follow-up (mean)	Authors
	6	34	45%	360 180/180 180	50%	3–19 mon	Goldberg, 1985
	2	N/A	N/A	360	50%	15.3 mon	Lieberman et al., 1983
	4	21.8	23%	360 180/180	75%	8.7 mon	Thomas et al., 1982
	3	N/A	N/A	360	33%	2 yr	Schwartz & Kopelman, 1983
	2	N/A	N/A	360	0%	5 yr	Schwartz et al., 1985
	11	39	2%	90 180	27% 27%	1 yr 1.5 yr	Fukuchi et al., 1983
	2	N/A	N/A	360 180	50%	1 yr	Horns et al., 1983
ARG (Angle cleavage)	8	25.3	28%	360	63%	4.6 mon	Spaeth et al., 1983
ARG (Trauma)	4	32	12.5%	360	0%	14 mon	Goldmann & Mellin, 1987
	7	N/A	N/A	180 180/180	86% 43%	1 yr 3 yr	Brooks et al., 1988
LTG	67	N/A	N/A	360 270 180/180 180 90 × 4	46%	2.5 yr	Sharpe & Simmons, 1985
	4	15.5	40%	360 180/180 180	50%	4–14 mon	Goldberg, 1985
	29	18.2	16% (1 mon)	360 180	82%	4 yr	Eendebak et al., 1990

Diagnosis	N		%	Degrees	%	Follow-up	Reference
	6	15.3	33%	360 / 180	86%	1 yr	Horns et al., 1983
Sturge-Weber syndrome	22	16.95	26% (2 mon)	360	73%	1.8 yr	Schwartz et al., 1984
	3	N/A	N/A	360	0%	N/A	Lieberman et al., 1983
	2	24	17%	360	0%	N/A	Spaeth et al., 1983
	2	31	45%	360	100%	6 mon	Robin & Pollack, 1983
Marfan syndrome	1	29	72% ↑	360	0%	N/A	Spaeth et al., 1983
ICE syndrome	2	21	14% ↑	360	50%	5.5 mon	Spaeth et al., 1983
	3	23	22%	360 / 180/180	33%	2 mon	Thomas et al., 1982a
Trabeculodys-genesis	5	24.8	56% ↑	360	40%	4.3 mon	Spaeth et al., 1983
Neovascular G	2	38	29%	360	50%	3.5 mon	Spaeth et al., 1983
	5	N/A	N/A	180 / 180/180	40%	N/A	Brooks et al., 1988
Iridocorneal mesodermal dysgenesis	1	N/A	N/A	360 / 180/180	0%	N/A	Thomas et al., 1982a
Combined-mechanism	1	N/A	N/A	360	100%	10.5 mon	Forbes & Bansal, 1981
	20	26.7	26% (1 wk)	360 / 180/180 / 180	70%	1 d to 12+ mon	Goldberg, 1985
	16	25	22% (1 mon)	180	N/A	6–12 mon	Hitchings, 1984
Essential iris atrophy	1	20	5% (1–2 mon)	360	0%	1–2 mon	Lichter, 1982
Aniridia	2	26.5	41% (1–2 mon)	360	100%	1–2 mon	Lichter, 1982

Table continued on following page

361

Table 7–12 Effectiveness of ALT with Secondary Glaucomas *Continued*

Type of Glaucoma	Number of ALTs	IOP Before (mm Hg)	Decrease in IOP	Amount of Angle Treated	Success	Follow-up (mean)	Authors
Elevated episcleral venous pressure	1	N/A	N/A	360	0%	10.5 mon	Forbes & Bansal, 1981
Narrow angle	26	25.9	32% (1 mon)	360 180	87% 76% 51%	1 yr 3.5 yr 4.5 yr	Eendebak et al., 1990
Angle-closure G	6	N/A	N/A	180 180/180	50%	1 yr	Brooks et al., 1988
Angle closure after LPI	4	33	52%	360	100%	7 mon	Robin & Pollack, 1983
Steroid-induced	2	N/A	N/A	360 180/180	0%	3.2 mon	Thomas et al., 1982a
Aphakia	7	31.3	38%	360 180/180 180	71%	6–12 mon	Goldberg, 1985
	3	25.7	26.6%	360	67%	1–2 mon	Lichter, 1982
	7	22.7	22%	360	86%	15.3 mon	Lieberman et al., 1983
	37	22.3	13%	360 180/180	62%	5 mon	Thomas et al., 1982a
	36	24.7	28%	360 180	83%	10.1 mon	Horns et al., 1983
	1	N/A	N/A	360	17%	10 yr	Ticho & Nesher, 1989
	6	N/A	N/A	180 180/180	33%	1 yr	Brooks et al., 1988
	15	21.9	10%	360	47%	5.1 mon	Spaeth et al., 1983

Group	N	Age	%	Degrees	Success	Follow-up	Reference
Aphakic G	22	34	21%	360	45%	18 mon	Goldmann & Mellin, 1987
	9	27.7	13%	360	22%	5.1 mon	Spaeth et al., 1983
	6	34	50%	360	100%	7 mon	Robin & Pollack, 1983
	2	28.5	16%	360	N/A	5.5 mon	Thomas et al., 1984
	126	N/A	N/A	360	44%	1.5 mon	Lund, 1988
	41			180	88%	1 yr	
	16				75%	2 yr	
	6				66%	3 yr	
	6	N/A	N/A	N/A	17%	1 mon	Brooks & Gillies, 1984
Aphakic with prior filtering	5	28	41%	360	100%	9 mon	Robin & Pollack, 1983
Pseudophakia	24	28.2	33%	180	75%	3 yr	Dreyer & Gorla, 1993
	10	30.6	30%	180 / 180/180	80%	1.3 yr	Van Meter et al., 1988
	3	N/A	N/A	180 / 180/180	33%	1 yr	Brooks et al., 1988
					33%	2 yr	
Phakic	82	26.8	30%	360	87%	≥12 mon	Scrivanti et al., 1988
	60	28	35%		82%	≥12 mon	
	45	27.5	26%	360	100%	11 mon	Wilensky & Jampol, 1981
	28	30.5	35%	360	N/A	7.6 mon	Thomas et al., 1984
	263	24.4	31%	360 / 180/180	87.5%	5.2 mon	Thomas et al., 1982a
	226	25.5	30%	360 / 180	82%	9 mon	Horns et al., 1983
	159	N/A	N/A	360 / 180/180	81%	1 yr	Moulin & Haut, 1993
					70%	2 yr	
					59%	3 yr	
					52%	4 yr	
					48%	5 yr	
					17%	8 yr	
					11%	10 yr	

Table continued on following page

Table 7-12 Effectiveness of ALT with Secondary Glaucomas *Continued*

Type of Glaucoma	Number of ALTs	IOP Before (mm Hg)	Decrease in IOP	Amount of Angle Treated	Success	Follow-up (mean)	Authors
	82	24.8	39%	360	77% / 46%	2 yr / 5 yr	Schwartz et al., 1985
	32	25.6 (calc.)	35% (calc.)	360	50%	5 yr	Tuulonen et al., 1987
	110	29.6	42% (6 yr)	360	61% / 56%	5 yr / 6 yr	Wise, 1987
	43	N/A	N/A	360	39%	3.65 yr	Searle et al., 1990
	61	26	33% (6 mon)	180	74%	4.4 yr	Amon et al., 1990
	112	27.1	32% (1 yr)	360	79% / 69% / 59%	1 yr / 2 yr / 3 yr	Grinich et al., 1987
After filtering	9	26.5	25%	180	89%	3.8 mon	Elsas & Harstad, 1983
	7	29	38%	360	86%	6 mon	Robin & Pollack, 1983
	25	20.0	14%	360 / 180	67%	14.3 mon	Fellman et al., 1984
	20	26.5	30%	360 / 180/180	70%	4.1 mon	Thomas et al., 1982a
	34	29	31%	360	71%	20 mon	Goldmann & Mellin, 1987
After penetrating keratoplasty	10	30.6	30%	180 / 180/180	80%	1.9 yr	Van Meter et al., 1988

LTG = Low-tension glaucoma
ARG = Angle-recession glaucoma
NAG = Narrow angle glaucoma

4. **Angle-closure glaucoma/narrow angle glaucoma** (see Tables 7–10 and 7–12)
   a. Success rates in angle-closure glaucoma patients with follow-up of 7 to 12 months ranged from 50% to 100% with a mean of 79% (three studies).
   b. The mean IOP reduction was 42% in 2 studies.
5. **Pigmentary glaucoma (PIG)** (see Tables 7–9 to 7–11)
   a. Success rates in PIG patients with follow-up of 7 to 15.3 months ranged from 44% to 100% with a mean of 77% (9 studies). The mean IOP reduction was 34% in six studies.
   b. Mean success rate in PIG patients with a follow-up of 2 years was 65.5% in four studies with a range of 50% to 100%.
   c. Mean success rate in PIG patients with a mean follow-up of 5 years was 69.5% in two studies with a range of 50% to 89%.
   d. Success rate in PIG patients with a follow-up of 10 years was 50% in one study.
6. **Glaucoma after failed filtering surgery** (see Tables 7–10 and 7–12)
   a. Success rates in glaucoma patients after failed filtering surgery with follow-up of 3.8 to 20 months ranged from 67% to 89% with a mean of 77% (five studies).
   b. The mean IOP reduction was 28% in five studies.
7. **POAG** (see Tables 7–9 to 7–11)
   a. Most of the patients in the larger studies have had primary open-angle glaucoma.
   b. Success rates in POAG patients with follow-up of 9 to 18 months ranged from 57% to 94% with a mean of 76% (17 studies). The mean IOP reduction was 28% in 18 studies where the IOP reduction was measured from 1 to 15.3 months post-ALT.
   c. Mean success rate in POAG patients with a mean follow-up of 2 years was 69% in 14 studies with a range of 40% to 100%.
   d. Mean success rate in POAG patients with a mean follow-up of 3 years was 65% in 6 studies with a range of 50% to 79%.
   e. Mean success rate in POAG patients with a follow-up of 5 years was 62.5% in six studies with a range of 46% to 80%.
   f. Mean success rate in POAG patients with a mean follow-up of 10.1 years was 34% in four studies with a range of 11% to 54%.
8. **Low-tension glaucoma** (see Tables 7–10 and 7–12)
   a. Success rates in low-tension glaucoma patients with follow-up of 1 to 4 years ranged from 46% to 86% with a mean of 67% (five studies).
   b. The mean IOP reduction was 29% in four studies.
9. **Neovascular glaucoma** (see Tables 7–10 and 7–12)
   a. Success rates in neovascular glaucoma patients ranged from 40% to 50% with a mean of 45% (two studies). The mean follow-up time was not mentioned in one of the studies and was 3.5 months in the other.
   b. The mean IOP reduction was 29% in one study.

10. **Iridocorneal endothelial (ICE) syndrome glaucoma** (see Tables 7–10 and 7–12)
    a. Success rates in ICE glaucoma patients with a follow-up of 2 to 5.5 months ranged from 33% to 50% with a mean of 41.5% (two studies).
    b. The mean IOP reduction was 4% in two studies.

11. **Trabeculodysgenesis glaucoma** (see Tables 7–10 and 7–12)
    a. The success rate for trabeculodysgenesis glaucoma patients was 40% in one study with a mean follow-up time of 4.3 months.
    b. The mean IOP change was an increase of 56% in the one study.

12. **Angle-recession glaucoma** (see Tables 7–10 and 7–12)
    a. Success rates in angle-recession glaucoma patients with follow-up of 4.6 to 18 months ranged from 0% to 75% with a mean of 39% (11 studies). The mean IOP reduction was 26% in seven studies.
    b. Success in angle-recession glaucoma patients with a mean follow-up of 1.75 years was 30% in two studies with a range of 27% to 33%.
    c. Success rate in angle-recession glaucoma patients with a follow-up of 5 years was 0% in one study.

13. **Uveitic glaucoma** (see Tables 7–10 and 7–12)
    a. Success rates in uveitic glaucoma patients with follow-up of 3 to 17 months ranged from 0% to 75% with a mean of 33.5% (seven studies).
    b. The mean IOP reduction was 14% in six studies.

14. **Sturge-Weber syndrome glaucoma** (see Tables 7–10 and 7–12)
    a. Success rates in Sturge-Weber glaucoma patients ranged from 0% to 100% with a mean of 33% (three studies).
    b. The mean IOP reduction was 31% in two studies.

15. **Congenital glaucoma** (see Tables 7–10 and 7–12)
    a. Success rates in congenital glaucoma patients with follow-up of 5 to 12 months ranged from 0% to 50% with a mean of 25% (two studies).
    b. The mean IOP reduction was 16.8% in two studies.

16. **Juvenile glaucoma** (see Tables 7–10 and 7–12)
    a. Success rates in juvenile glaucoma patients with follow-up of 1.5 to 24 months ranged from 0% to 40% with a mean of 23% (five studies).
    b. The mean IOP reduction was 5.6% in three studies.

17. **Steroid-induced glaucoma** (see Tables 7–10 and 7–12)
    a. The success rate in steroid-induced glaucoma was 0% in one study involving two patients and a follow-up of 3.2 months. No information was given on the mean IOP reduction.
    b. In one study of 94 normal patients with myopia who had radial keratotomy performed, it was found that laser trabeculoplasty did not prevent the IOP increase induced by steroid drops (Galin et al., 2000).

18. **Essential atrophy glaucoma** (see Tables 7–10 and 7–12)
    a. The success rate in essential iris atrophy glaucoma patients was 0% in one study with one patient.
    b. No information was given on the mean IOP reduction.

19. **Marfan syndrome glaucoma** (see Tables 7–10 and 7–12)
    a. The success rate in Marfan syndrome glaucoma patients was 0% in one study with one patient.
    b. The mean IOP change was an increase of 72% in the one patient.

20. **Glaucoma with elevated episcleral venous pressure** (see Tables 7–10 and 7–12)
    a. The success rate for glaucoma patients with elevated episceral venous pressure was 0% in one study with one patient.
    b. No information was given on the mean IOP change.

21. **Phakia** (see Tables 7–10 and 7–12)
    a. Success rates in phakic glaucoma patients with follow-up of 5.2 to 12 months ranged from 81% to 100% with a mean of 87% (three large studies and three smaller studies). The mean IOP reduction was 31% in six studies.
    b. In one of these large studies, the success rate was 90% at 2 years, 48% at 5 years, and 11% at 10 years.

22. **Pseudophakia** (see Tables 7–10 and 7–12)
    a. Success rates in pseudophakic glaucoma patients with follow-up of 1 to 3 years ranged from 33% to 80% with a mean of 63% (three studies).
    b. The mean IOP reduction was 31.5% in two studies.

23. **Aphakia** (see Tables 7–10 and 7–12)
    a. Success rates in aphakic glaucoma patients with follow-up of 1 to 18 months ranged from 17% to 100% with a mean of 63% (13 studies).
    b. The mean IOP reduction was 25% in 11 studies.
    c. In a study comparing 25 aphakic eyes to 38 pseudophakic eyes, pseudophakic eyes had a better response than aphakic eyes (Schwartz et al., 1997). Over an average follow-up period of 21.8 months, ALT was successful in 57.9% of pseudophakes and 40% of aphakes at the latest follow-up examination.

24. **Mixture of glaucomas** (see Tables 7–9 to 7–11)
    a. A number of studies lumped different types of glaucoma patients together. Most of these had a large percentage of patients with POAG.
    b. Success rates in these groups of patients with follow-up from 7.5 months to 12+ months ranged from 65% to 100% with a mean of 82% (18 studies). The mean IOP reduction was 33% in 19 studies.
    c. Mean success rate in these groups with a mean follow-up of 2 years was 68.5% in eight studies with a range of 57% to 85%.

  d. Mean success rate in these groups with a mean follow-up of 5.1 years was 48% in nine studies with a range of 35% to 56%.

  e. Mean success rate in these groups with a mean follow-up of 10 years was 44.5% in two studies with a range of 32% to 57%.

E. Repeat Trabeculoplasty (Table 7–13)

1. Consider repeat trabeculoplasty in patients who have initial success with their first trabeculoplasty. A repeat procedure could lower the IOP again and delay the need for a filtering operation.

2. Success rates for retreatment with follow-up of 3 to 6 months ranged from 21% to 100% with a mean of 56% (seven studies). The mean IOP reduction was 21% in 11 studies.

3. Mean success rate for retreatment for a mean follow-up of 1 year was 50% in seven studies with a range of 21% to 73%.

4. Mean success rate for retreatment for a mean follow-up of 2 years was 23% in five studies with a range of 11% to 47%.

XI. Complications (Table 7–14).

A. Transient IOP Elevation

1. The most common of the potentially serious complications after ALT is the transient IOP elevation, the IOP spike. This pressure spike can usually be detected in the first hour post-ALT and usually peaks within the first 3 to 6 hours. In a small percentage of patients, the spike can be detected at, or persist to, 24 hours (Hoskins et al., 1983; Thomas et al., 1982a).

2. The mechanisms responsible for this early elevation of pressure are not known.

3. Treating 180° leads to fewer and smaller IOP spikes than treating 360° (Eguchi et al., 1985; Heijl, 1984; Hoskins et al., 1983; Krupin et al., 1992; Thomas et al., 1982a; Weinreb et al., 1983b). The data from Heijl (1984) were smaller percentages than those of the other studies because the IOP was not measured within the first few hours but from the first day to 1 month after the ALT. In one study there was a tendency for fewer spikes, but the difference did not reach the level of statistical significance (Schwartz et al., 1983). In another study, the early IOP elevations were similar in the 180° and the 360° groups (Lustgarten et al., 1984). Krupin and colleagues (1984) reported that the magnitude of the spike is not correlated with the number of laser burns. However, they only treated 360° of the angle with 78 ± 7 (mean $\pm$ SD) laser burns.

4. The peak of the early IOP spike occurs significantly earlier when 180° is treated than when 360° is treated (Eguchi et al., 1985; Weinreb et al., 1983a).

Table 7–13 Effectiveness of Repeat ALT

Number of ALTs	IOP Before (mmHg)	Decrease in IOP After Tx	Success	Follow-up (mean) or Kaplan-Meier Analysis Times	Authors
26	25.1	7%	38%	5 mon	Brown et al., 1985
50	22.6	16% (3 mon)	35%	6 mon	Feldman et al., 1991
			21%	12 mon	
			11%	24 mon	
			5%	48 mon	
38	24 (from graph)	23% (3 mon)	78%	3 mon	Grayson et al., 1988
			73%	12 mon	
37	23.9	27% (1 mon)	70%	12 mon	Weber et al., 1989
			47%	20 mon	
			15%	24 mon	
12	28	36% (1.5 mon)	73%	40 mon	Jorizzo et al., 1988
40	26	22% (1 mon)	33%	12 mon	Richter et al., 1987
			14%	21 mon	
20	28.9	25% (2 mon)	60%	6 mon	Bergea, 1986a
			50%	12 mon	
			30%	30 mon	
16	21.7	21% (8 mon)	37.5%	8 mon	Lieberman et al., 1983
40	26	17% (3 mon)	32%	12 mon	Richter et al., 1987
17	22.5	14% (3 mon)	59%	3 mon	Starita et al., 1984
37	23.9	27% (1 mon)	100%	3 mon	Weber et al., 1989
			91%	6 mon	
			77%	9 mon	
			70%	12 mon	
			47%	16 mon	
			47%	20 mon	
14	N/A	N/A	36%	1.5 mon	Messner et al., 1987
			21%	6 mon	

Table 7–14 Complications of Laser Trabeculoplasty

Transient IOP elevation
Peripheral anterior synechiae
Inflammation
  Persistent iritis
  Severe trabeculitis
Hemorrhage/hyphema
Corneal burns
Keratopathy
Corneal edema/decompensation
Mild ocular pain
Syncope
Transient blurred vision
Loss of visual field
Generalized seizure
Iris burns
Sector palsy of the iris sphincter muscle
Herpes simplex keratitis
Cystoid macular edema
Persistent elevated IOP
Early failure of IOP-lowering effect
Encapsulated blebs/filtering surgery failure
Suprachoroidal effusion
Membrane formation in the chamber angle

5. Without added prophylaxis, IOP spikes of greater than 5 mm Hg have been reported in a mean of about 28% of patients that had 180° ALT and a mean of about 36% of patients that had 360° ALT.

6. Placement of the laser burns more anteriorly in the trabecular meshwork results in fewer and smaller IOP elevations immediately after treatment (Eguchi et al., 1985; Schwartz et al., 1983; Thomas, 1984; Traverso et al., 1984). Another study found a tendency for eyes with more than 10% of laser burns anterior to the ideal site to have IOP elevations (GLTRG, 1989). This difference was not statistically significant.

7. There is some controversy concerning the effect of laser energy on the early IOP spikes. Some studies report that the magnitude of the IOP spike is not correlated with the laser power or the total energy delivered (GLTRG, 1989; Krupin et al., 1984; Tuulonen et al, 1985). Others report that the transient IOP spikes may be correlated positively with the power level (Rosenblatt & Lutz, 1987; Rouhiainen et al., 1987), and the total energy delivered (Weinreb et al., 1984).

8. One study reports that there is a correlation between IOP spike and moderate or heavy angle pigmentation measured at 12 o'clock (GLTRG, 1989). Another study reports that there is no statistically significant correlation between the early IOP elevation and the amount of angle pigmentation (Rouhiainen et al, 1987).

9. The long-term effect of ALT on IOP apparently does not correlate with the occurrence of early IOP spikes (Krupin et al., 1984; Rosenblatt & Luntz, 1987).

10. There is no correlation between the transient inflammation and the IOP elevation post-treatment (Krupin et al., 1984; Thomas et al., 1982a). This conclusion is supported by the finding that steroids and nonsteroidal anti-inflammatory drugs do not significantly affect the early IOP elevation following ALT (Ascaso et al, 1992; Gelfand & Wolpert, 1985; Hotchkiss et al., 1984; Pappas et al., 1985; Ruderman et al., 1983; Shin et al., 1996).

11. There is apparently no correlation between the early IOP elevation and the patient's age (GLTRG, 1989; Robin et al., 1987; Rosenblatt & Luntz, 1987), race (GLTRG, 1989; Pappas et al., 1985; Robin et al., 1987), gender (GLTRG, 1989; Robin et al., 1987; Rosenblatt & Luntz, 1987), or eye color (GLTRG, 1989; Robin et al., 1987).

12. There is also apparently no correlation between the early IOP spikes and the pre-ALT IOP (GLTRG, 1989; Robin et al., 1987; Rouhiainen et al., 1987).

13. The magnitudes and frequencies of the IOP spikes can be reduced by prophylactic drug use. Apraclonidine and another relatively selective α-adrenoceptor agonist, brimonidine, are the most effective of the tested agents (Table 7–15). The pressure-lowering response to most of the other topical agents is not as great and many of the patients undergoing ALT are already on these other medications.

14. A single dose of 1% apraclonidine is comparable to two doses in preventing IOP spikes (Birt et al., 1995; Holmwood et al., 1992). The same is true for 0.5% brimonidine (David et al., 1993).

15. In terms of preventing the IOP spike, giving a single dose of 0.5% apraclonidine before and after ALT is apparently as equally effective as a single dose of 1% apraclonidine before and after ALT (Threlkeld et al., 1996a). Likewise, giving a single administration of 0.5% apraclonidine is apparently as effective as a single administration of 1% apraclonidine (Rosenberg et al., 1995).

16. For glaucoma patients receiving chronic apraclonidine therapy, the prophylactic use of 1% apraclonidine is relatively ineffective (Chung et al., 1997; Ren et al., 1999). These patients should be monitored closely, and, if they develop IOP spikes, should be treated with medications other than apraclonidine. Pilocarpine works well in these patients (Ren et al., 1999).

17. In addition to medical management, the IOP elevation may also require surgical treatment.

Text continued on page 376

Table 7–15 Management of Transient IOP Spikes Post-ALT

Placebo Spikes (>5 mm Hg)	Placebo Spikes (>10 mm Hg)	Prophylaxis Spikes (>5 mm Hg)	Prophylaxis Spikes (>10 mm Hg)	Prophylactic Agent; Degrees of Angle Treated	Authors
21% (19)	5% (19)			after 180	Bergea & Svedbergh, 1992
37% (19)	10% (19)			after 2nd 180	
0%	0%			after 360	Brancato et al., 1991
>4 mm Hg					Eguchi et al., 1985
83% (36)				after 360	
60% (84)				after 180 (posterior TM)	
30% (37)				after 180 (anterior TM)	
22% (269)	7% (269)			after 180	GLTRG, 1989
17% (269)	4% (269)			after 2nd 180	
10% (41)				after 360	Heijl, 1984
0% (35)				after 180	
29% (41)				after 360	Hoskins et al., 1983
9% (33)				after 180	
19% (62)				after 180	Klein et al., 1985
33% (57)	16% (57)			after 360	Krupin et al., 1984
33% (106)	22% (106)			after 360	Lieberman et al., 1983
19% (21)				after 180	Moriarty et al., 1993b
13% (15)	40% (15)			500 mW	Rouhiainen et al., 1987
27% (15)				700 mW	
53% (15)				900 mW (after 180)	
57% (35)	37% (35)			after 360	Thomas et al., 1982a
35% (26)	11.5% (26)			after180	
55% (20)	45% (20)			after 360	Weinreb et al., 1983b
15% (20)	0% (20)			after 180	

Table continued on following page

Reference	Medication (follow-up, days)				
Leung & Gillies, 1986	4% pilocarpine (after 180; after 2nd 180)	48% (31)			42% (33)
Dapling et al., 1994	4% pilocarpine (after 180)				0% (23)
Elsas et al., 1991	2% pilocarpine (after 360)		52% (25)		12% (25)
Robin, 1991	3% pilocarpine (after 360)			33% (37)	3% (37)
Ren et al., 1999	4% pilocarpine chronic use / no chronic use (after 180)			9% (46) / 1.5% (64)	1% (114)
Barnebey et al., 1993	0.5% brimonidine before & after / before only / after only (after 360)	38% (60)	23% (60)	3% (62) / 7% (57) / 9% (53)	2% (62) / 2% (57) / 2% (53)
Brimonidine-ALT Study Group, 1995	0.5% brimonidine before & after / before only / after only (after 360)	40% (116)	23% (116)	3% (122) / 5% (119) / 7% (114)	1% (122) / 2% (119) / 1% (114)
David et al., 1993	0.5% brimonidine (after 360)	41% (56)	23% (56)	4% (183)	0.5% (183)
Barnes et al., 1999	0.2% brimonidine (after 360)			0% (23)	0% (23)
Chevrier et al., 1999	0.2% brimonidine (after 180)			11% (27)	0% (27)
Odberg, 1990	0.5% timolol (after 180)			0% (27)	0% (27)
Robin, 1991	0.5% timolol (after 360)			32% (35)	15% (35)
Robin, 1991	250 mg acetazolamide (after 360)			39% (31)	13% (31)
Hoskins et al., 1983	500 mg acetazolamide (360, 180)		18% (55)		25% (20)
Brooks et al., 1987	500 mg acetazolamide (after 180)	42% (38)	12% (65)		2% (65)
Hartenbaum et al., 1999	2% dorzolamide (after 180)		9% (23)		0% (17)

Table 7–15 Management of Transient IOP Spikes Post-ALT *Continued*

Placebo Spikes (>5 mm Hg)	Placebo Spikes (>10 mm Hg)	Prophylaxis Spikes (>5 mm Hg)	Prophylaxis Spikes (>10 mm Hg)	Prophylactic Agent; Degrees of Angle Treated	Authors
		38% (32)	16% (32)	0.1% dipivefrin (after 360)	Robin, 1991
		3% (125)	1% (125)	1% apraclonidine (after 360)	Robin, 1991
		8% (407)	2% (407)	1% apraclonidine (after 180, 180/180, 360)	Mittra et al., 1995
		0% (72)	0% (72)	1% apraclonidine (after 180)	Birt et al., 1995
		19% (26)	0% (26)	1% apraclonidine (after 180)	Dapling et al., 1994
		7% (30)	0% (30)	1% apraclonidine (after 360)	Holmwood et al., 1992
24% (42)	19% (42)	10% (41)	5% (41)	1% apraclonidine (after 360)	Brown et al., 1988
38% (16) ≥3 mm Hg	38% (16) ≥3 mm Hg	0% (16) 19% (16)	0% (16)	1% apraclonidine (after 180)	Yalvac et al., 1996
17% (121) 23% (71) 8% (50)	12% (121) 17% (71) 4% (50)	6% (130) 10% (86) 0% (44)	3% (130) 5% (86) 0% (44)	1% apraclonidine overall (after 360) (after 180)	Krupin et al., 1992
		4% (28)	0% (28)	1% apraclonidine (after 180)	Chung et al., 1998

Study	Treatment		
Dapling et al., 1994	1% apraclonidine + 4% pilocarpine (after 180)	0% (26)	0% (26)
Chung et al., 1997	1% apraclonidine 1% apraclonidine in pxs on chronic 0.5% apraclonidine	0.6% (161) 1.4% (70)	3.1% (161) 12.9% (70)
Ren et al., 1999	1% apraclonidine	2% (114)	17% (42) 4% (72)
Barnes et al., 1999	1% apraclonidine chronic use no chronic use (after 180)	0% (23)	0% (23)
Robin et al., 1987	1% apraclonidine (after 360)	0% (39)	18% (34)
Rosenberg et al., 1995	1% apraclonidine 0.5% apraclonidine (after 360)	2% (44) 5% (39)	5% (44) 13% (39)
Englert et al., 1997	0.5% apraclonidine (after 180)	9% (11)	9% (11)
Chevier et al., 1999	0.5% apraclonidine (after 180)	0% (24)	0% (24)

18. Thus, **to minimize the frequency and magnitude of the early, transient IOP spikes**:
    a. **Treat 180° of the angle in a single session instead of 360°.**
    b. **Place the laser burns more anteriorly in the trabecular meshwork.**
    c. **Use minimal laser power.**
    d. **Use 1% apraclonidine (or 0.5% brimonidine) before and/or after the ALT session.**

B. *Peripheral Anterior Synechiae (PAS)*

1. The formation of synechial adhesion between the iris and the trabecular meshwork at a laser burn site can occur in from 0% to 52% of ALT-treated eyes (Table 7–16).

2. Reported values for the occurrence of PAS after ALT differ partly because of differences in the criteria for reporting. For example, Eguchi and colleagues (1985) reported fairly small percentages of patients with PAS. However, they used a stringent definition for PAS; the PAS had to reach the TM over more than 180° of the treated angle. Other studies reflect the development of any PAS in the angle (e.g., GLTRG, 1989).

3. These peripheral anterior synechiae have been noted as early as 1 week and as late as 4 months post-ALT (Schwartz et al., 1981).

4. Most are small, localized, and few in number (Rouhiainen et al., 1988; Schwartz et al., 1981; Thomas et al., 1982a). The amount of angle involved is usually small, but significant synechiae formation has been reported including PAS that involve more than 180° of the angle (Eguchi et al., 1985; Hoskins et al., 1983; Wilensky & Jampol, 1981).

5. PAS often involve discrete point foci of iris adhesions to the scleral spur and ciliary body band, but can also involve adhesions to the trabecular meshwork (Eguchi et al., 1985; Lieberman et al., 1983; Thomas et al., 1982a).

6. The prognostic implications of PAS are not entirely clear. Some studies report that PAS do not adversely affect the IOP control and are not clinically significant (GLTRG, 1990, 1995b; Pavan et al., 1992; Schwartz & Kopelman, 1983; Schwartz et al., 1981; Thomas et al., 1982b). However, other studies report that PAS formation can reduce the IOP-lowering effect of ALT (Rouhiainen et al., 1988; West, 1992).

7. Treating 180° of the angle at a single session instead of 360° leads to a reduction in the formation of PAS (Eguchi et al., 1985; Thomas et al., 1982a; Weinreb et al., 1983b).

8. PAS development is also decreased when the anterior rather than the posterior trabecular meshwork is treated (Eguchi et al., 1985; GLTRG, 1989; Hoskins et al., 1983; Rouhiainen et al., 1988; Schwartz et al., 1983; Traverso et al., 1984).

9. A brown iris is a risk factor for the development of PAS post-ALT (GLTRG, 1989). Pappas and colleagues (1985) also found a higher occurrence of PAS in black patients (91% of 11 eyes) than in white patients (13% of 38 eyes).

Table 7–16 Rate of Formation of Peripheral Anterior Synechiae

Occurrence (no. of ALTs)	Follow-up Time	Authors
18% (39)	≥2 mon	Bergea & Svedbergh, 1992
0% (10)	1 yr	Brancato et al., 1991
7.5% (133)	3 mon	Brooks & Gillies, 1984
6% (36) 360° Tx	39 mon	Eguchi et al., 1985
6% (84) 180° Tx	7.3 mon	
0% (37) 180° anterior Tx	8.1 mon	
17% (30)	14.3 mon	Fellman et al., 1984
46% (269)	3 mon	GLTRG, 1989
34% extended to TM		
5% (41) 360° Tx	≥3 mon	Heijl, 1984
9% (35) 180° Tx		
0% (54)	4–59 weeks	Higginbotham & Richardson, 1986
15% (137)	6 mon	Lieberman et al., 1983
19% (21)	2 mon	Moriarty et al., 1993b
20% (159)	15.3 mon	Moulin et al., 1991
32% (43)	1 mon	Pappas et al., 1985
19% (180)	18–42 mon	Pohjanpelto, 1983
19% (21)	6 mon	Pollack & Robin, 1982
22% (119)	6 mon	Rouhiainen et al., 1988
32% (82)	2 yr	Schwartz & Kopelman, 1983
29% (35)	18 mon	Schwartz et al., 1981
47% (70)	weeks to months	Thomas et al., 1982a
27% extended to TM		
52% (27)	weeks to months	Thomas et al., 1982b
0% (30)	7.5 mon	Thomas et al., 1984
28% (118)	4 mon	Traverso et al., 1984
12% anterior ALT		
43% posterior ALT		
4% (131)	≥12 mon	Tuulonen & Airaksinen, 1983
45% (51)–dexamethasone	35 days	West, 1992
22% (58)–fluoromethalone		
22.5% (44)–fluoromethalone		
23% (31)–naphazoline HCl		
10.7% (28)	3 mon	Chung et al., 1998

10. There does not appear to be a statistically significant correlation between PAS formation and age (Rouhiainen et al., 1988), gender (Rouhiainen et al., 1988; Traverso et al., 1984), pre-laser antiglaucoma medications (Rouhiainen et al., 1988), glaucoma type (Rouhiainen et al., 1988), anterior chamber angle pigmentation (Rouhiainen et al., 1988), width of the chamber angle (Thomas et al., 1982a; Traverso et al., 1984), number of laser burns (Traverso et al., 1984), or laser burn effect criterion (GLTRG, 1989; Rouhiainen et al., 1988).

11. Some studies report that there is no significant correlation between PAS and laser power (GLTRG, 1989; Thomas et al., 1982b) while others note that increased laser power leads to more PAS formation (Rouhiainen et al., 1988).

12. There also does not appear to be an association of PAS formation with inflammation following ALT (Pappas et al., 1985) or the early IOP spike after ALT (GLTRG, 1989).

13. In one study that compared post-ALT treatments for inflammation, the formation of PAS occurred more frequently when dexamethasone was used than when fluorometholone or even straight naphazoline was used (West, 1992). This suggests that a weak steroid-like fluorometholone does not affect PAS development and is preferable.

14. Thus, **to minimize PAS formation post-ALT**:
    a. **treat 180°** of the angle instead of 360° at a single session
    b. **treat the anterior portion** of the pigmented trabecular meshwork
    c. **use minimal laser power** when performing ALT
    d. **use weak steroids** (e.g., fluorometholone) **or no steroids** unless significant inflammation occurs.

C. Inflammation

1. Perhaps the most common of the complications following ALT is ocular inflammation. It usually resolves within a week with or without steroid treatment (Thomas, 1984; Thomas et al., 1982b; Moriarty et al., 1993b).

2. In 100% of patients post-ALT, a mild, transient iritis occurs (Higginbotham & Richardson, 1986; Keightley et al., 1987; Schwartz & Kopelman, 1983; Schwartz et al., 1981; Weinreb & Wilensky, 1984).

3. By measuring the amount of flare in the anterior chamber with a laser flare-cell meter, Mermoud and colleagues (1992c) found clinically relevant inflammation in 100% of patients with pigmentary glaucoma, 69% of patients with exfoliation syndrome glaucoma, and 23% of patients with primary open-angle glaucoma. This inflammation peaked 2 days after the ALT procedure.

4. Moriarty and colleagues (1993b) also measured flare following ALT and found that the flare peaked at 1 hour after ALT and remained elevated for about 1 week. They also found that diode laser trabeculoplasty produced significantly less inflammation than ALT.

5. Clinically determined flare has been reported in 29% of patients with exfoliation syndrome glaucoma and primary open-angle glaucoma (Heijl, 1984). The group of patients who received a 360° treatment in one session had a 24% incidence of flare and the group who received two 180° treatments had a 34% occurrence of flare.

6. ALT disrupts the blood-aqueous barrier transiently with reestablishment of the barrier by 1 month (Diestelhorst et al., 1995; Feller & Weinreb, 1984).

7. The amount of inflammation (i.e., cells and flare) apparently does not correlate with the magnitude of the early IOP spike (GLTRG, 1989). The disruption of the blood-aqueous barrier also does not correlate with the long-term IOP-reducing effects of ALT (Diestelhorst et al., 1995; Feller & Weinreb, 1984).

8. Inflammatory cells, including lymphocytes and macrophages, have been identified in the intertrabecular and juxtacanalicular spaces following ALT (Greenidge et al., 1984). The inflammatory mediators, prostaglandins, are synthesized and released by cultured human trabecular cells (Weinreb et al., 1983).

9. **Persistent iritis** (i.e., inflammation requiring treatment more than 1 week post-ALT) occurred in 0.5% to 31% of patients following ALT (Table 7–17).

10. The incidence of long-lasting iritis is less with 180° treatment than with 360° treatment (Eguchi et al., 1985).

11. The persistent iritis cases may be difficult to treat in some cases. In one case, the inflammation finally cleared up in 3 months with a sub-Tenon's steroid injection (Wilensky & Jampol, 1981). In another case, the inflammation cleared up in 9 months having persisted even after topical, systemic, and sub-Tenon's steroid therapy (Wilensky & Jampol, 1981).

Table 7–17 Occurrence of Persistent Iritis Following ALT

Occurrence (no. of ALTs)	*Amount of Angle Treated*	*Authors*
31% (36) 5% (84) 3% (37)	360 (pigment band or its posterior aspect) 180 (pigment band or its posterior aspect) 180 (anterior aspect)	Eguchi et al., 1985
7% (270) after first 180° 5% (265) after second 180°	180/180	GLTRG, 1989
0.5% (380)	360 180/180 180	Horns et al., 1986
5% (65)	360	Pohjanpelto, 1981
6% (17)	360 (repeat ALT)	Starita et al., 1984
9% (22)	360	Wilensky & Jampol, 1981

12. There are also reports of a late reaction, a **severe trabeculitis**, occurring within 1 month following ALT in two patients (Fiore et al., 1989). Both of the patients had exfoliation syndrome glaucoma and developed an elevated IOP with large inflammatory precipitates on the trabecular meshwork. Both were treated promptly with topical steroids.

13. Most studies used topical steroids or nonsteroidal anti-inflammatory drugs on every patient post-ALT. Others only used these agents if there was a significant reaction. The routine use of these drugs is probably not indicated, reserving them for significant inflammatory reactions (Weinreb & Tsai, 1996).

14. A number of steroids (e.g., prednisolone acetate, dexamethasone phosphate, and fluorometholone) and a number of nonsteroidal anti-inflammatory drugs (e.g., indomethacin, flurbiprofen, and diclofenac) have been found to be effective in treating the post-ALT inflammation (Ascaso et al., 1992; Diestelhorst et al., 1995; Goethals et al., 1994; Herbort et al., 1993; Huk et al., 1991; Mermoud et al., 1992c; Shin et al., 1996; Weinreb et al., 1984; West, 1992). There is one report suggesting that flurbiprofen and indomethacin do not significantly affect the anterior chamber reaction compared to placebo (Hotchkiss et al., 1984). When the more objective laser flare-cell meter was used to measure the amount of cells and flare, flurbiprofen, diclofenac, and prednisolone acetate were shown to be very efficient at treating the post-ALT inflammation (Diestelhorst et al., 1995; Herbort et al., 1993; Huk et al., 1991; Mermoud et al., 1992c).

15. The use or nonuse of topical nonsteroidal anti-inflammatory agents or steroids did not significantly influence the IOP-lowering effect of ALT or its success rate (Herbort et al., 1993; Kim et al., 1998; Pappas et al., 1985; Ruderman et al., 1983; Shin et al., 1996; Thomas et al., 1982b; Ustundag & Diestelhorst, 1997; Weinreb et al., 1984). Hotchkiss and colleagues (1984) reported no significant influence of indomethacin on the IOP-lowering effect of ALT, but apparently did detect a significantly smaller decrease in IOP when using flurbiprofen compared to placebo. After pretreatment with indomethacin or placebo, Gelfand and Wolpert (1985) found no statistically significant difference in pressure lowering at 1 week post-ALT, but did find that the placebo group had a significantly larger IOP drop compared to the indomethacin group after 1 month. There is one report that fluorometholone significantly prolongs the duration of success post-ALT (Hollo, 1997), and there is another report that concludes that this steroid does not influence the long-term outcome (Kim et al., 1998).

16. Likewise, the use of nonsteroidal anti-inflammatory agents or steroids did not significantly affect the transient IOP spike following ALT (Ascaso et al., 1992; Pappas et al., 1985; Ruderman et al., 1983).

17. One study reported that the use of 1% apraclonidine resulted in a smaller magnitude and duration of flare compared to the use of a placebo (Shimizu et al., 1991).

18. Thus, **to minimize the inflammation after ALT**:
    a. **treat 180°** of the angle per session
    b. **use nonsteroidal anti-inflammatory drugs or steroids** when there is a significant inflammatory reaction or routinely.

D. *Hemorrhage/Hyphema*

1. The occurrence of hemorrhage during or after ALT ranges from 0% to 9% (Table 7–18).

2. The site of the hemorrhage appears to be the trabecular meshwork at the laser burn site or at an adjacent area (Thomas et al., 1982a,b). The blood may come from Schlemm's canal or from a blood vessel on the trabecular meshwork (Goldberg, 1985; Thomas et al., 1982b; Wise, 1981).

3. The blood usually clears fairly quickly (Pavan et al., 1992; Thomas et al., 1982b). Occasionally the blood may obscure the trabecular meshwork and necessitate postponement of the laser session until the blood clears.

4. No correlation has been found between the presence of hemorrhage and any effect on long-term IOP reduction (Thomas et al., 1982a).

Table 7–18 Occurrence of Hemorrhage Following ALT

Occurrence of Hemorrhage (no. of ALTs)	*Authors*
1.4% (143)	Atmaca & Karel, 1993
2.3% (154)	Belgrado et al., 1988
0% (10)	Brancato et al., 1991
2% overall (155) 6% 360° treatment (36) 1% 180° (pigment band & posterior) (84) 0% 180° (anterior) (37)	Eguchi et al., 1985
1.9% (54)	Elsas & Harstad, 1983
1% (237)	Goldberg, 1985
9% (159)	Moulin et al., 1991
5% (82)	Schwartz & Kopelman, 1983
6% (35)	Schwartz et al., 1981
2.3% (300)	Thomas et al., 1982a
2.6% (114)	Thomas et al., 1982b
3% (30)	Thomas et al., 1984
3.8% (131)	Tuulonen & Airaksinen, 1983
5% (56)	Wise & Witter, 1979 Wise, 1981

5. Occasionally small hyphemas occur (Belgrado et al., 1988; Brooks & Gillies, 1984; Horns et al., 1983; Hoskins et al., 1983; Thomas, 1984). When noted, hyphemas have been reported to occur in from 0.3% to as many as 2% of patients (Belgrado et al., 1988; Brooks & Gillies, 1984; Horns et al., 1983).

6. To prevent bleeding, focus accurately.

7. **If bleeding occurs:**
   a. **Tamponade** by applying gentle pressure on the globe **with the laser contact lens**.
   b. **Use low power, large spot size laser burns to coagulate** the blood vessel if the bleeding persists (e.g., 250 µm, 0.2 sec, 250 mW) (Thomas et al., 1982a,b).

E. Corneal Burns

1. Mild, transient corneal epithelial opacities have been reported to occur frequently (Pohjanpelto, 1981; Schwartz et al., 1981; Wilensky & Jampol, 1981; Wise, 1981). These burns heal very quickly with no sequelae. One study stated that these epithelial burns occurred in 25% of patients following ALT (Wilensky & Jampol, 1981). Thomas (1984) also noted large, transient opacities during ALT in a patient with severe map-dot-fingerprint epithelial dystrophy.

2. Endothelial damage has been reported but is very uncommon (Hoskins et al., 1983; Wise, 1981). However, one study noted endothelial lesions in 4.6% of patients after ALT (Belgrado et al., 1988).

3. No statistically significant difference in endothelial cell size was noted in two studies (Brubaker & Liesegang, 1983; Traverso et al., 1984). However, one study did note a significant increase in endothelial cell size both 6 months and 1 year after ALT (Hong et al., 1983).

4. To prevent corneal burns, use the minimum laser power necessary and focus accurately.

F. Keratopathy

1. Traumatic keratopathy has been reported in 3% of patients after ALT (Fellman et al., 1984). Corneal abrasion has also been seen in patients following ALT (Hoskins et al., 1983; Sherwood, 1990). These occurrences are probably associated with the use of the goniolens.

2. Keratitis was noted in 2.3% of post-ALT patients in another study (Belgrado et al., 1988).

3. Punctate keratopathy has also been reported in both the treated and untreated eyes from the use of topical anesthetic and the reduced blink rate (Horns et al., 1983).

G. *Corneal Edema/Decompensation*

1. Epithelial edema has been reported to occur in 3.1% (Belgrado et al., 1988) and 9% (Wilensky & Jampol, 1981) of patients following ALT. In the patients reported by Wilensky and Jampol (1981), one had Fuch's endothelial dystrophy and the other had Chandler's syndrome.

2. Severe corneal decompensation has been noted by Traverso and colleagues (1984) in four patients after ALT. These involved edema and persistent keratitis and were treated with a bandage contact lens. In all four cases, there was a pre-existing corneal problem, like Fuch's endothelial dystrophy or keratitis sicca.

3. Wise (1981) also noted a case of bullous keratopathy in a patient that had a unilateral post-traumatic endothelial dystrophy and developed the keratopathy 16 months following ALT.

4. To minimize the possibility of corneal decompensation, consider excluding patients with preexisting corneal problems.

H. *Mild Ocular Pain*

1. Occasionally ocular pain has been reported during and/or after ALT.

2. According to Goldberg (1985), this pain only occurred when the laser power was excessive or when the ciliary body or iris were accidentally treated. He reported minor tenderness in the globe of 20% of his patients 24 hours post-ALT.

3. When comparing diode laser trabeculoplasty to ALT, Moriarty and colleagues (1993b) found that pain occurred in 33% of eyes post-ALT and in 0% of eyes post-DLT. During DLT, a mild, pricking sensation was noted by some patients, although none complained of pain or discomfort after DLT (Moriarty et al., 1993a).

4. Thomas (1984) noted that ocular pain is rare and may be associated with laser treatments that involve the posterior trabecular meshwork more than the anterior. If the ciliary body is avoided, pain was also found to be minimal by Weinreb and Wilensky (1984).

5. Pohjanpelto (1981) also mentioned that some patients experienced mild sensations of pain during ALT.

6. To prevent ocular pain, focus accurately and avoid the iris, ciliary body, and posterior meshwork.

I. *Syncope*

1. Syncope has been noted as occurring in 1% (Hoskins et al., 1983) and 2% (Schwartz & Kopelman, 1983) of patients during ALT. Weinreb and Wilensky (1984) also noted its occurrence.

2. Syncope may be due to anxiety and/or to the ocular-cardiac reflex from pressure on the globe with the laser goniolens.

3. Counsel the patient to report any symptoms of lightheadedness or sweating.

4. Look for pallor and forehead perspiration as warning signs of impending syncope.

5. If the patient starts to become faint or actually faints during the procedure:
   a. Halt the procedure and place the patient in the supine position with feet elevated.
   b. Use an ammonia vial.
   c. Try resuming the treatment when the symptoms disappear.

J. Transient Blurred Vision

1. Transient blurred vision can occur for the first few hours post-ALT (Horns et al., 1986; Wise, 1981).

2. Transient blurred vision can occur due to:
   a. the goniolens solution
   b. punctate keratopathy from topical anesthetic and reduced blinking (Horns et al., 1986).

K. Loss of Visual Field

1. The IOP spike can go as high as 37 mm Hg above the pretreatment baseline IOP (Heijl, 1984). This kind of spike could lead to a loss of visual field in potentially susceptible patients (Hoskins et al., 1983; Levene, 1983; Spaeth, 1985; Thomas et al., 1982a; Weinreb et al., 1983b).

2. The occurrence of reported visual field loss after ALT has ranged from 0% to 60% (Table 7–19).

3. Progressive visual field loss could be a result of:
   a. the occurrence of IOP spikes
   b. inadequate IOP reduction
   c. factors unrelated to IOP

4. Some of the differences in reported occurrences of visual field loss are probably due to differences in:
   a. visual field testing techniques (e.g., Friedman versus Goldmann versus automated methods)
   b. types of glaucoma
   c. initial IOPs
   d. laser trabeculoplasty technique

5. Visual field deterioration has been noted in patients even when their response to ALT is good and their pressures are in the statistically normal region (Heijl & Bengtsson, 1984; Hoskins et al., 1983; Lieberman et al., 1983).

6. Gillies and colleagues (1994) found a correlation between the post-ALT IOP and the amount of visual field deterioration; the higher the post-ALT IOP, the more visual field loss was noted.

Table 7–19 Visual Field Loss Following ALT

Occurrence of Visual Field Loss (no. of patients)	Treatment	Authors
0% (61)	ALT	Elsas et al., 1994
13.6% (82)	ALT	Fink et al., 1988
26% (23)	ALT	Fellman et al., 1984
11% (44)–overall	ALT	Gillies et al., 1994
5% (16)–post-ALT IOP 10–15		
12% (20)–post-ALT IOP 16–20		
22% (8)–post-ALT IOP > 20		
23% (261)–noted at least once	ALT first	GLTRG, 1995
12% (261)–persistent		
60% (35)	ALT first	Hitchings et al., 1991
13% (54)	ALT	Hoskins et al., 1983
2.5% (159)	ALT	Levene, 1983
11% (53)	ALT	Lieberman et al., 1983
26% (19)	ALT	Schultz et al., 1987
23% (13)	ALT	Starita et al., 1984
19% (232)	ALT	Traverso et al., 1986
31% (261)–noted at least once	Medications first	GLTRG, 1995
15% (261)–persistent		
57% (38)	Medications first	Hitchings et al., 1991
40% (57)	Medications first	Jay & Allan, 1989
24.6% (61)	Medications first	Phelps, 1979
15.6% (64)	Medications maintained	
65% (49)	Filtering surgery first	Hitchings et al., 1991
10% (50)	Early filtering surgery	Jay & Allan, 1989
3.8% (52)	Early filtering surgery	Phelps, 1979
42% (24)	Filtering surgery	Werner et al., 1977

7. In patients with severe glaucomatous optic nerve damage, it is possible to snuff out the patient's vision. A few cases have been reported **involving loss of central vision** following ALT: 0.3% (Thomas et al., 1982a), 1.9% (Levene, 1983), and 2.5% (Weinreb et al., 1983b) of patients.

8. As can be seen from Table 7–19, the visual field loss after ALT is comparable to, or less than, the loss noted after medications or filtering surgery.

   a. The mean in 12 studies after ALT was 18%, in five studies after medication it was 30%, and in four studies after filtering surgery it was 30%.

   b. The Glaucoma Laser Trial Study Group (1995a) found that the persistent field deterioration occurred in 12% of ALT-first patients and in 31% of medications-first patients. Localized visual field improvement was noted more frequently than deterioration in both groups.

c. Hitchings and colleagues (1991) found visual field loss in 60% of ALT-first patients, 57% of medication-first patients, and 65% of filtering surgery-first patients. There was no significant difference among them even though the mean IOP of the surgery-first group was significantly lower than that of the other two groups.

L. Generalized Seizure

1. One case of generalized seizure has been reported (Pillai & Drack, 1991).

2. The patient had a history of two occasions of head trauma but no prior seizures. During ALT, the patient had a generalized, tonic-clonic seizure. This case was considered an example of photically evoked epilepsy.

M. Iris Burns

1. Wise and Witter (1979) initially reported one patient who had a few areas of minimal iris root atrophy after ALT. This patient had been treated with 2000 mW of laser power.

2. Hoskin and colleagues (1983), as well as Pohjanpelto (1981) also reported iris burns.

3. To prevent iris burns, focus accurately and avoid the iris.

N. Sector Palsy of the Iris Sphincter Muscle

1. One case of sector palsy of the iris sphincter muscle has been reported (Pfeiffer & Kommerell, 1991).

2. The palsy involved the sphincter muscle from the 2 o'clock to the 5 o'clock position. It was discovered the day after ALT and disappeared 15 months later.

3. The palsy apparently occurred because one of the parasympathetic trunks was hit by the laser near the trabecular meshwork.

O. Herpes Simplex Keratitis

1. One case has been reported of herpes simplex keratitis triggered by ALT (Reed et al., 1994).

2. Three days post-ALT, the patient developed symptoms and a classic dendritic keratitis. The patient was treated with trifluridine and vidarabine and then recovered.

P. Cystoid Macular Edema

1. Two cases have been reported in aphakes by Hoskins and colleagues (1983).

2. There is no evidence indicating a direct, causative role for ALT.

Q. Persistent Elevated IOP

1. It is possible to have persistent elevated intraocular pressure following ALT.

2. The reported occurrence of this condition ranges from 3% to 6% of patients (Atmaca & Karel, 1993; Hoskins et al., 1983; Thomas et al., 1982a).

R. Early Failure of IOP-Lowering Effect

1. Over a 1 year follow-up period, about 13% of patients experience a significant upward shift in IOP after ALT (Hoskins et al., 1983).

2. Emergency filtering surgery has been reported as necessary in 1.8% (Levene, 1983), 4.6% (Forbes & Bansal, 1981), and 11.1% (Levy & Bonney, 1982) of patients following ALT.

S. Encapsulated Blebs/Filtering Surgery Failure

1. There is a controversy in the literature as to whether ALT affects the success rate for filtering surgery as well as the rate of encapsulated bleb formation. Encapsulated blebs, also known as Tenon's capsule cysts, can lead to increased IOP.

2. A number of reports indicate that ALT does not affect the success rate for subsequent filtering surgery (Lavin et al., 1990; Oge et al., 1995; Schoenleber et al., 1987). In fact, one report found that the odds of an adverse outcome of glaucoma surgery were reduced after ALT (Coleman et al., 1998).

3. On the other hand, two reports suggest that ALT is a risk factor that decreases the success rate for subsequent filtering surgery (Johnson et al., 1994; Stuermer et al., 1993). Johnson and colleagues (1994) reported that long-term medical management and ALT were both risk factors for filtering surgery. It was not clear whether ALT is just a selection factor identifying patients that would have poor surgical outcomes (e.g., patients that had been on medical therapy) or whether the ALT treatment itself results in a poor outcome. ALT is apparently a major risk factor for filtering surgery in young (<50 years old) patients (Stuermer et al., 1993).

4. Two studies report that ALT is a risk factor for development of encapsulated blebs (Feldman et al., 1989; Richter et al., 1988). Another study suggests that ALT may be a risk factor for development of encapsulated blebs although there were a small number of cases (Oge et al., 1995).

5. However, four studies claim that ALT is not a risk factor for encapsulated blebs or at least that the data do not show a statistically significant increase in the risk (Campagna et al., 1995; Lavin et al., 1990; Schoenleber et al., 1987; Schwartz et al., 1999). Another study states that there is no increase in risk but the study had a small sample size and a low incidence of encapsulated bleb (Johnson et al., 1994).

T. Suprachoroidal Effusion

1. There is one reported case of suprachoroidal effusion following argon laser trabeculoplasty (Kennedy et al., 1996).

2. The effusion may have occurred because of the profound hypotony that developed in the first few days after the ALT.

3. Treatment involved withholding topical timolol from the involved eye for 5 weeks. By this time, the effusion had completely resolved.

U. Membrane Formation in the Chamber Angle

1. A frequent cause of ALT failure appears to be membrane formation in the chamber angle. In one study in which trabeculectomy was performed after one or more ALTs were done, 23 out of 46 eyes treated with ALT had a collagenous and cellular membrane that covered the entire trabecular meshwork (Koller et al., 2000).

2. The most important risk factor is the number of ALTs performed.

XII. Mechanism of Action

A. The mechanism of action and pathophysiology of ALT is not completely understood (Melamed, 1997).

B. Tonography studies have shown that ALT reduces IOP by increasing aqueous outflow facility (Brubaker & Liesegang, 1983; Eguchi et al., 1985; Lichter, 1982; Merte et al., 1985; Perez et al., 1992; Pohjanpelto, 1981; Pollack & Robin, 1982; Schrems et al., 1985; Schwartz et al., 1981; Thomas et al., 1982a; Wilensky & Jampol, 1981; Yablonski et al., 1985).

C. Fluorophotometric studies have shown that ALT does not significantly affect the rate of aqueous humor formation (Araie et al., 1984; Brubaker & Liesegang, 1983; Yablonski et al., 1985). Thus, the increase in aqueous outflow appears to be the most important determinant of the IOP reduction post-ALT.

D. There are two major sets of theories that attempt to explain the effect of ALT:

1. **Mechanical theories**
   a. Wise and Witter (1979) were the first to posit that thermal shrinkage of the collagen sheets at the site of the laser burn could pull open the intertrabecular spaces in between the burn sites.
   b. This thermal contraction of the collagen may open up Schlemm's canal or prevent its collapse (Moses & Arnzen, 1980; Van Buskirk, 1989; Van Buskirk et al., 1984; Wise & Witter, 1979). However, this effect may only be important at high pressures (Van Buskirk et al., 1984).

2. **Cellular and biochemical theories**
   a. There is an **initial decrease in trabecular cell density** followed by an **increase in the rate of trabecular cell division** and, thus, repopulation (Acott et al., 1989; Bylsma et al., 1988, 1994; Van Buskirk et al., 1984).
      1) There is a decrease in trabecular cells right after ALT (Alexander & Grierson, 1989; Melamed et al., 1985; Rodrigues et al., 1982; Van Buskirk, et al., 1984). There is also disruption of the trabecular beams, fibrinous exudate, and debris (Alexander et al., 1989; Koss et al., 1984; Melamed et al., 1985, 1986; Rodrigues et al., 1982; Weber et al., 1983). This debris may account for the immediate elevation in IOP often seen after ALT.

2) A population of cells in the anterior meshwork experience an increase in the rate of cell division, migrate, and then repopulate the ALT target sites (Acott et al., 1989). This involves an enhancement in DNA synthesis (Bylsma et al., 1994). The increased rate of cell division in the trabecular area has been seen in cats (Bylsma et al., 1994; Kimpel & Johnson, 1992), monkeys (Dueker et al., 1990), as well as in organ-cultured human eyes (Bylsma et al., 1988). The repopulation may be involved in an increase in meshwork function post-ALT.

3) At longer intervals after ALT, there are reports of a layer of atypical corneoendothelial cells that can occlude the meshwork (Alexander & Grierson, 1989; Melamed et al., 1986; Rodrigues et al., 1982; Van der Zypen & Fankhauser, 1984). The formation of this layer of cells appears to be even more marked when the laser burns are more posterior (Van der Zypen & Fankhauser, 1984). If this layer of cells continues to grow, it may form a physical barrier to aqueous outflow and thus help account for the loss of IOP-lowering effect with time.

b. There **are changes in the trabecular glycosaminoglycan (GAG) profiles** (Van Buskirk, 1984, 1989). GAGs line the surfaces of the trabecular cell surfaces and are a major component of the extracellular matrix in the intertrabecular spaces. The remodeling of the extracellular matrix involves matrix metalloproteinases, some of which have been shown to be increased following ALT (Parshley et al., 1995, 1996). Since much of the normal aqueous outflow resistance is mediated by the trabecular extracellular matrix, this laser-induced change may play a role in increasing the outflow facility.

c. There is **increased phagocytic activity of the trabecular cells** after ALT (Alexander & Grierson, 1989, 1992; Bylsma et al., 1988; Melamed et al., 1985; Van Buskirk et al., 1984). This increased phagocytic activity also may be involved in increasing aqueous flow through the meshwork.

d. There are **different vacuolization patterns at Schlemm's canal** (Melamed et al., 1986; Van der Zypen & Fankhauser, 1984).

e. In monkeys that were treated by ALT, there were significant **structural changes in the adjacent nonlasered areas** (Melamed et al., 1986). This included wide open intertrabecular spaces with herniations of juxtacanalicular trabecular meshwork and of inner wall endothelium across and into the lumen of Schlemm's canal. These herniations also contained large vacuoles and chronic inflammatory cells.

f. In rabbits treated by ALT, there is an immediate and short-term **increase in the concentration of endothelin-1** in the aqueous humor (Hollo & Lakatos, 1998). Endothelin-1 is a polypeptide derived from endothelium that may play a role in the IOP changes after ALT.

g. In human glaucomatous eyes, ALT **increases protein synthesis within 24 hours after treatment and inhibits it after 24 hours** (Babizhayev et al., 1990).

h. There is **accumulation of fibronectin deposits** in the aqueous drainage channels after ALT (Babizhayev et al., 1990). This increase in fibronectin adhesion proteins may play a role in the tightening process posited by Wise and Witter (1979).

i. There is an **inflammatory response** that is stimulated in the eye following ALT (see previous discussion on *Inflammation* in section XI: C).

References

Acott TS et al. Trabecular repopulation by anterior trabecular meshwork cells after laser trabeculoplasty. Am J Ophthalmol 107:1–6 (1989).

AGIS Investigators. The Advanced Glaucoma Intervention Study (AGIS): 4. Comparison of treatment outcomes within race. Seven-year results. Ophthalmology 105:1146–1164 (1998).

AGIS Investigators. The Advanced Glaucoma Intervention Study (AGIS): 9. Comparison of glaucoma outcomes in black and white patients within treatment groups. Am J Ophthalmol 132:311–320 (2001).

Alexander RA, Grierson I. Morphological effects of argon laser trabeculoplasty upon the glaucomatous human meshwork. Eye 3:719–726 (1989).

Alexander RA, Grierson I. Argon laser trabeculoplasty: morphologic effects on the trabecular meshwork. Glaucoma 14:48–56 (1992).

Alexander RA, Grierson I, Church WH. The effect of argon laser trabeculoplasty upon the normal human trabecular meshwork. Graefes Arch Clin Exp Ophthalmol 227:72–77 (1989).

Allf BE, Shields MB. Early intraocular pressure response to laser trabeculoplasty 180° without apraclonidine versus 360° with apraclonidine. Ophthalmic Surg 22:539–542 (1991).

Alvarado J, Murphy C, Juster R. Trabecular meshwork cellularity in primary open-angle glaucoma and nonglaucomatous normals. Ophthalmology 91:564–579 (1984).

American Academy of Ophthalmology. Laser trabeculoplasty for primary open-angle glaucoma. Ophthalmology 103:1706–1712 (1996a).

American Academy of Ophthalmology. Preferred Practice Patterns Committee Glaucoma Panel. Preferred practice pattern: Primary open-angle glaucoma. American Academy of Ophthalmology, San Francisco, 1996b.

Amon M et al. Long-term follow-up of argon laser trabeculoplasty in uncontrolled primary open-angle glaucoma. Ophthalmologica 200:181–188 (1990).

Araie M et al. Effects of laser trabeculoplasty on the human aqueous humor dynamics: a fluorophotometric study. Ann Ophthal 16:540–544 (1984).

Ascaso FJ et al. Effects of topical diclofenac sodium administered before argon laser trabeculoplasty: a double-blind comparison versus dexamethasone phosphate eye drops. Lasers Light Ophthalmol 5:29–33 (1992).

Atmaca LS, Karel F. Argon laser trabeculoplasty in primary open-angle glaucoma. Glaucoma 15:78–79 (1993).

Babizhayev MA et al. Clinical, structural and molecular phototherapy effects of laser irradiation on the trabecular meshwork of human glaucomatous eyes. Graefes Arch Clin Exp Ophthalmol 228:90–100 (1990).

Balacco Gabrieli C et al. Open clinical statistical study on the effects of argon laser trabeculoplasty. Glaucoma 15:90–94 (1993).

Barnebey HS et al. The efficacy of brimonidine in decreasing elevations in intraocular pressure after laser trabeculoplasty. Ophthalmology 100:1083–1088 (1993).

Barnes SD et al. Control of intraocular pressure elevations after argon laser trabeculoplasty. Comparison of brimonidine 0.2% to apraclonidine 1.0%. Ophthalmology 106:2033–2037 (1999).

Belgrado G et al. Comparison of argon and cw.Nd.YAG laser trabeculoplasty. Clinical results. In Marshall J, ed. Laser technology in ophthalmology. Amsterdam, Netherlands: Kugler & Ghedini Publications, 1988; 45–52.

Bergea B. Some factors affecting the intraocular pressure reduction after argon laser trabeculoplasty in open-angle glaucoma. Acta Ophthalmol 62:696–704 (1984).

Bergea B. Repeated argon laser trabeculoplasty. Acta Ophthalmol 64:246–250 (1986a).

Bergea B. Intraocular pressure reduction after argon laser trabeculoplasty in open-angle glaucoma. A two-year follow-up. Acta Ophthalmol 64:401–406 (1986b).

Bergea B, Bodin L, Svedbergh B. Primary argon laser trabeculoplasty vs pilocarpine. II: Long-term effects on intraocular pressure and facility of outflow. Study design and additional therapy. Acta Ophthalmol 72:145–154 (1994).

Bergea B, Svedbergh B. Primary argon laser trabeculoplasty vs. pilocarpine. Short-term effects. Acta Ophthalmol 70:454–460 (1992).

Birt CM et al. One vs. two doses of 1.0% apraclonidine for prophylaxis of intraocular pressure spike after argon laser trabeculoplasty. Can J Ophthalmol 30:266–269 (1995).

Blondeau P, Roberge JF, Asselin Y. Long-term results of low power, long duration laser trabeculoplasty. Am J Ophthalmol 104:339–342 (1987).

Blumenthal EZ, Serpetopoulos CN. On focusing the slit-lamp: Part I. An inaccurate ocular setting—what is there to lose? Surv ophthalmol 42:351–354 (1998).

Brancato R, Carassa R, Trabucchi G. Diode laser compared with argon laser for trabeculoplasty. Am J Ophthalmol 112:50–55 (1991).

Brimonidine-ALT Study Group. Effect of brimonidine 0.5% on intraocular pressure spikes following 360° argon laser trabeculoplasty. Ophthalmic Surg Lasers 26:404–409 (1995).

Brooks AMV et al. Preventing a high rise in intraocular pressure after laser trabeculoplasty. Aust NZ J Ophthalmol 15:113–117 (1987).

Brooks AMV, Gillies WE. Do any factors predict a favourable response to laser trabeculoplasty? Aust J Ophthalmol 12:149–153 (1984).

Brooks AMV, Gillies WE. Laser trabeculoplasty—argon or diode? Aust NZ J Ophthalmol 21:161–164 (1993).

Brooks AMV, West RH, Gillies WE. Argon laser trabeculoplasty five years on. Aust NZ J Ophthalmol 16:343–351 (1988).

Brown JD, Brubaker RF. A study of the relation between intraocular pressure and aqueous humor flow in the pigment dispersion syndrome. Ophthalmology 96:1468–1470 (1989).

Brown RH et al. ALO 2145 reduces the intraocular pressure elevation after anterior segment surgery. Ophthalmology 95:378–384 (1988).

Brown SVL, Thomas JV, Simmons RJ. Laser trabeculoplasty re-treatment. Am J Ophthalmol 99:8–10 (1985).

Brubaker RF, Liesegang TJ. Effect of trabecular photocoagulation on the aqueous humor dynamics of the human eye. Am J Ophthalmol 96:139–147 (1983).

Bylsma SS et al. Trabecular cell division after argon laser trabeculoplasty. Arch Ophthalmol 106:544–547 (1988).

Bylsma SS et al. DNA replication in the cat trabecular meshwork after laser trabeculoplasty in vivo. J Glaucoma 3:36–43 (1994).

Campagna JA, Munden PM, Alward WLM. Tenon's cyst formation after trabeculectomy with mytomycin C. Ophthalmic Surg 26:57–60 (1995).

Chevrier RL et al. Apraclonidine 0.5% versus brimonidine 0.2% for the control of intraocular pressure elevation following anterior segment laser procedures. Ophthalmic Surg Lasers 30:199–204 (1999).

Chung HS et al. Chronic use of apraclonidine decreases its moderation of post-laser intraocular pressure spikes. Ophthalmology 104:1921–1925 (1997).

Chung PY et al. Five-year results of a randomized, prospective, clinical trial of diode vs argon laser trabeculoplasty for open-angle glaucoma. Am J Ophthalmol 126:185–190 (1998).

Coleman AL, Yu F, Greenland S. Factors associated with elevated complication rates after partial-thickness or full-thickness glaucoma surgical procedures in the United States during 1994. Ophthalmology 105:1165–1169 (1998).

Damji KF et al. Selective laser trabeculoplasty *v* argon laser trabeculoplasty: a prospective randomised clinical trial. Br J Ophthalmol 83:718–722 (1999).

Dapling RB, Cunliffe IA, Longstaff S. Influence of apraclonidine and pilocarpine alone and in combination on post laser trabeculoplasty pressure rise. Br J Ophthalmol 78:30–32 (1994).

David R et al. Brimonidine in the prevention of intraocular pressure elevation following argon laser trabeculoplasty. Arch Ophthalmol 111:1387–1390 (1993).

de Heer LJ, Peperkamp E. Experiences with laser trabeculopuncture. Doc Ophthalmol 46:317–324 (1979).

Del Priore LV, Robin AL, Pollack IP. Long-term follow-up of neodymium:YAG laser angle surgery for open-angle glaucoma. Ophthalmology 95:277–281 (1988).

Dieckert JP, Mainster MA, Ho PC. Contact lenses for laser applications. Ophthalmology 91 (suppl):79–87 (1984).

Diestelhorst M, Thull D, Krieglstein GK. The effect of argon laser trabeculoplasty on the blood-aqueous barrier and intraocular pressure in human glaucomatous eyes treated with diclofenac 0.1%. Graefes Arch Clin Exp Ophthalmol 233:559–562 (1995).

Dreyer EB, Gorla M. Laser trabeculoplasty in the pseudophakic patient. J Glaucoma 2:313–315 (1993).

Dueker DK et al. Stimulation of cell division by argon and Nd:YAG laser trabeculoplasty in cynomolgus monkeys. Invest Ophthalmol Vis Sci 31:115–124 (1990).

Eendebak GR, Boen-tan TN, Bezemer PD. Long-term follow-up of laser trabeculoplasty. Doc Ophthalmol 75:203–214 (1990).

Eguchi S et al. Methods of argon laser trabeculoplasty, complications and long-term follow-up of the results. Jpn J Ophthalmol 29:198–211 (1985).

Elsas T et al. Pressure increase following primary laser trabeculoplasty. Effect on the visual field. Acta Ophthalmol 72:297–302 (1994).

Elsas T, Harstad HK. Laser trabeculoplasty in open angle glaucoma. Acta Ophthalmol 61:991–997 (1983).

Elsas T, Johnsen H. Long-term efficacy of primary laser trabeculoplasty. Br J Ophthalmol 75:34–37 (1991).

Elsas T, Johnsen H, Stang O. Pilocarpine to prevent acute pressure increase following primary laser trabeculoplasty. Eye 5:390–394 (1991).

Englert JA et al. Argon vs diode laser trabeculoplasty. Am J Ophthalmol 124:627–631 (1997).

Epstein DL et al. Neodymium:YAG laser trabeculopuncture in open-angle glaucoma. Ophthalmology 92:931–937 (1985).

Fankhauser F. The Q-switched laser: principles and clinical results. In: Trokel SL, ed. YAG laser ophthalmic microsurgery. Norwalk, CT: Appleton-Century-Crofts, 1983:127.

Farrar SK et al. Optical properties of human trabecular meshwork in the visible and near-infrared region. Lasers Surg Med 25:348–362 (1999).

Feldman RM et al. Risk factors for the development of tenon's capsule cysts after trabeculectomy. Ophthalmology 96:336–341 (1989).

Feldman RM et al. Long-term efficacy of repeat argon laser trabeculoplasty. Ophthalmology 98:1061–1065 (1991).

Feller DB, Weinreb RN. Breakdown and reestablishment of blood-aqueous barrier with laser trabeculoplasty. Arch Ophthalmol 102:537–538 (1984).

Fellman RL et al. Argon laser trabeculoplasty following failed trabeculectomy. Ophthalmic Surg 15:195–198 (1984).

Fink AI et al. Therapeutic limitations of argon laser trabeculoplasty. Br J Ophthalmol 72:263–269 (1988).

Fiore PM, Melamed S, Epstein DL. Trabecular precipitates and elevated intraocular pressure following argon laser trabeculoplasty. Ophthalmic Surg 20:697–701 (1989).

Follmann P et al. Changes in the fine structure of the rabbit trabeculum following argon and Nd:YAG laser trabeculoplasty. Ophthalmologica Hungarica 131:17–21 (1994).

Forbes M, Bansal RK. Argon laser goniophotocoagulation of the trabecular meshwork in open-angle glaucoma. Trans Am Ophthalmol Soc 79:257–272 (1981).

Frenkel REP et al. Laser trabeculoplasty: how little is enough? Ophthalmic Surg Lasers 28:900–904 (1997).

Fukuchi T et al. Nd:YAG laser trabeculopuncture (YLT) for glaucoma with traumatic angle recession. Graefes Arch Clin Exp Ophthalmol 231:571–576 (1993).

Gaasterland D, Kupfer C. Experimental glaucoma in the rhesus monkey. Invest Ophthalmol 13:455–457 (1974).

Galin MA et al. Does laser trabeculoplasty prevent steroid glaucoma? Ophthalmic Surg Lasers 31:107–110 (2000).

Gelfand YA, Wolpert M. Effects of topical indomethacin pretreatment on argon laser trabeculoplasty: a randomized, double-masked study on black South Africans. Br J Ophthalmol 69:668–672 (1985).

Ghosh B et al. Argon laser trabeculoplasty for uncontrolled open-angle glaucoma in Indian eyes. Ann Ophthalmol 28:263–266 (1996).

Gilbert CM, Brown RH, Lynch MG. The effect of argon laser trabeculoplasty on the rate of filtering surgery. Ophthalmology 93:362–365 (1986).

Gillies WE, Dallison IW, Brooks AMV. Long-term results with argon laser trabeculoplasty. Aust NZ J Ophthalmol 22:39–43 (1994).

Glaucoma Laser Trial Research Group. The Glaucoma Laser Trial I. Acute effects of argon laser trabeculoplasty on Intraocular pressure. Arch Ophthalmol 107:1135–1142 (1989).

Glaucoma Laser Trial Research Group. The Glaucoma Laser Trial (GLT) 2. Results of argon laser trabeculoplasty versus topical medicines. Ophthalmology 97:1403–1413 (1990).

Glaucoma Laser Trial Research Group. The Glaucoma Laser Trial (GLT): 6. Treatment group differences in visual field changes. Am J Ophthalmol 120:10–22 (1995a).

Glaucoma Laser Trial Research Group. The Glaucoma Laser Trial (GLT) and Glaucoma Laser Trial Follow-up Study: 7. Results. Am J Ophthalmol 120:718–731 (1995b).

Goethals M, Missotten L. The Belgian Study Group on Glaucoma. Efficacy and safety of indomethacin 0.1% versus flurbiprofen 0.03% eyedrops in inflammation after argon laser trabeculoplasty. Doc Ophthalmol 85:287–293 (1994).

Goldberg I. Argon laser trabeculoplasty and the open-angle glaucomas. Aust NZ J Ophthalmol 13:243–248 (1985).

Goldmann DB, Mellin KB. Die Argon-Laser-trabekuloplastik bei speziellen Formen des Offenwinkel-Glaukoms. Klin Mbl Augenheilk 191:13–15 (1987).

Gracner T. Intraocular pressure response to selective laser trabeculoplasty in the treatment of primary open-angle glaucoma. Ophthalmologica 215:267–270 (2001).

Grayson D et al. Initial argon laser trabeculoplasty to the inferior vs. superior half of trabecular meshwork [letter]. Arch Ophthalmol 112:446–447 (1994).

Grayson DK et al. Long-term reduction of intraocular pressure after repeat argon laser trabeculoplasty. Am J Ophthalmol 106:312–321 (1988).

Grayson DK et al. Influence of treatment protocol on the long-term efficacy of argon laser trabeculoplasty. J Glaucoma 2:7–12 (1993).

Greenidge KC et al. Acute intraocular pressure elevation after argon laser trabeculoplasty and iridectomy: a clinicopathologic study. Ophthalmic Surg 15:105–110 (1984).

Greenidge KC, Spaeth GL, Fiol-Silva Z. Effect of argon laser trabeculoplasty on the glaucomatous diurnal curve. Ophthalmology 90:800–804 (1983).

Grinich NP, Van Buskirk EM, Samples JR. Three-year efficacy of argon laser trabeculoplasty. Ophthalmology 94:858–861 (1987).

Guzey M et al. Effects of frequency-doubled Nd:YAG laser trabeculoplasty on diurnal intraocular pressure variations in primary open-angle glaucoma. Ophthalmologica 213:214–218 (1999).

Hartenbaum D et al. A randomized study of dorzolamide in the prevention of elevated intraocular pressure after anterior segment laser surgery. J Glaucoma 8:273–275 (1999).

Heijl A. One- and two-session laser trabeculoplasty. A randomized, prospective study. Acta Ophthalmol 62:715–724 (1984).

Heijl A, Bengtsson B. The short-term effect of laser trabeculoplasty on the glaucomatous visual field. A prospective study using computerized perimetry. Acta Ophthalmol 62:705–714 (1984).

Herbort CP et al. Anti-inflammatory effect of diclofenac drops after argon laser trabeculoplasty. Arch Ophthalmol 111:481–483 (1993).

Higginbotham EJ, Richardson TM. Response of exfoliation glaucoma to laser trabeculoplasty. Br J Ophthalmol 70:837–839 (1986).

Higgins RA. Two years' experience with laser trabeculoplasty. Aust NZ J Ophthalmol 13:237–241 (1985).

Hitchings RA. Combined dye and argon laser treatment for narrow angle glaucoma. Trans Ophthalmol Soc UK 104:52–54 (1984).

Hitchings RA, Migdal CM, Fitzke F. Intraocular pressure control: does it protect the visual fields? In Krieglstein GK, ed. Glaucoma update IV. Berlin, Germany: Springer-Verlag, 1991; 179–182.

Hollo G. Argon and low energy, pulsed Nd:YAG laser trabeculoplasty. Acta Ophthalmol Scand 74:126–131 (1996).

Hollo G. Effect of topical anti-inflammatory treatment on the outcome of laser trabeculoplasty [letter]. Am J Ophthalmol 123:570–571 (1997).

Hollo G, Lakatos P. Increase of endothelin-1 concentration in aqueous humour induced by argon laser trabeculoplasty in the rabbit. A preliminary study. Acta Ophthalmol Scand 76:289–293 (1998).

Holmwood PC et al. Apraclonidine and argon laser trabeculoplasty. Am J Ophthalmol 114:19–22 (1992).

Hong C, Kitazawa Y, Tanishima T. Influence of argon laser treatment of glaucoma on corneal endothelium. Jpn J Ophthalmol 27:567–574 (1983).

Honrubia FM et al. Long term follow-up of the argon laser trabeculoplasty in eyes treated 180° and 360° of the trabeculum. Intl Ophthalmol 16:375–379 (1992).

Horns DJ et al. Argon laser trabeculoplasty for open angle glaucoma. A retrospective study of 380 eyes. Trans Ophthalmol Soc UK 103:288–295 (1983).

Hoskins HD et al. Complications of laser trabeculoplasty. Ophthalmology 90:796–799 (1983).

Hotchkiss ML et al. Nonsteroidal anti-inflammatory agents after argon laser trabeculoplasty. A trial with flurbiprofen and indomethacin. Ophthalmology 91:969–976 (1984).

Hugkulstone CE. Two-year follow-up of intra-ocular pressure control with long duration argon laser trabeculoplasty. Acta Ophthalmol 71:327–331 (1993).

Hugkulstone CE. Argon laser trabeculoplasty with standard and long duration. Acta Ophthalmol 68:579–581 (1990).

Huk B, Garus H-J, Bleckmann H. Antiinflammatorische Behandlung nach Argonlasertrabekuloplastik. Ophthalmologica 20:24–29 (1991).

Jampel HD. Initial treatment for open-angle glaucoma—medical, laser, or surgical? Laser trabeculoplasty is the treatment of choice for chronic open-angle glaucoma. Arch Ophthalmol 116:240–241 (1998).

Jay JL, Allan D. The benefit of early trabeculectomy versus conventional management in primary open angle glaucoma relative to severity of disease. Eye 3:528–535 (1989).

Johnson DH et al. The effect of long-term medical therapy on the outcome of filtration surgery. Am J Ophthalmol 117:139–148 (1994).

Jorizzo PA, Samples JR, Van Buskirk EM. The effect of repeat argon laser trabeculoplasty. Am J Ophthalmol 106:682–685 (1988).

Kajiya S, Hayakawa K, Sawaguchi S. Clinical results of selective laser trabeculoplasty. Jpn J Ophthalmol 44:574–575 (2001).

Kass MA et al. The ocular hypertensive effect of 0.25% fluorometholone in corticosteroid responders. Am J Ophthalmol 102:159–163 (1986).

Keightley SJ, Khaw PT, Elkington AR. The prediction of intraocular pressure rise following argon laser trabeculoplasty. Eye 1:577–580 (1987).

Kennedy CJ, Roden DM, McAllister IL. Suprachoroidal effusion following argon laser trabeculoplasty. Aust NZ J Ophthalmol 24:279–282 (1996).

Kim YY et al. Effect of topical anti-inflammatory treatment on the long-term outcome of laser trabeculoplasty. Fluorometholone-Laser Trabeculoplasty Study Group. Am J Ophthalmol 126:721–723 (1998).

Kimpel MW, Johnson DH. Factors influencing in vivo trabecular cell replication as determined by ^{3}H-thymidine labelling; an autoradiographic study in cats. Curr Eye Res 11:297–306 (1992).

Klein HZ, Shields MB, Ernest T. Two-stage argon laser trabeculoplasty in open-angle glaucoma. Am J Ophthalmol 99:392–395 (1985).

Koller T et al. Membrane formation in the chamber angle after failure of argon laser trabeculoplasty: analysis of risk factors. Br J Ophthalmol 84:48–53 (2000).

Koss MC et al. Acute intraocular pressure elevation produced by argon laser trabeculoplasty in the cynomolgus monkey. Arch Ophthalmol 102:1699–1703 (1984).

Krasnov MM. Laseropuncture of anterior chamber angle in glaucoma. Am J Ophthalmol 75:674–678 (1973).

Krasnov MM. Q-switched laser goniopuncture. Arch Ophthalmol 92:37–41 (1974).

Krupin T et al. Intraocular pressure the day of argon laser trabeculoplasty in primary open-angle glaucoma. Ophthalmology 91:361–365 (1984).

Krupin T et al. Argon laser trabeculoplasty in black and white patients with primary open-angle glaucoma. Ophthalmology 93:811–816 (1986).

Krupin T, Stank T, Feitl ME. Apraclonidine pretreatment decreases the acute intraocular pressure rise after laser trabeculoplasty or iridotomy. J Glaucoma 1:79–86 (1992).

Kwasniewska S et al. The efficacy of cw Nd:YAG laser trabeculoplasty. Ophthalmic Surg 24:304–308 (1993).

Kwasniewska S, Fankhauser F. Goniotomy Nd:YAG laser in developmental glaucoma. In Marshall J, ed. Laser technology in ophthalmology. Amsterdam, Netherlands: Kugler & Ghedini Publications, 1988; 67–73.

Lanzetta P, Menchini U, Virgili G. Immediate intraocular pressure response to selective laser trabeculoplasty. Br J Ophthalmol 83:29–32 (1999).

Latina MA et al. Q-switched 532-nm Nd:YAG laser trabeculoplasty (selective laser trabeculoplasty). A Multicenter, pilot, clinical study. Ophthalmology 105:2082–2090 (1998).

Latina MA, Park C. Selective targeting of trabecular meshwork cells: In vitro studies of pulsed and cw laser interactions. Exp Eye Res 60:359–372 (1995).

Lavin MJ et al. The influence of prior therapy on the success of trabeculectomy. Arch Ophthalmol 108:1543–1548 (1990).

Lehto I. Long-term follow up of argon laser trabeculoplasty in pigmentary glaucoma. Ophthalmic Surg 23:614–617 (1992).

Leske MC et al. Early Manifest Glaucoma Trial: design and baseline data. Ophthalmology 106:2144–2153 (1999).

Leung KW, Gillies WE. The detection and management of the acute rise in intraocular pressure following laser trabeculoplasty. Aust NZ J Ophthalmol 14:259–262 (1986).

Levene R. Major early complications of laser trabeculoplasty. Ophthalmic Surg 14:947–953 (1983).

Levy NS, Bonney RC. Argon laser therapy in advanced open-angle glaucoma. Glaucoma 4:25–29 (1982).

Lichter PR. Argon laser trabeculoplasty. Trans Am Ophthalmol 80:288–296 (1982).

Lieberman MF, Hoskins HD, Hetherington J Jr. Laser trabeculoplasty and the glaucomas. Ophthalmology 90:790–795 (1983).

Logan P et al. Laser trabeculoplasty in the pseudo-exfoliation syndrome. Trans Ophthalmol Soc UK 103:586–587 (1983).

Lotti R et al. Argon laser trabeculoplasty: Long-term results. Ophthalmic Surg 26:127–129 (1995).

Lund O-E. Laserbehandlund des Glaukoms. Fortschr Ophthalmol 85:583–592 (1988).

Lunde MW. Argon laser trabeculoplasty in pigmentary dispersion syndrome with glaucoma. Am J Ophthalmol 96:721–725 (1983).

Lustgarten J et al. Laser trabeculoplasty. A prospective study of treatment variables. Arch Ophthalmol 102:517–519 (1984).

Martenet A-C, Schwarzenbach N. Trabeculoplastie au laser. Klin Abl Augenheilk 188:515–518 (1986).

Mattox C, Schuman JS. Laser trabeculoplasty. Seminars in Ophthalmology 7:163–171 (1992).

McHugh D et al. Diode laser trabeculoplasty (DLT) for primary open-angle glaucoma and ocular hypertension. Br J Ophthalmol 74:743–747 (1990).

McMillan TA et al. Comparison of diode and argon laser trabeculoplasty in cadaver eyes. Invest Ophthalmol Vis Sci 35:706–710 (1994).

Melamed S. Argon laser trabeculoplasty—how does it work? In Epstein DL, Allingham RR, Schuman JS, eds. Chandler and Grant's glaucoma. Baltimore, MD: William & Wilkins, 1997; 54:466–469.

Melamed S. Nd:YAG laser trabeculopuncture: obstacles and hopes on the way to glaucoma treatment. Ophthalmic Laser Therapy 2:227–237 (1987).

Melamed S et al. Q-switched neodymium-yAG laser trabeculopuncture in monkeys. Arch Ophthalmol 103:129–133 (1985).

Melamed S et al. Nd:YAG laser trabeculopuncture in angle-recession glaucoma. Ophthalmic Surg 23:31–35 (1992).

Melamed S, Latina MA, Epstein DL. Neodymium:YAG laser trabeculopuncture in juvenile open-angle glaucoma. Ophthalmology 94:163–170 (1987).

Melamed S, Pei J, Epstein DL. Short-term effect of argon laser trabeculoplasty in monkeys. Arch Ophthalmol 103:1546–1552 (1985).

Melamed S, Pei J, Epstein DL. Delayed response to argon laser trabeculoplasty in monkeys. Morphological and morphometric analysis. Arch Ophthalmol 104:1078–1083 (1986).

Mermoud A et al. Comparison of argon and Nd:YAG laser trabeculoplasty. Invest Ophthalmol Vis Sci 33 (suppl.):1159 (1992a).

Mermoud A et al. Comparaison des effets de la trabeculoplastie effectuee avec le laser Nd-yAG et le laser argon. Klin Mbl Augenheilk 200:404–406 (1992b).

Mermoud A, Pittet N, Herbort CP. Inflammation patterns after laser trabeculoplasty measured with the laser flare meter. Arch Ophthalmol 110:368–370 (1992c).

Merte HJ, von Denffer H, Hirsch B. [Aqueous humor outflow capacity after argon laser trabeculoplasty. preliminary report.] Klin Monatsbl Augenheilkd 186:220–223 (1985).

Messner D et al. Repeat argon laser trabeculoplasty. Am J Ophthalmol 103:113–115 (1987).

Migdal C. Rational choice of therapy in established open angle glaucoma. Eye 6:346–347 (1992).

Migdal C, Gregory W, Hitchings R. Long-term functional outcome after early surgery compared with laser and medicine in open-angle glaucoma. Ophthalmology 101:1651–1657 (1994).

Migdal C, Hitchings R. Primary therapy for chronic simple glaucoma. The role of argon laser trabeculoplasty. Trans Ophthalmol Soc UK 104:62–66 (1984).

Migdal C, Hitchings R. Control of chronic simple glaucoma with primary medical, surgical and laser treatment. Trans Ophthalmol Soc UK 105:653–656 (1986).

Mittra RA, Allingham RR, Shields MB. Follow-up of argon laser trabeculoplasty: Is a day-one postoperative IOP check necessary? Ophthalmic Surg Lasers 26:410–413 (1995).

Mohan H, Jain RB, Kakar SK. Laser trabeculoplasty in dark brown eyes. In Marshall J, ed. Laser technology in ophthalmology. Amsterdam, Netherlands: Kugler & Ghedini Publications, 1988; 63–65.

Moriarty AP et al. Comparison of the anterior chamber inflammatory response to diode and argon laser trabeculoplasty using a laser flare meter. Ophthalmology 100:1263–1267 (1993a).

Moriarty AP et al. Long-term follow-up of diode laser trabeculoplasty for primary open-angle glaucoma and ocular hypertension. Ophthalmology 100:1614–1618 (1993b).

Moses RA, Arnzen RJ. The trabecular mesh: a mathematical analysis. Invest Ophthalmol Vis Sci 19:1490–1497 (1980).

Moulin F, Haut J. Argon laser trabeculoplasty: a 10-year follow-up. Ophthalmologica 207:196–201 (1993).

Moulin F, Le Mer Y, Haut J. Five-year results of the first 159 consecutive phakic chronic open-angle glaucomas treated by argon laser trabeculoplasty. Ophthalmologica 202:3–9 (1991).

Nesterov AP et al. Copper vapor laser prospects in glaucoma treatment. Proc SPIE Ophthalmic Technologies VI 2673:157–162 (1996).

Odberg T. Primary argon laser trabeculoplasty after pretreatment with timolol. A safe and economic therapy of early glaucoma. Acta Ophthalmol 68:317–319 (1990).

Odberg T, Sandvik L. The medium and long-term efficacy of primary argon laser trabeculoplasty in avoiding topical medication in open angle glaucoma. Acta Ophthalmol Scand 77:176–181 (1999).

Oge I et al. The effects of argon laser trabeculoplasty on trabeculectomy. Ann Ophthalmol 27:369–373 (1995).

Pappas HR et al. Topical indomethacin therapy before argon laser trabeculoplasty. Am J Ophthalmol 99:571–575 (1985).

Parshley DE et al. Early changes in matrix metalloproteinases and inhibitors after in vitro laser treatment to the trabecular meshwork. Curr Eye Res 14:537–544 (1995).

Parshley DE et al. Laser trabeculoplasty induces stromelysin expression by trabecular juxtacanalicular cells. Invest Ophthalmol Vis Sci 37:795–804 (1996).

Pavan PR et al. Complications of laser photocoagulation. In: Weingeist TA, greed SR, eds. Laser Surgery in Ophthalmology. Practical Applications. Norwalk, CT: Appleton & Lange, 1992:185–199.

Perez DA, Vila PCF, Martin PB. Study on the aqueous humor flow measured by fluorophotometry after argon laser trabeculoplasty. Intl Ophthalmol 16:315–319 (1992).

Pfeiffer N, Kommerell G. Sector palsy of the sphincter pupillae muscle after argon laser trabeculoplasty [letter]. Am J Ophthalmol 111:511–512 (1991).

Phelps CD. Visual field defects in open-angle glaucoma: progression and regression. Doc Ophthalmol Proc Series 19:187–196 (1979).

Pillai S, Drack AV. Generalized seizure occurring during argon laser trabeculoplasty. Glaucoma 13:141–142 (1991).

Pirnazar JR et al. The efficacy of 532 nm laser trabeculoplasty. Invest Ophthalmol Vis Sci 39:S5 (1998).

Pohjanpelto P. Argon laser treatment of the anterior chamber angle for increased intraocular pressure. Acta Ophthalmol 59:211–220 (1981).

Pohjanpelto P. Late results of laser trabeculoplasty for increased intraocular pressure. Acta Ophthalmol 61:998–1008 (1983).

Pollack IP, Robin AL. Argon laser trabeculoplasty: its effect on medical control of open-angle glaucoma. Ophthalmic Surg 13:637–643 (1982).

Pollack IP, Robin AL, Sax H. The effect of argon laser trabeculoplasty on the medical control of primary open-angle glaucoma. Ophthalmology 90:785–789 (1983).

Quigley HA, Hohman RM. Laser energy levels for trabecular meshwork damage in the primate eye. Invest Ophthalmol Vis Sci 24:1305–1307 (1983).

Reed SY et al. Herpes simplex keratitis following argon laser trabeculoplasty. Ophthalmic Surg 25:640 (1994).

Reiss GR, Wilensky JT, Higginbotham EJ. Laser trabeculoplasty. Surv Ophthalmol 35:407–428 (1991).

Ren J et al. Efficacy of apraclonidine 1% versus pilocarpine 4% for prophylaxis of intraocular pressure spike after argon laser trabeculoplasty. Ophthalmology 106:1135–1139 (1999).

Richter CU. How I do laser trabeculoplasty. In Epstein DL, Allingham RR, Schuman JS, eds. Chandler and Grant's glaucoma. Baltimore, MD: Williams & Wilkins, 1997; 53:464–465.

Richter CU et al. Retreatment with argon laser trabeculoplasty. Ophthalmology 94:1085–1089 (1987).

Richter CU et al. The development of encapsulated filtering blebs. Ophthalmology 95:1163–1168 (1988).

Ritch R. A new lens for argon laser trabeculoplasty. Ophthalmic Surg 16:331–332 (1985).

Ritch R et al. Argon laser trabeculaoplasty in pigmentary glaucoma. Ophthalmology 100:909–913 (1993).

Robin AL. Argon laser trabeculoplasty medical therapy to prevent the intraocular pressure rise associated with argon laser trabeculoplasty. Ophthalmic Surg 22:31–37 (1991).

Robin AL et al. Effects of ALO 2145 on intraocular pressure following argon laser trabeculoplasty. Arch Ophthalmol 105:646–650 (1987).

Robin AL, Pollack IP. Argon laser trabeculoplasty in secondary forms of open-angle glaucoma. Arch Ophthalmol 101:382–384 (1983).

Robin AL, Pollack IP. Q-switched neodymium-yAG laser angle surgery in open-angle glaucoma. Arch Ophthalmol 103:793–795 (1985).

Rodrigues MM, Spaeth GL, Donohoo P. Electron microscopy of argon laser therapy in phakic open-angle glaucoma. Ophthalmology 89:198–210 (1982).

Rol P, Fankhauser F, Kwasniewska S. Evaluation of contact lenses for laser therapy. Part I. Lasers in Ophthalmology 1:1–20 (1986).

Rosenberg LF et al. Apraclonidine and anterior segment laser surgery. Comparison of 0.5% versus 1.0% apraclonidine for prevention of postoperative intraocular pressure rise. Ophthalmology 102:1312–1318 (1995).

Rosenblatt MA, Luntz MH. Intraocular pressure rise after argon laser trabeculoplasty. Br J Ophthalmol 71:772–775 (1987).

Rosenthal AR, Chaudhuri PR, Chiapella AP. Laser trabeculoplasty primary therapy in open-angle glaucoma. A preliminary report. Arch Ophthalmol 102:699–701 (1984).

Rouhiainen H, Leino M, Terasvirta M. The effect of some treatment variables on long-term results of argon laser trabeculoplasty. Ophthalmologica 209:21–24 (1995).

Rouhiainen H, Terasvirta M. The laser power needed for optimum results in argon laser trabeculoplasty. Acta Ophthalmol 64:254–257 (1986).

Rouhiainen H, Terasvirta ME, Tuovinen EJ. Laser power and postoperative intraocular pressure increase in argon laser trabeculoplasty. Arch Ophthalmol 105:1352–1354 (1987).

Rouhiainen H, Terasvirta ME, Tuovinen EJ. Peripheral anterior synechiae formation after trabeculoplasty. Arch Ophthalmol 106:189–191 (1988).

Roussel P, Fankhauser F. Contact glass for use with high power lasers—geometrical and optical aspects. Solution for the angle of the anterior chamber. Intl Ophthalmology 6:183–190 (1983).

Ruderman JM et al. Effects of corticosteroid pretreatment on argon laser trabeculoplasty. Am J Ophthalmol 96:84–89 (1983).

Safran MJ, Robin AL, Pollack IP. Argon laser trabeculoplasty in younger patients with primary open-angle glaucoma. Am J Ophthalmol 97:292–295 (1984).

Savitt ML, Wilensky JT. Should laser trabeculoplasty be the initial mode of treatment in open-angle glaucoma? Seminar in Ophthalmology 7:92–96 (1992).

Schoenleber DB, Bellows AR, Hutchinson BT. Failed laser trabeculoplasty requiring surgery in open-angle glaucoma. Ophthalmic Surg 18:796–799 (1987).

Schrems W et al. [Demonstration of the tonographic effect in YAG laser trabeculoplasty in chronic glaucoma.] Klin Monatsbl Augenheilkd 187:170–172 (1985).

Schultz JS et al. Intraocular pressure and visual field defects after argon laser trabeculoplasty in chronic open-angle glaucoma. Ophthalmology 94:553–557 (1987).

Schuman JS. Laser trabeculoplasty. In Epstein DL, Allingham RR, Schuman JS, eds. Chandler and Grant's glaucoma. Baltimore, MD: William & Wilkins, 1997; 52:456–463.

Schwartz AL et al. Argon laser trabecular surgery in uncontrolled phakic open angle glaucoma. Ophthalmology 88:203–212 (1981).

Schwartz AL. Argon laser trabeculoplasty in glaucoma: what's happening (survey of results of American Glaucoma Society members). J Glaucoma 2:329–335 (1993).

Schwartz AL et al. The Advanced Glaucoma Intervention Study (AGIS): 5. Encapsulated bleb after initial trabeculectomy. Am J Ophthalmol 127:8–19 (1999).

Schwartz AL, Kopelman J. Four-year experience with argon laser trabecular surgery in uncontrolled open-angle glaucoma. Ophthalmology 90:771–780 (1983).

Schwartz AL, Love DC, Schwartz MA. Long-term follow-up of argon laser trabeculoplasty for uncontrolled open-angle glaucoma. Arch Ophthalmol 103:1482–1484 (1985).

Schwartz AL, Perman KI, Whitten M. Argon laser trabeculoplasty in progressive low-tension glaucoma. Ann Ophthalmol 16:560–566 (1984).

Schwartz AL, Wilson MC, Schwartz LW. Efficacy of argon laser trabeculoplasty in aphakic and pseudophakic eyes. Ophthalmic Surg Lasers 28:215–218 (1997).

Schwartz LW et al. Variation of techniques on the results of argon laser trabeculoplasty. Ophthalmology 90:781–784 (1983).

Scrivanti M et al. Is argon laser trabeculoplasty a reliable procedure in the treatment of open-angle glaucoma? In Marshall J, ed. Laser technology in ophthalmology. Amsterdam, Netherlands: Kugler & Ghedini Publications; 1988; 57–61.

Searle AET, Rosenthal AR, Chaudhuri PR. Argon laser trabeculoplasty as primary therapy in open-angle glaucoma: a long-term follow-up. Glaucoma 12:70–75 (1990).

Sharma A, Gupta A. Primary argon laser trabeculoplasty vs pilocarpine 2% in primary open angle glaucoma: two years follow-up study. Indian J Ophthalmol 45:109–113 (1997).

Sharpe ED, Simmons RJ. Argon laser trabeculoplasty as a means of decreasing intraocular pressure from "normal" levels in glaucomatous eyes. Am J Ophthalmol 99:704–707 (1985).

Sherwood MB. Complications of argon laser trabeculoplasty. In Sherwood MB, Spaeth GL, eds. Complications of glaucoma therapy. Thorofare, NJ: Slack Incorporated, 1990; 7:89–99.

Sherwood MB, Lattimer J, Hitchings RA. Laser trabeculoplasty as supplementary treatment for primary open angle glaucoma. Br J Ophthalmol 71:188–191 (1987).

Shields MB. Textbook of glaucoma. 3rd ed. Baltimore, MD: Williams and Wilkins, 1992.

Shimizu U, Inoue T, Kitazawa Y. Quantitative measurement of the inflammatory reaction to argon laser trabeculoplasty (ALT). In Khoo CY, Ang BC, Cheah WM, Chew PTK, Lim ASM, eds. New frontiers in ophthalmology. Amsterdam, Netherlands: Elsevier Science Publishers, 1991; 929–931.

Shin DH et al. Effect of topical anti-inflammatory treatment on the outcome of laser trabeculoplasty. Am J Ophthalmol 122:349–354 (1996).

Shingleton BJ et al. Long-term efficacy of argon laser trabeculoplasty. Ophthalmology 94:1513–1518 (1987).

Shingleton BJ et al. Long-term efficacy of argon laser trabeculoplasty. A 10-year follow-up study. Ophthalmology 100:1324–1329 (1993).

Smith J. Argon laser trabeculoplasty: comparison of bichromatic and monochromatic wavelengths. Ophthalmology 91:355–360 (1984).

Spaeth GL. The effect of change in intraocular pressure on the natural history of glaucoma: lowering intraocular pressure in glaucoma can result in improvement of visual fields. Trans Ophthalmol Soc UK 104:256–264 (1985).

Spaeth GL, Baez KA. Argon laser trabeculoplasty controls one third of cases of progressive, uncontrolled, open angle glaucoma for 5 years. Arch Ophthalmol 110:491–494 (1992).

Spaeth GL et al. Argon laser trabeculoplasty in the treatment of secondary glaucoma. Trans Am Ophthalmol Soc 81:325–330 (1983).

Spurny RC, Lederer CM Jr. Krypton laser trabeculoplasty. A clinical report. Arch Ophthalmol 102:1626–1628 (1984).

Starita RJ et al. The effect of repeating full-circumference argon laser trabeculoplasty. Ophthalmic Surg 15:41–43 (1984).

Stuermer J, Broadway DC, Hitchings RA. Young patient trabeculectomy. Assessment of risk factors for failure. Ophthalmology 100:928–939 (1993).

Tabak S, deWaard PWT, Lemij HG et al. Selective laser trabeculoplasty in glaucoma. Invest Ophthalmol Vis Sci 39:S472 (1998).

Thomas JV. Laser trabeculoplasty. In Belcher CD, Thomas JV, Simmons RJ, eds. Photocoagulation in glaucoma and anterior segment disease. Baltimore, MD: Williams & Wilkins, 1984; 5:61–86.

Thomas JV et al. Argon laser trabeculoplasty as initial therapy for glaucoma. Arch Ophthalmol 102:702–703 (1984).

Thomas JV, Simmons RJ, Belcher CD III. Argon laser trabeculoplasty in the presurgical glaucoma patient. Ophthalmology 89:187–197 (1982a).

Thomas JV, Simmons RJ, Belcher CD III. Complications of argon laser trabeculoplasty. Glaucoma 4:50–52 (1982b).

Thorpe HE. A new four-mirror gonioscope. Trans Am Acad Ophthalmol Otolaryngol 70:850–851 (1966).

Threlkeld AB et al. Apraclonidine 0.5% versus 1% for controlling intraocular pressure elevation after argon laser trabeculoplasty. Ophthalmic Surg Lasers 27:657–660 (1996a).

Threlkeld AB et al. Comparative study of the efficacy of argon laser trabeculoplasty for exfoliation and primary open-angle glaucoma. J Glaucoma 5:311–316 (1996b).

Ticho U et al. Argon laser trabeculotomies in primates: evaluation by histological and perfusion studies. Invest Ophthalmol Vis Sci 17:667–674 (1978).

Ticho U, Nesher R. Laser trabeculoplasty in glaucoma. Ten-year evaluation. Arch Ophthalmol 107:844–846 (1989).

Traverso C et al. Central corneal endothelial cell density after argonlaser trabeculoplasty. Arch Ophthalmol 102:1322–1324 (1984).

Traverso CE et al. Factors affecting the results of argon laser trabeculoplasty in open-angle glaucoma. Ophthalmic Surg 17:554–559 (1986).

Traverso CE, Greenidge KC, Spaeth GL. Formation of peripheral anterior synechiae following argon laser trabeculoplasty. A prospective study to determine relationship to position of laser burns. Arch Ophthalmol 102:861–863 (1984).

Tuulonen A. Laser trabeculoplasty as primary therapy in chronic open angle glaucoma. Acta Ophthalmol 62:150–155 (1984).

Tuulonen A, Airaksinen PJ. Laser trabeculoplasty I in simple and capsular glaucoma. Acta Ophthalmol 61:1009–1015 (1983).

Tuulonen A, Airaksinen PJ, Kuulasmaa K. Factors influencing the outcome of laser trabeculoplasty. Am J Ophthalmol 99:388–391 (1985).

Tuulonen A, Niva A-K, Alanko HI. A controlled five-year follow-up study of laser trabeculoplasty as primary therapy for open-angle glaucoma. Am J Ophthalmol 104:334–338 (1987).

Tuulonen A et al. Laser trabeculoplasty versus medication treatment as primary therapy for glaucoma. Acta Ophthalmol 67:275–280 (1989).

Ustundag C, Diestelhorst M. Efficacy of argon laser trabeculoplasty: 3-year preliminary results of a prospective placebo-controlled study. Graefes Arch Clin Exp Ophthalmol 235:354–358 (1997).

Van Buskirk EM. Pathophysiology of laser trabeculoplasty. Surv Ophthalmol 33:264–272 (1989).

Van Buskirk EM. The laser step in early glaucoma therapy. Am J Ophthalmol 112:89–90 (1991).

Van Buskirk EM et al. Argon laser trabeculoplasty. Studies of mechanism of action. Ophthalmology 91:1005–1010 (1984).

Van der Zypen E et al. Morphology of the trabecular meshwork within monkey (Macaca speciosa) eyes after irradiation with the free-running Nd:YAG laser. Ophthalmology 94:171–179 (1987).

Van der Zypen E, Fankhauser F. Ultrastructural changes of the trabecular meshwork of the monkey (Macaca speciosa) following irradiation with argon laser light. Graefes Arch Clin Exp Ophthalmol 221:249–261 (1984).

Van Meter WS et al. Laser trabeculoplasty for glaucoma in aphakia and pseudophakic eyes after penetrating keratoplasty. Arch Ophthalmol 106:185–188 (1988).

Watson PG et al. Argon laser trabeculoplasty or trabeculectomy. A prospective randomized block study. Trans Ophthalmol Soc UK 104:55–61 (1984).

Weber PA, Burton GD, Epitropoulos AT. Ophthalmic Surg 20:702–706 (1989).

Weber PA, Davidorf FH, McDonald C. Scanning electron microscopy of argon laser trabeculoplasty. Ophthalmic Forum 1:26–29 (1983).

Weinreb RN et al. Influence of the number of laser burns administered on the early results of argon laser trabeculoplasty. Am J Ophthalmol 95:287–292 (1983a).

Weinreb RN et al. Immediate intraocular pressure response to argon laser trabeculoplasty. Am J Ophthalmol 95:271–286 (1983b).

Weinreb RN et al. Flurbiprofen pretreatment in argon laser trabeculoplasty for primary open-angle glaucoma. Arch Ophthalmol 102:1629–1632 (1984).

Weinreb RN, Tsai CS. Laser trabeculoplasty. In Ritch R, Shields MB, Krupin T, eds. The glaucomas. St Louis, MO: Mosby, 1996; 77:1575–1590.

Weinreb RN, Wilensky JT. Clinical aspects of argon laser trabeculoplasty. Int Ophthalmol Clin 24:79–95 (1984).

Werner EB. Surgical management of glaucomas. In Lewis TL, Fingeret M, eds. The primary care of the glaucomas. Norwalk, CT: Appleton & Lange, 1993; 15:277–294.

Werner EB, Drance SM, Schulzer M. Trabeculectomy and the progression of glaucomatous visual field loss. Arch Ophthalmol 95:1374–1377 (1977).

West RH. The effect of topical corticosteroids on laser-induced peripheral anterior synechiae. Aust NZ J Ophthalmol 20:305–309 (1992).

Wickham MG, Worthen DM. Argon laser trabeculotomy: long-term follow-up. Ophthalmology 86:495–503 (1979).

Wilensky JT. Laser trabeculoplasty. Technique. In Wilensky JT, ed. Laser therapy in glaucoma. Norwalk, CT: Appleton-Century-Crofts, 1985; 2:15–23.

Wilensky JT. Laser trabeculoplasty. In Kaufman PL, Mittag TW, eds. Glaucoma. St. Louis, MO: Mosby, 1994; III:9.31–9.36.

Wilensky JT, Jampol LM. Laser therapy for open angle glaucoma. Ophthalmology 88:213–217 (1981).

Wilensky JT, Weinreb RN. Early and late failures of argon laser trabeculoplasty. Arch Ophthalmol 101:895–897 (1983a).

Wilensky JT, Weinreb RN. Low-dose trabeculoplasty. Am J Ophthalmol 95:423–426 (1983b).

Wise JB. Long-term control of adult open angle glaucoma by argon laser treatment. Ophthalmology 88:197–202 (1981).

Wise JB. Errors in laser spot size in laser trabeculoplasty. Ophthalmology 91:186–190 (1984).

Wise JB. Ten year results of laser trabeculoplasty. Does the laser avoid glaucoma surgery or merely defer it? Eye 1:45–50 (1987).

Wise JB, Witter SL. Argon laser therapy for open-angle glaucoma. A pilot study. Arch Ophthalmol 97:319–322 (1979).

Witschel BM, Rassow B. Laser trabeculopuncture. II. Scanning electron microscopic findings. Ophthalmologica 72:45–51 (1976).

Worthen DM, Wickham MG. Laser trabeculotomy in monkeys. Invest Ophthalmol Vis Sci 12:707–711 (1973).

Worthen DM, Wickham MG. Argon laser trabeculotomy. Trans Am Acad Ophthalmol Otolaryngol 78:OP-371–375 (1974).

Yablonski ME, Cook DJ, Gray J. A fluorophotometric study of the effect of argon laser trabeculoplasty on aqueous humor dynamics. Am J Ophthalmol 99:579–582 (1985).

Yalvac IS et al. Prophylactic use of apraclonidine for intraocular pressure increase after 180-degree argon laser trabeculoplasty. Ann Ophthalmol 28:240–243 (1996).

Yumita A et al. Goniotomy with Q-switched Nd-yAG laser in juvenile developmental glaucoma: a preliminary report. Jpn J Ophthalmol 28:349–355 (1984).

Zborowski L et al. Prognostic features in laser trabeculoplasty. Acta Ophthalmol 62:142–149 (1984).

Chapter 8
Other Glaucoma Therapeutic Uses

Charles M. Wormington

I. Cyclophotocoagulation

A. Introduction

1. The usual methods for decreasing the intraocular pressure in glaucoma patients involve increasing the outflow facility of aqueous humor. This is often accomplished by laser trabeculoplasty, laser iridotomy, or by filtering surgery.

2. Cyclophotocoagulation is a procedure of last resort because of its higher complication rate. When the usual methods are not adequate, cyclodestructive procedures can be used to decrease production of aqueous humor. These procedures are used to ablate a portion of the ciliary body. In addition to laser cyclophotocoagulation, other methods such as penetrating cyclodiathermy, cyclocryotherapy, electrolysis, beta irradiation, and ultrasound therapy have been used (Mastrobattista & Luntz, 1996; Schuman, 1997; Shields, 1985; Stewart et al., 1996).

3. As its name implies, cyclophotocoagulation is a thermal method of destroying a portion of the ciliary body (Figure 8–1).
   a. The mechanisms involved in decreasing aqueous production probably involve destruction of the ciliary epithelium and destruction of ciliary vascular tissue with limited revascularization (Assia et al., 1991; Fankhauser et al., 1993; Feldman et al., 1997; Ferry et al., 1995; Hennis et al., 1991; Marsh et al., 1993; Stewart et al., 1996; Stroman et al., 1996; van der Zypen et al., 1989b).
   b. The laser radiation is absorbed by melanin in the pigmented epithelial cells of the ciliary body and in the melanocytes of the stroma (Coleman et al., 1991; Ferry et al., 1995; Fankhauser et al., 1993; Gabel et al., 1979). Some radiation is also absorbed by the blood (Fankhauser et al., 1993; Marshall & Fankhauser, 1972).
   c. Nd:YAG laser lesions have more effect on the ciliary epithelium than the ciliary muscle, whereas it is the reverse with diode lasers (Simmons et al., 1994).
   d. In addition to reduction of aqueous secretion, this laser technique may also enhance uveoscleral outflow (Liu et al., 1994).

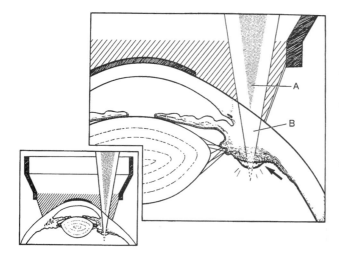

Figure 8–1 Trans-scleral cyclophotocoagulation involves focusing the beam from a thermal laser (e.g., a CW Nd:YAG laser) through the conjunctiva and sclera onto the ciliary body. (Reprinted with permission from Shields MB. Textbook of glaucoma. Baltimore, MD: Williams & Wilkins, 1998:552.)

    e. About 3% to 5% of the laser power output during transscleral cyclophotocoagulation reaches the posterior pole (Myers et al., 1998). The laser energy at the level of the posterior pole approaches or exceeds the American Conference of Governmental Industrial Hygienists guidelines. The clinical significance of this exposure is not clear.

4. Because it can visualize the ciliary body, **ultrasound biomicroscopy** may have a role to play in determining the correct position for placement of the laser probe (Brancato & Carassa, 1996). It may also be useful for assessment of both early and late changes in the ciliary body after the laser treatment, determination of ciliary body residuals before focal retreatment, and evaluation for scleral damage after the treatment.

5. Because of its ability to visualize photothermal visual changes, spectrum analysis of radio frequency (RF) ultrasound may be useful in helping to control cyclophotocoagulation (Rosenow et al., 1999).

B. Indications (Samples, 1995; Schuman, 1997). Cyclophotocoagulation is indicated in the following cases:

1. Refractory glaucomas that have failed prior filtration surgery, or for which it is expected that further filtering surgery will fail

2. Glaucomas that are likely to fail filtering surgery (e.g., inflammatory, neovascular, post-penetrating keratoplasty, or post-scleral buckling)

3. Glaucomas for which there is a high risk of complications for filtering surgery (e.g., vitrectomized aphakic eye)

4. Eyes with very poor visual prognosis, for which the treatment is basically intended to maintain comfort and prevent visual loss

5. Patients who are not surgical candidates for filtering surgery because of general medical reasons or who refuse to undergo the surgery

C. *Contraindications* (Samples, 1995). Cyclophotocoagulation is contraindicated in patients with:

1. marked uveitis

2. uncooperative attitudes

3. phakic eyes and elevated intraocular pressures with no sign of visual impairment or with well controlled pressures on tolerated medical therapy

4. blepharospasm, limbus deformation, or thinned sclera

D. *Techniques*

1. Informed consent must be obtained from the patient.

2. All preoperative anti-glaucoma medications should be continued prior to treatment.

3. Retrobulbar or peribulbar anesthesia should be administered.

4. For contact cyclophotocoagulation, the patient is in the recumbent position, and for noncontact cyclophotocoagulation, the patient is in the sitting position.

5. The total energy delivered and a treatment diagram should be documented.

6. **Transpupillary cyclophotocoagulation** (Fankhauser et al., 1993; Herschler, 1980; Kawahara et al., 1990; Kim & Moster, 1999; Lee, 1979; Lee & Pomerantzeff, 1971; March, 1986; Mastrobattista & Luntz, 1996; McDonnell et al., 1988; Shields, 1985; Shields et al., 1988b; Stewart et al., 1996; Strasser, 1985)

   a. Clinical results with this method of energy delivery have been somewhat unpredictable and disappointing.

   b. The **argon laser** (0.1 to 0.2 sec, 50 to 200 μm, 300 to 1000 mW) and the **Nd:YAG laser** (free-running mode: 20 msec, 0.2 to 0.8 J; continuous-wave mode: 0.2 to 0.4 sec, 10 W) have been used for this technique.

7. **Trans-scleral cyclophotocoagulation (TSCPC).** This is the treatment of choice by most glaucoma specialists. **Noncontact** methods involve slit-lamp delivery of the laser energy through the air. **Contact** methods involve fiberoptic probe delivery directly to the ocular surface. Transscleral delivery of radiation can be performed by any of the following laser systems:

   a. **Noncontact Nd:YAG laser** (Al-Ghamdi et al., 1993; Assia et al., 1991; Barraquer & Kargacin, 1991; Blasini et al., 1990; Blomquist et al., 1990; Cantor et al., 1989; Cohen et al., 1989; Crymes & Gross, 1990; Dickens et al., 1995; Eid et al., 1997; Fankhauser et al., 1986; Ferry et al., 1995; Fiore & Latina, 1989; Fiore et al., 1989; Geyer et al., 1993; Hampton et al., 1990; Hampton & Shields, 1988; Hardten & Brown, 1993; Klapper et al., 1988; March & Shaver, 1989; Marsh et al., 1993; Mastrobattista & Luntz, 1996; Maus & Katz, 1990; Miyazaki & Hoya, 1994; Noureddin et al., 1992; Oguri et al., 1998; Prum et al., 1992; Samples, 1995;

Schubert, 1989; Schubert et al., 1990; Schuman, 1997; Shields, 1992; Shields & Shields, 1994; Shields et al., 1988a, 1993; Simmons et al., 1990, 1991; Stewart et al., 1996; Suzuki et al., 1991; Threlkeld & Shields, 1995; Ulbig et al., 1995; Van der Zypen et al., 1989a,b; Wheatcroft et al., 1992; Youn et al., 1996, 1998; Zaidman & Wandel, 1988) (Figure 8–2)

1) The free-running mode with settings of 20 msec and 4 to 8 J has been used. For CW mode, 7 W of power for 1.5 sec has been used. Other settings have also been tried. Some advocate increasing the output until an audible "pop" is heard and then backing off (Prum et al., 1992, 1993). Others are more conservative (Schubert, 1993).

2) The beam was centered 1.0 to 1.5 mm posterior to the limbus.

3) 32 spots have been placed over 360° with 8 spots per quadrant. The 3 o'clock and 9 o'clock positions were spared in order to avoid destruction of the long posterior ciliary arteries. The treatment of 180° has been successful although the risk-to-benefit ratio may be better with an initial 360° treatment (Hardten & Brown, 1993).

4) A special contact lens has been designed for this procedure (Shields et al., 1989).

b. **Contact Nd:YAG laser** (Allingham et al., 1990; Ando & Kawai, 1993; Ayyala et al., 1998; Bechrakis et al., 1994; Benning & Pfeiffer, 1995; Bloom & Weber, 1992; Brancato et al., 1987, 1989, 1990, 1991, 1994; Coleman et al., 1991; Echelman et al., 1994, 1995; Fankhauser et al., 1992a; Higginbotham et al., 1991; Immonen et al., 1993; Iwach et al., 1991; Kermani et al., 1992; Kwasniewska et al., 1988; Latina et al., 1989; Liu et al., 1994; Mastrobattista & Luntz, 1996; Nasisse et al., 1992; Oguri et al., 1998; Phelan & Higginbotham, 1995; Preussner et al., 1997; Prum et al., 1992; Samples, 1995; Schubert, 1989; Schubert & Federman, 1989; Schuman et al., 1990b, 1992, 1997; Stewart et al., 1996; Stolzenburg et al., 1990; Takahashi & Okisaka, 1991; Van der Zypen et al., 1989a; Wei et al., 1999) (see Figure 8–2)

1) The CW mode has been used with settings of 0.7 to 1.0 sec and 7 Watts. Other variations have also been used.

2) The anterior edge of the probe should be 0.5 to 1.0 mm posterior to the limbus. This will ensure that the probe is centered 1.5 to 2.0 mm posterior to the limbus.

3) Gentle pressure should be applied with the probe against the sclera.

4) 32 spots were applied over 360° with 8 spots per quadrant (3 o'clock and 9 o'clock were spared). Other regimens have also been used.

c. **Noncontact diode laser** (Assia et al., 1991; Hawkins & Stewart, 1993; Hennis & Stewart, 1992a; Mastrobattista & Luntz, 1996; Stewart et al., 1996; Stroman et al., 1996)

1) The slit-lamp mounted CW laser has been applied with a 100-μm to 400-μm spot diameter, a 900-msec or 1-sec pulse duration, and with a power of

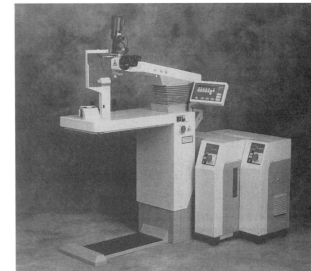

Figure 8–2 The Meridian/LASAG Microruptor III is a multi-laser system that contains a CW (thermal) Nd:YAG laser that can be used for both contact and noncontact cyclophotocoagulation. (Reprinted with permission from Samples JR. Laser cyclophotocoagulation for refractory glaucomas. Ophthalmol Clin North Am 8:401–411 (1995).)

1200 mW to 1500 mW. One study used 2 sec exposures with power between 1750 mW and 3000 mW.

2) The laser is then aimed parallel to the visual axis at the sclera 1 to 1.2 mm from the corneal limbus.

3) Thirty to 45 spots are distributed 360° around the limbus.

d. **Contact diode laser** (Aventuro et al., 1998; Bloom et al., 1997; Bock et al, 1997; Brancato et al., 1991, 1994, 1995; Chen et al., 1999; El-Harazi et al., 1998; Feldman et al., 1997; Fishbaugh, 1994; Flaxel et al., 1997; Gaasterland & Pollack, 1992; Immonen et al., 1996; Johnson, 1998; Kosoko et al., 1996; Mastrobattista & Luntz, 1996; Montanari et al., 1997; Munoz & Rebolleda, 1999; Oguri et al., 1998; Pablo et al., 1997; Palmer et al., 1997; Preussner et al., 1997; Pueyo et al., 1998; Schuman, 1997; Schuman et al., 1990a, 1991; Stewart et al., 1996; Stroman et al., 1995, 1996; Threlkeld & Johnson, 1999; Tsai et al., 1996; Ulbig et al., 1994, 1995; Walland, 1998; Walland & McKelvie, 1998; Wei et al., 1999; Wong et al., 1997; Yap-Veloso et al., 1998; Youn et al., 1998) (Figure 8–3)

1) The laser has been applied for 0.3 to 0.5 sec at 1.3 to 2.0 W, 1.3 sec at 3 W, 1.5 sec at 1.5 W, and for 2 sec at 1.25 to 3 W. It has been suggested that the power be set at the level where an audible "pop" is heard occasionally.

2) The fiberoptic has been centered 1.0 to 1.2 mm posterior to the limbus.

3) Gentle pressure is applied with the probe against the sclera.

4) 13 to 25 spots have been distributed over 270° while sparing the inferonasal quadrant (3 o'clock and 9 o'clock spared). Other studies have used 16 to 18,

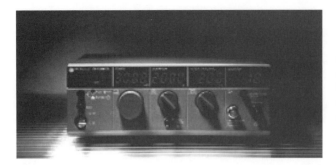

Figure 8–3 The Iris Medical Oculight SLx unit is a diode laser that can be used for contact cyclophotocoagulation. (Courtesy of Iris Medical Instruments, Mountain View, CA.)

30, and 40 spots over 360°. Treating only 270° is insufficient in many patients (Youn et al., 1998).

5) In addition to the usual 810 nm diode laser, a diode laser with a significant output at 670 nm is also being explored for cyclophotocoagulation (Immonen et al., 1996).

6) Audible "pops" can occur involving choroidal vaporization (Rebolleda et al., 1999). These pops occur more commonly in patients with higher IOPs and are associated with more severe postoperative inflammation as well as with a greater risk of postoperative hyphema.

e. **Contact krypton laser** (Di Staso et al., 1997; Immonen et al., 1993, 1994; Kivela et al., 1995)

1) The laser has been applied via a fiberoptic probe for 10 sec at 4 to 5 J per application or 350 mW (3.5 J) per application.

2) 17 to 20 applications have been made between the 5-o'clock and 9-o'clock meridians.

f. **Argon laser** (Lee et al., 1980)

g. **Ruby laser** (Beckman et al., 1972; Beckman & Waeltermann, 1984)

1) A pulsed ruby laser was delivered through a Zeiss operating microscope at either 7.5 J or 6J per pulse.

2) 32 applications were made 360° 3.5 mm from the corneo-scleral limbus.

8. **Endocyclophotocoagulation** (Haller, 1996; Uram, 1995b). This method involves the use of an intraocular laser probe to treat the ciliary processes. Most often it has been performed as an adjunct to pars plana vitrectomy in diabetic patients with neovascular glaucoma (Patel et al., 1986; Uram, 1992; Zarbin et al., 1988). An instrument has also been developed that combines an endolaser, endoscope, and light source that allows direct observation of the ciliary processes during treatment (Uram, 1992, 1995a,b). In addition to the pars plana approach, the procedure can also be carried out through a limbal cataract incision or a limbal incision in phakic patients (Chen

et al., 1997; Gayton et al., 1999; Uram, 1995a,b). Good results have been obtained with the following lasers:
  a. **Argon laser** (Lim et al., 1996; Patel et al., 1986; Shields, 1985, 1986; Shields et al., 1985; Zarbin et al., 1988)
  b. **Diode laser** (Chen et al., 1997; Gayton, 1998, 1999; Mora et al., 1997; Plager & Neely, 1999; Uram, 1992, 1994; Wallace et al., 1998)

9. **Immediate postoperative medications**
  a. Prednisolone acetate 1% and atropine sulfate 1% should be instilled after the procedure.
  b. The eye should be patched for 4 to 6 hours.
  c. An appropriate analgesic can be given for pain and discomfort.

E. *Postoperative Follow-up* (Mastrobattista & Luntz, 1996; Schuman, 1997)

1. Atropine sulfate 1% is continued BID and then tapered as the inflammation subsides.

2. Prednisolone acetate 1% is continued QID and then tapered.

3. All preoperative anti-glaucoma medications should be continued except for miotics. After the inflammation resolves, preoperative miotics may be resumed if necessary.

4. The intraocular pressure should be checked at 1 hour, 1 day, and 1 week following treatment.

5. Further follow-up will depend on the patient's response to treatment.

6. If the intraocular pressure response is inadequate at 1 month, retreatment can be performed (Figure 8–4).

F. *Complications* (Azuara-Blanco & Dua, 1999; Beadles & Smith, 1994; Bechrakis et al., 1994; Bloom et al., 1997; Edward et al., 1989; Fiore et al., 1989; Gayton, 1998; Gayton et al., 1999; Geyer et al., 1993; Gupta & Weinreb, 1997; Haller, 1996; Hardten & Brown, 1991; Jennings & Mathews, 1999; Johnson, 1998; Mastrobattista & Luntz, 1996; Maus & Katz, 1990; Mora et al., 1997; Oguri et al., 1998; Samples, 1995; Schuman, 1997; Shields & Shields, 1994; Stewart et al, 1996; Threlkeld & Johnson, 1999; Youn et al., 1996)

1. Routine
  a. Conjunctival burns and edema
  b. Mild intraocular inflammation

2. Frequent (10% to 45% of cases)
  a. Mild to severe pain
  b. Moderate to severe intraocular inflammation
  c. Reduction of visual acuity
  d. Transient intraocular pressure elevation

3. Infrequent anterior segment (less than 10% of cases)
  a. Corneal epithelial defect

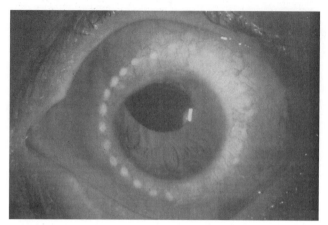

Figure 8–4 Noncontact trans-scleral Nd:YAG cyclophoto-coagulation produces conjunctival burns (white spots). Treatment with a special contact lens (Shields, 1989) results in smaller burns (lesions on the right side) compared to the larger burns on the left that result from treatment without the lens. (Reprinted with permission from Shields MB. Textbook of glaucoma. Baltimore, MD: Williams & Wilkins, 1998:556; Klapper RM, Wandel T, Donnenfeld E, Perry HD. Transscleral neodymium:YAG thermal cyclophotocoagulation in refractory glaucoma. A preliminary report. Ophthalmology 95:719–722 (1988).)

    b. Corneal graft failure
    c. Focal scleral thinning
    d. Hemorrhagic infarction of the iris
    e. Hyphema
    f. Hypopyon
    g. Posterior capsule fibrosis in pseudophakia

4. Infrequent posterior segment (less than 10% of cases)
    a. Cystoid macular edema
    b. Hypotony
    c. Malignant glaucoma
    d. Phthisis bulbi
    e. Retinal dialysis
    f. Retinal detachment
    g. Suprachoroidal hemorrhage
    h. Suprachoroidal serous effusion
    i. Transient choroidal detachment
    j. Vitreous hemorrhage

5. Rare
   a. Cataract
   b. Sympathetic ophthalmia
   c. Inadvertent sclerostomy
   d. Neurotrophic keratitis
   e. Traumatic aniridia

II. Laser Iridoplasty (Laser Gonioplasty, Laser Peripheral Iridoplasty)

A. Introduction

1. Laser iridoplasty is an alternative means for opening an appositionally closed angle when a laser iridotomy cannot be accomplished or when medical treatment fails (Chew & Yeo, 1995; Lim et al., 1993; Ritch, 1982, 1992; Ritch & Liebmann, 1996; Simmons & Simmons, 1984). Unlike iridotomy, it is not a treatment for pupillary block. It is a treatment for situations in which structural and mechanical factors in the peripheral iris and in the angle contribute to the increase in intraocular pressure.

2. The procedure involves the placement of laser burns on the peripheral iris. These burns cause contraction of the iris, hence pulling the iris away from the angle. This opens the angle, reestablishes aqueous outflow, and rapidly lowers the intraocular pressure (Ritch, 1992; Ritch & Liebmann, 1996).

3. This method was first described as **gonioplasty** (Kimbrough et al., 1979) and then evolved into the current procedure (Ritch, 1982, 1992; Ritch & Liebmann, 1996).

4. **Immediate laser iridoplasty** has also been explored as a first-line treatment for acute primary angle-closure glaucoma (Lai et al., 1999; Lam et al., 1998; Tham et al., 1999). This appears to be a safe and effective substitute for systemic medications. It helps control IOP and restore corneal clarity, allowing a subsequent laser iridotomy to be performed. Limiting the treatment to 180° also appears to be effective and safe (Lai et al., 1999).

B. Indications (Chew et al., 1991; Fu & Liaw, 1987; Ritch, 1982, 1992; Ritch & Liebmann, 1996; Schwartz, 1990; Simmons & Simmons, 1984; Weiss et al., 1992)

1. **Angle-closure glaucoma unresponsive to medical therapy**
   a. This category includes eyes where excessive corneal edema, marked inflammation, or a shallow anterior chamber preclude a laser iridotomy.
   b. This group also includes eyes that do not respond to a patent iridotomy.

2. **Angle-closure due to the size or position of the lens**
   a. An enlarged lens (i.e., in phacomorphic glaucoma) or a lens that has been pushed forward (i.e., in malignant glaucoma) can close the angle and be unresponsive to a laser iridotomy.

  b. An iridotomy should still be attempted because an element of pupil block may exist concomitantly.

3. **Nanophthalmos**
   a. Anterior chamber crowding exists in nanophthalmic eyes because of the small corneal diameter, thickened sclera, and narrow angles.
   b. When angle-closure glaucoma occurs under these conditions, laser iridotomy is not usually successful. But good pressure control usually occurs when iridoplasty is combined with an iridotomy.

4. **Plateau iris syndrome**
   a. In this syndrome the ciliary processes are anteriorly positioned. This allows the iris root to remain in contact with the angle structures even after an iridotomy.
   b. In order to make this diagnosis, an iridotomy must be done first to eliminate any pupillary block component (Figure 8–5).

5. **Retinopathy of prematurity** (ROP)
   a. The lens-iris diaphragm may shift forward in children with ROP. This can result in angle-closure that is resistant to laser iridotomy.
   b. An element of pupillary block may be present in young adults with angle-closure, so an iridotomy should still be performed.

6. **Adjunct to laser trabeculoplasty**
   a. Laser trabeculoplasty may be difficult to perform if the angle is narrow although open. There could be general narrowing because of angle crowding or a plateau iris, or there could be focal narrowing because of intraepithelial cysts or irregularities of the iris.

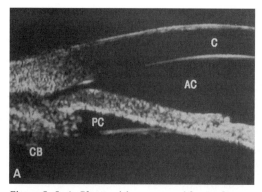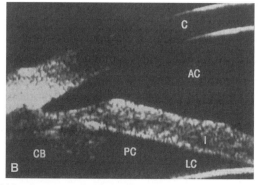

Figure 8–5 A. Plateau iris as seen with an ultrasound biomicroscope. B. Plateau iris in a similar eye after laser iridoplasty. Note how the compression of the iris root creates a space between it and the trabecular meshwork. AC = anterior chamber; C = cornea; CB = ciliary body; I = iris; LC = lens capsule; PC = posterior chamber. (Reprinted with permission from Ritch R, Liebmann JM. Argon laser peripheral iridoplasty. Ophthalmic Surg Lasers 27:289–300 (1996).)

b. As soon as the iridoplasty opens the angle enough to make the trabecular meshwork target visible, laser trabeculoplasty can be accomplished.

C. Contraindications (Ritch, 1992; Ritch & Liebmann, 1996; Simmons & Simmons, 1984)

1. **Advanced corneal edema or opacification**
   a. Corneal edema only becomes a problem when it is advanced. Because of the absorption of laser energy by the edematous or opacified cornea, the cornea may be injured during the attempt to produce iris contraction.
   b. Glycerin may be used to promote clearing of the cornea.

2. **Flat anterior chamber**
   a. When the iris is in apposition to the cornea, an attempt to contract the iris will result in heating of the aqueous just anterior to the iris and, hence, heating of the corneal endothelium. This can lead to thermal lesions of the corneal endothelium.
   b. If the iris is fairly close to the cornea, as in a very shallow anterior chamber, there should be enough time between laser applications for heat dissipation.

3. **Synechial angle closure**
   a. Often iridoplasty will not relieve synechial angle closure. This appears to be more evident in eyes with iridocorneal endothelial syndrome, neovascular glaucoma, and uveitis (Ritch & Liebmann, 1996; Schuman, 1997; Weiss et al., 1992). In these situations, iridoplasty may be harmful due to inflammation as a result of the procedure. Also, if the synechiae have been present for more than a year, it is unlikely that iridoplasty will be effective (Weiss et al., 1992).
   b. However, in chronic angle-closure glaucoma where more than three quarters of the angle revealed synechial angle closure, iridoplasty has been successful at lowering the intraocular pressure by opening at least half of the angle (Chew & Yeo, 1995; Wand, 1992). Iridoplasty is most effective if it is performed within 6 months of the formation of the synechiae (Fu & Liaw, 1987; Simmons & Simmons, 1984; Weiss et al., 1992).

D. Technique (Ritch, 1982, 1992; Ritch & Liebmann, 1996; Simmons & Simmons, 1984; Wand, 1992; Weiss et al., 1992)

1. **Pre-treatment regimen**
   a. Administer apraclonidine about 45 min prior to the procedure to blunt any intraocular pressure increase that might occur following the procedure.
   b. About 30 min or less before the treatment, 2% to 4% pilocarpine is administered to stretch the iris.
   c. A topical anesthetic is applied to the eye.
   d. A contact lens (e.g., a mirrored goniolens or an Abraham lens) can be used to position the laser beam at the periphery of the iris. A mirrored goniolens can also allow immediate evaluation of the effectiveness of the treatment.

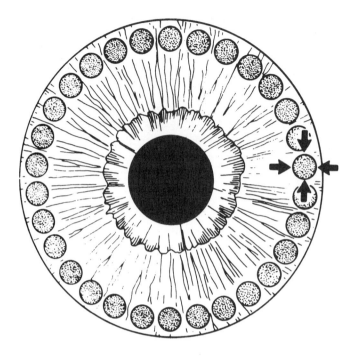

Figure 8–6 Contraction burns are placed around the iris as peripherally as possible. As indicated by the arrows, the iris stroma contracts toward the burn site from all directions. The contraction peripheral to the burn pulls the iris away from the trabecular meshwork. (Reprinted from Ritch R. Argon laser treatment for medically unresponsive attacks of angle-closure glaucoma. Am J Ophthalmol 94:197–204 (1982), with permission from Ophthalmic Publishing Company.)

2. **Treatment**
   a. Initially, the **argon** or **diode** laser is set to produce contraction burns: 500-μm spot size, 0.5 sec duration, and 200 mW of power for dark irides or 300 mW for light irides. The power is adjusted to obtain a visible contraction of the iris. If a bubble is formed at the iris or if pigment is released into the anterior chamber, then the power should be decreased.
   b. Either 20 to 24 spots (Ritch & Liebmann, 1996) or 30 to 40 spots (Schuman, 1997) are placed 360° around the iris at the extreme periphery to maximize iris contraction away from the trabecular meshwork. Visible radial blood vessels should be avoided to prevent bleeding or iris necrosis.
   c. When used as first-line treatment for an acute attack of primary angle-closure glaucoma, Lam et al. (1998) used 200- to 500-μm spot size, 0.2 to 0.3 sec duration, and 280 to 400 mW of power. They placed 40 to 211 contraction burns around the iris. Following this procedure the patients would receive a laser iridotomy as the definitive treatment (Figure 8–6).

3. **Post-treatment regimen**
   a. Perform gonioscopy to determine if the treatment was effective.
   b. Apply another drop of apraclonidine to the eye.
   c. Apply a drop of topical steroid and prescribe steroids for 3 to 5 days four to six times daily.

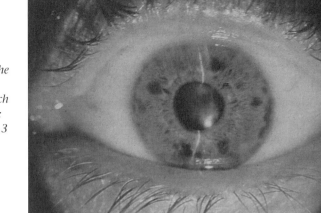

Figure 8–7 Clinical appearance of the eye following laser iridoplasty. (Reprinted with permission from Ritch R. Argon laser peripheral iridoplasty: and overview. J Glaucoma 1:206–213 (1992).)

    d. Monitor intraocular pressure 1 to 2 hours after the treatment and treat appropriately.

    e. Miotics should be discontinued (Figure 8–7).

E. Complications (Ritch, 1992; Ritch & Liebmann, 1996; Schuman, 1997; Schwartz, 1990; Simmons & Simmons, 1984; Tanihara & Nagata, 1991; Weiss et al., 1992)

1. **Intraocular inflammation.** This is very common and can be treated with topical steroids. Pigment dispersion occurs immediately after the treatment, but the diagnosis of iritis is made if cells and flare persist for more than 24 hours.

2. **Irritation or pain.** As the thermal contraction stretches the iris, the pain receptors may be stimulated. The pain or irritation is usually mild and can be treated with an analgesic.

3. **Corneal burns.** Corneal endothelial burns can occur in eyes with very shallow anterior chambers and usually disappear in a few days. Corneal epithelial burns could occur in edematous or opacified corneas. Clearing of the cornea can be facilitated by the use of glycerin and/or reduction of the intraocular pressure medically.

4. **Corneal decompensation.** This has been reported in a patient with Fuchs' endothelial dystrophy.

5. **Transient intraocular pressure spike.** As with any anterior segment laser treatment, there may be a rise in pressure a few hours after the treatment.

6. **Need for retreatment.** Regular follow-ups with gonioscopy should be performed.

7. **Pupil distortion.** This is minimized if the treatment is limited to the extreme periphery of the iris.

8. **Failure to open the angle.** If the treatment does not open the angle and lower the pressure, other treatment techniques should be attempted.

III. Laser Sclerostomy (Sclerectomy)

A. Introduction

1. Conventional glaucoma filtration surgery is fairly successful, but the most common cause of failure is episcleral scarring due to fibroblastic proliferation (Addicks et al., 1983). The use of a laser holds out the promise of fewer intraoperative and post-operative complications. With minimal collateral tissue damage, the laser can create a fistula or channel through the sclera that is relatively predictable and reproducible while at the same time minimizing manipulation of the conjunctiva and episclera. This may minimize the inflammatory response and hence the scarring that can close the fistula. However, spontaneous fistula fibrosis still occurs and, hence, antimetabolites such as mitomycin C and 5-fluorouracil are used (Chi et al., 1995; Karp et al., 1994; Iliev et al., 1997a,b; Schmidt-Erfurth et al., 1997; Wang et al., 1992).

2. There are two main methods for using a laser to perforate the sclera forming a fistula between the anterior chamber and the subconjunctival space. One method is called **ab interno** (from the inside out) and the other is called **ab externo** (from the outside in).

3. Lasers that have been used for **ab interno** sclerostomies either through a paracentesis or through a goniolens include:
   a. **Argon laser** (Gaasterland et al., 1987; Jaffe et al., 1988, 1989; Shirato et al., 1990; Wetzel & Scheu, 1994)
   b. **CTE:YAG laser (Q-switched)** (Kermani et al., 1993b)
   c. **Diode laser** (Fankhauser et al., 1992b; Karp et al., 1993; van der Zypen et al., 1995; Wang et al., 1996)
   d. **Dye laser** (Grossman et al., 1993; Latina et al., 1990, 1992; March, 1988; Melamed et al., 1992a, 1993; Rabowsky et al., 1997; Ruben et al., 1993; Sarraf & Lee, 1993; Wetzel & Scheu, 1994)
   e. **Erbium:YAG laser** (Hill et al., 1992, 1993a; Mizota et al., 1995; Ozler et al., 1991; Shields et al., 1995)
   f. **Erbium:YSGG laser** (Ozler et al., 1991)
   g. **Excimer laser** (Berlin, 1988; Berlin et al., 1987, 1988; Traverso et al., 1994)
   h. **Holmium:YAG laser** (Chi et al., 1995; Fankhauser et al., 1992b; Kendrick et al., 1996; van der Zypen et al., 1995)
   i. **Holmium:YSGG laser** (Ozler et al., 1991)
   j. **Nd:YAG laser (CW or free-running mode)** (Fankhauser et al., 1992b; Federman et al., 1987; Higginbotham et al., 1988, 1990; Hill et al., 1992; Iliev et al., 1997a,b; Javitt et al., 1989; Ozler et al., 1991; Tawakol et al., 1988; van der Zypen et al., 1993, 1995; Wilson & Javitt, 1990)
   k. **Nd:YAG laser (frequency-doubled CW mode)** (Shahinian et al., 1992)

l. **Nd:YAG laser (Q-switched mode)** (Gherezghiher et al., 1985; March, 1986; March et al., 1984, 1985, 1987a,b,c,d; Wetzel & Scheu, 1994)

m. **Nd:YLF laser** (Oram et al., 1995)

4. Lasers that have been used for **ab externo** sclerostomies under a conjunctival flap include:

a. **Argon laser** (Gaasterland et al., 1987; Litwin, 1979; March & Shaver, 1987)

b. **Carbon dioxide laser** (Beckman & Fuller, 1979; L'Esperance & Mittl, 1982; Ticho et al., 1979; Zhou-Wei et al., 1996)

c. **CTE:YAG laser (Q-switched)** (Kermani et al., 1993b)

d. **Diode laser** (Brinkmann et al., 1997; Karp et al., 1993, 1994; Rodrigues et al., 1998)

e. **Erbium:YAG laser** (Brinkmann et al., 1997; Haring et al., 1997–1998; Jacobi et al., 1997; McHam et al., 1997a; Schmidt-Erfurth et al., 1997; Wetzel & Scheu, 1993a,b; Wetzel et al., 1994, 1995a,b)

f. **Excimer laser** (Allan et al., 1993a,b, 1994; Aron-Rosa et al., 1990; Brooks et al., 1995; Campos et al., 1994; Seiler et al., 1989; Traverso et al., 1992, 1994)

g. **Holmium:YAG laser** (Ah-Fat & Canning, 1994; Bachman & Conto, 1994; Bonomi et al., 1993; Bray & Allen, 1994; Brinkmann et al., 1997; Di Meo et al., 1999; Feldman et al., 1993; Ferguson et al., 1994; Fliegler et al., 1994; Friedman et al., 1998; Hoskins et al., 1990, 1991; Iwach et al., 1993, 1994; Iwach et al., 1996; Luntz et al., 1996; Mannino et al., 1998; Mansour, 1992; McAllister & Watts, 1993; Onda et al., 1992, 1997; Saheb, 1993; Schmidt-Erfurth et al., 1997; Schuman et al., 1993; Terry, 1992a; Trible et al., 1998; Wang et al., 1992; Watts & McAllister, 1994; Wetzel & Scheu, 1993b; Wetzel et al., 1995b; Wong et al., 1993)

h. **Nd:YAG laser: CW** (Fankhauser et al., 1992b; Tawakol et al., 1989)

i. **Nd:YAG laser: giant-pulse** (Barak et al., 1995)

j. **Nd:YAG laser: Q-switched** (March & Shaver, 1987)

k. **Nd:YLF laser** (Cooper et al., 1993; Park et al., 1993)

5. Allen et al. (1992) have reviewed and discussed the pros and cons of the various types of lasers and delivery systems.

B. Indications. The indications for laser sclerostomy are fairly conservative placing it as a second or third option after conventional filtering surgery (Higginbotham, 1995, 1997). Some surgeons will not perform a full-thickness laser sclerostomy for any reason at this point in the procedure's development (Schuman, 1997).

1. Failed previous filtration surgery

2. Prior to shunt placement

3. Prior to cyclophotocoagulation

C. Techniques

1. **Ab interno procedures**
   a. **Noninvasive approach** (Berlin & Ahn, 1996; Higginbotham, 1997; Schuman, 1997). This involves delivery of the laser energy gonioscopically with no incision in the conjunctiva or cornea.
   b. **Invasive approach** (Berlin & Ahn, 1996; Higginbotham, 1997; Schuman, 1997). This involves delivery of the laser energy via a probe inserted into the anterior chamber.

2. **Ab externo procedures**
   a. **Subconjunctival approach** (Berlin & Ahn, 1996; Schuman, 1997). This involves a conjunctival incision. The usual technique includes the advancement of a fiberoptic probe through the incision to the target sclerostomy site. Another technique entails sliding the conjunctiva to the side, using a nonfiberoptic delivery system through an incision in the conjunctiva, and then sliding the conjunctiva back over the sclerostomy site.
   b. **Subconjunctival approach with a partial-thickness corneal flap** (Fliegler et al., 1994; Luntz et al., 1996). This is similar to the subconjunctival approach except that a corneo-sclera flap is used to create a "guarded" sclerostomy.

3. **Post-treatment regimen.** This varies somewhat depending on the technique, but it generally involves the following:
   a. Apply a topical antibiotic and steroid ointment.
   b. Patch the eye overnight.
   c. Apply topical steroid drops and antibiotic daily after the patch is removed.
   d. Use subconjunctival injections of 5-fluorouracil or mitomycin C to minimize scarring and closure of the fistula.
   e. Follow-up is similar to that after a full-thickness filtering operation.
   f. Ultrasound biomicroscopy may be of benefit during follow-up examination (Haring et al., 1997–98; Mannino et al., 1998). Follow-up of fistular paths and filtering blebs may make it possible to reoperate at an early stage before clinical manifestations occur.

D. Complications (Bachman & Conto, 1994; Bergsma & McCaa, 1996; Berlin & Ahn, 1996; Berlin et al., 1995; Bray & Allen, 1994; Di Meo et al., 1999; Ferguson et al., 1994; Friedman et al., 1998; Iwach et al., 1993, 1994, 1996; Jacobi et al., 1997; Onda et al., 1997; Schmidt-Erfurth et al., 1997; Schuman et al., 1993; Shields, 1998; Terry, 1992b; Trible et al., 1998; Watts & McAllister, 1994; Wong et al., 1993). The types of complications seen after the procedure depend to some extent on whether an ab interno or ab externo technique was used and on which type of laser was employed. But in general, the following complications can be seen:

1. Severe hypotony (IOP below 6 mm Hg)

2. Hypotony-induced maculopathy

3. Shallow or flat anterior chamber

4. Cataract formation

5. Choroidal effusion

6. Suprachoroidal hemorrhage. This is often identified by an acute onset of pain in the operated eye, possible severe visual loss, shallowing of the anterior chamber, and by dark reddish choroidal elevations.

7. Early or late iris incarceration. This is usually releasable using a Q-switched Nd:YAG laser or an argon laser.

8. Iris adherence

9. Failure to penetrate sclera

10. Descemet's membrane detachment and flaps

11. Conjunctival buttonhole (perforation) intraoperatively

12. Conjunctival burn

13. Hyphema

14. Peripheral anterior synechiae

15. Anterior chamber inflammation

16. Transient corneal changes (e.g., edema, striae, and dellen formation)

17. Induced astigmatism

18. Subconjunctival hemorrhage beneath the bleb

19. Endophthalmitis

20. Corneal toxicity associated with 5-fluorouracil or mitomycin C

21. Bleb leak

22. Prominent circular bleb

23. Cyclodialysis cleft

IV. Laser Revision of Failing Filter Bleb

A. Introduction

1. Postoperative success of glaucoma filtration surgery requires a patent fistula to maintain a constant flow of aqueous and an elevated bleb. Failure of a filtering bleb can occur due to extraocular, scleral, or intraocular occlusion (Azuara-Blanco & Katz, 1998; Latina & Shields, 1993; Maumenee, 1960; Van Buskirk, 1988). Externally, episcleral

membranes can stop or decrease aqueous outflow, but even more commonly, intrableb fibrosis and subconjunctival scarring can obstruct aqueous outflow. Additionally, tight scleral flap sutures can impede outflow. Scleral occlusion can occur due to an ingrowth of fibrous or gelatinous tissue. Internal obstruction of the fistula opening can occur due to movement or proliferation of tissue derived from ciliary body, cornea, iris, lens, sclera, or vitreous.

2. Both the **argon** and the **Nd:YAG** lasers have been used to revise hypofunctioning or failing filters either from a transconjunctival (external) or an internal approach (Budenz et al., 1986; Cohn et al., 1989; Cohn & Aron-Rosa, 1983; Dailey et al., 1986; De Alwis, 1993; Kandarakis et al., 1996; Kurata et al., 1984; Latina & Rankin, 1991; Oh & Katz, 1993; Praeger, 1984; Rankin & Latina, 1990; Shingleton et al., 1990; Ticho & Ivry, 1977; Van Buskirk, 1982; Van Rens, 1988; Weber et al., 1999). The picosecond **Nd:YLF** laser has also been used to open an occluded Molteno tube shunt via an internal approach (Oram et al., 1994). Similarly, the Nd:YAG laser has been used to open an occluded Ahmed tube shunt (Tessler et al., 1997).

3. A **laser-cured fibrinogen glue** is being explored as a way to close bleb leaks (Wright et al., 1998).

B. Indication: Failing or Hypofunctional Glaucoma Filtration Fistula. The best prognosis occurs in patients who had a well-established filtering bleb before the failure.

C. Techniques

1. **Pretreatment examination** (Latina & Shields, 1993; Van Buskirk, 1988)
   a. Careful **gonioscopic examination** of the internal fistula site
      1) Determine whether an unguarded or guarded fistula is present.
      2) Look for any internal obstruction of the fistula.
      3) If an internal obstruction is present, determine whether it is pigmented or nonpigmented.
   b. **Slit-lamp biomicroscope examination** of the bleb and external fistula site
      1) Look for any external obstruction of the fistula
      2) If an external obstruction is present, determine whether it is pigmented or nonpigmented.
      3) Check for membranes, fibrosis, and/or bleb encapsulation.
      4) Determine whether there is or is not a bleb.
      5) If there is a bleb, note whether it is localized or diffuse.
      6) Determine whether the fistula site is clearly visible through the bleb.
   c. **IOP response to digital pressure**
      1) Apply digital pressure for 15 sec.
      2) Examine the bleb for a change in size.
      3) Measure IOP before and after the digital pressure.
      4) If no reduction in IOP occurs, complete occlusion exists, and the prognosis for laser revision is poor.

    5) If a reduction of IOP greater than 3 mm Hg occurs, a partial occlusion exists, and the prognosis for laser revision is better.

2. **Transconjunctival (external) argon laser treatment** (Kurata et al., 1984; Pannu, 1991; Schultz, 1996)
   a. Laser suture lysis for tight scleral flap (see Chapter 9)
   b. Pigmented obstruction
     1) Topical anesthetic
     2) Abraham iridotomy lens over the bleb
     3) Spot size: 50 to 100 μm
     4) Power: 200 to 1000 mW
     5) Duration: 0.1 to 0.2 sec
     6) One variation of treatment involved 500 μm, 125 mW, for 1 sec (Pannu, 1991).
     7) Endpoints: spontaneous elevation of bleb and reduction of IOP

3. **Transconjunctival (external) Nd:YAG laser treatment** of pigmented or nonpigmented obstructions (Latina & Rankin, 1991; Rankin & Latina, 1990; Schultz, 1996; Shingleton et al., 1990; Van Rens, 1988; Weber et al., 1999)
   a. Topical anesthetic
   b. Abraham iridotomy lens over the bleb
   c. Energy: 2 to 17 mJ
   d. Number of shots in single burst mode: 4 to 200
   e. Focus slightly deeper than the obstructing tissue
   f. Endpoints: spontaneous elevation of bleb and reduction of IOP

4. **Internal argon laser treatment** of pigmented obstructions (Budenz et al., 1986; Schultz, 1996; Ticho & Ivry, 1977; Van Buskirk, 1982)
   a. Topical anesthetic
   b. Goniolens (e.g., Goldmann three-mirror lens)
   c. Spot size: 50 μm
   d. Power: 700 to 1500 mW
   e. Duration: 0.1 to 0.5 sec
   f. Endpoint: spontaneous elevation of bleb and reduction of IOP

5. **Internal Nd:YAG laser treatment** of pigmented or nonpigmented obstructions (Budenz et al., 1986; Cohn et al., 1989; Cohn & Aron-Rosa, 1983; Dailey et al., 1986; De Alwis, 1993; Kandarakis et al., 1996; Oh & Katz, 1993; Praeger, 1984; Schultz, 1996)
   a. Topical anesthetic
   b. Goniolens
   c. Energy: 1 to 10 mJ
   d. Number of pulses: 16 to 2800; 1 to 5 pulses/burst
   e. Endpoint: spontaneous elevation of bleb and reduction of IOP

6. **Internal Nd:YLF laser treatment** of membrane occluding a Molteno tube (Oram et al., 1994)

  a. Topical anesthetic
  b. Goniolens
  c. Energy: 300 µJ per pulse
  d. Repetition rate: 1000 pulses per second
  e. Number of pulses: 5005
  f. Endpoint: spontaneous elevation of bleb and reduction of IOP

7. **Post-treatment regimen** (Latina & Shields, 1993; Schultz, 1996)
  a. Perform ocular massage to encourage flow through fistula and reestablish the bleb.
  b. Use topical steroids: BID to QID for 4 to 7 days. If significant inflammation occurs, a cycloplegic drug can also be added.
  c. Monitor IOP at 1 hour, 1 day, 1 week, and appropriate intervals after treatment.
  d. Use 5-fluorouracil or mitomycin C to minimize scarring and closure of the fistula.

D. *Complications* (Azuara-Blanco & Katz, 1998; Cohn et al., 1989; De Alwis, 1993; Latina & Rankin, 1991; Latina & Shields, 1993; Prywes & Lopinto, 1986; Rankin & Latina, 1990; Van Buskirk, 1988; Weber et al., 1999)

1. **Transient IOP increase.** Monitor well and use anti-glaucoma medications if necessary.

2. **Mild inflammation.** The postoperative steroids usually suffice.

3. **Hemorrhaging.** Tamponade can be applied during treatment. Avoid blood vessels, especially with the Nd:YAG laser. Pretreatment with an argon laser to cauterize the vessels can be of value.

4. **Mild pain.** Topical anesthesia is usually sufficient.

5. **Conjunctival perforation (buttonholing).** This may require patching, contact lens application, or suturing.

6. **Ciliary body detachment**

7. **Failure to reopen the fistula**

V. Laser Closure of Overfiltering, Leaking Blebs

A. *Introduction*

1. After filtering surgery, overfiltering blebs and/or leaking blebs can occur. Overfiltering can lead to hypotony, which in turn can lead to cataract, choroidal hemorrhage, ciliochoroidal detachment, corneal edema, decreased aqueous production, gradual failure of the bleb, and hypotony maculopathy (Azuara-Blanco & Katz, 1998; Gass, 1972). Bleb leaks can result in bleb collapse, bleb infections, endophthalmitis, epithelial downgrowth, flattened anterior chamber, serous choroidal detachment, and conjunctival-scleral scarring (Ashkenazi et al., 1991; Brown et al., 1994). If the bleb is large and overhanging, corneal dellen and foreign body sensation can occur (Pannu, 1991; Soong & Quigley, 1983).

2. The **argon** and **Nd:YAG** lasers have been used to treat overfiltering and/or leaking blebs. A **diode** laser has been used in a rabbit model.

B. Indications

1. Leaking blebs
2. Overfiltering blebs
3. Large, overhanging, irritating blebs

C. Techniques

1. **Argon laser treatment** (Azuara-Blanco & Katz, 1998; Baum & Weiss, 1993; Fink et al., 1986; Hennis & Stewart, 1992b; Pannu, 1991)
   a. Apply topical anesthesia.
   b. Apply Rose bengal or methylene blue to the area to enhance absorption of the argon beam.
   c. Spot size: 200 to 500 μm
   d. Power: 300 to 1800 mW
   e. Duration: 0.1 to 0.2 sec
   f. One variation of the treatment involved 500 μm and 125 mW for 1 sec (Pannu, 1991).
   g. Focus the beam on the conjunctiva around the leak site
   h. Use enough shots to contract the tissue, form a clot, and close the leak. Then place another row of conjunctival burns around the leak site to induce more inflammation.
   i. Perform the Seidel test with topical fluorescein to confirm closure of the leak.
   j. Use a topical antibiotic and steroid for a few days.
   k. Examine the patient 1 day after the treatment and perform slit-lamp biomicroscopy, applanation tonometry, and another Seidel test. If a leak is noted, reapply the laser treatment.

2. **Nd:YAG laser treatment** (Azuara-Blanco & Katz, 1998; Bettin et al., 1999; Geyer, 1998; Lynch et al., 1996)
   a. Administer retrobulbar or peribulbar anesthesia
   b. Thermal mode is used.
   c. Energy: is initially set at 2.5 to 4 J, and the focus offset is placed at 0.9 to 1.5 mm.
   d. The area of the bleb can be "painted" with methylene blue to increase laser absorption.
   e. The aiming beam is focused on the conjunctival epithelium, and 20 to 50 spots are applied over the bleb.
   f. Energy and offset are adjusted to obtain epithelial whitening and wrinkling.
   g. The eye is patched and strong oral analgesics are prescribed with appropriate follow-up.

h. An alternative technique involves the induction of bleeding in conjunctival and episcleral vessels in the bleb area (Bettin et al., 1999). This results in the local delivery of autologous blood.

3. **Diode laser treatment** (Leen et al., 1999). A diode laser (810 nm) has been used to revise blebs in rabbits. A power setting of 3000 mW for 2000 ms achieved a positive initial response. The potential of using the diode laser for bleb revision in humans was demonstrated.

D. Complications

1. **Corneal edema** (Lynch et al., 1996). Marked corneal stromal edema can occur in eyes with a compromised corneal endothelium (e.g., Fuchs corneal dystrophy). Topical steroid therapy can be used.

2. **Corneal opacities** (Hennis & Stewart, 1992b). Application of the laser at the conjunctival-corneal interface may result in corneal stromal opacities. These usually resolve in a day.

3. **Creation of a bleb leak** (Fink et al., 1986; Geyer, 1998; Hennis & Stewart, 1992b; Lynch et al., 1996). Perforation and a new bleb leak can be created with the laser, and this could even lead to hypotony. The perforation may be due to excessive laser energy. Patching and aqueous suppression can be used to seal the leaks.

4. **Transient rise in IOP** (Geyer, 1998; Lynch et al., 1996). IOP can increase after the treatment. Anti-glaucoma medications and topical steroids can be used to treat.

5. **Retreatment** (Geyer, 1998; Lynch et al., 1996). Laser retreatment of the bleb may be necessary. Consider using higher energy levels than during the first treatment.

6. **Peaking of the pupil** (Geyer, 1998; Lynch et al., 1996). Flattening or peaking of the pupil can occur in the same quadrant as the bleb. This can occur without the formation of peripheral anterior synechiae.

7. **Failure to close the leak** (Hennis & Stewart, 1992b). Some leaks may not be closable with the laser even after multiple treatment sessions.

8. **Intraocular inflammation** (Geyer, 1998). As with most laser procedures, intraocular inflammation usually occurs.

9. **Loss of vision** (Geyer, 1998). A cataract developed in one patient due to prolonged hypotony induced by the laser treatment.

VI. Laser Hyaloidectomy/Hyaloidotomy/Vitreolysis (Treatment for Malignant Glaucoma)

A. Introduction

1. Malignant glaucoma (aqueous misdirection syndrome, ciliary block glaucoma, ciliovitreal block glaucoma, vitreociliary block glaucoma) is a rare and severe form of angle-closure glaucoma. It can be a complication of anterior segment surgery or can

occur in eyes that have not undergone surgery. It can occur in an aphakic, phakic, or pseudophakic form.

2. A patent iridectomy does not relieve the problem, and medical therapy is rarely successful. However, in addition to surgical vitrectomy, this form of glaucoma can be treated with the **Nd:YAG laser**.

3. The anterior hyaloid acts as a barrier to fluid movement into the anterior chamber, so the goal of the laser therapy is to disrupt that barrier. This can be accomplished using the photodisruption mechanism of the **Nd:YAG laser**.

B. *Indication: Malignant Glaucoma*

C. *Technique*

1. Apply topical anesthesia.

2. **Aphakic malignant glaucoma treatment** (Epstein et al., 1984; Little, 1994; Starita & Klapper, 1985)
   a. Use of a capsulotomy contact lens can be helpful.
   b. The Nd:YAG laser energy is set from 1 to 11 mJ using 1 to 3 pulses per burst.
   c. The Nd:YAG laser is focused just behind the anterior hyaloid face through the pupillary margin or through an iridotomy hole.
   d. One or more bursts may be necessary to disrupt the anterior hyaloid face.
   e. The anterior chamber should deepen within minutes.
   f. A goniolens can then be used to check the angle.

3. **Pseudophakic malignant glaucoma treatment** (Brown et al., 1986; Cinotti et al., 1986; Halkias et al., 1992; Little & Hitchings, 1993; Lockie, 1987; Melamed et al., 1991; Risco et al., 1989; Shrader et al., 1984; Tello et al., 1993; Tomey et al., 1987; Zacharia & Abboud, 1998)
   a. The Nd:YAG laser energy is set for 3 to 10 mJ and may take as many as 40 pulses total.
   b. The laser is focused just behind the anterior hyaloid.
   c. Effective treatment has included firing through the center of the pupil, through one of the positioning holes in the optic, or more peripheral than the optic through a large iridectomy. Most often the latter choices have been encouraged.
   d. Effective treatments have involved capsulotomy and hyaloidotomy as well as hyaloidotomy with the capsule remaining intact.
   e. The anterior chamber should deepen within minutes.
   f. A goniolens is then used to check the angle.

D. *Complications* (Epstein et al., 1984; Little & Hitchings, 1993; Tsai et al., 1997; Zacharia & Abboud, 1998)

1. **Failure of treatment.** Even though the initial treatment appears to be successful, the anterior chamber may flatten again (e.g., through fibrotic recondensation of the

hyaloid). Surgical vitrectomy and anterior segment reconstruction may then be necessary. Adequate disruption of the hyaloid face may need to be performed during the vitrectomy.

2. **Iris hemorrhage**.

VII. Laser Trabecular Ablation (Laser Trabeculopuncture)

A. *Introduction*

1. The first attempts at laser ablation of the trabecular tissue were made using a **ruby laser** (Krasnov, 1973; Krasnov, 1974). Subsequently, the **argon** (Dannheim & Rassow, 1976; Spitznas & Kreiger, 1974; Ticho et al., 1978; Witschel & Rassow, 1976), **Er:YSGG** (Hill et al., 1991), **Holmium:YAG** (Hill et al., 1991), **Nd:YAG** (Dutton et al., 1989; Epstein et al., 1985; Jacobi et al., 1996b; Melamed et al., 1985, 1987), **Nd:glass** (van der Zypen & Fankhauser, 1979, 1982), **Q-switched ruby** (Gaasterland et al., 1985), **CTE:YAG** (Kermani et al., 1993a), and **excimer** lasers (Vogel et al., 1990, 1996) have been used to perforate the trabecular tissue allowing direct access to Schlemm's canal.

2. For this kind of treatment, the **Er:YAG laser** was first demonstrated by Tsubota (1990) and then developed by Hill and colleagues (Hill et al., 1991, 1993b). They called their procedure **Laser trabecular ablation (LTA)**. Others have also used the Er:YAG laser (Dietlein et al., 1996, 1997a,b, 1998; Jacobi et al., 1996a, 1999; Jacobi & Dietlein, 2000; McHam et al., 1997b).

3. In addition to LTA, this type of procedure has been termed: laser **trabeculopuncture**, laser trabecular puncture, laseropuncture, laser trabeculotomy, laser trabeculectomy, laser trabeculopexy, laser trabeculoperforation, or internal ablative sinostomy (Jacobi & Dietlein, 2000; Kermani et al., 1993a; Moulin et al., 1985).

4. Most of the initial attempts in animals had high rates of failure due to closure of the perforations with scar tissue (Bonney et al., 1982; Dietlein et al., 1997b; Gaasterland et al., 1985; Krasnov, 1974; Melamed et al., 1985; Ticho, 1977; van der Zypen & Fankhauser, 1979, 1982; Witschel et al., 1977).

B. *Indications*

1. This type of procedure is being explored for patients with **high-IOP open-angle glaucoma** by the group using the Er:YAG laser (Dietlein et al., 1998). Micro-endoscopic trabecular ablation can also be used to treat open-angle glaucoma when *corneal opacification* has made it difficult to visualize the anterior segment (Jacobi et al., 1999).

2. Other groups using the Nd:YAG laser have reported success with glaucoma patients with **traumatic angle recession** (Fukuchi et al., 1993; Melamed et al., 1992b).

3. **Uncontrolled juvenile open-angle glaucoma** has also been suggested as an indication.

C. *Technique*

1. **Er:YAG laser** (Dietlein et al., 1997a, 1998; Jacobi et al., 1999)
   a. The Er:YAG laser has been used with a quartz fiber endoprobe attached to a zirconium fluoride fiber.
   b. The pulses have a duration of 200 μs and a pulse energy of 5 to 7 mJ at the fiber tip.
   c. Para- or retrobulbar anesthesia is administered.
   d. A miotic is instilled, mannitol (250 ml) is infused intravenously, and manometric oculopression is administered for 10 minutes.
   e. A viscoelastic is injected into the anterior chamber through a point at 9 o'clock OD or 3 o'clock OS on the peripheral cornea.
   f. The quartz endoprobe is then inserted and moved transcamerally to the trabecular meshwork on the opposite side of the eye.
   g. Under gonioscopic control, the probe is used to deliver 11 to 30 adjacent, but non-overlapping, pulses.
   h. The chamber is then irrigated and the corneal incision closed with a single suture.
   i. Topical pilocarpine 1% and steroid are started.
   j. The patients are followed-up at 1 day, 6 days, and then 1, 3, 6, and 12 months.

2. **Nd:YAG laser** (angle-recession glaucoma)
   a. The Nd:YAG laser was used with energy levels of 1 to 2.5 mJ by one group (Fukuchi et al., 1993) and levels averaging 5.8 mJ by another group (Melamed et al., 1992b).
   b. Topical anesthesia was administered.
   c. Using a three-mirror contact lens, an average of 65 exposures was applied to the lower angle by one group (Fukuchi et al., 1993). The endpoint was minimal blanching or a small bubble, just as in ALT. Another group attempted to expose Schlemm's canal for at least 1 hour (Melamed et al., 1992b).
   d. Steroid was only used in cases of marked iritis by Fukuchi et al. (1993). Whereas, Melamed et al. (1992b) administered steroid drops for 5 days after the procedure.
   e. Follow-up visits occurred at 1 week, 2 weeks, 1 month, 2 months, 3 months, and then every 3 months for Fukuchi et al. (1993).

3. **Nd:YAG laser** (juvenile open-angle glaucoma)
   a. For confluent exposure of Schlemm's canal, an average of 59 pulses with a mean energy of 5.5 mJ was used (Melamed et al., 1987).
   b. For focal treatment, four punctate holes were created with an average of 36 pulses with a mean energy of 4.97 mJ (Melamed et al., 1987).

D. Results

1. **Er:YAG**
   a. Eleven patients with chronic open-angle glaucoma were treated initially (Dietlein et al., 1997a; Dietlein et al., 1998). The preoperative mean maximum IOP was 36 mm Hg and the mean maximum IOP at the end of follow-up was 22 mm Hg. Thus a 39% decrease in mean maximum IOP was achieved at an average follow-up time of 12.5 months.
   b. Subsequently, seven patients with uncontrolled open-angle glaucoma and corneal opacification were treated (Jacobi et al., 1999). The preoperative mean maximum IOP was 35.1 mm Hg and the mean maximum IOP at the end of follow-up was 18.9 mm Hg. Thus a 46% decrease in mean maximum IOP was achieved at an average follow-up time of 20.7 months.

2. **Nd:YAG** (angle-recession glaucoma)
   a. For seven patients, the mean IOP was 31 mm Hg before Nd:YAG laser trabeculo-puncture (YLT) and 15 mm Hg after 6 to 12 months of follow-up (Fukuchi et al., 1993). Thus a 52% drop in mean IOP was achieved in the successful cases. In four other patients who had YLT after an ineffective ALT, the drop was 38%. The Kaplan-Meier analysis for both groups combined indicated a probability of success of 91% at 1 year.
   b. For 12 patients in another study, the mean IOP was 34.3 mm Hg before YLT and 26.8 mm Hg just after (22% drop) (Melamed et al., 1992b). With a mean follow-up of 12 months, the success rate was 41.7%.

3. **Nd:YAG** (juvenile open-angle glaucoma) (Melamed et al., 1987)
   a. For confluent treatment, there was a success rate of 80% in eight eyes with a mean follow-up of 6 months.
   b. For focal treatment, there was a success rate of 50% in four eyes.

E. Complications

1. IOP spikes (Melamed et al., 1987, 1992b)
2. Hyphema (Melamed et al., 1992b)
3. Inflammation (Melamed et al., 1987, 1992b)
4. Peripheral anterior synechiae (Dietlein et al., 1998)

VIII. Laser Goniopuncture (Mermoud et al., 1999)

A. Introduction

1. In the 1970s, initial attempts to treat open-angle glaucoma with a laser involved the creation of a fistula between the anterior chamber and Schlemm's canal (see *Laser Trabecular Ablation*).

2. Recently the laser has been used to allow passage of the aqueous humor from the anterior chamber to the subconjunctival space via a trabeculo-Descemet's membranotomy following a deep sclerectomy with collagen implant.

B. *Technique*

1. The **Nd:YAG laser** was used in the free-running Q-switched mode.

2. The goniopunctures were made in Descemet's membrane, the anterior trabeculum, or at the junction between the two.

3. Perforation was obtained with 2 to 4 mJ of energy and 2 to 15 pulses.

C. *Results*

1. The goniopuncture was performed an average of 9.9 months after deep sclerectomy.

2. The mean follow-up time after the goniopunctures was 10.3 months (range: 1 to 24 months).

3. The mean IOP before the laser procedure was 22.2 mm Hg and 12.5 mm Hg immediately after.

4. The Kaplan-Meier survival curve success rate was 83% immediately after the procedure and 68% at 24 months.

D. *Complications*

1. **Choroidal detachment** occurred in two patients (5%).

2. **Ocular hypotony** occurred in two patients (5%). This led to the choroidal detachments.

IX. Intrastromal Holmium Laser Keratostomy (ILK)

A. ILK is a new filtering procedure that is based on modifications to the subconjunctival holmium laser sclerostomy (SLS) procedure (Kessing et al., 2000). The poor success rates with SLS prompted the changes.

B. In ILK the laser canal has been moved so that it is now placed intrastromally in the cornea in front of Schwalbe's line. A knife is used to create a corneo-scleral tunnel incision, and then the laser probe is inserted in the floor of the incision from the corneal side. This technique can thus be accomplished without opening the conjunctiva, because the tunnel incision opens into the subconjunctival space.

C. The holmium laser is continuously applied until the keratostomy is complete. The perforation is accomplished within 5 to 6 seconds using 80 mJ per pulse.

D. No iridectomy is done, and regulation of the postoperative IOP is accomplished by Nd:YAG laser photodisruption of the internal laser ostium.

E. The Kaplan-Meier survival analysis success rate was 88% with a mean observation time of 23 months. Complete surgical success (no medications, no reoperations, peak IOP ≤ 20 mm Hg) was obtained in 63% of the eyes and qualified success in an additional 25%.

F. Complications (16 eyes; Kessing et al., 2000)
1. Early hypotony: 75%
2. Transient shallow anterior chamber: 25%
3. Late hypotony: 19%
4. Hypotension maculopathy: 6%
5. Early iris incarceration: 13%
6. Late lens changes: 13%
7. Transient corneal changes: 38%
8. Induced refractive astigmatism: 13%
9. Cystic bleb: 38%
10. Late laser canal fibrosis: 13%
11. Hyphema: 19%
12. Infected bleb: 6%

X. Photoablative Laser-Grid Trabeculectomy

A. In an attempt to minimize overfiltration and hypotony in the standard trabeculectomy procedure, a new technique is being developed (Jacobi et al., 2000). This new procedure involves the preparation of the standard scleral flap, but the penetration of the globe is accomplished using a mid-IR laser.

B. The pulsed **Er:YAG laser** is used for transscleral photoablation. The laser energy (6 mJ/pulse) is delivered through an optical fiber to a lateral-aiming probe with a quartz-fiber tip.

C. A laser-grid pattern of 10 single craters is used to penetrate the scleral bed. The full-thickness scleral perforations are very small, and aqueous flow through them is reduced compared to the flow through the standard trabeculectomy in porcine cadaver eyes.

D. This new procedure may decrease the incidence of hypotony-related complications.

References

Addicks EM et al. Histologic characteristics of filtering blebs in glaucomatous eyes. Arch Ophthalmol 101:795–798 (1983).

Ah-Fat FG, Canning CR. A comparison of the efficacy of holmium laser sclerostomy ab externo versus trabeculectomy in the treatment of glaucoma. Eye 8:402–405 (1994).

Al-Ghamdi S et al. Transscleral neodymium:YAG laser cyclophotocoagulation for end-stage glaucoma, refractory glaucoma, and painful blind eyes. Ophthalmic Surg 24:526–529 (1993).

Allan BDS et al. Laser microsclerostomy for primary open angle glaucoma: a review of laser mechanisms and delivery systems. Eye 6:257–266 (1992).

Allan BDS et al. Excimer laser sclerostomy: the in vivo development of a modified open mask delivery system. Eye 7:47–52 (1993a).

Allan BDS et al. Excimer laser sclerostomy: tissue damage and dimensional reproducibility in vitro. Lasers Light Ophthalmol 5:121–130 (1993b).

Allan BDS et al. 193 nm excimer laser sclerostomy in pseudophakic patients with advanced open angle glaucoma. Br J Ophthalmol 78:199–205 (1994).

Allingham RR et al. Probe placement and power levels in contact transscleral neodymium:YAG cyclophotocoagulation. Arch Ophthalmol 108:738–742 (1990).

Ando F, Kawai T. Transscleral contact cyclophotocoagulation for refractory glaucoma: comparison of the results of pars plicata and pars plana irradiation. Lasers Light Ophthalmol 5:143–147 (1993).

Aron-Rosa D et al. Preliminary study of argon fluoride (193 nm) excimer laser trabeculectomy. Scanning electron microscopy at five months. J Cataract Refract Surg 16:617–620 (1990).

Ashkenazi I et al. Risk factors associated with late infection of filtering blebs and endophthalmitis. Ophthalmic Surg 22:570–574 (1991).

Assia EI et al. A comparison of neodymium: yttrium aluminum garnet and diode laser transscleral cyclophotocoagulation and cyclocryotherapy. Invest Ophthalmol Vis Sci 32:2774–2778 (1991).

Aventuro JA, Gaasterland DE, Buzawa D. Effect of fiberoptic diameter in diode laser transscleral cyclophotocoagulation in human autopsy eyes. J Glaucoma 7:349–352 (1998).

Ayyala RS et al. Comparison of mitomycin C trabeculectomy, glaucoma drainage device implantation, and laser neodymium:YAG cyclophotocoagulation in the management of intractable glaucoma after penetrating keratoplasty. Ophthalmology 105:1550–1556 (1998).

Azuara-Blanco A, Dua HS. Malignant glaucoma after diode laser cyclophotocoagulation. Am J Ophthalmol 127:467–469 (1999).

Azuara-Blanco A, Katz LJ. Dysfunctional filtering blebs. Surv Ophthalmol 43:93–126 (1998).

Bachman JA, Conto JE. Postoperative complications of subconjunctival THC-YAG (holmium) laser sclerostomy. J Am Optom Assoc 65:311–320 (1994).

Barak A et al. Use of the giant-pulse Nd:YAG laser for ab-externo sclerostomy in rabbits and humans. Ophthalmic Surg 26:68–72 (1995).

Barraquer RI, Kargacin M. Nd:YAG laser diascleral cyclophotocoagulation: survival analysis after four years. Dev Ophthalmol 22:132–137 (1991).

Baum M, Weiss HS. Argon laser closure of conjunctival bleb leak. Arch Ophthalmol 111:438 (1993).

Beadles KA, Smith MF. Inadvertent sclerostomy during transscleral Nd:YAG cyclophotocoagulation [letter]. Am J Ophthalmol 118:669–670 (1994).

Bechrakis NE et al. Sympathetic ophthalmia following laser cyclocoagulation. Arch Ophthalmol 112:80–84 (1994).

Beckman H et al. Transsceral ruby laser irradiation of the ciliary body in the treatment of intractable glaucoma. Trans Am Acad Ophthalmol Otolaryngol 76:423–436 (1972).

Beckman H, Fuller TA. Carbon dioxide laser scleral dissection and filtering procedure for glaucoma. Am J Ophthalmol 88:73–77 (1979).

Beckman H, Waeltermann J. Transscleral ruby laser cyclophotocoagulation. Am J Ophthalmol 98:788–795 (1984).

Benning H, Pfeiffer N. Therapeutic range in transscleral contact cyclophotocoagulation. Ger J Ophthalmol 4:11–15 (1995).

Bergsma DR, McCaa CS. Extensive detachment of Descemet membrane after holmium laser sclerostomy. Ophthalmology 103:678–680 (1996).

Berlin MS. Excimer laser applications in glaucoma surgery. Ophthalmol Clin North Am 1:255–263 (1988).

Berlin MS, Ahn RJH. Current options in laser sclerostomy. In Ritch R, Shields MB, Krupin T, eds. The glaucomas. St Louis, MO: Mosby, 1996:1591–1604.

Berlin MS, Yoo PH, Ahn RJH. The role of laser sclerostomy in glaucoma surgery. Curr Opin Ophthalmol 6:102–114 (1995).

Berlin MS et al. Excimer laser photoablation in glaucoma filtering surgery. Am J Ophthalmol 103:713–714 (1987).

Berlin MS et al. Goniophotoablation: excimer laser glaucoma filtering surgery. Lasers Light Ophthalmol 2:17–24 (1988).

Bettin P et al. Treatment of hyperfiltering blebs with Nd:YAG laser-induced subconjunctival bleeding. J Glaucoma 8:380–383 (1999).

Blasini M, Simmons R, Shields MB. Early tissue response to transscleral neodymium:YAG cyclophotocoagulation. Invest Ophthalmol Vis Scie 31:1114–1118 (1990).

Blomquist PH, Gross RL, Koch DD. Effect of transscleral neodymium:YAG cyclophotocoagulation on intraocular lenses. Ophthalmic Surg 21:223–226 (1990).

Bloom M, Weber PA. Probe orientation in contact Nd:YAG laser cyclophotocoagulation. Ophthalmic Surg 23:364–366 (1992).

Bloom PA et al. "Cyclodiode." Trans-scleral diode laser cyclophotocoagulation in the treatment of advance refractory glaucoma. Ophthalmology 104:1508–1519 (1997).

Bock CJ et al. Transscleral diode laser cyclophotocoagulation for refractory pediatric glaucomas. J Pediatr Ophthalmol Strabismus 34:235–239 (1997).

Bonney CH et al. Short-term effects of Q-switched ruby laser on monkey anterior chamber angle. Invest Ophthalmol Vis Sci 22:310–318 (1982).

Bonomi L et al. Subconjunctival THC:YAG laser sclerostomy for the treatment of glaucoma: preliminary data. Ophthalmic Surg 24:300–303 (1993).

Brancato R, Carassa RG. Value of ultrasound biomicroscopy for ciliodestructive procedures. Curr Opin Ophthalmol 7:87–92 (1996).

Brancato R, Trabucchi G, Verdi M, Carassa RG, Gobbi PG. Diode and Nd:YAG laser contact transscleral cyclophotocoagulation in a human eye: a comparative histopathologic study of the lesions produced using a new fiber optic probe. Ophthalmic Surg 25:607–611 (1994).

Brancato R et al. Transscleral contact cyclophotocoagulation with Nd:YAG laser CW: experimental study on rabbit eyes. Int J Tissue React 9:493–498 (1987).

Brancato R et al. Contact transscleral cyclophotocoagulation with Nd:YAG laser in uncontrolled glaucoma. Ophthalmic Surg 20:547–551 (1989).

Brancato R et al. Probe placement and energy levels in continuous wave neodymium-YAG contact transscleral cyclophotocoagulation. Arch Ophthalmol 108:679–683 (1990).

Brancato R et al. Histopathology of continuous wave neodymium: yttrium aluminum garnet and diode laser contact transscleral lesions in rabbit ciliary body. A comparative study. Invest Ophthalmol Vis Sci 32:1586–1592 (1991).

Brancato R et al. Contact transscleral cyclophotocoagulation with the diode laser in refractory glaucoma. Eur J Ophthalmol 5:32–39 (1995).

Bray LC, Allen ED. Holmium laser sclerostomy. Eye 8:370–371 (1994).

Brinkmann R et al. Ablation dynamics in laser sclerostomy ab externo by means of pulsed lasers in the mid-infrared spectral range. Ophthalmic Surg Lasers 28:853–865 (1997).

Brooks AMV et al. Excimer laser filtration surgery. Am J Ophthalmol 119:40–47 (1995).

Brown RH et al. Neodymium-YAG vitreous surgery for phakic and pseudophakic malignant glaucoma. Arch Ophthalmol 104:1464–1466 (1986).

Brown RH et al. Treatment of bleb infection after glaucoma surgery. Arch Ophthalmol 112:57–61 (1994).

Budenz DL et al. Laser therapy for internally failing glaucoma filtration surgery. Ophthalmic Laser Ther 1:169–176 (1986).

Campos M et al. Transconjunctival sinusotomy using the 193-nm excimer laser. Acta Ophthalmol (Copenh) 72:707–711 (1994).

Cantor LB et al. Neodymium-YAG transscleral cyclophotocoagulation. The role of pigmentation. Invest Ophthalmol Vis Sci 30:1834–1837 (1989).

Chen J et al. Endoscopic photocoagulation of the ciliary body for treatment of refractory glaucomas. Am J Ophthalmol 124:787–796 (1997).

Chen TC et al. Diode laser transscleral cyclophotocoagulation. Int Ophthalmol Clin 39:169–176 (1999).

Chew P, Chee C, Lim A. Laser treatment of severe acute angle closure glaucoma in dark Asian irides: the role of iridoplasty. Laser Light Ophthalmol 4:129–132 (1991).

Chew PTK, Yeo LMW. Argon laser iridoplasty in chronic angle closure glaucoma. Int Ophthalmol 19:67–70 (1995).

Chi TS, Berrios RR, Netland PA. Holmium laser sclerostomy via corneal approach with transconjunctival mitomycin-C in rabbits. Ophthalmic Surg 26:353–357 (1995).

Cinotti DJ et al. Neodymium:YAG laser therapy for pseudophakic pupillary block. J Cataract Refract Surg 12:174–179 (1986).

Cohen EJ et al. Neodymium:YAG laser transscleral cyclophotocoagulation for glaucoma after penetrating kerato-plasty. Ophthalmic Surg 20:713–716 (1989).

Cohn HC, Aron-Rosa D. Reopening blocked trabeculectomy sites with the YAG laser. Am J Ophthalmol 95:293–294 (1983).

Cohn HC, Whalen WR, Aron-Rosa D. YAG laser treatment in a series of failed trabeculectomies. Am J Ophthal-mol 108:395–403 (1989).

Coleman AL et al. Transscleral cyclophotocoagulation of human autopsy and monkey eyes. Ophthalmic Surg 22:638–643 (1991).

Cooper HM et al. Picosecond neodymium:yttrium lithium fluoride laser sclerectomy. Am J Ophthalmol 115:221–224 (1993).

Crymes BM, Gross RL. Laser placement in noncontact Nd:YAG cyclophotocoagulation. Am J Ophthalmol 110:670–673 (1990).

Dailey RA, Samples JR, Van Buskirk EM. Reopening filtration fistulas with the neodymium-YAG laser. Am J Ophthalmol 102:491–495 (1986).

Dannheim F, Rassow B. Laser trabeculopuncture. III. Experiments with rhesus monkeys. Ophthalmologica 173:40–48 (1976).

De Alwis TV. The long-term follow-up of patients treated with YAG laser to re-open closed or closing fistulae following glaucoma surgery. Eye 7:444–445 (1993).

Dickens CJ et al. Long-term results of noncontact transscleral neodymium:YAG cyclophotocoagulation. Ophthalmology 102:1777–1781 (1995).

Dietlein TS, Jacobi PC, Krieglstein GK. Erbium:YAG laser ablation on human trabecular meshwork by contact delivery endoprobes. Ophthalmic Surg Lasers 27:939–945 (1996).

Dietlein TS, Jacobi PC, Krieglstein GK. Ab interno infrared laser trabecular ablation: preliminary short-term results in patients with open-angle glaucoma. Graefes Arch Clin Exp Ophthalmol 235:349–353 (1997a).

Dietlein TS et al. Experimental erbium:YAG laser photoablation of trabecular meshwork in rabbits: an in-vivo study. Exp Eye Res 64:701–706 (1997b).

Dietlein TS, Jacobi PC, Krieglstein GK. Erbium:YAG laser trabecular ablation (LTA) in the surgical treatment of glaucoma. Lasers Surg Med 23:104–110 (1998).

Di Meo A et al. Ab externo sclerostomy with holmium laser: 24 months follow-up. Ann Ophthalmol 31:180–183 (1999).

Di Staso S et al. Trans-scleral krypton laser cyclophotocoagulation: our experience of its use on patients with neovascular glaucoma. Act Ophthalmol Scand Suppl 224 75:37–38 (1997).

Dutton GN, Allan D, Cameron SA. Pulsed neodymium-YAG laser trabeculotomy: energy requirements and replicability. Br J Ophthalmol 73:177–181 (1989).

Echelman DA et al. Influence of exposure time on inflammatory response to neodymium:YAG cyclophotocoagulation in rabbits. Arch Ophthalmol 112:977–981 (1994).

Echelman DA et al. Variability of contact transscleral neodymium:YAG cyclophotocoagulation. Invest Ophthalmol Vis Sci 36:497–502 (1995).

Edward DP et al. Sympathetic ophthalmia following neodymium:YAG cyclotherapy. Ophthalmic Surg 20:544–546 (1989).

Eid TE et al. Tube-shunt surgery versus neodymium:YAG cyclophotocoagulation in the management of neovascular glaucoma. Ophthalmology 104:1692–1700 (1997).

El-Harazi SM, Kellaway J, Feldman RM. Semiconductor diode laser transscleral cyclophotocoagulation in a patient with glaucoma secondary to metastatic tumor to the iris. J Glaucoma 7:317–318 (1998).

Epstein DL et al. Neodymium:YAG laser trabeculopuncture in open-angle glaucoma. Ophthalmology 92:931–937 (1985).

Epstein DL, Steinert RF, Puliafito CA. Neodymium-YAG laser therapy to the anterior hyaloid in aphakic malignant (ciliovitreal block) glaucoma. Am J Ophthalmol 98:137–143 (1984).

Fankhauser F et al. Transscleral cyclophotocoagulation using a neodymium YAG laser. Ophthalmic Surg 17:94–100 (1986).

Fankhauser F et al. A new instrument for controlling pressure exerted on the sclera during contact Nd:YAG laser cyclodestruction. Ophthalmic Surg 23:465–468 (1992a).

Fankhauser F et al. Optical principles related to optimizing sclerostomy procedures. Ophthalmic Surg 23:752–761 (1992b).

Fankhauser F et al. Laser cyclophotocoagulation in glaucoma therapy. Ophthalmol Clin North Am 6:449–471 (1993).

Federman JL et al. Contact laser: thermal sclerostomy ab interna. Ophthalmic Surg 18:726–727 (1987).

Feldman RM et al. Histopathologic characteristics of failed holmium laser sclerostomy [letter]. Am J Ophthalmol 116:766–767 (1993).

Feldman RM et al. Histopathologic findings following contact transscleral semiconductor diode laser cyclophotocoagulation in a human eye. J Glaucoma 6:139–140 (1997).

Ferguson JG Jr, McGrath DJ, Stevens G Jr. Iris incarceration after holmium sclerostomy [letter]. Ophthalmology 101:219–220 (1994).

Ferry AP, King MH, Richards DW. Histopathologic observations on human eyes following neodymium:YAG laser cyclophotocoagulation for glaucoma. Trans Am Ophthalmol Soc 93:315–331 (1995).

Fink AJ, Boys-Smith JW, Brear R. Management of large filtering blebs with the argon laser. Am J Ophthalmol 101:695–699 (1986).

Fiore PM, Latina MA. A technique for precise placement of laser applications in transscleral Nd:YAG cyclophotocoagulation. Am J Ophthalmol 107:292–293 (1989).

Fiore PM, Melamed S, Krug JH Jr. Focal scleral thinning after transscleral Nd:YAG cyclophotocoagulation. Ophthalmic Surg 20:215–216 (1989).

Fishbaugh J. Overview and new technology in cyclodestructive procedures. Insight 19:26–29 (1994).

Flaxel CJ et al. Peripheral transscleral retinal diode laser for rubeosis iridis. Retina 17:421–429 (1997).

Fliegler RJ, Mastrobattista J, Luntz MH. Subconjunctival THC:YAG laser sclerostomy under a partial-thickness corneal flap. Ophthalmic Surg 25:28–33 (1994).

Friedman DS et al. Holmium laser sclerostomy in glaucomatous eyes with prior surgery: 24-month results. Ophthalmic Surg Lasers 29:17–22 (1998).

Fu Y-A, Liaw Z-C. Argon laser gonioplasty with trabeculoplasty for chronic angle-closure glaucoma. Ann Ophthalmol 19:419–422 (1987).

Fukuchi T et al. Nd:YAG laser trabeculopuncture (YLT) for glaucoma with traumatic angle recession. Graefes Arch Clin Exp Ophthalmol 231:571–576 (1993).

Gaasterland DE et al. Long-term effects of Q-switched ruby laser on monkey anterior chamber angle. Invest Ophthalmol Vis Sci 26:129–135 (1985).

Gaasterland DE et al. Ab interno and ab externo filtering operations by laser contact surgery. Ophthalmic Surg 18:254–257 (1987).

Gaasterland DE, Pollack IP. Initial experience with a new method of laser transscleral cyclophotocoagulation for ciliary ablation in severe glaucoma. Trans Am Ophthalmol Soc 90:225–243 (1992).

Gabel VP, Birngruber R, Hillenkamp F. Visible and near infrared light absorption in pigment epithelium and choroid. In Shimizu K, ed. International Congress Series No. 450, XXIII Concilium Ophthalmologicum, Kyoto, 1978. Amsterdam, Netherlands: Excerpta Medica Elsevier, 1979:658–662.

Gass JDM. Hypotony maculopathy. In Bellows JG, ed. Contemporary ophthalmology honoring Sir Stewart Duke-Elder. Baltimore, MD: Williams and Wilkins, 1972:343–366.

Gayton JL. Traumatic aniridia during endoscopic laser cycloablation. J Cataract Refract Surg 24:134–135 (1998).

Gayton JL, Van Der Karr M, Sanders V. Combined cataract and glaucoma surgery: trabeculectomy versus endoscopic laser cycloablation. J Cataract Refract Surg 25:1214–1219 (1999).

Geyer O. Management of large, leaking, and inadvertent filtering blebs with the neodymium:YAG laser. Ophthalmology 105:983–987 (1998).

Geyer O, Neudorfer M, Lazar M. Retinal detachment as a complication of neodymium: yttrium aluminum garnet laser cyclophotocoagulation. Ann Ophthalmol 25:170–172 (1993).

Gherezghiher T et al. Neodymium-YAG laser sclerostomy in primates. Arch Ophthalmol 103:1543–1545 (1985).

Grossman RE, Sarraf D, Lee DA. Iontophoresis of methylene blue for gonioscopic pulsed dye laser sclerostomy. J Ocul Phamacol 9:277–285 (1993).

Gupta N, Weinreb RN. Diode laser transscleral cyclophotocoagulation. J Glaucoma 6:426–429 (1997).

Halkias A, Magauran DM, Joyce M. Ciliary block (malignant) glaucoma after cataract extraction with lens implant treated with YAG laser capsulotomy and anterior hyaloidotomy. Br J Ophthalmol 76:569–570 (1992).

Haller JA. Transvitreal endocyclophotocoagulation. Trans Am Ophthalmol Soc 94:589–676 (1996).

Hampton C, Shields MB. Transscleral neodymium-YAG cyclophotocoagulation. A histologic study of human autopsy eyes. Arch Ophthalmol 106:1121–1123 (1988).

Hampton C et al. Evaluation of a protocol for transscleral neodymium:YAG cyclophotocoagulation in one hundred patients. Ophthalmology 97:910–917 (1990).

Hardten DR, Brown JD. Malignant glaucoma after Nd:YAG cyclophotocoagulation [letter]. Am J Ophthalmol 111:245–247 (1991).

Hardten DR, Brown JD. Transscleral neodymium:YAG cyclophotocoagulation: comparison of 180-degree and 360-degree initial treatments. Ophthalmic Surg 24:181–184 (1993).

Haring G, Behrendt S, Wetzel W. Evaluation of laser sclerostomy fistulas using ultrasound biomicroscopy. Int Ophthalmol 21:261–264 (1997–98).

Hawkins TA, Stewart WC. One-year results of semiconductor transscleral cyclophotocoagulation in patients with glaucoma. Arch Ophthalmol 111:488–491 (1993).

Hennis HL et al. Transscleral cyclophotocoagulation using a semiconductor diode laser in cadaver eyes. Ophthalmic Surg 22:274–278 (1991).

Hennis HL, Stewart WC. Semiconductor diode laser transscleral cyclophotocoagulation in patients with glaucoma. Am J Ophthalmol 113:81–85 (1992a).

Hennis HL, Stewart WC. Use of the argon laser to close filtering bleb leaks. Graefe's Arch Clin Exp Ophthalmol 230:537–541 (1992b).

Herschler J. Laser shrinkage of the ciliary processes. A treatment for malignant (ciliary block) glaucoma. Ophthalmology 87:1155–1159 (1980).

Higginbotham EJ. Is laser sclerostomy surgery ready for "prime time"? [editorial] Arch Ophthalmol 113:1243–1244 (1995).

Higginbotham EJ. Ab interno laser sclerectomy. In Epstein DL, Allingham RR, Schuman JS, eds. Chandler and Grant's glaucoma. Baltimore, MD: Williams & Wilkins, 1997:500–503.

Higginbotham EJ, Harrison M, Zou XL. Cyclophotocoagulation with the transscleral contact neodymium:YAG laser versus cyclocryotherapy in rabbits. Ophthalmic Surg 22:27–30 (1991).

Higginbotham EJ, Kao G, Peyman G. Internal sclerostomy with the Nd:YAG contact laser versus thermal sclerostomy in rabbits. Ophthalmology 95:385–390 (1988).

Higginbotham EJ, Zou X, Edward D. Internal sclerostomy with the Nd:YAG contact laser versus thermal sclerostomy in cynomolgus monkeys. Laser Light Ophthalmol 3:281–286 (1990).

Hill RA et al. Laser trabecular ablation (LTA). Lasers Surg Med 11:341–346 (1991).

Hill RA et al. Ab-interno neodymium:YAG versus erbium:YAG laser sclerostomies in a rabbit model. Ophthalmic Surg 23:192–197 (1992).

Hill RA et al. Ab-interno erbium (Er):YAG laser sclerostomy with iridotomy in Dutch cross rabbits. Lasers Surg Med 13:559–564 (1993a).

Hill RA et al. Effects of pulse width on erbium:YAG laser photothermal trabecular ablation (LTA). Lasers Surg Med 13:440–446 (1993b).

Hoskins HD Jr et al. Subconjunctival THC:YAG laser limbal sclerostomy ab externo in the rabbit. Ophthalmic Surg 21:589–592 (1990).

Hoskins HD Jr et al. Subconjunctival THC:YAG laser thermal sclerostomy. Ophthalmology 98:1394–1399 (1991).

Iliev ME et al. Spontaneous and pharmacologically modulated wound healing after Nd:YAG laser sclerostomy ab interno in rabbits. Eur J Ophthalmol 7:24–28 (1997a).

Iliev ME et al. Transconjunctival application of mitomycin C in combination with laser sclerostomy ab interno: a long-term morphological study of the postoperative healing process. Exp Eye Res 64:1013–1026 (1997b).

Immonen IJR et al. Energy levels needed for cyclophotocoagulation: a comparison of transscleral contact cw-YAG and krypton lasers in the rabbit eye. Ophthalmic Surg 24:530–533 (1993).

Immonen IJR, Puska P, Raitta C. Transscleral contact krypton laser cyclophotocoagulation for treatment of glaucoma. Ophthalmology 101:876–882 (1994).

Immonen IJR, Viherkoski E, Peyman GA. Experimental retinal and ciliary body photocoagulation using a new 670-nm diode laser. Am J Ophthalmol 122:870–874 (1996).

Iwach AG et al. A new contact neodymium:YAG laser for cyclophotocoagulation. Ophthalmic Surg 22:345–348 (1991).

Iwach AG et al. Subconjunctival THC:YAG ("holmium") laser thermal sclerostomy ab externo. A one-year report. Ophthalmology 100:356–366 (1993).

Iwach AG et al. Update of the subconjunctival THC:YAG (holmium) laser sclerostomy ab externo clinical trial: 30 month report. Ophthalmic Surg 25:13–21 (1994).

Iwach AG et al. Update on the subconjunctival THC:YAG (holmium) laser sclerostomy ab externo clinical trial: a 4-year report. Ophthalmic Surg Lasers 27:823–831 (1996).

Jacobi PC, Dietlein TS. Endoscopic surgery in glaucoma management. Curr Opin Ophthalmol 11:127–132 (2000).

Jacobi PC, Dietlein TS, Krieglstein GK. Effects of Er:YAG laser trabecular ablation on outflow facility in cadaver porcine eyes. Graefes Arch Clin Exp Ophthalmol 234 (Suppl 1):S204–S208 (1996a).

Jacobi PC, Dietlein TS, Krieglstein GK. Photoablative Nd:YAG-laser goniotomy enhancing trabecular outflow facility in porcine cadaver eyes. Ger J Ophthalmol 5:154–159 (1996b).

Jacobi PC, Dietlein TS, Krieglstein GK. Prospective study of ab externo erbium:YAG laser sclerostomy in humans. Am J Ophthalmol 123:478–486 (1997).

Jacobi PC, Dietlein TS, Krieglstein GK. Microendoscopic trabecular surgery in glaucoma management. Ophthalmology 106:538–544 (1999).

Jacobi PC et al. Photoablative laser-grid trabeculectomy in glaucoma filtering surgery: histology and outflow facility measurements in porcine cadaver eyes. Ophthalmic Surg Lasers 31:49–54 (2000).

Jaffe GJ et al. Ab interno sclerostomy with a high-powered argon endolaser. Am J Ophthalmol 106:391–396 (1988).

Jaffe GJ et al. Ab interno sclerostomy with a high-powered argon endolaser. Clinicopathologic correlation. Arch Ophthalmol 107:1183–1185 (1989).

Javitt JC et al. Laser sclerostomy ab interno using a continuous wave Nd:YAG laser. Ophthalmic Surg 20:552–556 (1989).

Jennings BJ, Mathews DE. Complications of neodymium:YAG cyclophotocoagulation in the treatment of open-angle glaucoma. Optom Vis Sci 76:686–691 (1999).

Johnson SM. Neurotrophic corneal defects after diode laser cycloablation. Am J Ophthalmol 126:725–727 (1998).

Kandarakis A et al. Reopening of failed trabeculectomies with ab interno Nd:YAG laser. Eur J Ophthalmol 6:143–146 (1996).

Karp CL et al. Diode laser surgery. Ab interno and ab externo versus conventional surgery in rabbits. Ophthalmology 100:1567–1573 (1993).

Karp CL, Higginbotham EJ, Griffin EO. Adjunctive use of transconjunctival mitomycin-C in ab externo diode laser sclerostomy surgery in rabbits. Ophthalmic Surg 25:22–27 (1994).

Kawahara J et al. Effect of transpupillary argon laser cyclophotocoagulation on anterior chamber oxygen tension in rabbit eyes. Jpn J Ophthalmol 34:450–462 (1990).

Kendrick R, Kollarits CR, Khan N. The results of ab interno laser thermal sclerostomy combined with cataract surgery versus trabeculectomy combined with cataract surgery 6 to 12 months postoperatively. Ophthalmic Surg Lasers 27:583–586 (1996).

Kermani O et al. Contact cw-Nd:YAG laser cyclophotocoagulation for treatment of refractory glaucoma. Ger J Ophthalmol 1:74–78 (1992).

Kermani O et al. Internal ablative sinostomy using a fiber delivered Q-switched CTE:YAG laser (2.69 μm). Intl Ophthalmol 17:211–215 (1993a).

Kermani O et al. Q-switched CTE:YAG laser sclerostomies on human autopsy eyes. Ger J Ophthalmol 2:100–106 (1993b).

Kessing SV, Boberg-Ans J, Heegaard S. Intrastromal holmium laser keratostomy: long-term results. Ophthalmic Surg Lasers 31:13–23 (2000).

Kim DD, Moster MR. Transpupillary argon laser cyclophotocoagulation in the treatment of traumatic glaucoma. J Glaucoma 8:340–341 (1999).

Kimbrough RL et al. Angle-closure in nanophthamos. Am J Ophthalmol 88:572–579 (1979).

Kivela T et al. Clinically successful contact transscleral krypton laser cyclophotocoagulation. Long-term histopathologic and immunohistochemical autopsy findings. Arch Ophthalmol 113:1447–1453 (1995).

Klapper RM et al. Transscleral neodymium:YAG thermal cyclophotocoagulation in refractory glaucoma. A preliminary report. Ophthalmology 95:719–722 (1988).

Kosoko O et al. Long-term outcome of initial ciliary ablation with contact diode laser transscleral cyclophotocoagulation for severe glaucoma. The Diode Laser Ciliary Ablation Study Group. Ophthalmology 103:1294–1302 (1996).

Krasnov MM. Laseropuncture of anterior chamber angle in glaucoma. Am J Ophthalmol 75:674–678 (1973).

Krasnov MM. Q-switched laser goniopuncture. Arch Ophthalmol 92:37–41 (1974).

Kurata F, Krupin T, Kolker AE. Reopening filtration fistulas with transconjunctival argon laser photocoagulation. Am J Ophthalmol 98:340–343 (1984).

Kwasniewska S et al. Acute effects following transscleral contact irradiation of the ciliary body and the retina/choroid with the cw Nd:YAG laser. Lasers Light Ophthalmol 2:25–34 (1988).

Lai JS, Tham CC, Lam DS. Limited argon laser peripheral iridoplasty as immediate treatment for an acute attack of primary angle closure glaucoma: a preliminary study. Eye 13:26–30 (1999).

Lam DS, Lai JS, Tham CC. Immediate argon laser peripheral iridoplasty as treatment for acute attack of primary angle-closure glaucoma: a preliminary study. Ophthalmology 105:2231–2236 (1998).

Latina MA et al. Transscleral cyclophotocoagulation using a contact laser probe: a histologic and clinical study in rabbits. Lasers Surg Med 9:465–470 (1989).

Latina MA et al. Laser sclerostomy by pulsed-dye laser and goniolens. Arch Ophthalmol 108:1745–1750 (1990).

Latina MA et al. Gonioscopic ab interno laser sclerostomy. A pilot study in glaucoma patients. Ophthalmology 99:1736–1744 (1992).

Latina MA, Rankin GA. Internal and transconjunctival neodymium:YAG laser revision of late failing filters. Ophthalmology 98:215–221 (1991).

Latina MA, Shields SR. Laser revision of failing filters. Ophthalmol Clin North Am 6:437–447 (1993).

Lee P-F. Argon laser photocoagulation of the ciliary processes in cases of aphakic glaucoma. Arch Ophthalmol 97:2135–2138 (1979).

Lee P-F, Pomerantzeff O. Transpupillary cyclophotocoagulation of rabbit eyes. An experimental approach to glaucoma surgery. Am J Ophthalmol 71:911–920 (1971).

Lee P-F, Shihab Z, Eberle M. Partial ciliary process laser photocoagulation in the management of glaucoma. Lasers Surg Med 1:85–92 (1980).

Leen MM et al. Mitotic effect of autologous blood injection and diode laser bleb revision on rabbit filtration blebs. Arch Ophthalmol 117:77–83 (1999).

L'Esperance FA Jr, Mittl RN. Carbon dioxide laser trabeculostomy for the treatment of neovascular glaucoma. Trans Am Ophthalmol Soc 80:262–287 (1982).

Lim ASM et al. Laser iridoplasty in the treatment of severe acute angle closure glaucoma. Int Ophthalmol 17:33–36 (1993).

Lim JI et al. Ciliary body endophotocoagulation during pars plana vitrectomy in eyes with vitreoretinal disorders and concomitant uncontrolled glaucoma. Ophthalmology 103:1041–1046 (1996).

Little BC. Treatment of aphakic malignant glaucoma using Nd:YAG laser posterior capsulotomy. Br J Ophthalmol 78:499–501 (1994).

Little BC, Hitchings RA. Pseudophakic malignant glaucoma: Nd:YAG capsulotomy as a primary treatment. Eye 7:102–104 (1993).

Litwin RL. Successful argon laser sclerostomy for glaucoma. Ophthalmic Surg 10:22–24 (1979).

Liu GJ, Mizikawa A, Okisaka S. Mechanism of intraocular pressure decrease after contact transscleral continuous-wave Nd:YAG laser cyclophotocoagulation. Ophthalmic Res 26:65–79 (1994).

Lockie P. Ciliary-block glaucoma treated by posterior capsulotomy. Aust NZ J Ophthalmol 15:207–209 (1987).

Luntz MH, Flieger RD, Mastrobattista J. Subconjunctival THC:YAG laser sclerostomy under a partial thickness flap. Lasers and Light 7:85–90 (1996).

Lynch MG, Roesch M, Brown RH. Remodeling filtering blebs with the neodymium:YAG laser. Ophthalmology 103:1700–1705 (1996).

Mannino G et al. Ultrasound biomicroscopy in the clinical evaluation of ab externo holmium:YAG laser sclerostomies. Ophthalmic Surg Lasers 29:157–161 (1998).

Mansour AM. THC:YAG laser sclerostomy: the resident experience. Ophthalmic Surg 23:801–803 (1992).

March WF. Indentation funnel use in transpupillary argon laser cyclophotocoagulation and neodymium:YAG sclerostomy [letter]. Arch Ophthalmol 104:972 (1986).

March WF. The principles of laser sclerostomy. Ophthalmol Clin North Am 1:239–244 (1988).

March WF, Shaver RP. Fluorescein in laser sclerostomy. Am J Ophthalmol 104:432–433 (1987).

March WF, Shaver RP. Histologic effects of cyclophotocoagulation [letter]. Ophthalmology 96:925 (1989).

March WF et al. Experimental YAG laser sclerostomy. Arch Ophthalmol 102:1834–1836 (1984).

March WF et al. Histologic study of a neodymium-YAG laser sclerostomy. Arch Ophthalmol 103:860–863 (1985).

March WF et al. Safety of high-energy neodymium:YAG laser pulses in YAG sclerostomy. Lasers Surg Med 6:584–587 (1987a).

March WF, LaFuente H, Rol P. Improved goniolens for YAG sclerostomy. Ophthalmic Surg 18:513 (1987b).

March WF, Shaver RP, Adams RL. Specialized needle for laser sclerostomy. Ophthalmic Surg 18:621–622 (1987c).

March WF et al. Silver oxide in YAG sclerostomy. Lasers Surg Med 7:353–354 (1987d).

Marsh P et al. A clinicopathologic correlative study of noncontact transscleral Nd:YAG cyclophotocoagulation. Am J Ophthalmol 115:597–602 (1993).

Marshall J, Fankhauser F. The effect of light radiation on blood vessels and membranes. Trans Ophthalmol Soc UK 92:469–478 (1972).

Mastrobattista JM, Luntz M. Ciliary body ablation: where are we and how did we get here? Surv Ophthalmol 41:193–213 (1996).

Maumenee AE. External filtering operations for glaucoma: the mechanism of function and failure. Trans Am Ophthalmol Soc 58:319–328 (1960).

Maus M, Katz LJ. Choroidal detachment, flat anterior chamber, and hypotony as complications of neodymium:YAG laser cyclophotocoagulation. Ophthalmology 97:69–72 (1990).

McAllister JA, Watts PO. Holmium laser sclerostomy: a clinical study. Eye 7:656–660 (1993).

McDonnell PJ et al. Molteno implant for control of glaucoma in eyes after penetrating keratoplasty. Ophthalmology 95:364–369 (1988).

McHam ML et al. Erbium:YAG laser sclerectomy with a sapphire optical fiber. Ophthalmic Surg Lasers 28:55–58 (1997a).

McHam ML et al. Erbium:YAG laser trabecular ablation with a sapphire optical fiber. Exp Eye Res 65:151–155 (1997b).

Melamed S, Ashkenazi I, Blumenthal M. Nd-YAG laser hyaloidotomy for malignant glaucoma following one-piece 7 mm intraocular lens implantation. Br J Ophthalmol 75:501–503 (1991).

Melamed S, Latina MA, Epstein DL. Neodymium:YAG laser trabeculopuncture in juvenile open-angle glaucoma. Ophthalmology 94:163–170 (1987).

Melamed S et al. Q-switched neodymium-YAG laser trabeculopuncture in monkeys. Arch Ophthalmol 103:129–133 (1985).

Melamed S et al. Goniopscopic sclerostomy using laser ablation of dyed sclera in refractory glaucoma. Lasers Light Ophthalmol 4:181–189 (1992a).

Melamed S et al. Nd:YAG laser trabeculopuncture in angle-recession glaucoma. Ophthalmic Surg 23:31–35 (1992b).

Melamed S et al. Internal sclerostomy using laser ablation of dyed sclera in glaucoma patients: a pilot study. Br J Ophthalmol 77:139–144 (1993).

Mermoud A et al. Nd:YAG goniopuncture after deep sclerectomy with collagen implant. Ophthalmic Surg Lasers 30:120–125 (1999).

Miyazaki M, Hoya T. Effect of transscleral Nd:YAG laser cyclophotocoagulation: research for a new manner of treatment. Ophthalmologica 208:122–130 (1994).

Mizota A et al. Internal contact sclerostomy with an erbium laser and intraocular fiberscope. Lasers Light Ophthalmol 7:57–64 (1995).

Montanari P et al. Diode laser trans-scleral cyclophotocoagulation in refractory glaucoma treatment. Acta Ophthalmol Scand Suppl 224 75:38 (1997).

Mora JS et al. Endoscopic diode laser cyclophotocoagulation with a limbal approach. Ophthalmic Surg Lasers 28:118–123 (1997).

Moulin F, Haut J, Abboud E. Trabeculoperforation? Trabeculoretraction? Trabeculoplasty? Review of the various designations used for laser treatment in primary open-angle glaucoma. Ophthalmologica 191:75–83 (1985).

Munoz FJ, Rebolleda G. Cyclophotocoagulation for glaucoma after penetrating keratoplasty [letter]. Ophthalmology 106:644–645 (1999).

Myers JS et al. Laser energy reaching the posterior pole during transscleral cyclophotocoagulation. Arch Ophthalmol 116:488–491 (1998).

Nasisse MP et al. Inflammatory effects of continuous-wave neodymium: yttrium aluminum garnet laser cyclophotocoagulation. Invest Ophthalmol Vis Sci 33:2216–2223 (1992).

Noureddin BN et al. Advanced uncontrolled glaucoma. Nd:YAG cyclophotocoagulation or tube surgery. Ophthalmology 99:430–436 (1992).

Oguri A et al. Transscleral cyclophotocoagulation with the diode laser for neovascular glaucoma. Ophthalmic Surg Lasers 29:722–727 (1998).

Oh Y, Katz LJ. Indications and technique for reopening closed filtering blebs using the Nd:YAG laser – a review and case series. Ophthalmic Surg 24:617–622 (1993).

Onda E et al. Determination of an appropriate laser setting for THC-YAG laser sclerostomy ab externo in rabbits. Ophthalmic Surg 23:198–202 (1992).

Onda E et al. Holmium YAG laser sclerostomy ab externo for refractory glaucoma. Int Ophthalmol 20:309–314 (1997).

Oram O et al. Opening an occluded Molteno tube with the picosecond neodymium—yttrium lithium fluoride laser [letter]. Arch Ophthalmol 112:1023 (1994).

Oram O et al. Gonioscopic ab interno Nd:YLF laser sclerostomy in human cadaver eyes. Ophthalmic Surg 26:136–138 (1995).

Ozler SA et al. Infrared laser sclerostomies. Invest Ophthalmol Vis Sci 32:2498–2503 (1991).

Pablo LE et al. Semiconductor diode laser transscleral cyclophotocoagulation versus filtering surgery with mitomycin C. Int Ophthalmol 20:11–14 (1997).

Palmer DJ et al. Transscleral diode laser cyclophotocoagulation on autopsy eyes with abnormally thinned sclera. Ophthalmic Surg Lasers 28:495–500 (1997).

Pannu JS. Laser treatment of a filtration bleb [letter]. J Cataract Refract Surg 17:110 (1991).

Park SB, Kim JC, Aquavella JV. Nd:YLF laser sclerostomy. Ophthalmic Surg 24:118–120 (1993).

Patel A et al. Endolaser treatment of the ciliary body for uncontrolled glaucoma. Ophthalmology 93:825–830 (1986).

Phelan MJ, Higginbotham EJ. Contact transscleral Nd:YAG laser cyclophotocoagulation for the treatment of refractory pediatric glaucoma. Ophthalmic Surg Lasers 26:401–403 (1995).

Plager DA, Neely DE. Intermediate-term results of endoscopic diode laser cyclophotocoagulation for pediatric glaucoma. J Aapos 3:131–137 (1999).

Praeger DL. The reopening of closed filtering blebs using the neodymium:YAG laser. Ophthalmology 91:373–377 (1984).

Preussner P-R et al. Real-time control for transscleral cyclophotocoagulation. Graefes Arch Clin Exp Ophthalmol 235:794–801 (1997).

Prum BE Jr et al. The influence of exposure duration in transscleral Nd:YAG laser cyclophotocoagulation. Am J Ophthalmol 114:560–567 (1992).

Prum BE Jr et al. The influence of exposure duration in transscleral Nd:YAG laser cyclophotocoagulation [letter reply]. Am J Ophthalmol 115:685 (1993).

Prywes AS, LoPinto RJ. Temporary visual loss with ciliary body detachment and hypotony after attempted YAG laser repair of failed filtering surgery. Am J Ophthalmol 101:305–307 (1986).

Pueyo M et al. Long-term results of transscleral contact cyclophotocoagulation by semiconductor diode laser. Ann Ophthalmol 30:296–300 (1998).

Rabowsky JH, Dukes AJ, Lee DA. Gonioscopic laser sclerostomy versus filtration surgery in a rabbit model. Eye 11:830–837 (1997).

Rankin GA, Latina MA. Transconjunctival Nd:YAG laser revision of failing trabeculectomy. Ophthalmic Surg 21:365–367 (1990).

Rebolleda G, Munoz FJ, Murube J. Audible pops during cyclodiode procedures. J Glaucoma 8:177–183 (1999).

Risco JM, Tomey KF, Perkins TW. Laser capsulotomy through intraocular lens positioning holes in anterior aqueous misdirection. Arch Ophthalmol 107:1569 (1989).

Ritch R. Argon laser treatment for medically unresponsive attacks of angle-closure glaucoma. Am J Ophthalmol 94:197–204 (1982).

Ritch R. Argon laser peripheral iridoplasty: and overview. J Glaucoma 1:206–213 (1992).

Ritch R, Liebmann JM. Argon laser peripheral iridoplasty. Ophthalmic Surg Lasers 27:289–300 (1996).

Rodrigues M et al. Histologic effect of diode laser sclerostomy in human cadaver eyes. Ophthalmic Surg Lasers 29:758–761 (1998).

Rosenow S-E et al. Cyclophotocoagulation: experimental investigations of dosage problems. Graefes Arch Clin Exp Ophthalmol 237:583–592 (1999).

Ruben S, Migdal C, De Vivero C. Ab interno pulsed dye laser sclerostomy for the treatment of glaucoma: preliminary results of a new technique. Eye 7:436–439 (1993).

Saheb NE. Short-term results of holmium laser sclerostomy in patients with uncontrolled glaucoma. Can J Ophthalmol 28:317–319 (1993).

Samples JR. Laser cyclophotocoagulation for refractory glaucomas. Ophthalmol Clin North Am 8:401–411 (1995).

Sarraf D, Lee DA. Iontophoresis of reactive black 5 for pulsed dye laser sclerostomy. J Ocul Pharmacol 9:25–33 (1993).

Schmidt-Erfurth U et al. Mitomycin-C in laser sclerostomy: benefit and complications. Ophthalmic Surg Lasers 28:14–20 (1997).

Schubert HD. Noncontact and contact pars plana transscleral neodymium:YAG laser cyclophotocoagulation in postmortem eyes. Ophthalmology 96:1471–1475 (1989).

Schubert HD. The influence of exposure duration in transscleral Nd:YAG laser cyclophotocoagulation [letter]. Am J Ophthalmol 115:684–685 (1993).

Schubert HD, Agarwala A, Arbizo V. Changes in aqueous outflow after in vitro neodymium: yttrium aluminum garnet laser cyclophotocoagulation. Invest Ophthalmol Vis Sci 31:1834–1838 (1990).

Schubert HD, Federman JL. A comparison of CW Nd:YAG contact transscleral cyclophotocoagulation with cyclocryopexy. Invest Ophthalmol Vis Sci 30:536–542 (1989).

Schultz JS. Additional uses of laser therapy in glaucoma. In Ritch R, Shields MB, Krupin T, eds. The glaucomas. St Louis, MO: Mosby, 1996:1621–1630.

Schuman JS. Cyclodestruction. In Epstein DL, Allingham RR, Schuman JS, eds. Chandler and Grant's Glaucoma. Baltimore, MD: Williams & Wilkins, 1997; 57:484–494.

Schuman JS. Laser sclerectomy. In Epstein DL, Allingham RR, Schuman JS, eds. Chandler and Grant's Glaucoma. Baltimore, MD: Williams & Wilkins, 1997:495–499.

Schuman JS et al. Experimental use of semiconductor diode laser in contact transscleral cyclophotocoagulation in rabbits. Arch Ophthalmol 108:1152–1157 (1990a).

Schuman JS et al. Contact transscleral continuous wave neodymium:YAG laser cyclophotocoagulation. Ophthalmology 97:571–580 (1990b).

Schuman JS et al. Energy levels and probe placement in contact transscleral semiconductor diode laser cyclophotocoagulation in human cadaver eyes. Arch Ophthalmol 109:1534–1538 (1991).

Schuman JS et al. Contact transscleral Nd:YAG laser cyclophotocoagulation. Midterm results. Ophthalmology 99:1089–1095 (1992).

Schuman JS et al. Holmium laser sclerostomy. Success and complications. Ophthalmology 100:1060–1065 (1993).

Schwartz LW. Complications of argon laser iridoplasty and coreoplasty. In Sherwood MB, Spaeth GL, eds. Complications of glaucoma therapy. Thorofare, NJ: SLACK Inc, 1990:113–121.

Seiler T, Kriegerowski M, Bende T. Partial external trabeculectomy (PET) with the excimer laser [abstract]. Lasers Light Ophthalmol 2:196 (1989).

Shahinian L Jr, Egbert PR, Williams AS. Histologic study of healing after ab interno laser sclerostomy. Am J Ophthalmol 114:216–219 (1992).

Shields MB. Cyclodestructive surgery for glaucoma: past, present, and future. Trans Am Ophthalmol Soc 83:285–303 (1985).

Shields MB. Intraocular cyclophotocoagulation. Trans Ophthalmol Soc UK 105 (Pt. 2):237–241 (1986).

Shields MB. Transscleral Nd:YAG cyclophotocoagulation. In Minckler DS, Van Buskirk EM, eds. Color atlas of ophthalmic surgery: glaucoma. Philadelphia, PA: JB Lippincott, 1992; 19:209–219.

Shields MB. Textbook of glaucoma. Baltimore, MD: Williams & Wilkins, 1998.

Shields MB et al. Intraocular cyclophotocoagulation. Histopathologic evaluation in primates. Arch Ophthalmol 103:1731–1735 (1985).

Shields MB et al. A contact lens for transscleral Nd:YAG cyclophotocoagulation [letter]. Am J Ophthalmol 108:457–458 (1989).

Shields MB, Shields SE. Noncontact transscleral Nd:YAG cyclophotocoagulation: a long-term follow-up of 500 patients. Trans Am Ophthalmol Soc 92:271–283 (1994).

Shields S, Stewart WC, Shields MB. Transpupillary argon laser cyclophotocoagulation in the treatment of glaucoma. Ophthalmic Surg 19:171–175 (1988b).

Shields MB, Wilkerson MH, Echelman DA. A comparison of two energy levels for noncontact transscleral neodymium-YAG cyclophotocoagulation. Arch Ophthalmol 111:484–487 (1993).

Shields SM et al. Histopathologic findings after Nd:YAG transscleral cyclophotocoagulation [letter]. Am J Ophthalmol 106:100–101 (1988a).

Shields SR et al. Transcorneal erbium laser sclerostomy: towards a guarded laser sclerostomy technique. J Glaucoma 4:391–397 (1995).

Shingleton BJ et al. Management of encapsulated filtration blebs. Ophthalmology 97:63–68 (1990).

Shirato S, Adachi M, Yamashita H. Internal sclerostomy with argon contact laser—animal experiment using 5-fluorouracil. Jpn J Ophthalmol 34:381–387 (1990).

Shrader CE et al. Pupillary and iridovitreal block in pseudophakic eyes. Ophthalmology 91:831–837 (1984).

Simmons RJ, Simmons RB. Gonioplasty. In Belcher CD III, Thomas JV, Simmons RJ, eds. Photocoagulation in glaucoma and anterior segment disease. Baltimore, MD: Williams & Wilkins, 1984:122–140.

Simmons RB et al. Comparison of transscleral neodymium:YAG cyclophotocoagulation with and without a contact lens in human autopsy eyes. Am J Ophthalmol 109:174–179 (1990).

Simmons RB et al. Transscleral Nd:YAG laser cyclophotocoagulation with a contact lens. Am J Ophthalmol 112:671–677 (1991).

Simmons RB et al. Videographic and histologic comparison of Nd:YAG and diode laser contact transscleral cyclophotocoagulation. Am J Ophthalmol 117:337–341 (1994).

Soong HK, Quigley HA. Dellen associated with filtering blebs. Arch Ophthalmol 101:385–387 (1983).

Spitznas M, Kreiger AE. Experimental argon laser trabeculopuncture in rhesus monkeys. Klin Monatsbl Augenheilkd 165:165–170 (1974).

Starita RJ, Klapper RM. Neodymium:YAG photodisruption of the anterior hyaloid face in aphakic flat chamber: a diagnostic and therapeutic tool. Int Ophthalmol Clin 25:119–123 (1985).

Stewart WC, Brindley GO, Schields MB. Cyclodestructive procedures. In Ritch R, Shields MB, Krupin T, eds. The glaucomas. St. Louis, MO: Mosby, 1996:1605–1620.

Stolzenburg S, Kresse S, Muller-Stolzenburg NW. Thermal side reactions during in vitro contact cyclophotocoagulation with the continuous wave Nd:YAG laser. Ophthalmic Surg 21:356–358 (1990).

Strasser G. Unsuccessful laser cyclophotocoagulation for glaucoma in aniridia [letter]. Arch Ophthalmol 103:890 (1985).

Stroman GA et al. Use of indocyanine green with diode laser transscleral cyclophotocoagulation in a cadaver eye model. Ophthalmic Surg Lasers 26:582–583 (1995).

Stroman GA et al. Contact versus noncontact diode laser transscleral cyclophotocoagulation in cadaver eyes. Ophthalmic Surg Lasers 27:60–65 (1996).

Suzuki Y et al. Transscleral Nd:YAG laser cyclophotocoagulation versus cyclocryotherapy. Graefes Arch Clin Exp Ophthalmol 229:33–36 (1991).

Takahashi H, Okisaka S. Safety and effectiveness of contact transscleral cyclophotocoagulation with continuous-wave Nd:YAG laser. Jpn J Clin Ophthalmol 45:1233–1237 (1991).

Tanihara H, Nagata M. Argon-laser gonioplasty following goniosynechialysis. Graefe's Arch Clin Exp Ophthalmol 229:505–507 (1991).

Tawakol ME et al. External limbal sclerostomy with contact Nd:YAG laser versus surgical knife. Int Ophthalmol 13:205–208 (1989).

Tawakol ME, Peyman GA, Abou-Steit M. Internal pars plana sclerotomy with the contact Nd:YAG laser: an experimental study. Int Ophthalmol 11:175–180 (1988).

Tello C et al. Ultrasound biomicroscopy in pseudophakic malignant glaucoma. Ophthalmology 100:1330–1334 (1993).

Terry S. Combined no-stitch phacoemulsification cataract extraction with foldable silicone intraocular implant and holmium laser sclerostomy followed by 5-FU injections. Ophthalmic Surg 23:218–219 (1992a).

Terry SA. Cyclodialysis cleft following holmium laser sclerostomy, treated by argon laser photocoagulation. Ophthalmic Surg 23:825–826 (1992b).

Tessler Z, Jluchoded S, Rosenthal G. Nd:YAG laser for Ahmed tube shunt occlusion by the posterior capsule. Ophthalmic Surg Lasers 28:69–70 (1997).

Tham CC, Lai JSM, Lam DSC. Immediate argon laser peripheral iridoplasty for acute attack of PACG (Addendum to previous report) [letter]. Ophthalmology 106:1042–1043 (1999).

Threlkeld AB, Johnson MH. Contact transscleral diode cyclophotocoagulation for refractory glaucoma. J Glaucoma 8:3–7 (1999).

Threlkeld AB, Shields MB. Noncontact transscleral Nd:YAG cyclophotocoagulation for glaucoma after penetrating keratoplasty. Am J Ophthalmol 120:569–576 (1995).

Ticho U. Laser application to the angle structures in animals and in human glaucomatous eyes. Adv Ophthalmol 34:210 (1977).

Ticho U et al. Argon laser trabeculotomies in primates: evaluation by histological and perfusion studies. Invest Ophthalmol Vis Sci 17:667–674 (1978).

Ticho U et al. Carbon dioxide laser filtering surgery in hemorrhagic glaucoma. Glaucoma 1:114–118 (1979).

Ticho U, Ivry M. Reopening of occluded filtering blebs by argon laser photocoagulation. Am J Ophthalmol 84:413–418 (1977).

Tomey KF et al. Aqueous misdirection and flat chamber after posterior chamber implants with and without trabeculectomy. Arch Ophthalmol 105:770–773 (1987).

Traverso CE et al. Photoablative filtration surgery with the excimer laser for primary open-angle glaucoma: a pilot study. Int Ophthalmol 16:363–365 (1992).

Traverso CE, Corazza M, Murialdo U. Excimer laser filtering surgery. In Benson WE, Coscas G, Katz LJ, eds. Current techniques in ophthalmic laser surgery. Philadelphia, PA: Current Medicine, 1994; 19:190–197.

Trible JR, Olander KW, Koenig SB. Corneal refractive and endothelial changes following THC:YAG (holmium) laser sclerostomy. Ophthalmic Surg Lasers 29:733–737 (1998).

Tsai JC et al. Combined transscleral diode laser cyclophotocoagulation and transscleral retinal photocoagulation for refractory neovascular glaucoma. Retina 16:164–166 (1996).

Tsai JC et al. Surgical results in malignant glaucoma refractory to medical or laser therapy. Eye 11:677–681 (1997).

Tsubota K. Application of erbium:YAG laser in ocular ablation. Ophthalmologica 200:117–122 (1990).

Ulbig MW et al. Contact diode laser cyclo-photocoagulation for refractory glaucoma. A pilot study. Ger J Ophthalmol 3:212–215 (1994).

Ulbig MW et al. Clinical comparison of semiconductor diode versus neodymium:YAG noncontact cyclophoto-coagulation. Br J Ophthalmol 79:569–574 (1995).

Uram M. Ophthalmic laser microendoscope ciliary process ablation in the management of neovascular glaucoma. Ophthalmology 99:1823–1828 (1992).

Uram M. Diode laser endocyclodestruction [letter]. Ophthalmic Surg 25:268–269 (1994).

Uram M. Combined phacoemulsification, endoscopic ciliary process photocoagulation, and intraocular lens implantation in glaucoma management. Ophthalmic Surg 26:346–352 (1995a).

Uram M. Endoscopic cyclophotocoagulation in glaucoma management. Curr Opinion Ophthalmol 6:19–29 (1995b).

Van Buskirk EM. Reopening filtration fistulas with the argon laser. Am J Ophthalmol 94:1–3 (1982).

Van Buskirk EM. Laser revision of filtering surgery. Ophthalmol Clin North Am 1:245–254 (1988).

Van der Zypen E et al. Cyclophotocoagulation in glaucoma therapy. Int Ophthalmol 13:163–166 (1989a).

Van der Zypen E et al. The effect of transscleral laser cyclophotocoagulation on rabbit ciliary body vasculariza-tion. Graefes Arch Clin Exp Ophthalmol 227:172–179 (1989b).

Van der Zypen E et al. Nd:YAG laser sclerostomy ab interno: morphological findings in cadaver pig eyes. Lasers Light Ophthalmol 5:131–142 (1993).

Van der Zypen E et al. Sclerostomy ab interno using long-wave laser modalities: acute morphological effects. Ger J Ophthalmol 4:7–10 (1995).

Van der Zypen E, Fankhauser F. The ultrastructural features of laser trabeculopuncture and cyclodialysis. Problems related to successful treatment of chronic simple glaucoma. Ophthalmologica 179:189–200 (1979).

Van der Zypen E, Fankhauser F. Lasers in the treatment of chronic simple glaucoma. Trans Ophthalmol Soc UK 102:147–153 (1982).

Van Rens GHMB. Transconjunctival reopening of an occluded filtration fistula with the Q-switched neodymium-YAG laser. Doc Ophthalmol 70:205–208 (1988).

Vogel M et al. Ablation of the trabecular meshwork. Klin Monatsbl Augenheilkd 197:250–253 (1990).

Vogel M, Lauritzen K, Quentin CD. Targeted ablation of the trabecular meshwork with excimer laser in primary open-angle glaucoma. Ophthalmologe 93:565–568 (1996).

Wallace DK et al. Surgical results of secondary glaucomas in childhood. Ophthalmology 105:101–111 (1998).

Walland MJ. Diode laser cyclophotocoagulation: dose-standardized therapy in end-stage glaucoma. Aust NZ J Ophthalmol 26:135–139 (1998).

Walland MJ, McKelvie PA. Diode laser cyclophotocoagulation: histopathology in two cases of clinical failure. Ophthalmic Surg Lasers 29:852–856 (1998).

Wand M. Argon laser gonioplasty for synechial angle closure. Arch Ophthalmol 110:363–367 (1992).

Wang Y, Cohen RE, Schuman JS. Iontophoresis of indocyanine green and monastral blue B for gonioscopic diode laser sclerectomy. Ophthalmic Surg Lasers 27:484–487 (1996).

Wang TH, Hung PT, Ho TC. THC:YAG laser sclerostomy with mitomycin subconjunctival injection in rabbits. J Ocul Pharmacol 8:325–332 (1992).

Watts P, McAllister J. Holmium laser sclerostomies. How well do they work? A two-year follow-up. Lasers Light Ophthalmol 6:99–105 (1994).

Weber PA, Jones JH, Kapetansky F. Neodymium:YAG transconjunctival laser revision of late-failing filtering blebs. Ophthalmology 106:2023–2026 (1999).

Wei Z, Guohua Y, Junzhong M. Long-term results of diode versus Nd:YAG contact transscleral laser cyclophoto-coagulation for refractory glaucoma. Lasers Light 9:29–35 (1999).

Weiss HS et al. Argon laser gonioplasty in the treatment of angle-closure glaucoma. Am J Ophthalmol 114:14–18 (1992).

Wetzel W et al. Laser sclerostomy ab externo using the erbium:YAG laser. First results of a clinical study. Ger J Ophthalmol 3:112–115 (1994).

Wetzel W et al. Development of a new Er:YAG laser conception for laser sclerostomy ab externo: experimental and first clinical results. Ger J Ophthalmol 4:283–288 (1995a).

Wetzel W et al. Laser sclerostomy ab externo using two different infrared lasers: a clinical comparison. Ger J Ophthalmol 4:1–6 (1995b).

Wetzel W, Scheu M. A new application system for laser sclerostomy ab externo. Lasers Light Ophthalmol 5:193–198 (1993a).

Wetzel W, Scheu M. Laser sclerostomy ab externo using mid infrared lasers. Ophthalmic Surg 24:6–12 (1993b).

Wetzel W, Scheu M. Laser sclerostomy ab externo using continuos wave and pulsed lasers in a rabbit model. Int Ophthalmol 18:71–75 (1994).

Wheatcroft S et al. Treatment of glaucoma following penetrating keratoplasty with transscleral YAG cyclophoto-coagulation. Int Ophthalmol 16:397–400 (1992).

Wilson RP, Javitt JC. Ab interno laser sclerostomy in aphakic patients with glaucoma and chronic inflammation. Am J Ophthalmol 110:178–184 (1990).

Witschel B, Dannheim F, Rassow B. Experimental studies on laser trabeculo-puncture. Adv Ophthalmol 34:197–200 (1977).

Witschel B-M, Rassow B. Laser trabeculopuncture. II. Scanning electron microscope findings. Ophthalmologica 172:45–51 (1976).

Wong EY et al. Diode laser contact transscleral cyclophotocoagulation for refractory glaucoma in Asian patients. Am J Ophthalmol 124:797–804 (1997).

Wong VK et al. Late detachment of Descemet's membrane after subconjunctival THC:YAG (holmium) laser thermal sclerostomy ab externo [letter]. Am J Ophthalmol 116:514–515 (1993).

Wright MM et al. Laser-cured fibrinogen glue to repair bleb leaks in rabbits. Arch Ophthalmol 116:199–202 (1998).

Yap-Veloso MI et al. Intraocular pressure control after contact transscleral diode cyclophotocoagulation in eyes with intractable glaucoma. J Glaucoma 7:319–328 (1998).

Youn J et al. Factors associated with visual acuity loss after noncontact transscleral Nd:YAG cyclophotocoagulation. J Glaucoma 5:390–394 (1996).

Youn J et al. A clinical comparison of transscleral cyclophotocoagulation with neodymium:YAG and semi-conductor diode lasers. Am J Ophthalmol 126:640–647 (1998).

Zaidman GW, Wandel T. Transscleral YAG laser photocoagulation for uncontrollable glaucoma in corneal patients. Cornea 7:112–114 (1988).

Zarbin MA et al. Endolaser treatment of the ciliary body for severe glaucoma. Ophthalmology 95:1639–1648 (1988).

Zhou-Wei et al. Ab-externo carbon dioxide laser sclerostomy in rabbits. Laser and Light 7:197–202 (1996).

Chapter 9
Other Anterior Segment Therapeutic Uses

Charles M. Wormington

I. Phototherapeutic Keratectomy (PTK)

A. Introduction

1. Phototherapeutic keratectomy (PTK) involves the removal of anterior corneal pathology using the excimer laser. Thus, this technique includes the removal of corneal opacities and surface irregularities. It was approved by the U.S. FDA in 1995 for the excimer lasers made by both Summit Technology, Inc. (Waltham, MA) and VISX, Inc. (Santa Clara, CA).

2. The excimer laser makes PTK possible because of the ability of the laser to remove very thin layers of tissue (ca. 0.25 μm) per pulse with minimal damage to adjacent tissue (Aron-Rosa et al., 1986; Marshall et al., 1985; Puliafito et al., 1987; Steinert & Puliafito, 1988). The postablation surface is very smooth and thus enhances re-epithelialization (Krueger et al., 1985; Marshall et al., 1986).

3. The frequency-quintupled Nd:YAG laser (213 nm) is also being investigated as an alternative to the use of the excimer laser (Shen et al., 1997).

4. Goals for PTK can include improvement of visual acuity, alleviation of discomfort, reduction of glare, improved contact lens fitting, wound healing, cosmesis, and treatment of recurrent corneal erosions (Fagerholm et al., 1993; Sher et al., 1993).

5. PTK can be used alone or as an adjunctive strategy in the more traditional mechanical superficial keratectomy techniques. Prior to the advent of PTK, the main techniques for treating anterior corneal pathology were superficial keratectomy, penetrating keratoplasty, and lamellar keratoplasty.

B. Indications and Contraindications

1. Good candidates for PTK include patients with visually significant pathology in the anterior 100 μm of the cornea where the corneal thickness is greater than 400 μm in the treatment area (Thompson, 1995).

2. **The Food and Drug Administration** (FDA) has **approved** the following **indications** for PTK:
   a. superficial corneal dystrophies (e.g., granular, lattice, Reis-Bücklers', Schnyder's)
   b. epithelial basement membrane dystrophy
   c. corneal scars (e.g., postinfection, postsurgical, post-traumatic, or secondary to pathology)
   d. irregular corneal surfaces (e.g., band keratopathy, nodules)

3. **Indications** based on published reports: Success (%) (see Azar et al., 1997a)
   a. Corneal dystrophies
      1) Avellino: 100%
      2) Fuchs' endothelial: 100%
      3) Gelatinous droplike: 100%
      4) Granular: 70%
      5) Lattice: 92%
      6) Map-dot-fingerprint: 100%
      7) Meesmann's: 100%
      8) Reis-Bücklers': 100%
      9) Salzmann's nodular: 67%
      10) Schnyder's: 67%
   b. Corneal intraepithelial dysplasia: 100%
   c. Corneal irregularities
      1) Apical scars in keratoconus: 81%
      2) Band keratopathy: 91%
   d. Corneal scars
      1) Contact lens wear-related: 50%
      2) Herpetic: 71%
      3) Postinfectious: 50%
      4) Post-traumatic: 61%
      5) Pterygium: 80%
      6) Stevens-Johnson syndrome: 67%
      7) Trachomatous: 67%
      8) Unknown etiology: 50%
   e. Recurrent epithelial erosions: 77%

4. **Relative contraindications** (Azar et al., 1997a,c; Thompson, 1995) include:
   a. Anterior stromal scarring secondary to herpetic keratitis
   b. Hyperopia (due to possible additional flattening of the cornea during PTK)
   c. Keratoconjunctivitis

5. The **contraindications** (Azar et al., 1997a,c; Chamon et al., 1993; Thompson, 1995) include:
   a. Collagen vascular disease
   b. Lagophthalmos

c. Severe blepharitis

d. Severe dry eye

e. Systemic immunosuppression

f. Uncontrolled diabetes

g. Uncontrolled uveitis

C. Preprocedure Management (Azar et al., 1997a,c; Chamon et al., 1993; Clinch, 1996; Gallo & Raizman, 1997; Rapuano, 1997; Starr et al., 1996)

1. Thorough history: This includes an assessment for antihistamine use, collagen-vascular disease, diabetes, ocular herpetic disease, previous steroid responsiveness, seasonal allergy, and the use of medications that may affect the cornea.

2. Visual acuity (uncorrected and best corrected)

3. Potential vision (e.g., evaluation with pinhole, hard contact lens, potential acuity meter, or interferometer)

4. Pupil size (in light and dark)

5. Keratometry

6. Manifest and cycloplegic refraction (because of the hyperopic shift potential, a myope is preferable to a hyperope)

7. Slit-lamp biomicroscopy (include type, location and depth of pathology, precorneal tear film status, lid function, corneal status, presence of external disease or inflammation, presence of corneal vascularization)

8. Slit-lamp photography (optional)

9. Intraocular pressure

10. Dilated fundus examination (to exclude retinal disorders that may contribute to decreased vision)

11. Pachymetry (to measure corneal thickness and help estimate the depth of the pathology)

12. Corneal topography

13. Informed consent discussion

    a. Question patients about what they know about PTK and what their expectations are.

    b. Address any concerns the patient may have.

    c. Describe the procedure in detail.

    d. Explain the risks. This should also include a discussion of the possibility of a significant hyperopic shift and the possibility of wearing a contact lens after PTK. Cover the possible complications and the potential for decrease in vision, continued need for contact lenses or spectacles, or further surgery. Also inform the patient that the underlying pathology may recur (e.g., a corneal dystrophy).

e. Advise the patient that uncertainties exist, including unknown future long-term effects.

f. Give the patient sufficient time to make a decision.

D. Technique (Azar et al., 1997a,c; Durrie et al., 1995; Fong et al., 2000; Forster et al., 1997; Gallo & Raizman, 1997; Hersh et al., 1996; Kremer & Blumenthal, 1997; Sher et al., 1991; Stevens and Bowyer, 1996; Talamo et al., 1992; Thompson, 1995; Thompson et al., 1993)

1. The epithelium is removed either manually or by excimer laser ablation through the epithelium.

2. A masking fluid (e.g., 1% hydroxymethylcellulose) is used during the procedure to create a smooth surface and help minimize induced hyperopic shifts. Without the use of a masking fluid, any surface irregularities would be maintained as the relatively uniform excimer beam ablated the surface valleys and peaks equally. The masking fluid protects the valleys from the beam so that the peaks are ablated preferentially.

3. Stromal ablation is accomplished using either a small beam spot size, large spot size, or varying spot size depending on the nature of the lesion.

4. A smoothing of the corneal surface at the edges of the ablation is accomplished by various techniques. These include moving the patient's head or eye in a circular motion so the laser polishes or smoothes the cornea.

E. Post-Procedure Management (Azar et al., 1997a,c; Chamon et al., 1993; Clinch, 1996; Forster et al., 1997; Gallo & Raizman, 1997; Rapuano, 1997; Starr et al., 1996)

1. The point of post-procedure management is to monitor the ocular surface, facilitate healing of the corneal epithelium, minimize inflammation and scarring, avoid infection, and minimize pain and discomfort.

2. A bandage contact lens may be used immediately after PTK. This is useful in decreasing postoperative pain. The alternative is antibiotic ointment, a cycloplegic, and patching.

3. Antibiotic-steroid combination drops or a separate antibiotic (e.g., ofloxacin 0.3%) and steroid (e.g., fluorometholone 0.1% or, for more severe inflammation, prednisolone acetate 1%) can be given QID.

4. A nonsteroidal anti-inflammatory agent (e.g., diclofenac 0.1%) can be given TID or QID.

5. Oral analgesic agents (e.g., acetaminophen with codeine) can be given as necessary.

6. Preservative-free artificial tears can be used to increase patient comfort and enhance epithelial healing.

7. Have the patient return daily until re-epithelialization occurs. This usually occurs within 5 days. The antibiotic can then be discontinued.

8. After re-epithelialization, a mild steroid drop (e.g., fluorometholone 0.1%) can be prescribed QID and then tapered over 3 weeks to several months, depending on the amount of inflammation and/or corneal haze.

9. After re-epithelialization, the patient is usually seen at 1 month, 3 months, 6 months, 12 months, and 24 months.

10. Each visit should include an evaluation of:
    a. Symptoms
    b. Visual acuity
    c. Anterior segment examination
    d. Grading of corneal haze with slit lamp biomicroscopy
    e. Intraocular pressure

11. In a patient with a history of ocular herpes simplex, oral acyclovir 400 mg and topical antiviral (e.g., trifluridine) agents may be started 2 days before the procedure and then continued BID for 3 weeks after the procedure in order to avoid reactivation of the virus.

F. Complications (Azar et al., 1997b,c; Hersh et al., 1996)

1. **Delayed epithelialization and recurrent epithelial erosions.** Healing of the epithelium occurs within 3 to 7 days in most patients, but it may take up to a month for complete re-epithelialization in some patients (Chamon et al., 1993; Hersh et al., 1996; Migden et al., 1996; Rapuano, 1997; Sher et al., 1991; Stark et al., 1992; Zuckerman et al., 1996). Prolonged healing occurred in 3.5% of 255 patients in a Summit Technology study (1995) and in from 3% to 19% in other major studies. In some cases it may be useful to use nonpreserved ocular lubricants, bandage soft contact lenses, blepharitis management, punctal occlusion, or even tarsorrhaphy. Also consider the possibility of toxicity of one of the postoperative medications or of a previously undiagnosed systemic condition that may impair corneal healing. Recurrent epithelial erosions have also been reported following PTK (Dausch et al., 1993; Morad et al., 1998; O'Brart et al., 1993).

2. **Stromal haze/scarring.** Most patients will have trace to mild subepithelial stromal haze (Hersh et al., 1996). This haze tends to regress with time. Summit Technology reported 14% of 255 patients experienced scarring (Summit Technology, 1995). Overtreatment with subsequent corneal scarring can occur (Alaa et al., 1997). Usually hyaluronan is formed in the treatment area following PTK and may contribute to the formation of the haze (Weber & Fagerholm, 1998).

3. **Loss of best-corrected visual acuity.** Up to 17% of patients may lose two or more lines of best-corrected acuity following PTK and up to 20% may lose one or more lines

(Alaa et al., 1997; Campos et al., 1993; Durrie et al., 1995; Forster et al., 1997; Maloney et al., 1996; Migden et al., 1996; Rapuano, 1997; Sher et al., 1991; Starr et al., 1996). In a multicenter trial involving 103 eyes, 9% lost two or more lines of acuity at postoperative month 12 (Maloney et al., 1996). Causes for this loss include an increase in irregular corneal astigmatism and corneal opacification. Some of these patients can be treated with contact lenses and some may need penetrating keratoplasty.

4. **Glare.** In a large series of patients, Summit Technology (1995) reported 12.2% of patients experienced glare.

5. **Infection/ulceration.** Summit Technology (1995) noted that 2% of 255 patients had a corneal infection or ulceration after PTK. Fulton et al. (1996) reported a bacterial ulcer in an elderly patient with a corneal transplant, rheumatoid arthritis, and dry eye syndrome. Out of 22 eyes with corneal scars, Migden et al. (1996) reported bacterial keratitis in one eye of a patient that was found to be positive for herpes simplex by polymerase chain reaction (PCR). In a study of 258 eyes, Al-Rajhi et al. (1996) noted bacterial keratitis in 3 (1.2%). All three patients had climatic droplet keratopathy. Certainly, any postoperative eye where infection is suspected should be cultured and aggressively treated with appropriate antibiotics.

6. **Corneal graft rejection.** Rejection of a corneal graft has been noted in a few patients following PTK (Epstein & Robin, 1994; Hersh et al., 1993; Maloney et al., 1996). Intense medical therapy is indicated. If a rejection episode is recognized early, prompt treatment may prevent graft failure.

7. **Subsequent penetrating keratoplasty.** If the PTK does not result in an acceptable outcome or if the pathology recurs, it may be necessary to go on to penetrating keratoplasty (Azar et al., 1997c; Maloney et al., 1996).

8. **Recurrent herpes simplex keratitis.** There have been cases of reactivation of the herpes virus following PTK (Fagerholm et al., 1993; Maloney et al., 1996; Starr et al., 1996; Vrabec et al., 1994; Zuckerman et al., 1996). If herpes simplex keratitis occurs postoperatively, then oral acyclovir and topical antiviral agents can be used with modification of any steroid therapy.

9. **Pain.** Significant pain may occur during the first 24 to 48 hours post-procedure (Azar et al., 1997a; Forster et al., 1997; Rapuano, 1997). Usually the pain resolves by the time re-epithelialization is complete, but it may persist for a few days. Nonsteroidal anti-inflammatory agents have been shown to significantly reduce the pain. If necessary, cycloplegics, ice packs, narcotics, or peribulbar or retrobulbar anesthesia may be useful. Disposable soft contact lenses can also be helpful.

10. **Induced hyperopia.** Corneal flattening often occurs during PTK, resulting in a hyperopic shift (Amm & Duncker, 1997; Campos et al., 1993; Faschinger, 2000; Gartry et al., 1991; Maloney et al., 1996; Migden et al., 1996; O'Brart et al., 1993; Orndahl

& Fagerholm, 1998a; Rapuano, 1997; Sher et al., 1991; Stark et al., 1992; Starr et al., 1996; Zuckerman et al., 1996). The induced hyperopic shift increases with increasing ablation depth. This may be a problem for patients that are not myopic before the PTK. Various techniques have been proposed to minimize this shift (Amm & Duncker, 1997; Azar et al., 1997a: Hersh et al., 1996; Stark et al., 1992). If anisometropia is produced, it may be necessary to fit the patient with a contact lens, or in contact-lens-intolerant patients, refractive surgery or a lamellar or penetrating keratoplasty may ultimately be needed.

11. **Induced myopia.** Myopic shifts have occurred following PTK in from 3% to 30% of patients (Amm & Duncker, 1997; Campos et al., 1993; Orndahl & Fagerholm, 1998a; Sher et al., 1991).

12. **Induced astigmatism.** Summit Technology (1995) reported that 9% of 255 patients had astigmatism induced by PTK. Astigmatism after PTK has occurred in a number of studies (Amm & Duncker, 1997; Campos et al., 1993; Rapuano, 1997; Starr et al., 1996).

13. **Narrow angle glaucoma.** Angle-closure glaucoma can occur due to the use of a cycloplegic agent (Zuckerman et al., 1996).

14. **A Wessely-type immune ring.** Teichmann et al. (1996) reported a case of an incomplete corneal white ring that appeared on the fourth day following PTK and slowly faded over a period of 9 months.

15. **Increased intraocular pressure.** Some patients experience an increase in intraocular pressure due to the steroids used after PTK (Stark et al., 1992; Starr et al., 1996). This usually resolves following tapering and discontinuation of the steroid.

16. **Recurrence of underlying pathology.** The lesion treated by PTK can recur following the procedure (Dinh et al., 1999; Forster et al., 1997; Krag & Ehlers, 1992; Maloney et al., 1996; Orndahl & Fagerholm, 1998b; Rapuano, 1997; Starr, 1999; Talu et al., 1998).

17. **Retinal detachment.** A few patients who have undergone PTK or PRK have experienced a retinal detachment (Charteris et al., 1997). In two of the patients, symptoms of visual loss were initially attributed to corneal haze following the excimer procedure.

18. **Episcleritis.** An episode of episcleritis may occur following PTK (Zuckerman et al., 1996).

II. Laser Suture Lysis

A. Introduction

1. If dark nylon or proline sutures are used to secure the scleral flap in a trabeculectomy and they are too tight, a laser can be used to cut (lyse) the suture and increase filtra-

tion. This has evolved into an established procedure in the early post-procedure period.

2. The sutures can be more securely applied during surgery because of the availability of laser suture lysis (Blok et al., 1993; Melamed et al., 1990; Savage et al., 1988). This reduces the potential for hypotony and flat anterior chamber shortly after the surgery. It also allows titration of the filtration.

3. By using this technique, surgical manipulation of the scleral flap may be avoided with its associated risks.

4. Suture ligatures occluding Molteno drainage tubes can also be lysed with a laser (Liebmann & Ritch, 1992; Price & Whitson, 1989).

5. In addition to its use following glaucoma operations, lysis of selected sutures can be used to reduce residual astigmatism following cataract operations and to remove projecting suture ends.

6. Unless specifically noted, the following comments refer to laser suture lysis following trabeculectomy.

B. *Indications and Contraindications*

1. One indication is **inadequate filtration due to a tight suture following trabeculectomy** (Chopra et al., 1992; Hoskins & Migliazzo, 1984; Macken et al., 1996; Singh et al., 1996). The early use of laser suture lysis should be considered in an eye with increased risk of early subconjunctival fibrosis. This is especially true after combined procedures, reoperations, or eyes with significant post-procedure inflammation.

2. Another indication is **residual astigmatism due to a tight suture following cataract extraction** (Hayashi et al., 1993; Sachdev et al., 1990).

3. A further indication is **projecting suture ends following cataract surgery** (Talwar et al., 1991).

4. Still another indication is **incomplete removal of corneal sutures**, especially when the knot is buried well below the stromal surface (Bourne & Maguire, 1990).

5. **If the suture cannot be seen, laser suture lysis is contraindicated.**

C. *Technique* (Asomoto et al., 1995; Chopra et al., 1992; Hayashi et al., 1993; Keller & To, 1993; Lieberman, 1996; Macken et al., 1996; Schuman, 1997; Singh et al., 1996)

1. Tight sutures can be lysed 3 days to 3 weeks after the trabeculectomy. The procedure is usually done within 2 weeks of the surgery (Chopra et al., 1992). When an antimetabolite such as mitomycin C has been used, laser suture lysis may still be effective in the late (7 to 21 weeks) postoperative period (Morinelli et al., 1996; Pappa et al., 1993).

2. Lasers used to perform the lysis include:
   a. **Argon laser** (488 + 514 nm, 50-µm to 100-µm spot size, 0.05 to 0.1 sec duration, 200 to 1000 mW; most studies)
   b. **Diode laser** (810 nm, 75-µm spot size, 0.1 to 0.2 sec duration, 1000 mW; Lieberman, 1996)
   c. **Diode laser** (780 + 830 nm, 100-µm spot size, 0.1 sec, 1100 mW; Beck et al., 1995; McMillan et al., 1992)
   d. **Dye laser** (488 + 514 nm, 514 nm, 585 nm, 610 nm, 630 nm; 50-µm spot size, 0.1 sec duration, 200 to 250 mW in rabbits; McMillan et al., 1992; or 500 to 600 nm, 50-µm spot size, 0.2 sec duration, 400 to 500 mW in patients; Bardak et al., 1998)
   e. **Krypton laser** (647 nm, 50-µm to 100-µm spot size, 0.1 sec duration, 150 to 500 mW; Aktan & Mandelkorn, 1998; Keller & To, 1993; Kumar & Talwar, 1991)
   f. **Nd:YAG laser** [532 nm (frequency-doubled CW), 100-µm spot size, 0.1 sec duration, 350–1000 mW; Singh et al., 1996]

3. A **special lens** can be used to assist in focusing the laser onto the sutures. By using the lens to apply pressure to the overlying conjunctiva, thinning of the conjunctiva and blanching of the conjunctival vessels can be achieved. This allows laser focusing even in the presence of conjunctival edema or subconjunctival hemorrhage. The following lenses have been used:
   a. Hoskins laser suture lens (Hoskins & Migliazzo, 1984) (Figure 9–1)
   b. Goldmann goniolens (Lieberman, 1983)
   c. Zeiss four-mirror goniolens (Savage et al., 1988)
   d. Fiberoptic endolaser probe (Salamon, 1987)
   e. Glass micropipettes (Tomey, 1991)
   f. Glass blood-collecting tube (Temel & Sayin, 1996)
   g. Mandelkorn suture lysis lens (Mandelkorn et al., 1994)
   h. Laser suture lysis lens (Ritch et al., 1994)
   i. Laser lens holder for children (Beck et al., 1995)

4. Instead of using a special lens, an endolaser probe can also be used to lyse sutures (Salamon, 1987).

5. If seton implantation is used, a clear corneal graft can be placed over the tube in order to facilitate laser lysis (Rojanapongpun & Ritch, 1996).

6. Avoid delivering a large number of laser applications in the same location on the conjunctiva, especially when there is pigmentation present.

7. Do not cut more than one suture per day (Schuman, 1997).

8. Cutting of the suture with a laser is an effective technique to titrate filtration. If the bleb does not spontaneously form after the lysis, gentle ocular massage can be employed.

9. Argon laser suture lysis can also be used to reduce surgically induced astigmatism (Sachdev et al., 1990). One to two laser shots (50-µm spot size, 0.1 sec duration, 0.3

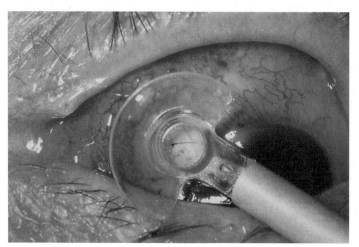

Figure 9–1 The Hoskins laser suture lens can be used to compress the conjunctiva overlying a suture. Using this lens, fluid from the overlying conjunctiva can be displaced and the overlying vessels can be blanched to enhance the view of the underlying suture. (Reprinted with permission from Dickens and Hoskins. Laser suteralysis. In Minckler DS, VanBuskiak EM, Wright KW, eds. Color Atlas of Ophthalmic Surgery: Glaucoma. Philadelphia: Lippincott Williams and Wilkins, 1992:102–103.)

to 0.6 W) can be applied to the suture in the steepest meridian and to two adjacent sutures about 6 or more weeks after surgery.

10. In the case of projecting suture ends following cataract surgery, the argon laser can be used to vaporize the suture ends (one to five applications of a 100-μm spot size, 0.1 sec duration, 0.2 to 0.3 W) (Talwar et al., 1991).

11. With corneal sutures that have large, deeply buried knots, the suture can be lysed on either side of the knot (50-μm spot size, 0.2 sec duration, 0.3 to 0.5 W), and then the suture can be removed with forceps (Bourne & Maguire, 1990).

D. Post-Procedure Management (Oh, 1994)

1. Measure the intraocular pressure 15 to 30 minutes after lysis.

2. If the pressure has not changed significantly, digital massage can be used to apply pressure to the scleral edge of the incision. This may increase filtration by separating the flap from the underlying sclera.

3. If massage does not decrease the intraocular pressure, consider lysing another suture.

4. Antibiotic-steroid drops can be started.

5. The patient can be followed the next day and as required thereafter. Since some of the complications arise 2 to 3 days after lysis, it would be prudent to maintain fairly close follow-up for the first few days.

6. Ultrasound biomicroscopy may be useful in evaluation of bleb function (Avitabile et al., 1998; McWhae & Crichton, 1996; Yamamoto et al., 1995).

E. Complications. Although laser suture lysis is considered a safe procedure, a number of complications can occur.

1. **Hypotony with a shallow anterior chamber.** This is probably the most common complication seen after laser suture lysis (Bardak et al., 1998; Blok et al., 1993; Geijssen et al., 1992; Melamed et al., 1990; Morinelli et al., 1996; Oh, 1994; Pappa et al., 1993; Savage & Simmons, 1986; Savage et al., 1988; Schwartz & Weiss, 1992; Singh et al., 1996; Zacharia et al., 1993). It can be minimized by delaying the suture lysis for at least 48 hours to allow the flap to heal sufficiently. Lysing only one suture per treatment and limiting pressure on the globe during the procedure may also be helpful.

2. **Flat anterior chamber** (iridocorneal touch up to the pupil margin). These cases often settle with conservative measures within a few days (Macken et al., 1996; Savage et al., 1988). In a pseudophakic eye, the intraocular lens can touch the cornea (Melamed et al., 1990).

3. **Conjunctival perforation/external aqueous leaks.** This can result from setting the power or energy too high or from using too many laser applications in the same location (Blok et al., 1993; Macken et al., 1996; Oh, 1994; Savage et al., 1988; Savage & Simmons, 1986; Singh et al., 1996). A very thin, ischemic bleb, as well as conjunctival hemorrhages, can increase the risk of perforation. A Seidel test can be performed after the lysis. If aqueous leak occurs, a bandage contact lens can be tried.

4. **Conjunctival laser burn.** These are usually superficial and do not cause a problem (Singh et al., 1996).

5. **Malignant glaucoma.** This can be precipitated by suture lysis (DiSclafani et al., 1989; Macken et al., 1996). It may be that a rapid ocular decompression in eyes that are predisposed can precipitate a forward displacement of the lens iris diaphragm and hence ciliary vitreous block.

6. **Iris incarceration.** Within 24 hours after lysis, the iris can become incarcerated, requiring surgical repair (Macken et al., 1996).

7. **Hyphema.** After suture lysis a hyphema can occur (Macken et al., 1996; Melamed et al., 1990). The blood can clear within 24 hours.

8. **Excessive bleb formation.** An elevation of the bleb can occur after lysis, especially in eyes treated with antimetabolites (Macken et al., 1996).

9. **Corneal dellen.** Persistence of excessive bleb formation can lead to the development of corneal dellen (Macken et al., 1996).

10. **Hypotonus maculopathy.** The decrease in intraocular pressure from excessive filtration can cause maculopathy (Jampel et al., 1992; Savage & Simmons, 1986).

11. **Progressive lens opacity.** This may occur after the lysis procedure (Savage et al., 1988; Singh et al., 1996).

12. **Failure to lyse the suture.** In a few cases, the laser was unable to lyse the suture (Blok et al., 1993).

III. Oculoplastic Surgery

A. Introduction

1. Over the past few years, a number of oculoplastic applications of lasers have been developed (Hornblass & Coden, 1995; Maus, 1995; Yeatts, 1996). These include:
   a. **Treatment of skin lesions**
   b. **Treatment of trichiasis**
   c. **Lacrimal obstruction surgery**
   d. **Miscellaneous uses**

2. One of the most prevalent applications is **laser skin resurfacing or dermablation** (American Academy of Ophthalmology, 1998; Bass, 1998; Biesman, 1998; Chernoff et al., 1995; Felder, 1996; Felder & Mayl, 1996; Fisher, 1996; Goldberg & Whitworth, 1997; Hrabovsky, 1998; Khan, 1997; Kopelman, 1998a; Perez et al., 1998; Teikemeier and Goldberg, 1997; Than & Spear, 1997; Weinstein, 1998a). This method was pioneered in the early 1990s and quickly generated interest within the medical community and the public. An indication of that interest is the large number of recent books on the subject (Alster & Apfelberg, 1999; Arndt et al., 1997; Backer et al., 1998; Carniol, 1998; Coleman & Lawrence, 1998; Cook and Cook, 1999; Goldman & Fitzpatrick, 1998; Lask and Lowe, 1999; Sarnoff & Swirsky, 1998). Using a laser to ablate a layer of skin a few micrometers thick is safer than conventional resurfacing techniques. Besides ablation of the skin, the laser thermal effect also shrinks the collagen in the skin, causing the skin to tighten and smooth.

3. The most extensively used lasers in this area include the CO_2 laser, the argon laser, and the Nd:YAG laser. More recently, a number of other lasers (e.g., Er:YAG lasers) have been employed for oculoplastic surgery.

4. Following is an abbreviated discussion of the different kinds of applications for each type of laser. Detailed discussions of the techniques, perioperative management, and complications can be found in the cited references. A review of complications of oculoplastic surgery was recently published (Nanni, 1998).

B. Argon Laser Applications. The CW argon laser is absorbed by chromophores in the skin, especially melanin and hemoglobin. It penetrates up to about 1 mm of dermis and can be used to photothermally ablate pigmented and vascular lesions.

1. **Benign eyelid tumors** (Wohlrab et al., 1998). Actinic keratosis, cysts, molluscum contagiosum, dermal nevus, papilloma, seborrheic keratosis, verruca vulgaris, and verruca plana juvenilis have all been treated with the argon laser.

2. **Blepharopigmentation** (Tanenbaum et al., 1988). In order to enhance eyelashes, iron oxide pigment can be implanted in the eyelid skin adjacent to the cilia. The argon laser can be used to treat misplacement or overcorrection of the pigment.

3. **Capillary hemangioma** (Gladstone & Beckman, 1983; Hobby, 1983). These benign vascular tumors can be treated with the argon laser.

4. **Chloasma gravidarum** (Hornblass & Coden, 1995). This periorbital hyperpigmentation occurs after pregnancy or the use of oral contraceptives. The laser can be used to decrease the pigmentation.

5. **Dacryocystorhinostomy** (DCR) (Bartley, 1994; Boush et al., 1994; Massaro et al., 1990). The blue green argon laser has been used to create an opening between the nasal cavity and the lacrimal sac as well as to identify the osteotomy site with a fiberoptic probe.

6. **Dry eye** (Benson et al., 1992; Cartwright, 1994; Hutnik & Probst, 1998; Murube & Murube, 1996; Vrabec et al., 1993). Punctal occlusion via photothermal coagulation can be used to treat dry eye. However, laser treatment may not be as effective as electrocautery treatment.

7. **Phthiriasis palperarum** (Awan, 1986). The crab louse can be treated by aiming the laser at the junction between the head and the body of each parasite.

8. **Port-wine stain** (Apfelberg et al., 1989; Carruth et al., 1992; Cosman, 1980; Wisnicki, 1984). This congenital vascular malformation, also called nevus flammeus, can be treated with some success by the argon laser.

9. **Punctal stenosis** (Awan, 1985). Argon laser punctoplasty can be used to form an opening in the canalicular medial wall to treat occlusion or stenosis of the lacrimal punctum.

10. **Trichiasis** (Bartley & Lowry, 1992; Campbell, 1990; Elder, 1996; Gossman et al., 1992; Ladas et al., 1993; Oshry et al., 1994; Sharif et al., 1991; Yung et al., 1994). The argon laser can be used to thermally ablate the misdirected cilia with less scarring, inflammation, and destruction of neighboring meibomian glands. Multiple treatments may be necessary.

C. Carbon Dioxide Laser Applications. The CO_2 laser is strongly absorbed by water, so it is absorbed essentially totally by 0.1 mm of soft tissue. This allows it to be used for precise delivery of laser energy and for minimizing damage to adjacent tissue (Goldbaum

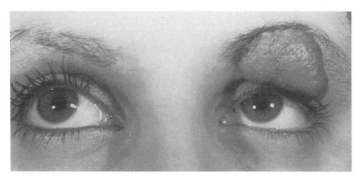

Figure 9–2 Vascular lid tumor before laser procedure. (Reprinted with permission from Hornblass A, Coden DJ. Lasers in ophthalmic plastic and orbital surgery. In Karlin DB, ed. Lasers in Ophthalmic Surgery. Cambridge, MA: Blackwell Science, 1995;11:214–226.)

& Woog, 1997). Its beam also seals small blood vessels and lymphatic vessels. Minimal adjacent tissue thermal damage can be achieved with short duration pulses (1 msec) or with continuous scanning of the beam. The latter techniques extend the applications to **laser skin resurfacing**, which has become increasingly popular as a technique for facial rejuvenation (Bernstein et al., 1997; Biesman, 1998; Chernoff et al., 1995; Cohen & Swartz, 1999; Felder, 1996; Felder & Mayl, 1996; Fisher, 1996; Goldbaum & Woog, 1997; Khan, 1997; Than & Spear, 1997; Weinstein, 1998a). It also allows treatment of lesions of the eyelids and periorbital region (Goldbaum & Woog, 1997; Kaplan et al., 1996) (Figures 9–2 and 9–3).

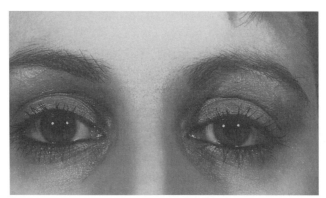

Figure 9–3 Vascular lid tumor excised with a CO_2 laser. (Reprinted with permission from Hornblass A, Coden DJ. Lasers in ophthalmic plastic and orbital surgery. In Karlin DB, ed. Lasers in Ophthalmic Surgery. Cambridge, MA: Blackwell Science, 1995;11:214–226.)

1. **Atrophic acne scars** (Alster & West, 1996; Apfelberg, 1997). Atrophic facial acne scars may be improved from 50% to 80%.

2. **Adenoma sebaceum** (Bellack & Shapshay, 1986). The CO_2 laser has been recommended to treat adenoma sebaceum.

3. **Basal cell carcinoma** (Adams & Price, 1979; Bandieramonte et al., 1997; Humphreys et al., 1998; Wheeland et al., 1987a). Primary superficial basal cell carcinomas of the eyelid margins have been treated by excision and posterior tumor-margin vaporization using the CO_2 laser.

4. **Blepharoplasty** (American Academy of Ophthalmology, 1998; Baker et al., 1984; Baskin, 1996; David & Goodman, 1995; Lessner & Fagien, 1998; Morrow & Morrow, 1992; Trelles et al., 1996a; Wesley & Bond, 1985). This involves an operation to restore a defect in an eyelid. The CO_2 laser incisions can be useful in minimizing bleeding, operating time, and postprocedure ecchymosis, swelling, and pain.

5. **Capillary hemangioma** (Wesley & Bond, 1985). By using the superb hemostatic capability of the CO_2 laser, congenital capillary hemangiomas can be vaporized effectively.

6. **Chalazion** (Korn, 1988; Wesley & Bond, 1985). The core of the chalazion has been vaporized with good results using the CO_2 laser.

7. **Dacryocystorhinostomy** (Bartley, 1994; Gonnering et al., 1991; Hartikainen et al., 1998). The CO_2 laser has been used in endoscopic laser-assisted DCR.

8. **Ectropion of the eyelid** (Korn & Glotzbach, 1988). Medial-eyelid ectropion has been successfully repaired using the laser.

9. **Eruptive vellus hair cysts** (Huerter & Wheeland, 1987). These well-encapsulated cystic structures in the periorbital and central face areas can be effectively removed with the CO_2 laser.

10. **Exenterations** (Wesley & Bond, 1985). The CO_2 laser is especially useful in exenterations (i.e., removal of an organ) in cancer surgery because of its ability to seal blood vessels and lymphatics. This can limit the spread of tumors.

11. **Hemangioma** (Wesley & Bond, 1985). Hemangiomas have been vaporized with the CO_2 laser.

12. **Lymphangioma** (Kennerdell et al., 1986; Jordan & Anderson, 1981; Wesley & Bond, 1985). These unencapsulated infiltrative tumors can be debulked with the CO_2 laser while maintaining superior hemostasis.

13. **Meningioma** (Takizawa et al., 1980). Neoplasms that originate in arachnoidal tissue (meningiomas) can adhere to the optic nerve and globe. These can be removed with the CO_2 laser.

14. **Periocular skin reshaping** (Trelles et al., 1996b). Overlaxness of the eyelid skin can be treated by thermally treating the skin.

15. **Photodamaged facial skin** (Apfelberg, 1997; Chernoff et al., 1995; Felder, 1996; Fitzpatrick et al., 1996). Resurfacing of skin damaged by sun (UV) exposure is a very promising technique.

16. **Rhytids** (wrinkles, also spelled rhytides; Apfelberg, 1997; Biesman, 1996; Felder, 1996; Gross & Rogers, 1998; Harris et al., 1999; Khatri et al., 1999; Shim et al., 1998; Waldorf et al., 1995). Cutaneous resurfacing with the CO_2 laser can be used to improve facial rhytids (periorbital, glabellar, perioral).

17. **Syringoma** (Apfelberg et al., 1987a; Nerad & Anderson, 1988; Wheeland et al., 1987b). Precise removal of this benign neoplasm of the sweat glands can be accomplished.

18. **Xanthalasma** (Apfelberg et al., 1987b; Gladstone et al., 1985). Satisfactory results have been obtained by employing the CO_2 laser to treat xanthelasma palperarum.

D. Nd:YAG Laser Applications

1. **Blepharopigmentation** (Watts et al., 1992). The Q-switched Nd:YAG laser has been used to precisely and safely reduce the level of blepharopigmentation.

2. **Blepharoplasty** (Mittelman, 1998). The frequency-doubled Nd:YAG laser has been used with a sculptured fiber tip. There is greater hemostasis with this laser than with the CW CO_2 laser.

3. **Dacryocystorhinostomy** (Bartley, 1994; Doyle et al., 2000; Flaharty et al., 1994; Gonnering et al., 1991; Hartikainen et al., 1998; Kong et al., 1994; Levin & Stormo-Gipson, 1992; Muellner et al., 2000; Patel et al., 1997; Reifler, 1993; Rosen et al., 1997; Tutton & O'Donnell, 1995; Woo et al., 1998). A frequency-doubled Nd:YAG laser has been used to create a lacrimal-nasal opening in laser-assisted DCR. It and the infrared Nd:YAG have also been used to revise failed DCRs using a transcanalicular approach.

4. **Facial hemangioma of infancy** (Achauer et al., 1996). The Nd:YAG (1064 nm) and the frequency-doubled Nd:YAG (532 nm) lasers have been used to improve volume, color, and texture in cases of capillary hemangioma of infancy.

5. **Laser skin resurfacing** (Cisneros et al., 1998; Goldberg & Whitworth, 1997). The Q-switched Nd:YAG laser may play a role in the treatment of rhytids, postacne patients, and pigmented lesions. Also, the frequency-doubled Nd:YAG laser along with topical application of an exogenous chromophore may be useful (Sumian et al., 1999).

6. **Trichiasis** (Oguz et al., 1999). A diode-pumped, frequency-doubled, Nd:YAG laser operating in the CW mode has been used to treat trichiasis caused by trachoma.

E. Ho:YAG Laser Applications: Dacryocystorhinostomy.

The Ho:YAG laser has been used in laser-assisted endonasal DCR (Bartley, 1994; Kong et al., 1994; Metson et al., 1994; Sadiq et al., 1997; Silkiss et al., 1992; Woog et al., 1993). It has also been used for primary endonasal laser DCR resulting in significantly quicker surgery performed as an outpatient procedure compared to conventional surgery (Sadiq et al., 1996).

F. Er:YAG Laser Applications. Because of the strong absorption by water of its 2940 nm wavelength, the Er:YAG laser can ablate and cut tissue with surgical precision and minimal collateral tissue damage.

1. **Skin resurfacing** (American Academy of Ophthalmology, 1998; Bass, 1998; Hughes, 1998; Kaufmann et al., 1994; Kaufmann & Hibst, 1996; Khatri et al., 1999; Kopelman, 1998b; Perez et al., 1998; Polnikorn et al., 1998; Teikemeier and Goldberg, 1997; Weinstein, 1998b). The laser has been used to treat rhytids, for facial rejuvenation, and for scar removal. It apparently produces less thermal damage than the CO_2 laser, less erythema, and faster healing. But because of the reduction in thermal damage, the laser provides limited hemostasis. The CO_2 laser has been used in combination with the Er:YAG laser for eyelid resurfacing (Millman & Mannor, 1999).

2. **Benign skin disorders** (Dmovsek-Olup & Vedlin, 1997). The laser has been found to be a useful tool for treating disorders like milia, warts, actinic keratosis, scars, xanthelasma palperarum, hidradenoma, chloasma, epidermal nevi, senile lentigo, and fibroepithelial papillomata.

3. **Endonasal laser dacryocystorhinostomy** (Haeusler et al., 1999). A custom-built laser has been used with very little thermal damage in the surrounding tissue.

G. Pulsed Dye Laser Applications. This tunable laser can be used at 580, 577, or 585 nm. This allows increased penetration of the skin tissue compared to the argon laser and minimizes the risk of pigment loss. These wavelengths are selectively absorbed by blood vessels allowing for selective photothermolysis. In the treatment of vascular lesions of the face, the pulse dye laser is apparently superior to the argon laser.

1. **Hemangiomas** (Garden et al., 1992; Scheepers & Quaba, 1995). The pulsed dye laser has been used to treat capillary and mixed hemangiomas with satisfactory lightening and thinning of the lesions.

2. **Port-wine stains** (Goldman et al., 1993; Holy & Geronemus, 1992; Tan, 1992; Tan et al., 1989; van der Horst et al., 1998). Both children and adults have been treated with good-to-excellent results.

3. **Telangiectases** (Boska et al., 1994; Gonzalez et al., 1992; Ross et al., 1993). Linear, spider, and matted vascular ectases have been treated with good-to-excellent results.

H. Copper Vapor Laser Applications. This laser produces a green (511 nm) and a yellow (578 nm) line. The 511-nm line is strongly absorbed by melanin, and the 578-nm line is strongly absorbed by hemoglobin. This makes the laser useful in lightening skin lesions and removing vascular lesions (Bosniak & Ginsberg, 1993; Dinehart et al., 1993; Key & Waner, 1992; Pickering et al., 1990).

1. **Obliteration of vascular lesions** (e.g., hemangiomas, port-wine stains, angiomas, telangiectases, and spider veins)
2. **Treatment of pigment lesions** (e.g., lentigines, freckles, café au lait spots, keratoses, age spots)

I. Krypton Laser Applications. The same laser used to treat the retina can also be used to treat superficial pigmented and vascular lesions (Patel, 1998).

J. Ruby Laser. Although it was the first laser developed, the Q-switched ruby laser (694 nm) is still used today to treat epidermal and dermal pigment (e.g., lentigines, melanocytic nevi, nevi of Ota, and tattoos) (Nanni, 1998).

K. Alexandrite Laser. The Q-switched alexandrite laser (755 nm) is also used for the treatment of dermal pigment (Moreno-Arias & Camps-Fresneda, 1999; Nanni, 1998).

L. Complications (Apfelberg, 1998; Blanco et al., 1999; Linsmeier-Kilmer, 1997; Nanni & Alster, 1998a,b; Weinstein et al., 1998a)
1. **Prolonged erythema** (Apfelberg, 1998; Bass, 1998; Linsmeier-Kilmer, 1998; Nanni & Alster, 1998b)
2. **Hyperpigmentation** (Khan, 1997; Linsmeier-Kilmer, 1997)
3. **Hypopigmentation** (Apfelberg, 1998; Laws et al., 1998; Linsmeier-Kilmer, 1997)
4. **Hypertrophic or keloidlike scarring** (Apfelberg, 1998; Khan, 1997; Nanni & Alster, 1998a)
5. **Bacterial, viral, or fungal infections** (Apfelberg, 1998; Jordan et al., 1998; Khan, 1997; Linsmeier-Kilmer, 1997; Nanni & Alster, 1998a; Weinstein et al., 1998a)
6. **Ectropion** (Apfelberg, 1998; Nanni & Alster, 1998a,b)
7. **Corneal injury** (Apfelberg, 1998)
8. **Ocular perforation** (Goldbaum & Woog, 1997)
9. **Severe burns** (Grossman et al., 1998)

IV. Anterior Stromal Puncture

A. Introduction. Most patients with recurrent corneal erosion respond to mechanical debridement, patching, topical lubrication, hypertonic drops, collagen shields, or therapeutic bandage contact lenses. If they do not respond to this conservative treatment, anterior stromal puncture with a needle has been performed. Because of the irregular depth and anterior scarring with the needle, anterior stromal puncture has been introduced with the laser instead of a needle (Geggel, 1990). The use of the laser has also been viewed critically (Rubinfeld et al., 1991).

B. *Indications*

1. Recurrent corneal erosion that does not respond to conservative treatment may be treated with the laser.

2. Retreatment may be necessary at a later time.

C. *Preprocedure Management*

1. Topical anesthetic (e.g., proparacaine hydrochloride) is applied.

2. Topical antibiotic drops are applied.

D. *Technique*

1. The corneal epithelium in the area of the erosion is debrided. This can be done, for example, with cellulose sponges. Debridement makes it easier to focus the laser just in front of the corneal basement membrane.

2. The aiming beam of the **Nd:YAG laser** is focused just in front of the corneal basement membrane in order to minimize damage to the corneal stroma and, hence, scarring. The slit-lamp biomicroscope can be used with medium magnification and white light or the cobalt blue filter can be used in conjunction with fluorescein dye to enhance contrast.

3. Laser applications are made in rows about 0.20 mm to 0.25 mm apart with an energy level between 1.8 mJ and 2.2 mJ. This may involve 100 to 200 spots depending on the area of the erosion.

4. The intended effect is to breach Bowman's membrane in order to produce stronger epithelial adhesion.

5. A **variant** of this treatment involves lower laser energies (0.4 mJ to 0.5 mJ) delivered through an intact epithelium with no attempt to create breaks in Bowman's layer (Katz et al., 1994). The authors call the method **"Nd:YAG laser photo-induced adhesion of the corneal epithelium."**

E. *Post-Procedure Management*

1. Topical steroid and cycloplegic drops are administered. An antibiotic ointment is used, and a pressure patch is applied.

2. The patient is examined daily until the epithelium is healed.

3. After the pressure patch is removed, topical steroid drops may be used for a week.

4. After healing of the epithelium, bland, nonpreserved eyedrops and ointment can be used throughout the day and at bedtime, respectively.

F. *Complications*

1. **Stromal scars** may occur; although they are smaller and less frequent than the scars that occur after use of the needle. Precise focus of the laser will minimize scarring.

2. **Focal endothelial or Descemet's membrane damage** may occur if the laser is misfocused (Geggel & Maza, 1990).

V. Pupilloplasty, Photomydriasis, and Sphincterotomy

A. Introduction

1. **Pupilloplasty** is a laser technique used to alter the size, shape, or position of the pupil.
2. **Photomydriasis** is a form of pupilloplasty that involves the enlargement of a miotic pupil using photothermal laser treatment.
3. Other terms that have been used to refer to pupilloplasty include **coreoplasty** (Schwartz et al., 1984) and **coreopexy** (Pollack, 1985).
4. **Sphincterotomy** refers to the incision of the iris sphincter muscle. This can be done with the Nd:YAG laser by photodisruption or with the argon laser by a photothermal mechanism (Sobel et al., 1986; Thomas, 1984; Wise, 1985).

B. Indications and Contraindications

1. **Indications**
   a. **Miotic pupil.** Causes of chronic miotic pupils include miotic therapy for glaucoma, seclusio-pupillae due to healed iritis, miosis during vitrectomy surgery, and pediatric aphakia with microophthalmia. In these cases, pupilloplasty/photomydriasis may be beneficial (James et al., 1976; L'Esperance & James, 1975; Mohan et al., 1991; Schwartz et al., 1984; Stern, 1985; Summers & Holland, 1991; Zimmerman & Wheeler, 1982). Very small pupils can compromise visual acuity and visual fields. They can also impede ophthalmoscopy or surgery (Fine, 1994; Miller & Keener, 1994; Sobel et al., 1986; Whitsett & Stewart, 1993).
   b. **Pupil block.** In cases of pupillary block where laser iridotomy is impractical because of corneal edema or iritis, a pupil block may be broken by photothermally dilating the pupil. This has been done not only in simple pupillary-block glaucoma, but also in cases of pseudophakic pupil block and aphakic pupil block (Blumenthal et al., 1982; Obstbaum et al., 1981; Palli & Cinotti, 1975; Ritch, 1982; Schwartz et al., 1984; Shin, 1982a,b; Theodossiadis, 1985). After breaking the angle closure attack, a laser iridotomy can be performed when the eye settles down.
   c. **Updrawn pupil.** Vision can also be compromised if the iris is covering the visual axis or if media opacities are obscuring vision. Enlarging the updrawn pupil or pulling it into the visual axis region may improve vision (L'Esperance & James, 1975; Schwartz et al., 1984; Thomas, 1984).

d. **Subluxated lens.** If impairment of vision occurs even with optical correction, and if pharmacologic mydriasis and aphakic correction improves vision, then pupilloplasty may be indicated (Straatsma et al., 1966; Thomas, 1984).

2. **Relative contraindications** (Schwartz et al., 1984)

   a. **Cloudy cornea.** In order for the laser energy to reach the iris, the cornea must be relatively clear. If the cornea absorbs the laser radiation, a corneal burn may form and not enough energy will reach the iris.

   b. **Cloudy anterior chamber.** If there is protein or cellular debris in the chamber, it can absorb part of the beam, thus raising the threshold for an iris burn. If there is too much debris, the procedure cannot be completed successfully.

   c. **Shallow anterior chamber.** There must be enough space between the iris and the corneal endothelium so that the photothermal change at the iris does not spread to the endothelium and cause damage. A gap of only a millimeter is usually enough.

C. Preprocedure Management (James et al., 1976; Obstbaum et al., 1981; Schwartz et al., 1984; Summers & Holland, 1991; Thomas, 1984)

1. An indication as to whether the procedure will be of benefit can usually be obtained by pharmacologically dilating the patient. If visual acuity and visual field improve, then the procedure will be of benefit. Sometimes the iris will not respond to mydriatic drugs and a determination will have to be made from available data.

2. Topical anesthetic is instilled. Rarely, retrobulbar anesthesia may be necessary if the patient has nystagmus or is uncooperative. Occasionally, a Goldmann or similar lens may be useful for inhibiting eye movements.

3. If the fundus cannot be adequately visualized because of the smallness of the pupil and the iris does not respond to mydriatics, ultrasound may need to be performed to rule out gross pathology.

4. Informed consent must be obtained.

D. Technique (James et al., 1976; Obstbaum et al., 1981; Ritch, 1982; Schwartz et al., 1984; Shin, 1982b; Sobel et al., 1986; Summers & Holland, 1991; Theodossiadis, 1985; Thomas, 1984; Zimmerman & Wheeler, 1982)

1. The **argon** laser can be set initially at a 200-μm spot size, 0.2 sec to 0.5 sec duration, and low power (e.g., 150 mW to 600 mW). An alternative is to use a 500-μm spot size, 0.05 sec to 0.2 sec duration, and 200 mW.

2. For a round, miotic pupil, a row of laser burns can be placed outside the pupil margin. The first burns should be placed just inside the iris collarette. Care must be taken with the first burns to make sure that the burn is not too close to the pupil. If they are too close, the laser beam may reach the retina if the iris shrinks from under the beam.

3. Select the power level that produces instantaneous iris shrinkage with no explosive event.

4. Another row of burns may be placed peripheral to the first row, if necessary.

5. In addition to iris tissue shrinkage, the goal of the procedure is to damage the iris sphincter muscle so the larger pupil can be maintained.

6. An updrawn pupil can also be treated in a similar manner. Larger spot sizes and more applications may be indicated.

7. Retreatment may be necessary in 2 to 3 weeks.

8. The initial or retreatment procedure may also be accomplished with an **Nd:YAG** laser either in the thermal or photodisruptive mode. An **Nd:YLF** laser has also been used for pupilloplasty (Geerling et al., 1998).

9. An argon laser sphincterotomy can be performed with a 50-μm spot size, 0.01 to 0.05 sec duration, and 800 to 1500 mW of power (Sobel et al., 1986; Wise, 1985). With a special iridotomy-sphincterotomy lens, low power levels can be used (Fankhauser, 1986; Wise et al., 1986).

E. Post-Procedure Management (James et al., 1976; Obstbaum et al., 1981; Schwartz et al., 1984; Summers & Holland, 1991; Thomas, 1984)

1. A steroid drop may be prescribed (e.g., prednisolone 1% or fluorometholone) four times a day for a week and then tapered. Intraocular inflammation should be assessed at each subsequent visit and managed appropriately.

2. Apraclonidine can be administered just before and after the procedure. Intraocular pressure is monitored during the first 3 hours, at 24 hours, at 1 week, and thereafter as required. An IOP spike may occur. Patients with glaucoma need to continue their medications and may require additional medication (e.g., a carbonic anhydrase inhibitor).

F. Complications. The complications are essentially the same as those following laser iridotomy or trabeculoplasty and are managed similarly (James et al., 1976; L'Esperance & James, 1975; Mohan et al., 1991; Schultz, 1996; Schwartz et al., 1984; Sobel et al., 1986; Theodossiadis, 1985; Thomas, 1984; Zimmerman & Wheeler, 1982). They include:

1. Intraocular pressure spikes

2. Transient plasmoid iritis with moderate pigment dispersion

3. Corneal burns

4. Lens opacities

5. Iris hemorrhage

6. Iris atrophy

7. Pigment dispersion

8. Retinal burn
9. Pain. This may occur if too high a power and duration are used, resulting in excessive stretching of the iris.

VI. Laser Phacolysis

A. Introduction

1. The fragmentation of a crystalline lens using a laser has been referred to as laserphaco, laser phacolysis, photophacofragmentation, laser photofragmentation, laser cataract ablation, phacofracture, laser phacoemulsification, laser photophacoablation, laser phakoablation, laser ablation of the lens, endocapsular phakoablation, laser phacovaporization, and laser lens lysis (Bath et al., 1987a; Beckman et al., 1980; Chambless, 1988; Dardenne et al., 1991; Dodick et al., 1993; Dodick & Sperber, 1996; Gailitis et al., 1993; Gwon et al., 1995; Kermani et al., 1990; Levin & Wyatt, 1990; Ryan & Logani, 1987; Sperber, 1996; Sperber & Dodick, 1995; Stevens et al., 1998; Tsubota, 1990; Zelman, 1987).

2. Interest in developing laser phacolysis developed from a concern to improve precision and safety of lens removal (Dodick & Sperber, 1996; Obstbaum et al., 1995; Snyder & Noecker, 1998).

B. Indications and Contraindications

1. **Aid to phacoemulsification.** Laser phacolysis has been suggested as a pretreatment of the lens nucleus prior to standard phacoemulsification (Chambless, 1988; Ryan & Logani, 1987; Zelman, 1987). This can increase the ease of phacoemulsification, decrease the ultrasound time, and allow phacoemulsification on dark, hard nuclei. The advisability of the technique has been debated (Chambless, 1990; Levin & Wyatt, 1990).

2. **Cataract.** Instead of the conventional methods of cataract extraction, laser phacolysis has been suggested as an alternative (Dodick, 1991; Dodick & Sperber, 1996; Snyder & Noecker, 1998). Lasers probably have a role to play in small incision cataract surgery. What is needed is the development of better fiberoptics, fluidics, and handpiece designs.

C. Technique

1. Various lasers have been used to fragment the lens. They include:
   a. **Carbon dioxide** laser (10,600 nm) (Beckman et al., 1980). There was an early attempt to explore the effect of the CO_2 laser on various ocular tissues, including the lens.
   b. **Erbium:YAG** laser (2940 nm)/**Er:YSSG** laser (2790 nm) (Berger et al., 1996; Brazitikos et al., 1998; Colvard & Kratz, 1996; Gailitis et al., 1993; Noecker et al.,

1994; Peyman & Katoh, 1987; Ross & Puliafito, 1994; Snyder et al., 1998; Stevens et al., 1998; Tsubota, 1990; Wetzel et al., 1996). The safety and efficacy of Er:YAG laser-assisted cataract surgery has been established (Stevens et al., 1998).

   c. **Excimer** laser (**XeCl**: 308 nm) (Bath et al., 1987a,b; Kermani et al., 1990; Maguen et al., 1989; Martinez et al., 1992; Mueller-Stolzenburg et al., 1991; Nanevicz et al., 1986; Peyman et al., 1986). This laser wavelength has aroused safety concerns and has not been approved for clinical trials (Marshall & Sliney, 1986; Sliney, 1990). Of the various excimer wavelengths, 308 nm seemed the most promising since it could be transmitted through a fiberoptic probe (Mueller-Stolzenberg and Mueller, 1989; Nanevicz et al., 1986).

   d. **Excimer** lasers (**ArF**: 193 nm and **KrF**: 248 nm) (Nanevicz et al., 1986; Puliafito et al., 1985).

   e. **Holmium:YAG** laser (2120 nm) (Ross & Puliafito, 1994).

   f. **Nd:YAG** laser (mode-locked: 1064 nm) (Levin & Wyatt, 1990).

   g. **Nd:YAG** laser (Q-switched: 1064 nm) (Chambless, 1988; Dodick, 1991; Dodick & Christiansen, 1991; Dodick & Sperber, 1996; Dodick et al., 1993; Eichenbaum, 1996; Kanellopoulos et al., 1999; Ryan & Logani, 1987; Sperber, 1996; Zelman, 1987).

   h. **Nd:YLF** laser (1053 nm) (Dardenne et al., 1991; Dodick & Sperber, 1996; Gwon et al., 1995; Hoppeler & Gloor, 1992).

2. The **Photon Laser Phacolysis system** is produced by Paradigm Medical Industries, Inc. (Figure 9–4). It uses a Q-switched Nd:YAG laser with a quartz clad silica fiber optic as well as irrigation and aspiration capability (Dodick & Sperber, 1996; Eichenbaum, 1996; Snyder & Noecker, 1998). It is designed to allow minimally invasive small incision cataract removal.

3. The **Laser Lens Lysis device** was produced by IOLAB (Dodick & Sperber, 1996; Dodick et al., 1993). Now the **Dodick Photolysis system** is produced by A.R.C. Laser AG, Jona, Switzerland (Kanellopoulos et al., 1999).

   a. At first, a scleral tunnel and a self-sealing, internal corneal lip incision were made. Then, two paracentesis sites were created. The anterior chamber was maintained by attaching a bottle of balanced saline to one of the sites. This system also supplemented infusion. A viscoelastic agent was insufflated into the anterior chamber.

   b. More recently, a 1.4-mm clear-cornea incision was made between the 9- and 12-o'clock positions to insert the laser-aspiration probe. And a 0.9-mm clear cornea incision was made between 12-o'clock and 3-o'clock in order to insert the irrigation probe.

   c. An anterior capsulorhexis was made and the probes were inserted into the anterior chamber.

   d. The system used a pulsed Q-switched Nd:YAG laser. The energy was transferred to the probe using a quartz fiber optic. The energy was then focused onto a tita-

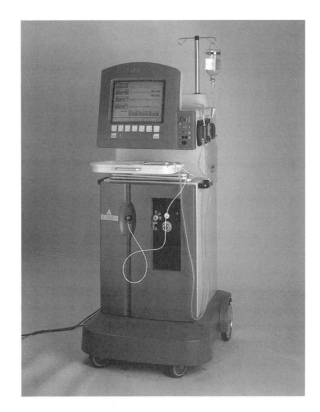

Figure 9–4 Photon Laser Phacolysis System. (Courtesy of Paradigm Medical Industries, Inc., San Diego, CA.)

     nium target within the probe tip. The shock wave fragmented the lens material into small particles.

  e. Phacolysis and aspiration of the lens fragments were accomplished initially with the Nd:YAG laser energy set at 4.0 mJ and a repetition rate of 20 Hz. More recently, the energy was increased to 12 mJ with a 14-nsec duration.

  f. The intraocular lens was inserted, the anterior chamber was re-formed, and the incision was closed.

4. Three companies (Aesculap-Meditec, Coherent, and Premier) are developing the **Er:YAG laser** for phacolysis (Colvard & Kratz, 1996; Snyder & Noecker, 1998). The handpieces for the systems are evolving.

5. When used as a preoperative procedure, the phacolysis has been done 16 hours to 12 weeks prior to the cataract extraction (Chambless, 1988; Zelman, 1987). In this case, the anterior chamber and capsule are not opened. The laser is focused toward the back of the nucleus first, then the center of the nucleus, and finally the anterior aspect of the nucleus. The Nd:YAG laser energy settings ranged from 1.6 mJ to 10 mJ with over 100 shots being used.

D. Post-Procedure Management. The standard cataract postoperative regimen is followed.

E. Complications. The usual complications of cataract surgery can occur. Used preoperatively, anterior and posterior capsule rupture have occurred due to misfocusing (Levin & Wyatt, 1990; Zelman, 1987). Used operatively, posterior capsule rupture has occurred (Kanellopoulos et al., 1999). In addition, the fiber optic can lose efficiency during the procedure (Stevens et al., 1998). An in vitro study showed that tissue heating does not occur with laser phacolysis (Alzner & Grabner, 1999).

VII. Miscellaneous Procedures

A. Laser Synechialysis (aka Synechiolysis, Synechiotomy)

1. **Posterior synechiae** can by lysed with the Q-switched Nd:YAG laser (Fankhauser et al., 1985; Flynn & Carlson, 1996; Hurvitz, 1992; Kumar et al., 1994a; Paylor, 1985; Wise, 1985). Using a Peyman wide-field or Abrahams-type contact lens, 1–2 mJ of energy is usually sufficient.

2. The posterior synechiae can occur after cataract surgery, after chronic granulomatous uveitis, or after long-term miotic therapy for glaucoma.

3. Visually disruptive pigmented cellular membranes can accumulate on the anterior surface of silicone intraocular lenses. By lysing the posterior synechiae with the laser, the recurrence of these membranes can be prevented (Flynn & Carlson, 1996).

4. A flat anterior chamber can lead to the development of **focal iridocorneal adhesions**. These can be lysed with a laser (Gross & Robin, 1985).

5. **Pupillary capture** has been treated using the Nd:YAG laser to cut synechia between the iris and the capsule (Bartholomew, 1997). The entrapment of the intraocular lens through the pupillary aperture can be reversed, especially if treated early.

6. **Goniosynechiae** can be lysed in addition (Wand, 1992).

7. Complications can include hemorrhage, pigment dispersal, and intraocular pressure spike.

8. The Nd:YLF laser has also been used for synechialysis (Geerling et al., 1998).

B. Anterior Capsulotomy

1. In the early 1970s, Krasnov (1975) described experiments and a clinical trial using a **Q-switched Nd:YAG laser** to perform a small anterior capsulotomy. He called the procedure "laser-phakopuncture." The procedure then involved the gradual absorption of the lens substance over several months.

2. The capsulorhexis opening after cataract extraction can contract due to capsular fibrosis and compromise vision (capsule contraction syndrome). The Q-switched Nd:YAG

laser can be used to enlarge the opening (Dahlhauser et al., 1998; Davison, 1993; Hurvitz, 1992; Reeves & Yung, 1998). A modification of the technique can be used in extreme capsule contraction syndrome (Chawla & Shaikh, 1999).

3. If a can-opener anterior capsulotomy is performed with the Nd:YAG laser to enlarge an opacified anterior capsule after cataract extraction, complications can occur. The detached opacified anterior lens capsule can induce inferior corneal endothelial cell loss (Chiba et al., 1995). Dislocations of foldable plate-haptic silicone intraocular lenses have also been reported (Dahlhauser et al., 1998; Tuft & Talks, 1998).

4. A preoperative Nd:YAG laser anterior capsulotomy before cataract extraction can also be done (Aron-Rosa, 1981; Manchester, 1984; Panda & Pattnaik, 1991). This procedure apparently decreased the incidence of posterior capsule opacification in a 10-year follow-up (Aron-Rosa, 1981; Aron-Rosa & Aron, 1992). However, complications like miosis, iritis, and intraocular pressure spikes, along with the need to perform the cataract extraction soon after the procedure, dampened enthusiasm for the procedure.

5. The **mode-locked** (picosecond) as well as the Q-switched (nanosecond) **Nd:YAG laser** can be employed to perform an anterior capsulotomy (Puliafito & Steinert, 1983).

6. The **holmium:YAG laser** can also be used to perform an anterior capsulotomy (Miyake, 1992).

7. Two companies are studying the use of the **Er:YAG laser** to generate a circular anterior capsulotomy (Brazitikos et al., 1998; Snyder & Noecker, 1998).

C. *Membranectomy and Deposit Removal*

1. Membranes can form in the anterior chamber and on the lens for various reasons. Persistent pupillary membranes are a common congenital anomaly and can occasionally disturb vision. Additionally, opacities and membranes can form on the anterior surface of intraocular lenses after surgery (e.g., cataract surgery or pars plana vitrectomy). Occasionally these membranes and/or opacities do not resolve with topical steroid treatment. Fibrovascular pupillary membranes can also occur after ocular injuries.

2. The Q-switched Nd:YAG laser can be used to treat the persistent pupillary membranes, the traumatic fibrovascular, and the postoperative membranes (Daus et al., 1991; Fankhauser & Kwasniewska, 1989; Gandham et al., 1995; Grene, 1990; Kovacs et al., 1993; Kozobolis et al., 1997; Ramakrishnan et al., 1993; Slomovic et al., 1985; Talks, 1997; Vega & Sabates, 1987; Virdi et al., 1997). Pulses with energies from 0.8 to 3.1 mJ are usually sufficient. The Nd:YAG laser, as well as the Nd:YLF laser, have also been used to open blocked glaucoma tube shunts via membranectomy (Oram et al., 1994; Singh et al., 1997).

3. Nd:YAG **laser "sweeping"** has been advocated to clear isolated, corticosteroid-resistant deposits from the anterior surface of the intraocular lens (Fankhauser & Kwasniewska, 1989, 1995; Kumar et al., 1994b; Kwasniewska & Fankhauser, 1985; Talks, 1997; Vajpayee et al., 1993). Energy levels ranging from 0.2 mJ to 1.6 mJ can be delivered by focusing the laser in the aqueous just anterior to the intraocular lens.

D. *Corneal Stromal Vascularization Treatment*

1. Corneal stromal vascularization can be caused by a number of conditions including: burns, contact lens wear, corneal graft rejection, infections, metabolic disorders, nutritional deficiency states, toxins, trauma, and vasculitides. Persistent corneal vascularization can lead to decreased vision by inducing edema, graft rejection, lipid keratopathy, and scarring. Vascularized lipid keratopathy is secondary to corneal inflammatory disease (e.g., herpes simplex and herpes zoster disciform keratitis).

2. When conventional therapy has failed, **laser photocoagulation** may be a useful tool in the treatment of corneal stromal vascularization. The main problems with the technique have been due to collateral thermal damage, blood vessel recanalization, and potential worsening of the neovascularization (Mendelsohn et al., 1986). An even more important alternative is photothrombosis (see the photodynamic therapy section below).

3. Laser photocoagulation can be accomplished by a number of lasers including: **argon** (514.5 nm), **CW Nd:YAG** (1064 nm), and **dye lasers** (570, 577 nm) (Baer & Foster, 1992; Cherry et al., 1973; Cherry & Garner, 1976; Hemady et al., 1993; Krasnick & Spigelman, 1995; Lim et al., 1993; Marsh, 1982, 1988; Marsh & Marshall, 1982; Mendelsohn et al., 1986; Nirankari, 1992; Nirankari et al., 1993; Park & Kim, 1994; Reed et al., 1975; Tommila et al., 1987).

4. Besides reestablishing corneal avascularity, the laser treatment may be useful in **reducing graft rejection following corneal transplant** (Nirankari, 1992; Nirankari & Baer, 1986).

5. Laser photocoagulation has also been used to treat **lipid keratopathy** (Marsh, 1982, 1988; Marsh & Marshall, 1982; Mendelsohn et al., 1986).

6. **Complications** from the laser treatment (Marsh, 1982, 1988; Marsh & Marshall, 1982; Mendelsohn et al., 1986; Nirankari, 1992; Parsa et al., 1994) include:
   a. Mild uveitis
   b. Iris atrophy
   c. Intracorneal hemorrhage
   d. Corneal thinning
   e. Descemetocele
   f. Temporary peaking of the pupil
   g. Vessel recanalization
   h. Worsening of neovascularization

      i. Adjacent tissue thermal damage with subsequent enhancement of the inflammatory response

E. *Closure of Cyclodialysis Clefts*

1. **Introduction**
   a. A cyclodialysis cleft involves the detachment of the ciliary body from the sclera at the scleral spur. This can result from trauma, a complication of surgery, or a planned procedure. It can lead to hypotony and, hence, to choroidal effusions, macular edema, and optic disk edema (Maumenee & Stark, 1971).
   b. The photothermal effect of the **argon** laser has been used to close cyclodialysis clefts. Recently, a contact trans-scleral **diode** laser and a transscleral **Nd:YAG** laser have been used (Brooks et al., 1996; Brown & Mizen, 1997). **Endolaser** photocoagulation with a **diode** laser has also been reported (Caronia et al., 1999).

2. **Indication: cyclodialysis cleft resulting in hypotony**

3. **Technique** (Alward et al., 1988; Bauer, 1995; Harbin, 1982; Joondeph, 1980; Ormerod et al., 1991; Partamian, 1985; Schultz, 1996)
   a. Apply topical anesthetic. Retrobulbar anesthesia may be necessary if high laser power is used.
   b. Place a goniolens on the eye.
   c. If the anterior chamber is very shallow, the chamber can be deepened by compression gonioscopy with a 4-mirror lens or by injection of a viscoelastic substance through a paracentesis.
   d. The argon laser can be set for a spot size of 50 μm to 200 μm, a power of 300 mW to 3000 mW, and a duration of 0.1 sec to 0.2 sec.
   e. The goal is to adjust the power to blanch the tissue in the depths of the cleft and at its edges. When high power is used (e.g., 1000 mW to 3000 mW), the goal would be gas-bubble formation on the scleral surface as well as marked blanching. If this does not close the cleft, the procedure can be repeated in 1 to 2 weeks.
   f. A steroid and a cycloplegic can be prescribed for a week. Most practitioners have avoided steroids.

4. **Complications** (Bauer, 1995; Brown & Mizen, 1997; Harbin, 1982; Joondeph, 1980; Kuechle & Naumann, 1995; Metrikin et al., 1994; Ormerod et al., 1991; Small et al., 1994)
   a. **Excessive intraocular pressure increase.** This is likely to occur in the first 2 weeks after the laser procedure and should be treated with anti-glaucoma medications. Pilocarpine should not be used since it could reopen the cleft. This situation is usually transient.
   b. **Failure to maintain closure.** Most clefts can be closed with the laser; however, it may take more than one treatment.

F. Photodynamic Therapy (PDT)

1. **Introduction.**

    a. Photodynamic therapy is a photochemical technique that may be useful in the treatment of ocular tumors and neovascularization (Oleinick & Evans, 1998). It involves the intravenous injection of a photosensitizing drug. These drugs, especially the newer-generation drugs, are selectively taken up by malignant, fast-growing cell populations and by neovascular endothelial cells. Then a laser, tuned to the maximum of the drug's absorption band, is focused on the lesion and irradiates the tissue.

    b. By absorbing the laser radiation, the photosensitizing drug is raised from its ground state to a higher excited triplet state. When the excited photosensitizer drops back to its ground state, it transfers energy to molecular oxygen or to other compounds. If the energy is transferred to compounds other than oxygen (Type I mechanism), radicals are formed that can generate reactive oxygen species (e.g., hydroxyl radicals, superoxides, or peroxides), and they subsequently can damage the tissue (Buettner & Oberly, 1980). If the energy is transferred to oxygen (Type II mechanism), the very reactive singlet oxygen is formed (Weishaupt et al., 1976). This damages tissue by reacting with lipid membranes, proteins, or nucleic acids. The predominant mechanism of damage in photodynamic therapy is via singlet oxygen formation.

    c. The response of tumors to PDT may involve three different processes (Fisher et al., 1995; Oleinick & Evans, 1998). First, the malignant cells may be damaged directly. Second, the radiation can cause the release of cytokines and other inflammatory mediators that generate an inflammatory response with recruitment of lymphocytes and phagocytic cells to the tumor. Third, the radiation may affect the tumor vasculature, producing vascular leakage, blood flow stasis, and/or vascular collapse. The relative contribution of each process is dependent on the tumor and the particular photosensitizer.

    d. The photosensitizers that have been used to treat ocular tumors and neovascularization are shown in Table 9–1. The applications of hematoporphyrin derivative (HPD) and porfimer sodium (a purified hematoporphyrin derivative; Photofrin) to PDT have been studied the most (Dougherty et al., 1998). Newer-generation photosensitizers have improved properties like higher absorption peaks at longer, more penetrating wavelengths and reduced phototoxicity.

    e. The use of photodynamic therapy is still under experimental investigation in the United States, although it has been approved for use in Canada and a number of European countries. While the early clinical trials in the 1980s were disappointing, the use of newer-generation photosensitizers and the employment of new knowledge about basic mechanisms of action have stimulated a new interest in ocular PDT (Dougherty et al., 1998; Fisher et al., 1995; Haimovici et al., 1994;

Table 9–1 Photosensitizers Used to Treat
Ocular Tumors and Neovascularization

Chlorins and bacteriochlorins
  ATX-s10
  Bacteriochlorin a
  Chlorine$_6$
  Tin ethyl etiopurpurin (SnET2)
Phthalocyanines
  Chloraluminum sulfonated phthalocyanine
    (CASPc)
Tetrapyrrole derivatives
  Benzoporphyrin derivative monoacid (BPD)
  Dihematoporphyrin ether (DHE)
  Hematoporphyrin derivative (HPD)
  Porfimer sodium (Photofrin; a commercial
    preparation of DHE)
Xanthene derivatives
Rose bengal

Husain & Miller, 1997; Husain et al., 1996; Ochsner, 1997; Young et al., 1996). In addition, new delivery systems (e.g., liposomes, low-density lipoproteins, microspheres, and monoclonal antibodies) have been used to enhance target cell killing and to minimize collateral tissue damage (Miller et al., 1995; Schmidt-Erfurth et al., 1994a; Young et al., 1996).

f. **Photothrombosis** is a primary mechanism used in PDT for treating neovascularization (Gohto et al., 1998; Joussen et al., 1998; Kliman et al., 1994a; Nanda et al., 1987; Peyman et al., 1997; Primbs et al., 1998; Royster et al., 1988; Schmidt-Erfurth et al., 1994b, 1995). In this process a photosensitizer is injected intravenously. There is increased uptake in the neovascular endothelial cells. Subsequent laser irradiation induces the formation of a thrombus with resultant occlusion of the vessel. Since this is a photochemical process, less energy is used than is needed for photocoagulation. Thus there is minimal thermal damage. In addition, recanalization is minimized since the thrombus is formed by platelet aggregation without activation of the extrinsic or intrinsic coagulation system.

g. Besides the indications mentioned below, the use of PDT is being investigated to:

  1) **Treat glaucoma by cyclodestruction** (Hill et al., 1997a; Tsilimbaris et al., 1997). The second-generation photosensitizing drug, phthalocyanine, along with diode laser transscleral irradiation is being used to destroy ciliary body via vascular thrombosis. By decreasing aqueous production, this treatment reduces the intraocular pressure.

2) **Inhibit fibrosis in glaucoma filtering surgery** (Hill et al., 1997b). The use of the photosensitizer, tin ethyl etiopurpurin, and diode laser irradiation are being explored as an alternative antifibrotic therapy.

3) **Treat lipid keratopathy** (Mendelsohn et al., 1987). Rose bengal dye and the argon laser have been used to create permanent photothrombotic occlusions in the corneal neovascularization of rabbits with experimentally induced lipid keratopathy. This technique works better than laser photocoagulation of the vessels.

4) **Close bleb leaks after filtration surgery** (Wright et al., 1998). Fibrinogen glue and indocyanine green dye activated by a diode laser have been used to repair bleb leaks in rabbits.

5) **Close corneal wounds after penetrating keratoplasty or radial keratotomy** (Goins et al., 1997, 1998; Khadem et al., 1994). Fibrinogen and riboflavin-5-phosphate activated by a blue green argon laser have been used to explore the possibility of using photodynamic biologic tissue glue as an alternative to sutures.

6) **Treat primary nonmelanomatous skin tumors** (Kuebler et al., 1999; Wang et al., 1999). The second generation photosensitizer, metatetrahydroxyphenylchlorin, has been used to treat basal cell and squamous cell cancers with a dye laser. Another photosensitizer, δ-aminolevulinic acid, has also been used.

2. **Indications**
   a. **Corneal neovascularization** (Corrent et al., 1989; Epstein et al., 1987, 1991; Gohto et al., 1998, 2000; Huang et al., 1988a,b; Joussen et al., 1998; Pallikaris et al., 1993, 1996; Primbs et al., 1998; Schmidt-Erfurth et al., 1995; Sobaci et al., 1998; Tsilimbaris et al., 1994; van Gool et al., 1995)
   b. **Iris melanoma** (Bruce & McCaughan, 1989; Chambers et al., 1986; Davidorf & Davidorf, 1992; Lewis et al., 1984; Panagopoulos et al., 1989; Schmidt-Erfurth et al., 1996; Sery et al., 1987; Tse et al., 1984)
   c. **Ciliary body melanoma** (Bruce & McCaughan, 1989; Lewis et al., 1984; Tse et al., 1984)
   d. **Choroidal melanoma** (Bruce, 1993; Bruce & McCaughan, 1989; Favilla et al., 1991; Gonzalez et al., 1995; Kim et al., 1996; Murphree et al., 1987; Schmidt-Erfurth et al., 1994a; Tse et al., 1984; Winward et al., 1990; Young et al. 1996)
   e. **Retinoblastoma** (Murphree, 1989; Murphree et al., 1987; Ohnishi et al., 1986)
   f. **Iris neovascularization** (Husain et al., 1997; Miller et al., 1991; Packer et al., 1984)
   g. **Choroidal neovascularization** (Asrani et al., 1997; Haimovici et al., 1997; Husain & Miller, 1997; Husain et al., 1996; Iliaki et al., 1996; Kliman et al., 1994a,b, 1989; Kramer et al., 1996; Lin et al., 1994; Miller & Miller, 1993; Miller

et al., 1995; Peyman et al., 1997; Schmidt-Erfurth et al., 1994b; Thomas & Langhofer, 1987; Wilson & Hatchell, 1991)

3. **Complications** (Bruce, 1993; Davidorf & Davidorf, 1992, Haimovici et al., 1994; Lewis et al., 1984; Ohnishi et al., 1986; Tse et al., 1984). These can include:
   a. Iris neovascularization
   b. Neovascular glaucoma
   c. Severe uveitis
   d. Skin photosensitivity
   e. Chemosis
   f. Vitritis
   g. Cataract
   h. Choroidal detachment
   i. Retinal detachment
   j. Choroidal hemorrhage
   k. Resumption of tumor growth

References

Achauer BM, Chang C-J, Kam VMV. Nd:YAG laser treatment for facial hemangioma of infancy. Lasers and Light 7:111–116 (1996).

Adams EL, Price NM. Treatment of basal-cell carcinomas with a carbon-dioxide laser. J Dermatol Surg Oncol 5:803–806 (1979).

Aktan SG, Mandelkorn RM. Krypton laser suture lysis. Ophthalmic Surg Lasers 29:635–638 (1998).

Alaa M et al. Increased corneal scarring after phototherapeutic keratectomy in Fuchs' corneal dystrophy. J Refract Surg 13:308–310 (1997).

Al-Rajhi AA et al. Bacterial keratitis following phototherapeutic keratectomy. J Refractive Surgery 12:123–127 (1996).

Alster TS, Apfelberg DB, eds. Cosmetic laser surgery: a practitioner's guide. New York, NY: Wiley-liss, 1999.

Alster TS, West TB. Resurfacing of atrophic facial acne scars with a high-energy, pulsed carbon dioxide laser. Dermatol Surg 22:151–155 (1996).

Alward WLM et al. Argon laser endophotocoagulator closure of cyclodialysis clefts. Am J Ophthalmol 106:748–749 (1988).

Alzner E, Grabner G. Dodick laser phacolysis: thermal effects. J Cataract Refract Surg 25:800–803 (1999).

American Academy of Ophthalmology. Ophthalmic procedure preliminary assessment. Laser blepharoplasty and skin resurfacing. Ophthalmology 105:2154–2159 (1998).

Amm M, Duncker GIW. Refractive changes after phototherapeutic keratectomy. J Cataract Refract Surg 23:839–844 (1997).

Apfelberg DB. Ultrapulse carbon dioxide laser with CPG scanner for full-face resurfacing for rhytids, photoaging, and acne scars. Plast Reconstr Surg 99:1817–1825 (1997).

Apfelberg DB. Summary of the 1997 ASAPS/ASPRS laser task force survey on laser resurfacing and laser blepharoplasty. Plast Reconstr Surg 101:511–518 (1998).

Apfelberg DB et al. Superpulse CO_2 laser treatment of facial syringomata. Lasers Surg Med 7:533–537 (1987a).

Apfelberg DB et al. Treatment of xanthelasma palpebrarum with the carbon dioxide laser. J Dermatol Surg Oncol 13:149–151 (1987b).

Apfelberg DB, Smith T, White J. Preliminary study of the vascular dynamics of the portwine hemangioma with therapeutic implications of argon laser treatment. Plastic and Reconstructive Surgery 83:820–827 (1989).

Arndt KA, Dover JS, Olbricht SM, eds. Lasers in cutaneous and aesthetic surgery. Philadelphia, PA: Lippincott-Raven Publishers, 1997.

Aron-Rosa DS. Use of a pulsed neodymium-YAG laser for anterior capsulotomy before extracapsular cataract extraction. American Intraocular Implant Society Journal 7:332–333 (1981).

Aron-Rosa DS et al. Excimer laser surgery of the cornea: qualitative and quantitative aspects of photoablation according to the energy density. J Cataract Refract Surg 12:27–33 (1986).

Aron-Rosa DS, Aron JJ. Effect of preoperative YAG laser anterior capsulotomy on the incidence of posterior capsule opacification: ten year follow-up. J Cataract Refract Surg 18:559–561 (1992).

Asomoto A, Yablonski ME, Matsushita M. A retrospective study of the effects of laser suture lysis on the long-term results of trabeculectomy. Ophthalmic Surg 26:223–227 (1995).

Asrani S, Zou S et al. Feasibility of laser-targeted photoocclusion of the choriocapillary layer in rats. Invest Ophthalmol Vis Sci 38:2702–2710 (1997).

Avitabile T et al. Ultrasound-biomicroscopic evaluation of filtering blebs after laser suture lysis trabeculectomy. Ophthalmologica 212 (Suppl 1):17–21 (1998).

Awan KJ. Laser punctoplasty for the treatment of punctal stenosis. Am J Ophthalmol 100:341–342 (1985).

Awan KJ. Argon laser phototherapy of phthiriasis palpebrarum. Ophthalmic Surg 17:813–814 (1986).

Azar DT, Jain S, Stark W. Phototherapeutic keratectomy. In Krachmer JH, Mannis MJ, Holland EJ, eds. Cornea, Vol III. Surgery of the cornea and conjunctiva. St. Louis, MO: Mosby, 1997a; 175:2211–2223.

Azar DT, Steinert RF, Stark WJ. Excimer laser phototherapeutic keratectomy: management of scars, dystrophies, and complications. Baltimore, MD: Williams & Wilkins, 1997b.

Azar DT et al. PTK: Indications, surgical techniques, postoperative care, and complications management. In Talamo JH, Krueger RR, eds. The excimer manual. A clinician's guide to excimer laser surgery. Boston, MA: Little, Brown and Company, 1997c:173–199.

Backer TJ, Stuzin JM, Baker TM. Facial skin resurfacing. St. Louis, MO: Quality Medical Publications, 1998.

Baer JC, Foster CS. Corneal laser photocoagulation for treatment of neovascularization. Efficacy of 577 nm yellow dye laser. Ophthalmology 99:173–179 (1992).

Baker SS et al. Carbon dioxide laser blepharoplasty. Ophthalmology 91:238–243 (1984).

Bandieramonte G et al. Laser microsurgery for superficial T1-t2 basal cell carcinoma of the eyelid margins. Ophthalmology 104:1179–1184 (1997).

Bardak Y et al. Ocular hypotony after laser suture lysis following trabeculectomy with mitomycin C. Int Ophthalmol 21:325–330 (1998).

Bartholomew RS. Incidence, causes, and neodymium:YAG laser treatment of pupillary capture. J Cataract Refract Surg 23:1404–1408 (1997).

Bartley GB. The pros and cons of laser dacryocystorhinostomy. Am J Ophthalmol 117:103–106 (1994).

Bartley GB, Lowry JC. Argon laser treatment of trichiasis. Am J Ophthalmol 113:71–74 (1992).

Baskin MA. How to do your first laser blepharoplasty. Rev Ophthalmol 3:112–117 (1996).

Bass LS. Erbium:YAG laser skin resurfacing: preliminary clinical evaluation. Ann Plast Surg 40:328–334 (1998).

Bath PE et al. Endocapsular excimer laser phakoablation through a 1-mm incision. Ophthalmic Laser Therapy 2:245–248 (1987a).

Bath PE et al. Excimer laser lens ablation [letter]. Arch Ophthalmol 105:1164–1165 (1987b).

Bauer B. Argon laser photocoagulation of cyclodialysis clefts after cataract surgery. Acta Ophthalmol Scand 73:283–284 (1995).

Beck AD et al. The use of a new laser lens holder for performing suture lysis in children. Arch Ophthalmol 113:140–141 (1995).

Beckman H et al. Carbon dioxide laser surgery of the eye and adnexa. Ophthalmology 87:990–1000 (1980).

Bellack GS, Shapshay SM. Management of facial angiofibromas in tuberous sclerosis: Use of the carbon dioxide laser. Otolaryngol Head Neck Surg 94:37–40 (1986).

Benson DR, Hemmady PB, Snyder RW. Efficacy of laser punctal occlusion. Ophthalmology 99:618–621 (1992).

Berger JW et al. Temperature measurements during phacoemulsification and erbium:YAG laser phacoablation in model systems. J Cataract Refract Surg 22:372–378 (1996).

Bernstein LJ et al. The short- and long-term side effects of carbon dioxide laser resurfacing. Dermatol Surg 23:519–525 (1997).

Biesman BS. Cutaneous facial resurfacing with the carbon dioxide laser. Ophthal Surg Lasers 27:685–698 (1996).

Biesman BS. Carbon dioxide laser skin resurfacing. Semin Ophthalmol 13:123–135 (1998).

Blanco G et al. The ocular complications of periocular laser surgery. Curr Opin Ophthalmol 10:264–269 (1999).

Blok MDW et al. Scleral flap sutures and the development of shallow or flat anterior chamber after trabeculectomy. Ophthalmic Surg 24:309–313 (1993).

Blumenthal A, Floman N, Treister G. Laser iris retraction for narrow-angle glaucoma. Glaucoma 4:47–49 (1982).

Boska P, Martinho E, Goodman MM. Comparison of the argon tunable dye laser with the flashlamp pulsed dye laser in the treatment of facial telangiectasia. Dermatol Surg Oncol 20:749–753 (1994).

Bosniak SL, Ginsberg G. Laser eyelid surgery. Evaluating the therapeutic options. Ophthalmol Clin North America 6:479–489 (1993).

Bourne WM, Maguire LJ. Use of the argon laser to avoid complications from incomplete removal of corneal sutures with deeply buried knots. Am J Ophthalmol 110:310–311 (1990).

Boush GA, Lemke BN, Dortzbach RK. Results of endonasal laser-assisted dacryocystorhinostomy. Ophthalmology 101:955–959 (1994).

Brazitikos PD et al. Experimental ocular surgery with a high-repetition-rate erbium:YAG laser. Invest Ophthalmol Vis Sci 39:1667–1675 (1998).

Brooks AMV, Troski M, Gillies WE. Noninvasive closure of a persistent cyclodialysis cleft. Ophthalmology 103:1943–1945 (1996).

Brown SVL, Mizen T. Transscleral diode laser therapy for traumatic cyclodialysis cleft. Ophthalmic Surg Lasers 28:313–317 (1997).

Bruce RA Jr. Photoradiation therapy for choroidal malignant melanoma. In McCaughan JS Jr, ed. A clinical manual: photodynamic therapy of malignancies. Austin, TX: RG Landes Co.; 1993.

Bruce RA Jr, McCaughan JS Jr. Lasers in uveal melanoma. Ophthalmol Clin North Am 2:597–604 (1989).

Buettner GR, Oberly LW. The apparent production of superoxide and hydroxyl radicals by hematoporphyrin and light as seen by spin-trapping. FEBS Lett 121:161–164 (1980).

Campbell DC. Thermoablation treatment for trichiasis using the argon laser. Aust NZ J Ophthalmol 18:427–430 (1990).

Campos M et al. Clinical follow-up of phototherapeutic keratectomy for treatment of corneal opacities. Am J Ophthalmol 115:433–440 (1993).

Carniol PJ, ed. Laser skin rejuvenation. Philadelphia, PA: Lippincott-Raven, 1998.

Caromia RM et al. Treatment of a cyclodialysis cleft by means of ophthalmic laser microendoscope endophoto-coagulation. Am J Ophthalmol 128:760–761 (1999).

Carruth JAS, van Gemert MJC, Shakespeare PG. The argon laser in the treatment of the port-wine stain birth-mark. In Tan OT, ed. Management and treatment of benign cutaneous vascular lesions. Philadelphia, PA: Lea and Febiger, 1992:53–67.

Cartwright MJ. A prospective, randomized comparison of thermal cautery and argon laser for permanent punctal occlusion [letter]. Am J Ophthalmol 117:414 (1994).

Chambers RB et al. Treatment of iris melanoma with dihematoporphyrin ether and an ophthalmic laser delivery system. Contemp Ophthalmic Forum 4:79–84 (1986).

Chambless WS. Neodymium:YAG laser phacofracture: an aid to phacoemulsification. J Cataract Refract Surg 14:180–181 (1988).

Chambless WS. Laser photophaco fragmentation [letter]. J Cataract Refract Surg 16:386–387 (1990).

Chamon W et al. Phototherapeutic keratectomy. Ophthalmol Clin North Am 6:399–413 (1993).

Charteris DG et al. Retinal detachment following excimer laser. Br J Ophthalmol 81:759–761 (1997).

Chawla JS, Shaikh MH. Neodymium:YAG laser parabolic anterior capsulotomy in extreme capsule contraction syndrome. J Cataract Refract Surg 25:1415–1417 (1999).

Chernoff WG et al. Cutaneous laser resurfacing. Int J Aesthet Restorative Surg 3:57–68 (1995).

Cherry PM et al. Argon laser treatment of corneal neovascularization. Ann Ophthalmol 5:911–920 (1973).

Cherry PM, Garner A. Corneal neovascularization treated with argon laser. Br J Ophthalmol 60:464–472 (1976).

Chiba K, Hara T, Hara T. Corneal endothelial cell loss caused by detached opacified anterior lens capsule in the anterior chamber. J Cataract Refract Surg 21:701–705 (1995).

Chopra H, Goldenfeld M, Krupin T, Rosenberg LF. Early postoperative titration of bleb function: argon laser suture lysis and removable sutures in trabeculectomy. J Glaucoma 1:54–57 (1992).

Cisneros JL, Rio R, Palou J. The Q-switched neodymium (Nd):YAG laser with quadruple frequency. Clinical histological evaluation of facial resurfacing using different wavelengths. Dermatol Surg 24:345–350 (1998).

Clinch TE. Therapeutic uses of the excimer laser photorefractive keratectomy. Seminars in Ophthalmology 11:269–275 (1996).

Cohen MS, Swartz NG. Esthetic laser surgery. In Yanoff M, Duker JS, eds. Ophthalmology. Philadelphia, PA: Mosby, 1999; 7:9.1–9.2.

Coleman WP, Lawrence N. Skin resurfacing. Baltimore, MD: Williams & Wilkins, 1998.

Colvard DM, Kratz RP. Cataract surgery utilizing the erbium laser. In Fine IH, ed. Phacoemulsification: new technology and clinical application. Thorofare, NJ: Slack Inc, 1996; 11:161–180.

Cook WR Jr, Cook KK. Manual of tumescent liposculpture and laser cosmetic surgery: including the weekend alternative to the facelift. Philadelphia, PA: Lippincott Williams & Wilkins, 1999.

Corrent G et al. Promotion of graft survival by photothrombotic occlusion of corneal neovascularization. Arch Ophthalmol 107:1501–1506 (1989).

Cosman B. Experience in the argon laser therapy of port-wine stains. Plast Reconstr Surg 65:119–129 (1980).

Dahlhauser KF, Wroblewski KJ, Mader TH. Anterior capsule contraction with foldable silicone intraocular lenses. J Cataract Refract Surg 24:1216–1219 (1998).

Dardenne CM et al. Lens liquefaction using a picosecond IR laser. Invest Ophthalmol Vis Sci 32 (Suppl): 797 (1991).

Daus W, Tetz M, Voelcker HE. Nd:YAG laser cellular cleansing of intraocular lenses: results of ten consecutive patients. Dev Ophthalmol 22:52–57 (1991).

Dausch D et al. Phototherapeutic keratectomy in recurrent corneal epithelial erosion. Refract Corneal Surg 9:419–424 (1993).

David L, Goodman G. Blepharoplasty for the laser dermatologic surgeon. Clin Derm 13:49–53 (1995).

Davidorf J, Davidorf F. Treatment of iris melanoma with photodynamic therapy. Ophthalmic Surg 23:522–527 (1992).

Davison JA. Capsule contraction syndrome. J Cataract Refract Surg 19:582–589 (1993).

Dinehart SM, Waner M, Flock S. The copper vapor laser for the treatment of cutaneous vascular and pigmented lesions. J Dermatol Surg Oncol 19:370–375 (1993).

Dinh R et al. Recurrence of corneal dystrophy after excimer laser phototherapeutic keratectomy. Ophthalmology 106:1490–1497 (1999).

DiSclafani M, Liebmann JM, Ritch R. Malignant glaucoma following argon laser release of scleral flap sutures after trabeculectomy. Am J Ophthalmol 108:597–598 (1989).

Dmovsek-Olup B, Vedlin B. Use of Er:YAG laser for benign skin disorders. Lasers Surg Med 21:13–19 (1997).

Dodick JM. Laser phacolysis of the human cataractous lens. Dev Ophthalmol 22:58–64 (1991).

Dodick JM et al. Neodymium-YAG laser phacolysis of the human cataractous lens [letter]. Arch Ophthalmol 111:903–904 (1993).

Dodick JM, Christiansen J. Experimental studies on the development and propagation of shock waves created by the interaction of short Nd:YAG laser pulses with a titanium target. Possible implications for Nd:YAG laser phacolysis of the cataractous human lens. J Cataract Refract Surg 17:794–797 (1991).

Dodick JM, Sperber LTD. Current techniques in laser cataract surgery. In Fine IH, ed. Phacoemulsification: New Technology and Clinical Application. Thorofare, NJ: Slack Inc, 1996; 9:145–153.

Dougherty TJ et al. Photodynamic therapy. J Natl Cancer Inst 90:889–905 (1998).

Doyle A, Russell J, O'Keefe M. Paediatric laser DCR. Acta Ophthalmol Scand 78:204–205 (2000).

Durrie DS, Schumer JD, Cavanaugh TB. Phototherapeutic keratectomy: the Summit experience. In Salz JJ, McDonnell PJ, McDonald MB, eds. Corneal laser surgery, St. Louis, MO: Mosby, 1995; 16:227–235.

Eichenbaum DM. Paradigm system: a laser probe for cataract removal. In Fine IH, ed. Phacoemulsification: new technology and clinical application. Thorofare, NJ: Slack Inc, 1996; 10:155–158.

Elder MJ. The true rate of success in argon laser eyelash thermoablation. Opthal Surg Lasers 27:888–890 (1996).

Epstein RJ et al. Corneal vascularization. Pathogenesis and inhibition. Cornea 6:250–257 (1987).

Epstein RJ, Hendricks RL, Harris DM. Photodynamic therapy for corneal neovascularization. Cornea 10:424–432 (1991).

Epstein RJ, Robin JB. Corneal graft rejection episode after excimer laser phototherapeutic keratectomy [letter]. Arch Ophthalmol 112:157 (1994).

Fagerholm P et al. Phototherapeutic keratectomy: long-term results in 166 eyes. Refract Corneal Surg (Suppl) 9:S76–S81 (1993).

Fankhauser F. A high-efficiency laser iridotomy-sphincterotomy lens. Am J Ophthalmol 102:670–671 (1986).

Fankhauser F, Kwasniewska S. Neodymium: yttrium-aluminum garnet laser. In L'Esperance FA Jr, ed. Ophthalmic lasers, Vol II. St Louis, MO: Mosby; 1989: 841–843.

Fankhauser F, Kwasniewska S. Nd:YAG laser sweeping of an intraocular lens [letter]. Ophthalmic Surg 26:169 (1995).

Fankhauser F, Kwasniewska S, Klapper RM. Neodymium Q-switched YAG laser lysis of iris lens synechiae. Ophthalmology 92:790–792 (1985).

Faschinger CW. Phototherapeutic keratectomy of a corneal scar due to presumed infection after photorefractive keratectomy. J Cataract Refract Surg 26:296–300 (2000).

Favilla I et al. Phototherapy of posterior uveal melanomas. Br J Ophthalmol 75:718–721 (1991).

Felder DS. CO_2 laser skin resurfacing in oculoplastic surgery. Curr Opinion Ophthalmol 7:32–37 (1996).

Felder DS, Mayl N. Peri-orbital CO_2 laser resurfacing. Seminar Ophthalmol 11:201–210 (1996).

Fine IH. Pupilloplasty for small pupil phacoemulsification. J Cataract Refract Surg 20:192–196 (1994).

Fisher AM, Murphree AL, Gomer CJ. Clinical and preclinical photodynamic therapy. Lasers Surg Med 17:2–31 (1995).

Fisher JC. Basic biophysical principles of resurfacing of human skin by means of the carbon dioxide laser. J Clin Laser Med Surg 14:193–210 (1996).

Fitzpatrick RE et al. Pulsed carbon dioxide laser resurfacing of photoaged facial skin. Arch Dermatol 132:395–402 (1996).

Flaharty PM, Patel BK, Anderson RL. Lasers in oculoplastic surgery. In Benson WE, Coscas G, Katz LJ, eds. Current techniques in ophthalmic laser surgery. Philadelphia, PA: Current Medicine, 1994; 3:26–34.

Flynn WJ, Carlson DW. Laser synechialysis to prevent membrane recurrence on silicone intraocular lenses. Am J Ophthalmol 122:426–428 (1996).

Fong Y-C et al. Phototherapeutic keratectomy for superficial corneal fibrosis after radial keratotomy. J Cataract Refract Surg 26:616–619 (2000).

Forster W et al. Topical diclofenac sodium after excimer laser phototherapeutic keratectomy. J Refract Surg 13:311–313 (1996).

Forster W et al. Therapeutic use of the 193-nm excimer laser in corneal pathologies. Graefes Arch Clin Exp Ophthalmol 235:296–305 (1997).

Fulton JC, Cohen EJ, Rapuano CJ. Bacterial ulcer 3 days after excimer laser phototherapeutic keratectomy. Arch Ophthalmol 114:626–627 (1996).

Gailitis RP et al. Comparison of laser phacovaporization using the Er-YAG and the Er-YSSG laser. Arch Ophthalmol 111:697–700 (1993).

Gallo JP, Raizman MB. Phototherapeutic keratectomy for superficial corneal disorders. Int Ophthalmol Clin 37:155–170 (1997).

Gandham SB et al. Neodymium:YAG membranectomy for pupillary membranes on posterior chamber intraocular lenses. Ophthalmology 102:1846–1852 (1995).

Garden JM, Bakus AD, Paller AS. Treatment of cutaneous hemangiomas by the flashlamp-pumped pulsed dye laser: prospective analysis. J Pediatr 120:555–560 (1992).

Gartry D, Muir MK, Marshall J. Excimer laser treatment of corneal surface pathology: a laboratory and clinical study. Br J Ophthalmol 75:258–269 (1991).

Geerling G et al. Initial clinical experience with the picosecond Nd:YLF laser for intraocular therapeutic applications. Br J Ophthalmol 82:504–509 (1998).

Geggel HS. Successful treatment of recurrent corneal erosion with Nd:YAG anterior stromal puncture. Am J Ophthalmol 110:404–407 (1990).

Geggel HS, Maza CE. Anterior stromal puncture with the Nd:YAG laser. Invest Ophthalmol Vis Sci 31:1555–1559 (1990).

Geijssen HC, Greve EL. Mitomycin, suture lysis and hypotony. Int Ophthalmol 16:371–374 (1992).

Gladstone GJ, Beckman H. Argon laser treatment of an eyelid margin capillary hemangioma. Ophthalmic Surg 14:944–946 (1983).

Gladstone GJ, Beckman H, Elson LM. CO_2 laser excision of xanthelasma lesions. Arch Ophthalmol 103:440–442 (1985).

Gohto Y et al. Photodynamic effect of a new photosensitizer ATX-s10 on corneal neovascularization. Exp Eye Res 67:313–322 (1998).

Gohto Y et al. Photodynamic therapy for corneal neovascularization using topically administered ATX-S10(Na). Ophthalmic Surg Lasers 31:55–60 (2000).

Goins KM et al. Photodynamic biologic tissue glue to enhance corneal wound healing after radial keratotomy. J Cataract Refract Surg 23:1331–1338 (1997).

Goins KM, Khadem J, Majmudar PA. Relative strength of photodynamic biologic tissue glue in penetrating keratoplasty in cadaver eyes. J Cataract Refract Surg 24:1566–1570 (1998).

Goldbaum AM, Woog JJ. The CO_2 laser in oculoplastic surgery. Surv Ophthalmol 42:255–267 (1997).

Goldberg DJ, Whitworth J. Laser skin resurfacing with the Q-switched Nd:YAG laser. Dermatol Surg 23:903–906 (1997).

Goldman MP, Fitzpatrick RE. Cutaneous laser surgery: the art and science of selective photothermolysis. St. Louis, MO: Mosby Year Book, 1998.

Goldman MP, Fitzpatrick RE, Ruiz-Esparza J. Treatment of port-wine stains (capillary malformation) with the flashlamp-pumped pulsed dye laser. J Pediatr 122:71–77 (1993).

Gonnering RS, Lyon DB, Fisher JC. Endoscopic laser-assisted lacrimal surgery. Am J Ophthalmol 111:152–157 (1991).

Gonzalez E, Gange RW, Momtaz KT. Treatment of telangiectases and other benign vascular lesions with the 577 nm pulsed dye laser. J Am Acad Dermatol 27:220–226 (1992).

Gonzalez VH et al. Photodynamic therapy of pigmented choroidal melanomas. Invest Ophthalmol Vis Sci 36:871–878 (1995).

Gossman MD et al. Prospective evaluation of the argon laser in the treatment of trichiasis. Ophthalmic Surg 23:183–187 (1992).

Grene RB. Use of the YAG laser to open a dense fibrovascular pupillary membrane [letter]. Ophthalmic Surg 21:159–160 (1990).

Gross EA, Rogers GS. A side-by-side comparison of carbon dioxide resurfacing lasers for the treatment of rhytides. J Am Acad Dermatol 39:547–553 (1998).

Gross JG, Robin AL. Argon laser iridocorneal adhesiolysis. Am J Ophthalmol 100:330–331 (1985).

Grossman AR, Majidian AM, Grossman PH. Thermal injuries as a result of CO_2 laser resurfacing. Plast Reconstr Surg 102:1247–1252 (1998).

Gwon A et al. Focal laser photophacoablation of normal and cataractous lenses in rabbits: preliminary report. J Cataract Refract Surg 21:282–286 (1995).

Haeusler R et al. External dacryocystaorhinostomy versus endonasal laser dacryocystorhinostomy [letter]. Ophthalmology 106:647–648 (1999).

Haimovici R et al. Localization of lipoprotein-delivered benzoporphyrin derivative in the rabbit eye. Curr Eye Res 16:83–90 (1997).

Haimovici R, Miller JW, Gragoudas ES. Photodynamic therapy for ocular tumors and neovascularization. In Benson WE, Coscas G, Katz LJ, eds. Current techniques in ophthalmic laser surgery. Philadelphia, PA: Current Medicine, 1994:135–146.

Harbin TS Jr. Treatment of cyclodialysis clefts with argon laser photocoagulation. Ophthalmology 89:1082–1083 (1982).

Harris DM et al. Eyelid resurfacing. Lasers Surg Med 25:107–122 (1999).

Hartikainen J et al. Prospective randomized comparison of external dacryocystorhinostomy and endonasal laser dacryocystorhinostomy. Ophthalmology 105:1106–1113 (1998).

Hayashi K, Nakao F, Hayashi F. Changes in corneal shape after suture cutting using the argon laser for postoperative astigmatism following cataract extraction. J Cataract Refract Surg 19:236–241 (1993).

Hemady RK, Baer JC, Foster CS. Biomicroscopic and histopathologic observations after corneal laser photocoagulation in a rabbit model of corneal neovascularization. Cornea 12:185–190 (1993).

Hersh PS et al. Excimer laser phototherapeutic keratectomy. Surgical strategies and clinical outcomes. Ophthalmology 103:1210–1222 (1996).

Hersh PS, Jordan AJ, Mayers M. Corneal graft rejection episode after excimer laser phototherapeutic keratectomy. Arch Ophthalmol 111:735–736 (1993).

Hill RA et al. Photodynamic therapy of the ciliary body with tin ethyl etiopurpurin and tin octaethyl benzochlorin in pigmented rabbits. Ophthalmic Surg Lasers 28:948–953 (1997a).

Hill RA et al. Photodynamic therapy for antifibrosis in a rabbit model of filtration surgery. Ophthalmic Surg Lasers 28:574–581 (1997b).

Hobby LW. Further evaluation of the potential of the argon laser in the treatment of strawberry hemangiomas. Plast Reconstr Surg 71:481–489 (1983).

Holy A, Geronemus RG. Treatment of periorbital port-wine stains with the flashlamp-pumped pulsed dye laser. Arch Ophthalmol 110:793–797 (1992).

Hoppeler T, Gloor B. Preliminary clinical results with the ISL laser. Proc SPIE Ophthalmic Technologies II 1644:96–99 (1992).

Hornblass A, Coden DJ. Lasers in ophthalmic plastic and orbital surgery. In Karlin DB, ed. Lasers in ophthalmic surgery. Cambridge, MA: Blackwell Science, 1995; 11:214–226.

Hoskins HD Jr, Migliazzo C. Management of failing filtering blebs with the argon laser. Ophthalmic Surg 15:731–733 (1984).

Hrabovsky SL. Preoperative and postoperative skin care with laser resurfacing. Semin Ophthalmol 13:115–122 (1998).

Huang AJ et al. Induction of conjunctival transdifferentiation on vascularized corneas by photothrombotic occlusion of corneal neovascularization. Ophthalmology 95:228–235 (1988a).

Huang AJ et al. Photothrombosis of corneal neovascularization by intravenous rose bengal and argon laser irradiation. Arch Ophthalmol 106:680–685 (1988b).

Huerter CJ, Wheeland RG. Multiple eruptive cysts treated with carbon dioxide laser vaporization. J Dermatol Surg Oncol 13:260–263 (1987).

Hughes PS. Skin contraction following erbium:YAG laser resurfacing. Dermatol Surg 24:109–111 (1998).

Humphreys TR et al. Treatment of superficial basal cell carcinoma and squamous cell carcinoma in situ with a high-energy pulsed carbon dioxide laser. Arch Dermatol 134:1247–1252 (1998).

Hurvitz LM. YAG anterior capsulectomy and lysis of posterior synechiae after cataract surgery. Ophthalmic Surg 23:103–107 (1992).

Husain D et al. Intravenous infusion of liposomal benzoporphyrin derivative for photodynamic therapy of experimental choroidal neovascularization. Arch Ophthalmol 114:978–985 (1996).

Husain D et al. Photodynamic therapy and digital angiography of experimental iris neovascularization using liposomal benzoporphyrin derivative. Ophthalmology 104:1242–1250 (1997).

Husain D, Miller JW. Photodynamic therapy of exudative age-related macular degeneration. Seminars in Ophthalmology 12:14–25 (1997).

Hutnik CML, Probst LE. Argon laser punctal therapy versus thermal cautery for the treatment of aqueous deficiency dry eye syndrome. Can J Ophthalmol 33:365–372 (1998).

Iliaki OE et al. Photothrombosis of retinal and choroidal vessels in rabbit eyes using chloroaluminum sulfonated phthalocyanine and a diode laser. Lasers Surg Med 19:311–323 (1996).

James WA et al. Argon laser photomydriasis. Am J Ophthalmol 81:62–70 (1976).

Jampel HD, Pasquale LR, Dibernardo C. Hypotony maculopathy following trabeculectomy with mitomycin C. Arch Ophthalmol 110:1049–1050 (1992).

Joondeph HC. Management of postoperative and post-traumatic cyclodialysis clefts with argon laser photocoagulation. Ophthalmic Surg 11:186–188 (1980).

Jordan DR, Anderson RL. Carbon dioxide laser therapy for conjunctival lymphangioma. Ophthalmic Surg 18:728–730 (1981).

Jordan DR, Mawn L, Marshall DH. Necrotizing fasciitis caused by a group A Streptococcus infection after laser blepharoplasty. Am J Ophthalmol 125:265–266 (1998).

Joussen AM et al. Photothrombosis of corneal neovascularization with photosensitizers coupled to macromolecules. Lasers Light Ophthalmol 8:211–219 (1998).

Kanellopoulos AJ et al. Dodick photolysis for cataract surgery. Early experience with the Q-switched neodymium:YAG laser in 100 consecutive patients. Ophthalmology 106:2197–2202 (1999).

Kaplan I, Kott I, Giler S. The CO2 laser in the treatment of lesions of the eyelids and periorbital region. J Clin Laser Med Surg 14:185–187 (1996).

Katz HR et al. Nd:YAG laser photoinduced adhesion of the corneal epithelium. Am J Ophthalmol 118:612–622 (1994).

Kaufmann R, Hartmann A, Hibst R. Cutting and skin-ablative properties of pulsed mid-infrared laser surgery. J Dermatol Surg Oncol 20:112–118 (1994).

Kaufmann R, Hibst R. Pulsed erbium:YAG laser ablation in cutaneous surgery. Lasers Surg Med 19:324–330 (1996).

Keller C, To K. Bleb leak with hypotony after laser suture lysis and trabeculectomy with mitomycin C [letter]. Arch Ophthalmol 111:427–428 (1993).

Kennerdell JS et al. Surgical management of orbital lymphangioma with the carbon dioxide laser. Am J Ophthalmol 102:308–314 (1986).

Kermani O et al. In-vitro investigations on 308 nm XeCl-excimer laser cataract ablation. Laser Light Ophthalmol 3:173–185 (1990).

Key MJ, Waner M. Selective destruction of facial telangiectasia using a copper vapor laser. Arch Otolaryngol Head Neck Surg 118:509–513 (1992).

Khadem J, Truong T, Ernest JT. Photodynamic biologic tissue glue. Cornea 13:406–410 (1994).

Khan JA. Millisecond CO_2 laser skin resurfacing. Intl Ophthalmol Clin 37:29–68 (1997).

Khatri KA et al. Comparison of erbium:YAG and carbon dioxide lasers in resurfacing of facial rhytides. Arch Dermatol 135:391–397 (1999).

Kim RY et al. Photodynamic therapy of pigmented choroidal melanomas of greater than 3-mm thickness. Ophthalmology 103:2029–2036 (1996).

Kliman GH et al. Angiography and photodynamic therapy of experimental choroidal neovascularization using phthalocyanine dye [abstract]. Invest Ophthalmol Vis Sci 30 (Suppl):371 (1989).

Kliman GH et al. Retinal and choroidal vessel closure using phthalocyanine photodynamic therapy. Lasers Surg Med 15:11–18 (1994a).

Kliman GH et al. Phthalocyanine photodynamic therapy: new strategy for closure of choroidal neovascularization. Lasers Surg Med 15:2–10 (1994b).

Kong Y, Kim T, Kong B. A report of 131 cases of endoscopic laser lacrimal surgery. Ophthalmology 101:1793–1800 (1994).

Kopelman JE. Aesthetic facial skin resurfacing. The erbium:YAG laser versus the ultrapulsed carbon dioxide laser. Ophthalmol Clin North Am 11:257–263 (1998a).

Kopelman J. Erbium:YAG laser—an improved periorbital resurfacing device. Semin Ophthalmol 13:136–141 (1998b).

Korn EL. Laser chalazion removal. Ophthalmic Surg 19:428–431 (1988).

Korn EL, Glotzbach RK. Carbon dioxide repair of medial ectropion. Ophthalmic Surg 19:653–657 (1988).

Kovacs B, Czeke I, Dobszai G. Nd:YAG laser treatment of a persistent pupillary membrane causing reduced visual acuity. Lasers Light Ophthalmol 6:37–40 (1993).

Kozobolis VP et al. Nd:YAG laser removal of pupillary membranes developed after ECCE with PC-IOL implantation. Acta Ophthalmol Scan 75:711–715 (1997).

Krag S, Ehlers N. Excimer laser treatment of pterygium. Acta Opthalmol 70:530–533 (1992).

Kramer M et al. Liposomal benzoporphyrin derivative verteporfin photodynamic therapy. Selective treatment of choroidal neovascularization in monkeys. Ophthalmology 103:427–438 (1996).

Krasnick NM, Spigelman AV. Comparison of yellow dye, continuous wave Nd:YAG, and argon green laser on experimentally induced corneal neovascularization. J Refract Surg 11:45–49 (1995).

Krasnov MM. Laser-phakopuncture in the treatment of soft cataracts. Br J Ophthalmol 59:96–98 (1975).

Kremer I, Blumenthal M. Combined PRK and PTK in myopic patients with recurrent corneal erosion. Br J Ophthalmol 81:551–554 (1997).

Krueger RR, Trokel SL, Schubert HD. Interaction of ultraviolet laser light with the cornea. Invest Ophthalmol Vis Sci 25:1455–1463 (1985).

Kuebler AC et al. Photodynamic therapy of primary nonmelanomatous skin tumours of the head and neck. Lasers Surg Med 25:60–68 (1999).

Kuechle M, Naumann GO. Direct cyclopexy for traumatic cyclodialysis with persisting hypotony. Report in 29 consecutive patients. Ophthalmology 102:322–333 (1995).

Kumar H, Ahuja S, Garg SP. Neodymium:YAG laser iridolenticular synechiolysis in uveitis. Ophthalmic Surg 25:288–291 (1994a).

Kumar H, Honavar SG, Vajpayee RB. Nd:YAG laser sweeping of the anterior surface of an intraocular lens: a new observation. Ophthalmic Surg 25:409–410 (1994b).

Kumar H, Sakhuja N, Sachdev MS. Hyperplastic pupillary membrane and laser therapy. Ophthalmic Surg 25:189–190 (1994).

Kumar H, Talwar D. Is krypton red better than argon blue-green for laser suturotomy [letter]? Ophthalmic Surg 22:303–304 (1991).

Kwasniewska S, Fankhauser F. Photodisruption of precipitates on the anterior surface of IOL implants. Cataract 1:23–25 (1985).

Ladas ID et al. Use of argon laser photocoagulation in the treatment of recurrent trichiasis: long-term results. Ophthalmologica 207:90–93 (1993).

Lask GP, Lowe NJ. Lasers in cutaneous and cosmetic surgery. Philadelphia, PA: Churchill Livingstone, 1999.

Laws RA et al. Alabaster skin after carbon dioxide laser resurfacing with histologic correlation. Dermatol Surg 24:633–636 (1998).

L'Esperance FA Jr, James WA Jr. Argon laser photocoagulation of iris abnormalities. Trans Am Acad Ophthalmol Otolaryngol 79:OP-321–329 (1975).

Lessner AM, Fagien S. Laser blepharoplasty. Semin Ophthalmol 13:90–102 (1998).

Levin ML, Wyatt KD. Prospective analysis of laser photophacofragmentation. J Cataract Refract Surg 16:96–98 (1990).

Levin PS, StormoGipson J. Endocanalicular laser-assisted dacryocystorhinostomy. Arch Ophthalmol 110:1488–1490 (1992).

Lewis RA et al. Neovascular glaucoma after photoradiation therapy for uveal melanoma. Arch Ophthalmol 102:839–842 (1984).

Lieberman MF. Suture lysis by laser and goniolens. Am J Ophthalmol 95:257–258 (1983).

Lieberman MF. Diode laser suture lysis following trabeculectomy with mitomycin [letter]. Arch Ophthalmol 114:364 (1996).

Liebmann J, Ritch R. Intraocular suture ligature to reduce hypotony following Molteno seton implantation. Ophthalmic Surg 23:51–52 (1992).

Lim KJ, Wee WR, Lee JH. Treatment of corneal neovascularization with argon laser. Korean J Ophthalmol 7:25–27 (1993).

Lin SC et al. The photodynamic occlusion of choroidal vessels using benzoporphyrin derivative. Curr Eye Res 13:513–522 (1994).

Linsmeier-Kilmer S. Laser resurfacing complications: how to treat them and how to avoid them. Int J Aesthetic Restorative Surg 5:41–45 (1997).

Macken P, Buys Y, Trope GE. Glaucoma laser suture lysis. Br J Ophthalmol 80:398–401 (1996).

Maguen E et al. Excimer laser ablation of the human lens at 308 nm with a fiber delivery system. J Cataract Refract Surg 15:409–414 (1989).

Maloney RK et al. A prospective multicenter trial of excimer laser phototherapeutic keratectomy for corneal vision loss. Am J Ophthalmol 122:149–160 (1996).

Manchester T. YAG laser anterior capsulotomy. Trans Am Ophthalmol Soc 82:176–186 (1984).

Mandelkorn RM et al. A new argon laser suture lysis lens [letter]. Ophthalmic Surg 25:480–481 (1994).

Marsh RJ. Lasering of lipid keratopathy. Trans Ophthalmol Soc UK 102:154–156 (1982).

Marsh RJ. Argon laser treatment of lipid keratopathy. Br J Ophthalmol 72:900–904 (1988).

Marsh RJ, Marshall J. Treatment of lipid keratopathy with the argon laser. Br J Ophthalmol 66:127–135 1982).

Marshall J et al. An ultrastructural study of corneal incisions induced by an excimer laser at 193 nm. Ophthalmology 92:749–758 (1985).

Marshall J et al. Photoablative reprofiling of the cornea using an excimer laser: photorefractive keratectomy. Lasers in Ophthalmology 1:21–48 (1986).

Marshall J, Sliney DH. Endoexcimer laser intraocular ablative photodecomposition [letter]. Am J Ophthalmol 101:130–131 (1986).

Martinez M et al. A comparison of excimer laser (308 nm) ablation of the human lens nucleus in air and saline with a fiber optic delivery system. Refract Corneal Surg 8:368–374 (1992).

Massaro BM, Gonnering RS, Harris GJ. Endonasal laser dacryocystorhinostomy: a new approach to nasolacrimal duct obstruction. Arch Ophthalmol 108:1172–1176 (1990).

Maumenee AE, Stark WJ. Management of persistent hypotony after planned or inadvertent cyclodialysis. Am J Ophthalmol 71:320–327 (1971).

Maus M. Lasers in oculoplastic surgery. Curr Opin Ophthalmol 6:37–42 (1995).

McMillan TA et al. The effect of varying wavelength on subconjunctival scleral laser suture lysis in rabbits. Acta Ophthalmol 70:758–761 (1992).

McWhae JA, Crichton ACS. The use of ultrasound biomicroscopy following trabeculectomy. Can J Ophthalmol 31:187–191 (1996).

Melamed S et al. Tight scleral flap trabeculectomy with postoperative laser suture lysis. Am J Ophthalmol 109:303–309 (1990).

Mendelsohn AD et al. Laser photocoagulation of feeder vessels in lipid keratopathy. Ophthalmic Surg 17:502–508 (1986).

Mendelsohn AD et al. Amelioration of experimental lipid keratopathy by photochemically induced thrombosis of feeder vessels. Arch Ophthalmol 105:983–988 (1987).

Metrikin DC, Allinson RW, Snyder RW. Transscleral repair of recalcitrant, inadvertent, postoperative cyclodialysis cleft. Ophthalmic Surg 25:406–408 (1994).

Metson R, Woog J, Puliafito C. Endoscopic laser dacryocystorhinostomy. Laryngoscope 104:269–274 (1994).

Migden M, Elkins BS, Clinch TE. Phototherapeutic keratectomy for corneal scars. Ophthalmic Surg Lasers 27:S503–s507 (1996).

Miller H, Miller B. Photodynamic therapy of subretinal neovascularization in the monkey eye. Arch Ophthalmol 111:855–860 (1993).

Miller KM, Keener GT Jr. Stretch pupilloplasty for small pupil phacoemulsification [letter]. Am J Ophthalmol 117:107–108 (1994).

Miller JW et al. Photodynamic therapy of experimental choroidal neovascularization using lipoprotein-delivered benzoporphyrin. Arch Ophthalmol 113:810–818 (1995).

Miller JW et al. Phthalocyanine photodynamic therapy of experimental iris neovascularization. Ophthalmology 98:1711–1719 (1991).

Millman AL, Mannor GE. Histologic and clinical evaluation of combined eyelid erbium:YAG and CO_2 laser resurfacing. Am J Ophthalmol 127:614–616 (1999).

Mittelman H. The use of lasers for blepharoplasty. Ophthalmol Clin North Am 11:267–275 (1998).

Miyake K. Anterior lens capsulotomy using the holmium YAG laser in pig cadaver eyes. Ophthalmic Surg 23:176–178 (1992).

Mohan H, Talwar R, Verma D. Combined argon/YAG laser pupilloplasty—a new technique. In Khoo CY et al., eds. New frontiers in ophthalmology. New York, NY: Excerpta Medica, 1991:922–924.

Morad Y et al. Excimer laser phototherapeutic keratectomy for recurrent corneal erosion. J Cataract Refract Surg 24:451–455 (1998).

Moreno-Arias GA, Camps-Fresneda A. Use of the Q-switched alexandrite laser (755 nm, 100 nsec) for eyebrow tattoo removal. Lasers Surg Med 25:123–125 (1999).

Morinelli EN et al. Laser suture lysis after mitomycin C trabeculectomy. Ophthalmology 103:306–314 (1996).

Morrow DM, Morrow LB. CO_2 laser blepharoplasty: a comparison with cold-steel surgery. J Dermatol Surg Oncol 18:307–313 (1992).

Mueller-Stolzenburg N, Mueller GJ. Transmission of 308 nm excimer laser radiation for ophthalmic microsurgery—medical, technical and safety aspects. Biomed Tech 34:131–138 (1989).

Mueller-Stolzenburg N, Stange N, Mueller GJ. Excimer laser lens ablation via quartz fiber. Dev Ophthalmol 22:11–15 (1991).

Muellner K et al. Endolacrimal laser assisted lacrimal surgery. Br J Ophthalmol 84:16–18 (2000).

Murphree AL. Retinoblastoma. In Ryan SJ, Ogden TE, eds. Retina, Vol. 1. St Louis, MO: Mosby; 1989, 544.

Murphree AL, Cote M, Gomer CJ. The evolution of photodynamic therapy techniques in the treatment of intraocular tumors. Photochem Photobiol 46:919–923 (1987).

Murube J, Murube E. Treatment of dry eye by blocking the lacrimal canaliculi. Surv Ophthalmol 40:463–480 (1996).

Nanevicz TM et al. Excimer laser ablation of the lens. Arch Ophthalmol 104:1825–1829 (1986).

Nanni C. Complications of laser surgery. Ophthalmol Clin North Am 11:277–291 (1998).

Nanni CA, Alster TS. Complications of carbon dioxide laser resurfacing: an evaluation of 500 patients. Dermatol Surg 24:315–320 (1998a).

Nanni CA, Alster TS. Complications of cutaneous laser surgery: a review. Dermatol Surg 24:209–219 (1998b).

Nerad JA, Anderson RL. CO2 laser treatment of eyelid syringomas. Ophthal Plast Reconstr Surg 4:91–94 (1988).

Nirankari VS. Laser photocoagulation for corneal stromal vascularization. Trans Am Ophthalmol Soc 90:595–669 (1992).

Nirankari VS, Baer JC. Corneal argon laser photocoagulation for neovascularization in penetrating keratoplasty. Ophthalmology 93:1304–1309 (1986).

Nirankari VS, Dandona L, Rodrigues MM. Laser photocoagulation of experimental corneal stromal vascularization. Efficacy and histopathology. Ophthalmology 100:111–118 (1993).

Noecker RJ et al. Endolenticular phacolysis using the erbium:YAG laser on human autopsy lenses: a histopathologic study. Proc SPIE Ophthalmic Technologies IV 2126:315–322 (1994).

O'Brart DPS et al. Treatment of band keratopathy by excimer laser phototherapeutic keratectomy: Surgical techniques and long term follow-up. Br J Ophthalmol 7:702–708 (1993).

Obstbaum SA et al. Laser photomydriasis in pseudophakic pupillary block. Intra-Ocular Implant Soc 7:28–30 (1981).

Obstbaum SA, To KW, Galler EL. Lasers in cataract surgery. In Karlin DB, ed. Lasers in ophthalmic surgery. Cambridge, MA: Blackwell Science, 1995; 4:80–91.

Ochsner M. Photophysical and photobiological processes in the photodynamic therapy of tumours. J Photochem Photobiol B 39:1–18 (1997).

Oguz H, Aras C, Ozdamar A. Thermoablation treatment for trichiasis in trachoma using the semiconductor diode pumped laser. Eur J Ophthalmol 9:85–88 (1999).

Oh YG. Revision of failing filtering bleb. In Benson WE, Coscas G, Katz LJ, eds. Current Techniques in Ophthalmic Laser Surgery. Philadelphia, PA: Current Medicine, 1994; 199–204.

Ohnishi Y, Yamana Y, Minei M. Photoradiation therapy using argon laser and a hematoporphyrin derivative for retinoblastoma: a preliminary report. Jpn J Ophthalmol 30:409–419 (1986).

Oleinick NL, Evans HH. The photobiology of photodynamic therapy: cellular targets and mechanisms. Radiat Res 150:S146–s156 (1998).

Oram O et al. Opening an occluded tube with the picosecond neodymium-yttrium lithium fluoride laser [case report]. Arch Ophthalmol 112:1023 (1994).

Ormerod LD et al. Management of the hypotonous cyclodialysis cleft. Ophthalmology 98:1384–1393 (1991).

Orndahl MJF, Fagerholm PP. Phototherapeutic keratectomy for map-dot-fingerprint corneal dystrophy. Cornea 17:595–599 (1998a).

Orndahl MJF, Fagerholm PP. Treatment of corneal dystrophies with phototherapeutic keratectomy. J Refract Surg 14:129–135 (1998b).

Oshry T et al. Argon green laser photoepilation in the treatment of trachomatous trichiasis. Ophthal Plast Reconstr Surg 10:253–255 (1994).

Packer AJ et al. Hematoporphyrin photoradiation therapy for iris neovascularization. A preliminary report. Arch Ophthalmol 102:1193–1197 (1984).

Palli JC, Cinotti AA. Iris photocoagulation therapy of aphakic pupillary block. Arch Ophthalmol 93:347–348 (1975).

Pallikaris IG et al. Effectiveness of corneal neovascularization photothrombosis using phthalocyanine and a diode laser (675 nm). Lasers Surg Med 13:197–203 (1993).

Pallikaris IG et al. Histological evaluation of phthalocyanine mediated photodynamic occlusion of corneal neovascularization by hyperbaric oxygenation. J Refract Surg 12:S313–s316 (1996).

Panagopoulos JA et al. Photodynamic therapy for experimental intraocular melanoma using chloroaluminum sulfonated phthalocyanine. Arch Ophthalmol 107:886–890 (1989).

Panda A, Pattnaik NK. Neodymium: yttrium aluminum garnet laser anterior capsulotomy. Ann Ophthalmol 23:334–336 (1991).

Pappa KS et al. Late argon laser suture lysis after mitomycin C trabeculectomy. Ophthalmology 100:1268–1271 (1993).

Park SC, Kim JH. Effects of laser photocoagulation on corneal neovascularization in rabbits. J Refract Corneal Surg 10:631–639 (1994).

Parsa CF et al. Hemorrhage complicating YAG laser feeder vessel coagulation of cornea vascularization. Cornea 13:264–268 (1994).

Partamian LG. Treatment of a cyclodialysis cleft with argon laser photocoagulation in a patient with a shallow anterior chamber. Am J Ophthalmol 99:5–7 (1985).

Patel BCK. The krypton yellow-green laser for the treatment of facial vascular and pigmented lesions. Semin Ophthalmol 13:158–170 (1998).

Patel BCK et al. Transcanalicular neodymium:YAG laser for revision of dacryocystorhinostomy. Ophthalmology 104:1191–1197 (1997).

Paylor R. Central retinal artery occlusion following YAG synechialysis [letter]. Arch Ophthalmol 103:325–326 (1985).

Perez MI, Bank DE, Silvers D. Skin resurfacing of the face with the erbium:YAG laser. Dermatol Surg 24:653–658 (1998).

Peyman GA et al. Effects of XeCl excimer laser on the eyelid and anterior segment structures. Arch Ophthalmol 104:118–122 (1986).

Peyman GA et al. Photodynamic therapy for choriocapillaris using tin ethyl etiopurpurin (SnET2). Ophthalmic Surg Lasers 28:409–417 (1997).

Peyman GA, Katoh N. Effects of an erbium:YAG laser on ocular structures. Int Ophthalmol 10:245–253 (1987).

Pickering JW, Walker PHB, Halewyn CN. Copper vapour laser treatment of port-wine stains and other vascular malformations. Br J Plast Surg 43:273–282 (1990).

Pollack IP. Photomydriasis and coreopexy. In Wilensky JT, ed. Laser therapy in glaucoma. Norwalk, CT: Appleton-Century-Crofts, 1985; 3:43–46.

Polnikorn N et al. Erbium:YAG laser resurfacing in Asians. Dermatol Surg 24:1303–1337 (1998).

Price FW Jr, Whitson WE. Polypropylene ligatures as a means of controlling intraocular pressure with Molteno implants. Ophthalmic Surg 20:781–783 (1989).

Primbs GB et al. Photodynamic therapy for corneal neovascularization. Ophthalmic Surg Lasers 29:832–838 (1998).

Puliafito CA et al. Excimer laser ablation of the cornea and lens. Ophthalmology 92:741–748 (1985).

Puliafito CA, Steinert RF. Laser surgery of the lens. Experimental studies. Ophthalmology 90:1007–1012 (1983).

Puliafito CA, Wong K, Steinert RF. Quantitative and ultrastructural studies of excimer laser ablation of the cornea at 193 nm and 248 nm. Lasers Surg Med 7:155–159 (1987).

Ramakrishnan R et al. Bilateral extensive persistent pupillary membranes treated with the neodymium-YAG laser. Arch Ophthalmol 111:28 (1993).

Rapuano CJ. Excimer laser phototherapeutic keratectomy: long-term results and practical considerations. Cornea 16:151–157 (1997).

Reed JW, Fromer C, Klintworth K. Induced corneal vascularization remission with argon laser therapy. Arch Ophthalmol 93:1017–1019 (1975).

Reeves PD, Yung C-W. Silicone intraocular lens encapsulation by shrinkage of the capsulorhexis opening. J Cataract Refract Surg 24:1275–1276 (1998).

Reifler DM. Results of endoscopic KTP laser-assisted dacryocystorhinostomy. Ophthalmic Plast Reconstr Surg 9:231–236 (1993).

Ritch R. Argon laser treatment for medically unresponsive attacks of angle-closure glaucoma. Am J Ophthalmol 94:197–204 (1982).

Ritch R, Potash SD, Liebmann JM. A new lens for argon laser suture lysis. Ophthalmic Surg 25:126–127 (1994).

Rojanapongpun P, Ritch R. Clear corneal graft overlying the seton tube to facilitate laser suture lysis. Am J Ophthalmol 122:424–425 (1996).

Rosen N, Barak A, Rosner M. Transcanalicular laser-assisted dacryocystorhinostomy. Ophthalmic Surg Lasers 28:723–726 (1997).

Ross BS, Puliafito CA. Erbium-YAG and holmium-YAG laser ablation of the lens. Lasers Surg Med 15:74–82 (1994).

Ross M, Watcher MA, Goodman MM. Comparison of the flashlamp pulsed dye laser with the argon tunable dye laser with robotized handpiece for facial telangiectasia. Lasers Surg Med 13:374–378 (1993).

Royster AJ et al. Photochemical initiation of thrombosis: Fluorescein angiographic, histologic, and ultrastructural alterations in the choroid, retinal pigment epithelium, and retina. Arch Ophthalmol 106:1608–1614 (1988).

Rubinfeld RS, MacRae SM, Laibson PR. Successful treatment of recurrent corneal erosion with Nd:YAG anterior stromal puncture [letter]. Am J Ophthalmol 111:252–254 (1991).

Ryan EH Jr, Logani S. Nd:YAG laser photodisruption of the lens nucleus before phacoemulsification. Am J Ophthalmol 104:382–386 (1987).

Sachdev MS, Kumar H, Dada VK, Mehta MR, Jain AK. Argon laser suturotomy: a technique for the correction of surgically induced astigmatism. Ophthalmic Surg 21:277–281 (1990).

Sadiq SA et al. Endoscopic holmium:YAG laser dacryocystorhinostomy. Eye 10:43–46 (1996).

Sadiq SA et al. Endonasal laser dacryocystorhinostomy—medium term results. Br J Ophthalmol 81:1089–1092 (1997).

Salamon SM. Trabeculectomy flap suture lysis with endolaser probe. Ophthalmic Surg 18:506–507 (1987).

Sarnoff DS, Swirsky J. Beauty and the beam: your complete guide to cosmetic laser surgery. St. Louis, MO: Quality Medical Publications, 1998.

Savage JA et al. Laser suture lysis after trabeculectomy. Ophthalmology 95:1631–1638 (1988).

Savage JA, Simmons RJ. Staged glaucoma filtration surgery with planned early conversion from scleral flap to full thickness operation using argon laser. Ophthalmic Laser Ther 1:201–210 (1986).

Scheepers J, Quaba A. Does the pulsed tunable dye laser have a role in the management of infantile hemangiomas? Observations based on 3 years' experience. Plast Reconstr Surg 95:305–312 (1995).

Schmidt-Erfurth U et al. Photodynamic therapy of experimental choroidal melanoma using lipoprotein-delivered benzoporphyrin. Ophthalmology 101:89–99 (1994a).

Schmidt-Erfurth U et al. Vascular targeting in photodynamic occlusion of subretinal vessels. Ophthalmology 101:1953–1961 (1994b).

Schmidt-Erfurth U et al. In vivo uptake of liposomal benzoporphyrin derivative and photothrombosis in experimental corneal neovascularization. Lasers Surg Med 17:178–188 (1995).

Schmidt-Erfurth U et al. Benzoporphyrin-lipoprotein-mediated photodestruction of intraocular tumors. Exp Eye Res 62:1–10 (1996).

Schultz JS. Additional uses of laser therapy in glaucoma. In Ritch R, Shields MB, Krupin T, eds. The glaucomas. St Louis, MO: Mosby, 1996:1621–1630.

Schuman JS. Miscellaneous laser procedures. In Epstein DL, Allingham RR, Schuman JS, eds. Chandler and Grant's glaucoma. Baltimore, MD: Williams & Wilkins, 1997:504–508.

Schwartz AL, Weiss HS. Bleb leak with hypotony after laser suture lysis and trabeculectomy with mitomycin C. Arch Ophthalmol 110:1049 (1992).

Schwartz L, Spaeth G, Brown G. Laser therapy of the anterior segment. A practical approach. Thorofare, NJ: Slack Inc., 1984.

Sery TW et al. Photodynamic therapy of human ocular cancer. Ophthalmic Surg 18:413–418 (1987).

Sharif KW, Arafat AFA, Wykes WC. The treatment of recurrent trichiasis with argon laser photocoagulation. Eye 5:591–595 (1991).

Shen JH, Joos KM et al. Ablation rate of PMMA and human cornea with a frequency-quintupled Nd:YAG laser (213 nm). Lasers Surg Med 21:179–185 (1997).

Sher NA, Demarchi J, Lindstrom RL. Use of the 193 nm excimer laser for photorefractive and phototherapeutic keratectomy. In Brightbill FS, ed. Corneal surgery. St. Louis, MO: Mosby, 1993:518–525.

Sher NA et al. Clinical use of the 193–nm excimer laser in the treatment of corneal scars. Arch Ophthalmol 109:491–498 (1991).

Shim E, Tse Y et al. Short-pulse carbon dioxide laser resurfacing in the treatment of rhytides and scars. A clinical and histopathological study. Dermatol Surg 24:113–117 (1998).

Shin DH. Argon laser iris photocoagulation to relieve acute angle-closure glaucoma. Am J Ophthalmol 93:348–350 (1982a).

Shin DH. Argon laser treatment for relief of medically unresponsive angle-closure glaucoma attacks. Am J Ophthalmol 94:821–822 (1982b).

Silkiss RZ et al. Transcanalicular THC:YAG dacryocystorhinostomy. Ophthalmic Surg 23:351–353 (1992).

Singh J et al. Enhancement of post trabeculectomy bleb formation by laser suture lysis. Br J Ophthalmol 80:624–627 (1996).

Singh K et al. Evaluation of Nd:YAG laser membranectomy in blocked tubes after glaucoma tube-shunt surgery. Am J Ophthalmol 124:781–786 (1997).

Sliney DH. Laser phacoemulsification: considerations of safety and effectiveness. Lasers Light Ophthalmol 3:267–276 (1990).

Slomovic AR, Parrish RK II, Sherman R. Corneal endothelial trauma after Descemet's membranotomy with the neodymium-YAG laser. Am J Ophthalmol 99:484–485 (1985).

Small EA, Solomon JM, Prince AM. Hypotonous cyclodialysis cleft following suture fixation of a posterior chamber intraocular lens. Ophthalmic Surg 25:107–109 (1994).

Snyder RW et al. Erbium:YAG laser for cataract extraction. Proc SPIE Ophthalmic Technologies VIII 3246:172–184 (1998).

Snyder RW, Noecker RJ. Laser cataract surgery. Ophthalmol Clin North Am 11:201–212 (1998).

Sobaci G et al. An investigation of the effects of photothrombosis and photocoagulation on corneal neovascularization. Ann Ophthalmol 30:388–391 (1998).

Sobel LI, Ritch R, Prince A. Argon laser sphincterotomy. Ophthalmic Laser Ther 1:87–92 (1986).

Sperber LT. Neodymium:YAG laser lens ablation in a rabbit model. J Cataract Refract Surg 22:485–489 (1996).

Sperber LTD, Dodick JM. Laser therapy in cataract surgery. Curr Opinion Ophthalmol 6:22–26 (1995).

Stark WJ et al. Clinical follow-up of 193–nm ArF excimer laser photokeratectomy. Ophthalmology 99:805–812 (1992).

Starr MB. Recurrent subepithelial corneal opacities after excimer laser phototherapeutic keratectomy. Cornea 18:117–120 (1999).

Starr M et al. Excimer laser phototherapeutic keratectomy. Cornea 15:557–565 (1996).

Steinert RF, Puliafito CA. Laser corneal surgery. Int Ophthalmol 28:150–154 (1988).

Stern WH. Argon laser photomydriasis during vitrectomy surgery. Am J Ophthalmol 99:366–367 (1985).

Stevens G Jr et al. Erbium:YAG laser-assisted cataract surgery. Ophthalmic Surg Lasers 29:185–189 (1998).

Stevens SX, Bowyer BL. Corneal modulators and their use in excimer laser phototherapeutic keratectomy. Int Ophthalmol Clinics 36:119–125 (1996).

Straatsma BR et al. Subluxation of the lens treated with iris photocoagulation. Am J Ophthalmol 61:1312–1324 (1966).

Sumian CC et al. Laser skin resurfacing using a frequency doubled Nd:YAG laser after topical application of an exogenous chromophore. Lasers Surg Med 25:43–50 (1999).

Summers CG, Holland EJ. Neodymium:YAG pupilloplasty in pediatric aphakia. J Pediatr Ophthalmol Strabismus 28:155–156 (1991).

Summit Technology Phototherapeutic Education Manual Document 711038, Waltham, MA: Summit Technology, Inc, 1995; section 5, 1–22.

Takizawa T et al. Laser surgery of basal, orbital and ventricular meningiomas which are difficult to extirpate by conventional methods. Neurol Med Chir (Tokyo) 20:729–737 (1980).

Talamo JH, Steinert RF, Puliafito CA. Clinical strategies for excimer laser therapeutic keratectomy. Refract Corneal Surg 8:319–324 (1992).

Talks SJ. Nd:YAG laser clearance of the anterior surface of posterior chamber intraocular lenses. Eye 11:479–484 (1997).

Talu H et al. Excimer laser phototherapeutic keratectomy for recurrent pterygium. J Cataract Refract Surg 24:1326–1332 (1998).

Talwar D et al. Argon laser vaporization for management of projecting suture ends after cataract surgery [letter]. Ophthalmic Surg 22:181–182 (1991).

Tan OT. Pulsed dye laser treatment of adult port-wine stains. In Tan OT, ed. Management and treatment of benign cutaneous vascular lesions. Philadelphia, PA: Lea and Febiger, 1992:83–99.

Tan OT, Sherwood K, Gilchrest BA. Treatment of children with port-wine stains using the flashlamp-pulsed tunable dye laser. N Eng J Med 320:416–421 (1989).

Tanenbaum M, Karas S, McCord CD Jr. Laser ablation of blepharopigmentation. Ophthal Plast Reconstr Surg 4:49–56 (1988).

Teichmann KD et al. Wessely-type immune ring following phototherapeutic keratectomy. J Cataract Refract Surg 22:142–146 (1966).

Teikemeier G, Goldberg DJ. Skin resurfacing with the erbium:YAG laser. Dermatol Surg 23:685–687 (1997).

Temel A, Sayin I. An inexpensive visualization method for laser suture lysis. Arch Ophthalmol 114:1301–1302 (1996).

Than TP, Spear CH Jr. Advanced primary care skills: An optometric primer to CO_2 laser skin resurfacing. Rev Optom 134(5):102–104 (1997).

Theodossiadis GP. Pupilloplasty in aphakic and pseudophakic pupillary block glaucoma. Trans Ophthalmol Soc UK 104:137–141 (1985).

Thomas EL, Langhofer M. Closure of experimental subretinal neovascular vessels with dihematoporphyrin ether augmented argon green laser photocoagulation. Photochem Photobiol 46:5881–5886 (1987).

Thomas JV. Pupilloplasty and photomydriasis. In Belcher CD, Thomas JV, Simmons RJ, eds. Photocoagulation in glaucoma and anterior segment disease. Baltimore, MD: Williams & Wilkins, 1984;11:150–157.

Tommila P, Summanen P, Tervo T. Cortisone, heparin and argon laser in the treatment of corneal neovascularization. Act Ophthalmol Suppl 182:89–92 (1987).

Thompson V, Durrie DS, Cavanaugh TB. Philosophy and technique for excimer laser phototherapeutic keratectomy. Refract Corneal Surg (Suppl) 9:S81–S85 (1993).

Thompson VM. Excimer laser phototherapeutic keratectomy: clinical and surgical aspects. Ophthalmic Surgery and Lasers 26:461–472 (1995).

Tomey KF. A simple device for laser suture lysis after trabeculectomy. Arch Ophthalmol 109:14–15 (1991).

Trelles MA et al. Carbon dioxide laser transconjunctival lower lid blepharoplasty complications. Ann Plast Surg 37:465–468 (1996a).

Trelles MA et al. Periocular skin reshaping by CO_2 laser coagulation. Aesthetic Plast Surg 20:327–131 (1996b).

Tse DT et al. Hematoporphyrin photoradiation therapy for intraocular and orbital malignant melanoma. Arch Ophthalmol 102:833–838 (1984).

Tsilimbaris MK et al. Phthalocyanine mediated photodynamic thrombosis of experimental corneal neovascularization: effect of phthalocyanine dose and irradiation onset time on vascular occlusion rate. Lasers Surg Med 15:19–31 (1994).

Tsilimbaris MK et al. Transscleral ciliary body photodynamic therapy using phthalocyanine and a diode laser: functional and morphologic implications in albino rabbits. Ophthalmic Surg Lasers 28:483–494 (1997).

Tsubota K. Application of erbium:YAG laser in ocular ablation. Ophthalmologica 200:117–122 (1990).

Tuft SJ, Talks SJ. Delayed dislocation of foldable plate-haptic silicone lenses after Nd:YAG laser anterior capsulotomy. Am J Ophthalmol 126:586–588 (1998).

Tutton MK, O'Donnell NP. Endonasal laser dacryocystorhinostomy under direct vision. Eye 9:485–487 (1995).

Vajpayee RB et al. Nd:YAG "sweeping"—an indirect technique for clearing intraocular lens deposits. Ophthalmic Surg 24:489–491 (1993).

van der Horst CMAM et al. Effect of the timing of treatment of port-wine stains with the flash-lamp-pumped pulsed-dye laser. N Engl J Med 338:1028–1033 (1998).

Van Gool CA, Schuitmaker HJ, Jager MJ. Corneal neovascularization in rats as a model for photothrombotic therapy using bacteriochlorin a and an argon laser. Graefes Arch Clin Exp Ophthalmol 233:435–440 (1995).

Vega LF, Sabates R. Neodymium:YAG laser treatment of persistent pupillary membrane. Ophthalmic Surg 18:452–454 (1987).

Virdi M, Beirouty ZAY, Saba SN. Neodymium:YAG laser discission of postoperative pupillary membrane: peripheral photodisruption. J Cataract Refract Surg 23:166–168 (1997).

Vrabec MP et al. Electron microscopic findings in a cornea with recurrence of herpes simplex keratitis after excimer laser phototherapeutic keratectomy. CLAO J 20:41–44 (1994).

Vrabec MP, Elsing SH, Aitken PA. A prospective, randomized comparison of thermal cautery and argon laser for permanent punctal occlusion. Am J Ophthalmol 116:469–471 (1993).

Waldorf HA, Kauvar ANB, Geronemus RG. Skin resurfacing of fine to deep rhytides using a char-free carbon dioxide laser in 47 patients. Dermatol Surg 21:940–946 (1995).

Wand M. Argon laser gonioplasty for synechial angle closure. Arch Ophthalmol 110:363–367 (1992).

Wang I et al. Photodynamic therapy utilising topical δ-aminolevulinic acid in non-melanoma skin malignancies of the eyelid and the periocular skin. Acta Ophthalmol Scand 77:182–188 (1999).

Watts MT et al. The use of Q-switched Nd:YAG laser for removal of permanent eyeliner tattoo. Ophthal Plast Reconstr Surg 8:292–294 (1992).

Weber B, Fagerholm P. Presence and distribution of hyaluronan in human corneas after phototherapeutic keratectomy. Acta Ophthalmol Scand 76:146–148 (1998).

Weinstein C. Carbon dioxide laser resurfacing. Long-term follow-up in 2123 patients. Clin Plast Surg 25:109–130 (1998a).

Weinstein C. Computerized scanning erbium:YAG laser for skin resurfacing. Dermatol Surg 24:83–89 (1998b).

Weinstein C, Ramirez O, Pozner J. Postoperative care following carbon dioxide laser resurfacing: avoiding pitfalls. Dermatol Surg 24:51–56 (1998).

Weishaupt KR, Gomer CJ, Dougherty TJ. Identification of singlet oxygen as the cytotoxic agent in photo-inactivation of a murine tumor. Cancer Res 36:2326–2329 (1976).

Wesley RE, Bond JB. Carbon dioxide laser in ophthalmic plastic and orbital surgery. Ophthalmic Surg 16:631–633 (1985).

Wetzel W et al. Photofragmentation of lens nuclei using the Er:YAG laser: preliminary report of an in vitro study. Ger J Ophthalmol 5:281–284 (1996).

Wheeland RG et al. Carbon dioxide laser vaporization and curettage in the treatment of large or multiple super-ficial basal cell carcinomas. J Dermatol Surg Oncol 13:119–125 (1987a).

Wheeland RG et al. Carbon dioxide (CO_2) laser vaporization of multiple facial syringomas. J Dermatol Surg Oncol 13:149–151 (1987b).

Whitsett JC, Stewart RH. A new technique for combined cataract/glaucoma procedures in patients on chronic miotics. Ophthalmic Surg 24:481–485 (1993).

Wilson CA, Hatchell DL. Photodynamic retinal vascular thrombosis. Rate and duration of vascular occlusion. Invest Ophthalmol Vis Sci 32:2357–2365 (1991).

Winward KE et al. Encircling photothrombotic therapy for choroidal Greene melanoma using rose bengal. Arch Ophthalmol 108:588–594 (1990).

Wise JB. Iris sphincterotomy, iridotomy, and synechiotomy by linear incision with the argon laser. Ophthalmol-ogy 92:641–645 (1985).

Wise JB, Munnerlyn CR, Erickson PJ. A high-efficiency laser iridotomy-sphincterotomy lens. Am J Ophthalmol 101:546–553 (1986).

Wisnicki JL. Hemangiomas and vascular malformations. Ann Plast Surg 12:41–59 (1984).

Wohlrab T-M et al. Argon laser therapy of benign tumors of the eyelid. Am J Ophthalmol 125:693–697 (1998).

Woo KI, Moon SH, Kim Y-d. Transcanalicular laser-assisted revision of failed dacryocystorhinostomy. Ophthalmic Surg Lasers 29:451–455 (1998).

Woog JJ, Metson R, Puliafito CA. Holmium:YAG endonasal laser dacryocystorhinostomy. Am J Ophthalmol 116:1–10 (1993).

Wright MM et al. Laser-cured fibrinogen glue to repair bleb leaks in rabbits. Arch Ophthalmol 116:199–202 (1998).

Yamamoto T, Sakuma T, Kitazawa Y. An ultrasound biomicroscopic study of filtering blebs after mitomycin C trabeculectomy. Ophthalmology 102:1770–1776 (1995).

Yeatts RP. Current concepts in lacrimal drainage surgery. Curr Opinion Ophthalmol 7:43–47 (1996).

Young LHY et al. Photodynamic therapy of pigmented choroidal melanomas using a liposomal preparation of benzoporphyrin derivative. Arch Ophthalmol 114:186–192 (1996).

Yung C, Massicotte SJ, Kuwabara T. Argon laser treatment of trichiasis: a clinical and histopathologic evaluation. Ophthal Plast Reconstr Surg 10:130–136 (1994).

Zacharia PT, Deppermann SR, Schuman JS. Ocular hypotony after trabeculectomy with mitomycin C. Am J Ophthalmol 116:314–326 (1993).

Zelman J. Photophaco fragmentation. J Cataract Refract Surg 13:287–289 (1987).

Zimmerman TJ, Wheeler TM. Miotics: side effects and ways to avoid them. Ophthalmology 89:76–80 (1982).

Zuckerman SJ, Aquavella JV, Park SB. Analysis of the efficacy and safety of excimer laser PTK in the treatment of corneal disease. Cornea 15:9–14 (1996).

Chapter 10
Laser Eye Safety

Felix Barker

I. Introduction

A. *Lasers Present a Special Hazard for the Eye*

Although the safety standards and regulations we will discuss in this chapter relate to more than just eye protection, the eye warrants special attention when it comes to protective measures. This is because of a number of characteristics of the eye and laser energy that make blinding injuries possible.

B. First, the optical components of the eye are essentially transparent (i.e., 90% transmittance over the visible range). This opens the potential for retinal damage due to light exposure, especially when such energy is intense, as in the case of a laser beam. In order to put lasers in proper perspective, it is useful to consider the sun, which is the most significant terrestrial vision hazard. It is well known that "sun gazing" can lead to retinal damage, but only after several minutes of exposure. In contrast to the sun, lasers are capable of producing a nearly ten times smaller retinal image with a much higher energy density, thus making it possible to produce instantaneous thermal damage within the retina.

C. In order to serve the visual function, the optical components of the eye also focus light onto the retina, thereby increasing dramatically the energy density striking the retina. Given that the human fovea, with its best acuity vision, is easily and quickly "fixated" by the observer to a point of interest such as a bright laser beam, the potential for dramatic vision loss by laser exposure is significant.

D. For laser energy falling within the ultraviolet (UV) and portions of the infrared (IR) range, there is often less retinal hazard, due to the lower penetration of these wavelengths. However, these spectral regions open up the possibility of damage to the lens, ocular surface, and skin, and the invisible nature of IR and UV make for special concerns in eye protection.

II. Laser Safety Standards and Regulations

A. *American National Standards Institute (ANSI)*

1. The establishment of safety standards for lasers started around 1968, 8 years after the first laser was introduced. These were voluntary guidelines for those working with this new and somewhat mysterious technology. In 1973, a national consensus document was developed by a volunteer panel of experts, and this was published as the first American National Standards Institute (ANSI) laser standard (ANSI Z-136). Since that time the standard has been revised a number of times, becoming two standards:
    a. **Z-136.1-2000: American National Standard for the Safe Use of Lasers** (American National Standards Institute, 2000)
    b. **Z-136.3-1996: American National Standard for the Safe Use of Lasers in Health Care Facilities** (American National Standards Institute, 1996)

2. Although voluntary, the ANSI standards attain the weight of law because they are used as a basis for regulatory activities of governmental agencies that are concerned with laser safety.

3. Updates and further information can be obtained on the ANSI Web site (http://www.ansi.org).

B. *Food and Drug Administration (FDA)*

1. FDA concern and action with regard to lasers is determined by the **Code of Federal Regulations, Title 21, Part 1040** and by the **Compliance Guide for Laser Products** (Food and Drug Administration, 1985, 1999). Under this mandate, the Center for Devices and Radiological Health (CDRH) of the FDA regulates the manufacture and use of all medical lasers manufactured after 1976. The regulations and other information can be obtained at the CDRH Web site: (http://www.fda.gov/cdrh/index.html).

2. The FDA approval scheme for new lasers involves the process of investigational device testing. FDA approval of new medical lasers is specific for each use. The FDA does not determine which category of medical practitioner may use a particular device, and leaves this determination as a matter of state licensure. The FDA utilizes the ANSI Standards 136.1 and 136.3 as a basis for its classification and labeling of lasers by hazard category.

C. *Occupational Safety and Health Administration (OSHA)*

1. The Department of Labor regulates safety in the workplace via its OSHA regulations (U.S. Department of Labor, 1999a–c). OSHA places the responsibility for safety in the workplace upon the employer, who must conduct safety assessments, prescribe protective measures, and ensure that they are followed. OSHA manages safety in the

workplace by responding to complaints and by making unannounced inspections. OSHA has the power to fine employers for noncompliance with regulations.

2. OSHA safety procedures for lasers in the workplace (manufacturing or medical) are a bit more specific than other safety issues, in that they require a Laser Safety Officer (LSO). This officer must establish and maintain a laser safety program for the facility.

3. Like the FDA regulations, OSHA regulations cite ANSI laser standards as a basis for many regulatory details.

4. In addition to its regulations, OSHA publishes many other documents that can be helpful to those interested in creating a safe laser work environment. These include OSHA Directives (e.g., Guidelines for Laser Safety and Hazard Assessment) and Standard Interpretations and Compliance Letters (e.g., laser standards applicable to a surgical laser program) (U.S. Department of Labor, 1987, 1991).

5. OSHA recently published a Technical Manual with a chapter on laser hazards (U.S. Department of Labor, 1999d).

6. All of the OSHA regulations and publications can be obtained at the OSHA Web site (http://www.osha.gov).

D. *State Regulation.* Some states do license the use of lasers for the purpose of safety, but such licensure is usually restricted to industrial and nonmedical uses.

E. *Laser Institute of America (LIA)*

1. The Laser Institute of America, an independent organization, is devoted to the promotion of laser safety in the workplace and the medical clinic.

2. LIA conducts a wide variety of laser safety educational programs throughout the country each year, including a comprehensive course for Medical Laser Safety Officers.

3. LIA also publishes the *LIA Guide to Medical Laser Safety,* the *LIA Guide to Non-Beam Hazards Associated with Laser Use,* the *Laser Safety Guide,* the *Guide for the Selection of Laser Eye Protection,* and the *Medical Laser Safety Reference Guide* (Laser Institute of America, 1990, 1993, 1996; Sliney, 1999; Trogel, 1997).

4. Information about LIA courses and publications can be obtained at the LIA Web site (http://www.LaserInstitute.org). Copies of the ANSI standards and OSHA Pub 8-1.7 can also be purchased on the Web site.

F. *American Conference of Governmental Industrial Hygienists (ACGIH)*

1. The American Conference of Governmental Industrial Hygienists is an association of health and safety professionals dedicated to protecting the health of the American worker.

2. ACGIH has established recommendations for threshold limit values (TLVs) for direct and diffuse laser exposures to the eye and skin (American Conference of Governmental Industrial Hygienists, 2000). It updates these TLVs annually.

3. In addition, ACGIH has issued a guide for control of laser hazards (American Conference of Governmental Industrial Hygienists, 1990).

4. More information about ACGIH and its publications can be obtained on the ACGIH Web site (http://www.acgih.org).

G. *The American Society for Laser Medicine and Surgery (ASLMS)*

1. The American Society for Laser Medicine and Surgery is a scientific organization that promotes education, research, and standards of clinical care for medical laser applications.

2. This society is made up of physicians, nurses, and other health professionals, as well as scientists and engineers. Its official journal is *Lasers in Surgery and Medicine*.

3. ASLMS suggests standards of physician training, credentialing, guidelines for office-based laser procedures, and standards of perioperative clinical practice. These can be found on the ASLMS Web site (http://www.aslms.org).

H. *International Standards*

1. The International Electrotechnical Commission (IEC) is the world organization that publishes international standards for all electronic, electrical, and related technologies. More than 50 countries participate in this organization.

2. IEC standards are normative documents involving a consensus of the IEC members. They can be adopted on a voluntary basis by any country. They have formed the basis for many of the standards of countries throughout the world.

3. The IEC 60825-1 (1998–2001) standard deals with the safety of laser products (International Electrotechnical Commission, 1998). It indicates safe working levels for laser exposure and provides a system of classification of lasers. The IEC has also published a guide for diagnostic and therapeutic laser applications in healthcare facilities (International Electrotechnical Commission, 1999).

4. More information about the IEC and its standards can be obtained from the IEC Web site (http://www.iec.ch).

5. Guidelines for the safe use of lasers in the United Kingdom were published in 1984 (United Kingdom Department of Health and Social Security, 1984).

I. *Books on Laser Safety*

1. In addition to the publications already mentioned, a number of books have been published on laser safety (Galoff & Sliney, 1990; Henderson, 1997; International

Radiation Protection Association, 1993; Matthews & Garcia, 1995; Rockwell, 1987; Sliney, 1995; Sliney & Trokel, 1993; Sliney & Wolbarsht, 1980; Winburn, 1990).

2. Many of the books include specific discussions of safety associated with ophthalmic uses of lasers.

III. Laser Hazard Classification

A. Introduction

1. Laser hazard classification guidelines for all lasers are published in the ANSI Z136.1–2000 Standard (American National Standards Institute, 2000) with explanatory notes regarding medical lasers being found in Z136.3–1996 (American National Standards Institute, 1996). In general, lasers are determined to fall within one of four hazard classifications depending mainly on their power within a number of specific wavelength ranges.

2. Table 10–1 provides a summary of these classification levels, where it can be seen that there are other factors such as wavelength and pulse duration that can ultimately affect the exact hazard class for any given laser. A general description of each hazard class follows.

B. Class 1

1. Class 1 lasers are **very low power lasers** and, by definition, **pose no hazard**.

2. The allowed power for this class varies with the spectral range, but, in the visible range, an exposure of 40 microwatts (μW) may not be exceeded.

3. Lasers that emit 40 μW or less are therefore included in this class. These include some of the lowest output diode lasers.

Table 10–1 Laser Hazard Classifications

	Near UV (302–400 nm)	*Visible (400–700 nm)*	*Near IR (700–1050 nm)*
Duration (s)	3×10^4	10	≥ 10
Class 1	$''3.2 \times 10^{-6}$ W	$''4.0 \times 10^{-4}$ W	$''4.0 \times 10^{-4}$ W to $''1.9 \times 10^{-3}$ W
Class 2	—	$>4.0 \times 10^{-4}$ to $''1.0 \times 10^{-3}$ W	—
Class 3a	$>3.2 \times 10^{-6}$ W to 1.6×10^{-5} W	$>1.0 \times 10^{-3}$ W to 5.0×10^{-3} W	$>1.90 \times 10^{-3}$ W to 9.5×10^{-3} W
Class 3b	$>1.6 \times 10^{-5}$ W to 5.0×10^{-1} W	$>5.0 \times 10^{-3}$ W to 5.0×10^{-1} W	$>9.5 \times 10^{-3}$ W to 5.0×10^{-1} W
Class 4	$>5.0 \times 10^{-1}$ W	$>5.0 \times 10^{-1}$ W	$>5.0 \times 10^{-1}$ W

4. However, most Class 1 lasers are devices containing higher-class lasers "embedded" in an internal location within an instrument. Examples would include laser disc players or laser printers. The lasers in these instruments are not intended to be externally exposed under normal use, so the user is protected by the housing(s) of the device. In such a case of an embedded Class 1 laser, service personnel would find inner warning labels of an appropriate higher classification upon opening the system.

C. *Class 2*

1. Class 2 lasers are **low power systems**.

2. Class 2 is a special classification that applies only to lasers working in the **visible range**. These are the types of lasers used as pointers and for alignment and price scanning and therefore may be visually accessible in supermarkets and other public areas. They are considered safe in these applications because an extended intrabeam viewing interval would be necessary to exceed the Class 1 limit, thus requiring staring on the part of the observer. When Class 2 lasers are very bright, such staring is usually impossible, and the natural aversion reflex is protective.

3. In the visible range, the Class 2 laser may not exceed 1 mW.

D. *Class 3*

1. Class 3 lasers are **medium power lasers**. They are rated for a number of wavelength ranges and pose a significant visual hazard under certain circumstances. This class of laser is divided into two subcategories.

2. **Class 3a**
   a. Class 3a CW lasers operate between 1 mW and 5 mW in the visible range. Depending on the actual irradiance, these levels are considered to be either an acute intrabeam viewing hazard or a chronic viewing hazard, and an acute viewing hazard if the beam is viewed with optical instruments (e.g., binoculars or microscopes).
   b. Many more powerful models of laser pointers fall in this class of lasers.

3. **Class 3b**
   a. Class 3b CW lasers operate in the visible range between 5 mW and 500 mW. Because of their higher power, they are considered **hazardous to skin and eyes from direct radiation exposures and specular reflections**.
   b. Limits for Class 3b pulsed lasers depend on the wavelength and pulse duration.
   c. Many Nd:YAG pulsed lasers (including ophthalmic devices) fall into this class.

E. *Class 4*

1. Class 4 lasers are **high-power, high-risk lasers**. These lasers may present an **eye and skin hazard from direct exposure, specular reflections, as well as diffuse reflections**.

2. Over each spectral range, Class 4 lasers are those that exceed Class 3b levels.

3. Because of their high power, Class 4 lasers may also constitute a **fire hazard**, especially in the surgical suite, where sources of 100% oxygen are present.

4. Most ophthalmic lasers are Class 4 lasers.

IV. Laser Safety Program

A. Introduction

1. Any organization utilizing lasers for manufacturing or medical purposes must establish and maintain a laser safety program. The purposes of such a program are to assess and to manage potential laser hazards, to promote the safe use of lasers, and to ensure compliance with applicable ANSI, CDRH, and OSHA requirements pertaining to laser use (Table 10–2).

2. This requirement is usually met by the appointment of a Laser Safety Officer (LSO) and possibly a laser safety committee of knowledgeable individuals to develop institutional laser use policies and standard operating procedures (SOPs) for various lasers and their specific uses.

B. Laser Safety Officer (LSO)

1. The laser safety officer is the individual within the organization who, by training or experience, is responsible for leading and for overseeing the Laser Safety Program of the organization (Rockwell Laser Industries, 1990).

2. The LSO is required whenever Class 3b and/or Class 4 lasers are in use. The LSO ensures the implementation of laser control measures in the work place, reviews and approves SOPs, and calculates Nominal Hazard Zones (NHZs). This person may be a health physicist or other safety manager within the organization. In the case of a hospital or other clinical setting, this person is usually one of the providers of care who works regularly with lasers as they are applied in that clinic. This can be an operating room nurse, optometrist, or other physician willing to keep abreast of the necessary standards and their application to ensure safety (American National Standards Institute, 2000; Rockwell Laser Industries, 1990).

C. Hazard Assessment

1. Under OSHA, all occupational activities in any workplace must be assessed to determine their potential for hazard and injury to the worker. Such hazards must then be addressed by the implementation of control measures sufficient to prevent injury (U.S. Department of Labor, 1999c).

2. Furthermore, it is the ongoing responsibility of the employer to ensure compliance by the employee(s) with the specified control measures via training and oversight (U.S. Department of Labor, 1999c).

Table 10–2 Outline of a Laser Safety Training Program for Laser Surgeons and Technical Staff

I. Operational Characteristics of the Laser
II. Bioeffects and Potential Hazards of the Laser
    Eye and skin hazards of direct and reflected beams
    Fire hazards
    Hazards with laser produced fumes and particulates
    Associated hazards (high pressure gas, anesthetics, etc.)
III. Requirements of Laser Safety Standards
IV. Practical Controls for Lasers in the Medical Environment
    Laser eye protection: Types and proper selection
    Methods to eliminate the possibility of explosion hazards
    Methods for smoke evacuation
    Methods to reduce fire hazards
    Reducing reflected beam hazards
    Standard operating procedures (SOP) for medical laser use
V. Methods and Procedures to Assure Safety
    Methods for surgical drapes in laser surgery procedures
    Techniques for safety while focusing the beam
    Proper laser system controls (foot switch, etc.)
    Proper laser area warning signs
    Entryway interlocks
    Control of unauthorized personnel

Reprinted with permission from Rockwell, RJ. Laser safety in surgery and medicine, 2nd ed., Cincinnati, OH: Rockwell Laser Industries, 1987:VI–19.

D. Control Measures. In the case of lasers, there is always the potential for eye injury (especially macular burn), skin damage, and fire (American National Standards Institute, 2000; Rockwell Laser Industries, 1990). The control measures that can be invoked fall within several categories. Table 10–3 illustrates the various categories of control measures typically used in laser safety.

1. **Engineering controls**
   a. Engineering controls for laser safety refer to the **various design features that are built into the laser system in order to prevent inadvertent injury**. Because engineering controls are inherent to the device and do not require any special knowledge or training on the part of the user to be active, they are considered to be a most important method of safety assurance. Knowledge of engineering controls, however, is critical for service personnel who may have to enter the interior of the device, thus defeating such controls.
   b. The first line of defense in engineering controls is the **laser enclosure (housing)** itself. In certain instruments, this may amount to the complete "embedding" of the laser within the device, thus enabling the laser to be com-

Table 10–3 Basic Laser Controls for Safe Laser Use

Protective housing	Fit & comfort
Interlocks housing	Clothing
Beam enclosures	Other
Beam shutter or attenuator	Administrative and Procedural Controls
Remote interlock connector	Laser safety officer
Key switch control	Written work practices (SOPs)
Viewing optics and windows	Output limitations
Service panels	Education and training
Emission delay	Maintenance
Warning system	Alignment procedures
Controlled areas	Personal protective devices
Indoor	Spectator limitations
Temporary	Warning signs (caution/danger)
Outdoor	Special Controls
Remote firing and	IR and UV requirements (nonvisible
monitoring	beams)
Equipment labels	Demonstrations involving the
Personal Protective Equipment	general public (laser shows)
Eyewear	Fiber optic systems
Factors	Responsibility of manufacturers
Optical density	Repair and maintenance
Transmission	Modification of laser systems
Identification	

Reprinted with permission form Rockwell, RJ. Laser safety in surgery and medicine, 2nd ed., Cincinnati, OH: Rockwell Laser Industries, 1987:VI–2.

pletely safe in any environment. More typically, there will be output at some position on the laser system, but the housing will, nevertheless, prevent unnecessary emissions at points other than the intended output. There is usually an internal interlock in the system that disables the operation of the laser when the housing is removed for service or any other reason.

c. **External interlock plugs** are also typically available on most units that enable safety personnel to disable the system automatically if a critical public doorway or other barrier is open or inoperable. However, these types of "interrupt" systems have fallen in disfavor in medical laser practice since the sudden turning off of a laser during a surgical procedure can have other negative consequences to the specific treatment of the patient while only marginally adding to safety. Perhaps the best use of such interlock protection is in the industrial application of lasers where an unaware individual might stumble into an area without protection while a very high power laser beam is operating.

d. A well-known FDA-mandated engineering control for Class 3b or Class 4 lasers is the **key switch**, which limits control of the use of any laser to a specified number of trained individuals. It is often desirable for a laser to run in a steady state mode long enough to become stable in its operation. This leaves open the possibility that a system may be left operating while it is not in direct use. Some lasers may therefore also have a standby mode whereby the laser is attenuated or blocked in its output to prevent injury while it is running but not actively in use.

2. **Administrative and procedural controls**
   a. These are **methods and instructions that regulate work practices in the interest of promoting and ensuring safety**. It is the responsibility of the employer, via the LSO, to establish and maintain an adequate program for the control of laser hazards (American National Standards Institute, 2000; Rockwell Laser Industries, 1990). All lasers except Classes 1 and 2a should be the subjects of training programs for employees. This training is required for Class 3b and Class 4 lasers.
   b. The employer appoints the **Laser Safety Officer (LSO)** as the critical basis for the program of laser safety. The LSO is responsible for the development, promulgation, and general compliance with SOPs and other protocols for use of lasers in the specified environment. Depending upon the complexity of the laser program, the LSO may function in conjunction with a laser safety committee.
   c. Administrative controls may include which personnel are authorized to use which lasers and for what procedures. Manufacturer's protocols, maintenance and service recommendations, and training programs also fall into this category of laser control. Procedures for storing and disabling a laser when not in use, incident management, and safety audits are also part of this requirement.
   d. **Educational and in-service training requirements** are other essential components of the administrative control of laser use. The employer must ensure the LSO has the requisite education and training for the highest laser class in use, and the LSO, in turn, must ensure that all employees and other persons using or coming into contact with laser operations are trained sufficiently to ensure safety. As with the general aspects of industrial safety programs, training in the general principles of laser safety along with the specifics of SOPs and protocols that have been adopted is considered a critical component of any safety program (see Table 10–3). The behavior of the employee in the work place can be positively affected by such training, and this helps combat one of the most important causes of accident and injury, human error. After engineering controls, the training of personnel working with lasers or in the area of lasers is considered one of the most important steps to be taken.

3. **Control of the laser use area**
   a. All Class 3b and 4 lasers must be used in areas that are controlled with regard to public access as well as in the arrangement of the laser(s) within the area.

    b. Limitation of public access to a laser area is by physical restriction or locking of the area when not in use.

    c. During use, the area must be under the direct control of authorized personnel trained in the safe use of the particular laser being used.

    d. Upon entry to the laser area, other personnel must encounter a doorway, blocking barrier, screen, or curtain that is designed to be protective and will further alert such persons to the hazardous nature of the area. The protective effect of such barriers must ensure that the maximum permissible exposure (MPE) for that device is not exceeded for a new person entering the area.

4. **Maximum permissible exposure (MPE)**

    a. MPEs are exposure levels below those known to cause damage to eye and skin.

    b. MPE levels are determined for each laser as a function of wavelength, total beam power, and delivery configuration of the beam. The addition of a condensing lens in the beam imparts significant focal characteristics to the beam that, in turn, causes the beam to diverge much more rapidly than would normally be the case. Such divergence creates a lower energy density, thus shortening significantly the distance over which an MPE can be exceeded.

5. **Design of the area**

    a. For persons working in the area of the laser, the laser area should be arranged in a way that minimizes direct exposure to the beam (American National Standards Institute, 2000). This can be achieved through directional positioning of the system and by the establishment of a **nominal hazard zone (NHZ)** (Figure 10–1).

    b. The NHZ is the area surrounding the laser in which the maximum permissible exposure (MPE) can be attained by direct, reflected, or by scattered laser energy from the system. Therefore, persons in the area of the laser but outside the NHZ are not subject to damaging effects by the laser. The NHZ is determined by the LSO from manufacturer's literature, safety standards, and/or physical measurements, and may be an area around the laser or, in some cases, may be the entire room.

    c. Typically, the ophthalmic Nd:YAG laser has an NHZ as short as a half a meter because of its very steep focal cone angle, while the ophthalmic argon laser's highly parallel beam propagation can establish an NHZ of several hundred meters.

6. **Signage**

    a. Control of an area is also established by the use of signage (American National Standards Institute, 2000).

    b. The format for laser warning signs is stipulated in the ANSI Z136.1 standard. Examples are given in Figures 10–2 and 10–3. These signs are easily recognizable by the presence of the laser beam "starburst" logo.

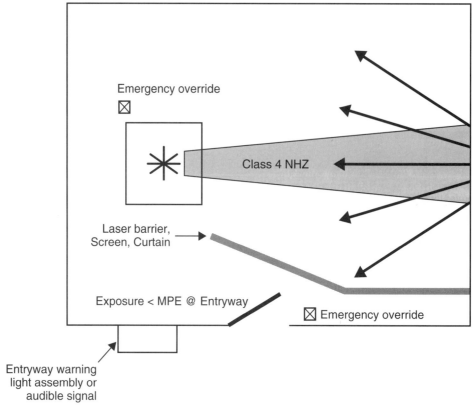

Emergency override

Class 4 NHZ

Laser barrier, Screen, Curtain

Exposure < MPE @ Entryway

Emergency override

Entryway warning light assembly or audible signal

Figure 10–1 Schematic diagram illustrating the concept of a Nominal Hazard Zone (NHZ). (Reprinted from ANSI Z136.1;2000:60, with permission from American National Standards Institute, Washington, DC.)

c. There are two basic levels of signage depending on whether the laser system in question requires special protection and/or training or not. Class 2 and certain Class 3a lasers require a "caution" sign (see Figure 10–2A), while other Class 3a, 3b, and Class 4 lasers warrant a "danger" sign (see Figure 10–2B).

d. There is also a special requirement for posting a "notice" sign (see Figure 10–3) in an area in which a laser repair is taking place and where a laser classified as nonhazardous may become hazardous upon opening the encasement of the system.

e. Of course, the problem with signage as a control measure is its effectiveness, especially since significant specific knowledge can be necessary on the part of the reader to understand the nature of the warning. For the average person, a sign is effective only if it simply strikes fear in the heart of the reader so that the reader does not trespass into the area. However, people become somewhat immune to

Figure 10–2 A. Sample warning signs for use with lasers. B. Sample warning signs for posting at entry of laser area. The classical laser "starburst" logo is prominently featured in each of these signs. Narrative comments are made in each of three positions—position 1: special precautionary instructions or applicable protective actions; position 2: type of laser including medium, wavelength, pulse duration, and maximum output; position 3: class of Laser; caution sign for Class 2 and certain Class 3a lasers; danger sign for certain Class 3a, Class 3b, and Class 4 lasers. (A, Reprinted from ANSI Z136.1;2000:55–56, with permission from American National Standards Institute, Washington, DC.)

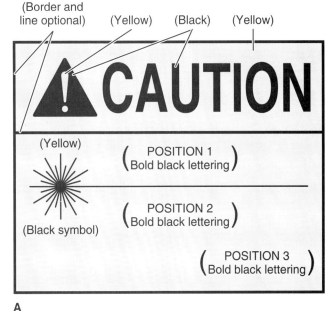

A

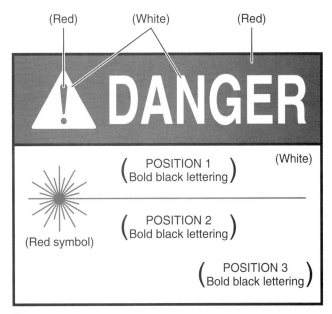

B

(White)   (Blue)

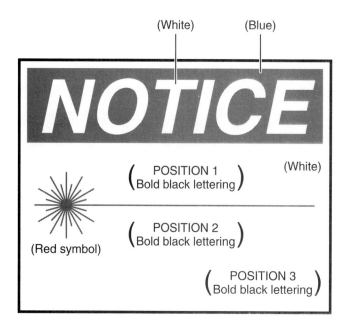

$$\left(\begin{array}{c}\text{POSITION 1}\\\text{Bold black lettering}\end{array}\right)$$ (White)

(Red symbol)

$$\left(\begin{array}{c}\text{POSITION 2}\\\text{Bold black lettering}\end{array}\right)$$

$$\left(\begin{array}{c}\text{POSITION 3}\\\text{Bold black lettering}\end{array}\right)$$

Figure 10–3 Sample notice sign for use outside a temporary laser-controlled area, such as during a repair. (Reprinted from ANSI Z136.1;2000:58, with permission from American National Standards Institute, Washington, DC.)

warning signs. The knowledgeable reader, who understands the details of the warning, may not need the sign at all to be safe. Thus, while laser-warning signs are deemed a necessary measure, they are not sufficient to ensure safety by themselves.

7. **Personal protective devices (PPD)**

   a. The use of laser protective eyewear is an important measure required by the ANSI Standards and OSHA for Class 3b and 4 lasers (American National Standards Institute, 1996, 2000; U.S. Department of Labor, 1999c).

   b. However, the LSO must be prepared to deal with several issues in stipulating the use of protective eyewear. First of all, **the correct laser PPD must be specified for each laser used**. The use of the wrong eyewear can be worse than no eyewear at all because it can impart a sense of security and protection that is unwarranted, thus leading to specific injury (Sliney & Wolbarsht, 1980). In fact, although it is necessary, the use of any PPD in the workplace is considered secondary to the engineering and training measures that are in place because it is important that the employee exercise due caution and follow procedures regardless of whether or not a PPD is worn. Unfortunately, many employees behave as if the mere wearing of a PPD, appropriate or not, will be sufficient to protect them, whatever their behavior.

   c. **Laser eyewear can be provided in a number of formats**, including spectacles with side shields, goggles, face shields, or in some cases as part of the instrument optics (e.g., a biomicroscope eyepiece) (American National Standards Institute, 2000; Sliney & Wolbarsht, 1980). This must be specifically selected by the LSO for each application.

d. The **laser eyewear used in any application must be specified for each laser as to its wavelength and density of absorbance**. These parameters must be printed into the surface of the lens.

e. Protective lenses may be totally protective or, in certain applications where at least some visibility of the beam is desirable, the PPD may be designed to reduce the exposure received by the wearer sufficiently to be below the MPE. Such partial-visibility PPDs have application in cases in which being able to see the beam is critical to the task at hand or if the complete invisibility of the beam constitutes a hazard in itself.

f. **Lenses can be made from glass, plastic, or polycarbonate materials.** Current trends in safety eyewear litigation would argue for at least using Z87.1 polycarbonate in the impact protective layer of the laser PPD (American National Standards Institute, 1989).

g. It is also important that the reduced transmittance afforded by many laser protective lenses be accounted for in terms of the user's mobility within the environment in which it is being used. Often, the room in which a laser is used is rather dimly lit and any reduction in light by the lenses can create a physical hazard for the wearer. Finally, the physical comfort of the wearer with the device selected should be good in order to ensure compliance.

8. **Medical surveillance**

a. Medical surveillance measures are also a part of the laser safety program of an organization (American National Standards Institute, 1996, 2000).

b. The purposes of medical surveillance evaluations are to determine whether an employee has any medical conditions, or is taking any medications, that might increase the risk of working with lasers (Table 10–4). These evaluations can also detect any pre-existing medical conditions that might be confused at the time of an incident with tissue damage.

c. An optometrist, ophthalmologist, or other qualified physician may conduct medical surveillance examinations.

d. There is no requirement in the standard for periodic re-examination beyond the preliminary examination described previously.

9. **Credentialing**

a. Although not a part of the formal standard, ANSI Z-136.3–1996 outlines the recommendations of the American Society for Laser Medicine and Surgery (American National Standards Institute, 1996).

b. These recommendations state that the physician shall meet all the requirements for hospital privileges and shall in addition take specific laser education and train-

Table 10–4 Partial Listing of Specific Drugs That Can Alter the Tissue Response of a Person Exposed to Laser Energy

Agent	Reaction
Sulfonamide	Phototoxic
	Photoallergic
Sulfonylurea	Phototoxic
Chlorothiazides	Papular and edematous eruptions
	Plaques
Phenothiazines	Exaggerates sunburn
	Urticaria
	Gray-blue hyperpigmentation
Tetracycline	Exaggerates sunburn
	Phototoxic
Griseofulvin	Exaggerates sunburn
	Phototoxic
	Photoallergic
Naladixic Acid	Erythema
	Bullae
Furocoumarins (Psoralen)	Erythema
	Bullae hyperpigmentation
Estrogens/Progesterones	Melasma
	Phototoxic
Chlordiazepoxide (Librium)	Eczema
Triacetyldiphenolisatin (laxative)	Eczematous photoallergy
Cyclamates	Phototoxic
	Photoallergic
Porphyrins (Porphyria)	Phototoxic
Retin-A (Retinoic Acid)	Exaggerates sunburn
	Photoallergic

Reprinted from ANSI Z136.1;2000:143, with permission from American National Standards Institute, Washington, DC.

ing of at least 16 hours duration. This is to be followed by from 8 to 16 hours of preceptorship with a practitioner experienced with the laser technology under consideration. In lieu of this additional training, completion of an accredited residency in which the laser technology in question was a part of the standard training would also suffice.

10. **Accidents**

   a. In spite of adherence to appropriate control measures, accidents may occur. These can involve physicians, assistants, patients, or observers. They may result from failure of one of the control measures, but they are usually caused by noncompliance with safety guidelines.

b. Accidents, especially those that cause significant harm, arc more commonly seen with systems of higher power, such as in operating room settings or in research labs. Ophthalmic lasers are typically of much lower power and hence, much safer.

c. In general surgery, the laser is also riskier because its beam is often invisible and is delivered via a hand piece that allows for a less controlled directionality during treatment. There is also significant risk of fire with higher power CO_2 lasers in the high oxygen environment of the operating room.

d. In research labs, the lasers used are also of a higher power, and there is frequently very little in the way of engineering safeguards. Many research accidents have involved macular burns that have occurred as a result of looking down the laser aperture while trying to align the system.

11. **Nonbeam hazards**

a. These include **fire, electrocution, and aerosol contaminants** generated in the conduct of a laser procedure.

b. The LSO needs to look carefully at the totality of the laser design, including its high voltage component, any combination of oxygen with the laser use, and the flammability of any surgical drapes or other materials that may be present in the laser field.

V. Conclusion

A. As our society increases in its technological sophistication, lasers and other potentially hazardous devices are becoming a more common part of our lives. Because lasers are used in such common applications as checking out groceries at the store, many people encounter them daily.

B. Ophthalmic practice is another area in which this technology is rapidly advancing. Eye surgical applications were some of the very first uses of lasers in medicine and surgery, and more treatments are continually being developed. Especially important is the burgeoning growth and development of solid-state lasers, which will undoubtedly supplant many of the classical systems in ophthalmic practice. They are cheaper and often have much more convenient delivery configurations, thus making them more attractive for a wider range of practitioners. All of this increases the risk of injury, and makes the understanding and application of safe practices a critical issue.

References

American Conference of Governmental Industrial Hygienists (ACGIH). A guide for control of laser hazards (Publication 0165). 4th ed. Cincinnati, OH: ACGIH, 1990.

American Conference of Governmental Industrial Hygienists, 2000 TLVs and BEIs (Publication 0100). Cincinnati, OH: American Conference of Governmental Industrial Hygienists, 2000.

American National Standards Institute (ANSI). Z87.1-1989 Practice for occupational and educational eye and face protection. New York, NY: American National Standards Institute, 1989. (Also available from the Laser Institute of America, Orlando, FL)

American National Standards Institute (ANSI). Z136.3-1996 American national standard for safe use of lasers in health care facilities. New York, NY: American National Standards Institute, 1996. (Also available from the Laser Institute of America, Orlando, FL)

American National Standards Institute (ANSI). Z136.1-2000 American national standard for safe use of lasers. New York, NY: American National Standards Institute, 2000. (Also available from the Laser Institute of America, Orlando, FL)

Food and Drug Administration. Compliance guide for laser products. Center for Devices and Radiological Health, Food and Drug Administration, HHS Publication FDA 86-8260, 1985.

Food and Drug Administration, Code of Federal Regulations, Title 21, Chapter I, Subchapter J, Part 1040 (21CFR1040). Performance standards for light-emitting products, Section 1040.10-Laser products, and Section 1040.11-Specific purpose laser products, 1999.

Galoff PK, Sliney DH, eds. Laser safety, eyesafe laser systems, and laser eye protection. Bellingham, WA: SPIE, 1990.

Henderson AR. A guide to laser safety. Boca Raton, FL: Chapman & Hall, 1997.

International Electrotechnical Commission. Safety of laser products—Part 1: Equipment classification, requirements and user's guide. IEC 60825-1 (1998-01). Geneva, Switzerland: International Electrotechnical Commission, 1998.

International Electrotechnical Commission. Safety of laser products—Part 8: Guidelines for the safe use of medical laser equipment. IEC/TR 60825-8 (1999-11). Geneva, Switzerland: International Electrotechnical Commission, 1999.

International Radiation Protection Association. International Non-Ionizing Radiation Committee. The use of lasers in the workplace: a practical guide. Geneva, Switzerland: International Labour Office, 1993.

Laser Institute of America. Medical laser safety reference guide. Orlando, FL: Laser Institute of America, 1990.

Laser Institute of America. Laser safety guide. Orlando, FL: Laser Institute of America, 1993.

Laser Institute of America, Guide for the selection of laser eye protection. Orlando, FL: Laser Institute of America, 1996.

Matthews L, Garcia G. Laser and eye safety in the laboratory. New York: IEEE Press; Bellingham, WA: SPIE Optical Engineering Press, 1995.

Rockwell Laser Industries. Medical laser safety officer course manual. Cincinnati, OH: Rockwell Laser Industries, 1990.

Rockwell RJ. Laser safety in surgery and medicine. 2nd ed. Cincinnati, OH: Rockwell Associates, 1987.

Sliney D. LIA guide to non-beam hazards associated with laser use. Orlando, FL: Laser Institute of America, 1999.

Sliney DH, ed. Selected papers on laser safety. Bellingham, WA: SPIE Optical Engineering Press, 1995.

Sliney DH, Trokel SL. Medical lasers and their safe use. New York: Springer-Verlag, 1993.

Sliney DH, Wolbarsht M. Safety with lasers and other optical sources: a comprehensive handbook. New York: Plenum Press, 1980.

Trogel SL, ed. LIA guide to medical laser safety. Orlando, FL: Laser Institute of America, 1997.

United Kingdom Department of Health and Social Security. Guidance on the safe use of lasers in medical practice. London: Her Majesty's Stationery Office, 1984.

U.S. Department of Labor. OSHA Standards Interpretation and Compliance Letters. 06/03/1987—Laser standards applicable to a surgical laser program, 1987.

U.S. Department of Labor. Guidelines for laser safety and hazard assessment. OSHA Instruction PUB 8-1.7, Directorate of Technical Support, 1991.

U.S. Department of Labor. OSHA Regulations (Standards–29 CFR) Eye and face protection—1926.102, 1999a.

U.S. Department of Labor. OSHA Regulations (Standards–29 CFR) Nonionizing radiation—1926.54, 1999b.

U.S. Department of Labor. OSHA Regulations (Standards–29 CFR), Part 1910 Subpart I—Personal Protective Equipment, 1999c.

U.S. Department of Labor. OSHA Technical Manual (TED 1-0.15A), Section III: Chapter 6. Laser hazards, 1999d.

Winburn DC. Practical laser safety. 2nd ed. New York, NY: M. Dekker, 1990.

Index

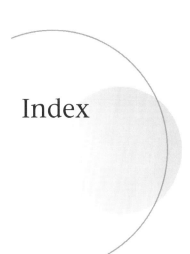

Note: Page numbers followed by f refer to figures; page numbers followed by t refer to tables.